Tumors of the Kidney, Bladder, and Related Urinary Structures

AFIP Atlas of Tumor Pathology

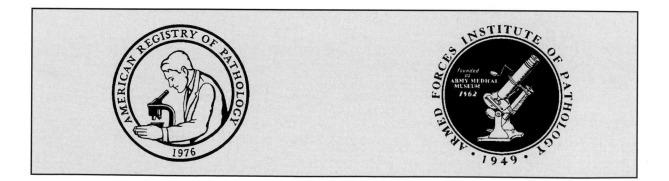

AFIP ATLAS OF TUMOR PATHOLOGY

Fourth Series
Fascicle 1

TUMORS OF THE KIDNEY, BLADDER, AND RELATED URINARY STRUCTURES

by

WILLIAM M. MURPHY, MD
Professor of Pathology
Department of Pathology
University of Florida
Gainesville, Florida

DAVID J. GRIGNON, MD
Professor and Chairman
Department of Pathology
Wayne State University and
the Detroit Medical Center
Detroit, Michigan

ELIZABETH J. PERLMAN, MD
Professor of Pathology
Northwestern University
Evanston, Illinois
Pathologist-in-Chief
Children's Memorial Medical Center
Chicago, Illinois

Published by the
AMERICAN REGISTRY OF PATHOLOGY
Washington, DC
2004

Available from the American Registry of Pathology
Armed Forces Institute of Pathology
Washington, DC 20306-6000
www.afip.org
ISBN 1-881041-88-3

AFIP ATLAS OF TUMOR PATHOLOGY

EDITORS' NOTE

The Atlas of Tumor Pathology has a long and distinguished history. It was first conceived at a Cancer Research Meeting held in St. Louis in September 1947 as an attempt to standardize the nomenclature of neoplastic diseases. The first series was sponsored by the National Academy of Sciences-National Research Council. The organization of this Sisyphean effort was entrusted to the Subcommittee on Oncology of the Committee on Pathology, and Dr. Arthur Purdy Stout was the first editor-in-chief. Many of the illustrations were provided by the Medical Illustration Service of the Armed Forces Institute of Pathology (AFIP), the type was set by the Government Printing Office, and the final printing was done at the Armed Forces Institute of Pathology (hence the colloquial appellation "AFIP Fascicles"). The American Registry of Pathology (ARP) purchased the Fascicles from the Government Printing Office and sold them virtually at cost. Over a period of 20 years, approximately 15,000 copies each of nearly 40 Fascicles were produced. The worldwide impact of these publications over the years has largely surpassed the original goal. They quickly became among the most influential publications on tumor pathology, primarily because of their overall high quality but also because their low cost made them easily accessible the world over to pathologists and other students of oncology.

Upon completion of the first series, the National Academy of Sciences-National Research Council handed further pursuit of the project over to the newly created Universities Associated for Research and Education in Pathology (UAREP). A second series was started, generously supported by grants from the AFIP, the National Cancer Institute, and the American Cancer Society. Dr. Harlan I. Firminger became the editor-in-chief and was succeeded by Dr. William H. Hartmann. The second series' Fascicles were produced as bound volumes instead of loose leaflets. They featured a more comprehensive coverage of the subjects, to the extent that the Fascicles could no longer be regarded as "atlases" but rather as monographs describing and illustrating in detail the tumors and tumor-like conditions of the various organs and systems.

Once the second series was completed, with a success that matched that of the first, UAREP and AFIP decided to embark on a third series. Dr. Juan Rosai was appointed as editor-in-chief, and Dr. Leslie H. Sobin became associate editor. A distinguished Editorial Advisory Board was also convened, and these outstanding pathologists and educators played a major role in the success of this series, the first publication of which appeared in 1991 and the last (number 32) in 2003.

The same organizational framework will apply to the current fourth series. New features will include a hardbound cover, illustrations almost exclusively in color, and an accompanying electronic version of each Fascicle. There will also be increased emphasis (wherever appropriate) on the cytopathologic (intraoperative, exfoliative, and/or fine needle aspiration) and molecular features that are important in diagnosis and prognosis. What will not change from the three previous series, however, is the goal of providing the practicing pathologist with thorough, concise, and up-to-date information on the nomenclature and classification; epidemiologic, clinical, and pathogenetic features; and, most importantly, guidance in the diagnosis of the tumors and tumorlike lesions of all major organ systems and body sites.

As in the third series, a continuous attempt will be made to correlate, whenever possible, the nomenclature used in the Fascicles with that proposed by the World Health Organization's Classification of Tumors, as well as to ensure a consistency of style throughout. Close cooperation between the various authors and their respective liaisons from the Editorial Board will continue to be emphasized in order to minimize unnecessary repetition and discrepancies in the text and illustrations.

Particular thanks are due to the members of the Editorial Advisory Board, the reviewers (at least two for each Fascicle), the editorial and production staff, and—first and foremost—the individual Fascicle authors for their ongoing efforts to ensure that this series is a worthy successor to the previous three.

Steven G. Silverberg, MD
Leslie H. Sobin, MD

PREFACE AND ACKNOWLEDGEMENTS

This atlas was created as a standard reference text for individuals interested in tumors of the kidneys, bladder, and urinary collecting system. We have documented the current state of the art, with emphasis on the pathologic features of the diseases as they appear through the light microscope. In a work of this scope, controversial issues are unavoidable and we have approached them with perspective as well as a point of view. Emerging information is included in separate sections on Special Techniques. Since most readers will use this atlas as an encyclopedia, referring to individual sections rather than to entire chapters, we have not hesitated to be repetitious when reiteration adds clarity, balance, and easy reference. References have been selected and cited for the convenience of the reader, with many clustered at the beginning of the discussion of a subject. Review articles and the current literature have been preferred. We claim no personal priority to the knowledge base and apologize if seminal contributions have been overlooked.

Any work of this scope reflects the collective efforts of investigators whose thoughts have directly contributed to the literature as well as pathologists whose consultation material has enriched the perspectives of the authors. Many of these contributions are acknowledged in the credits to the illustrations. We are especially grateful to our mentors, colleagues, and fellows. They include Drs. J. Bruce Beckwith, George M. Farrow, John N. Eble, and Wael A. Sakr. We are grateful for the support of our institutions, Children's Memorial Medical Center, Chicago, Illinois; Wayne State University and the Detroit Medical Center, Detroit, Michigan; and the University of Florida Department of Pathology, Immunology, and Laboratory Medicine, Gainesville, Florida. In addition to encouragement and personal support, the financial contributions of our institutions have been substantial and should be recognized. We are indebted to the reviewers, those anonymous experts whose efforts have added depth, perspective, and clarity to the final product. A great deal of effort has been expended to create the text and illustrations, and we are grateful to the production staff at the American Registry of Pathology (ARP) and Armed Forces Institute of Pathology (AFIP) as well as to Ms. Margaret Klein (DMC).

William M. Murphy, MD
David J. Grignon, MD
Elizabeth J. Perlman, MD

TUMORS OF THE KIDNEY, BLADDER, AND RELATED URINARY STRUCTURES

KIDNEY TUMORS IN CHILDREN

NORMAL ANATOMY

The anatomy of the kidney is detailed in several publications (4,11,14,15); therefore, only those features particularly relevant to the understanding of the development of renal tumors are emphasized here. The human kidney is derived from the nephric ridge, a longitudinal protrusion of primitive mesenchyme situated just lateral to the somites. Three successive stages are recognized in the embryonic development of the nephric ridge: from cephalad to caudad, the pronephros, mesonephros, and metanephros. The pronephros is transient and important in humans only because its proximal portion forms the mesonephric duct. The mesonephros develops as a series of solid cords that canalize to form tubules and enter the mesonephric duct. The proximal portion of each primitive tubule indents and receives a branch from the aorta to form a glomerulus. These nephrons first appear rostrally and new units are progressively added caudally. Ultimately, the primitive mesonephros regresses, preserved only as rudimentary parovarian tubules in females and components of the excretory duct system of the testis in males. The mesonephros is required for normal development of the nearby gonad (figs. 1-1, 1-2).

The human kidney is formed from the metanephros. On about day 28 of gestation, the ureteric bud emerges from the caudal end of the mesonephric duct due, in large part, to induction by the signaling molecule *GDNF* within the metanephric blastema and the concomitant expression of its receptor, *RET*, in the cells at the growing tip of the ureteric bud. As the ureteric bud grows into the nephric ridge, further reciprocal inductive signals from the ureteric bud initiate the series of morphologic steps that convert the metanephric mesenchyme into the mature nephron (6,12,16). One of the first events is the induction of *Pax2* and *WT1* genes within the mesenchyme; these genes are required for the transition from mesenchyme to epithelium. A potential target for both genes is *Bmp7*, which

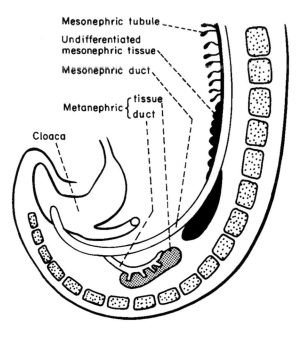

Figure 1-1

DEVELOPMENT OF THE METANEPHRIC KIDNEY

The ureteric bud arises from the caudal end of the mesonephric duct and gives rise to the ureter, renal pelvis, calices, and collecting ducts. The metanephric blastema, shown in fine gray stippling, is induced by the ureteric bud to form the nephrons and renal stroma. (Fig. 1-1 from Fascicle 11, 3rd Series.)

appears to suppress tubulogenesis and control the rate of nephrogenesis, and to thereby maintain an active nephrogenic zone. *Pax2* and *WT1* also appear to be important for the normal spatial patterning of the nephron described below.

The advancing end of the ureteric bud dilates and undergoes a series of dichotomous branchings, forming the pelvicaliceal system. The first 3 to 5 branches are resorbed to form the renal pelvis and calices. As each branch of the ureteric bud advances, its lumen dilates to form an ampulla; the corresponding apical blastema elongates and folds to form a tubular structure in the shape of the letter S. The proximal portion

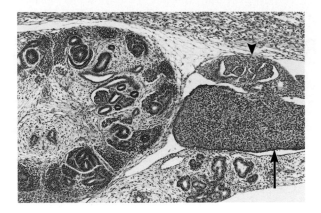

Figure 1-2

THE DIFFERENTIATING METANEPHROS, MESONEPHROS, AND GONADAL RIDGE

The mesonephros (arrowhead) induces the formation of the nearby gonadal ridge (arrow) and is required for normal gonadal development. At this point in gestation, the developing metanephros is identified cephalad to the gonadal ridge and mesonephros.

of this developing nephron then connects to the adjacent ampulla to establish a collecting duct, while the remaining blastema differentiates into other parts of the renal tubule (fig. 1-3).

The lobar pattern created by the branching ureteric bud is established early in renal development (fig. 1-4) (10). The formation of the first generations of nephrons between the 8th and 34th weeks of gestation results in constant elongation and branching of the ureteric bud, pushing the blastemal cells to the periphery of the lobes (fig. 1-5) (15). Approximately two thirds of the nephrons are generated in the last third of human gestation. When new nephrons cease to generate, blastemal cells are no longer apparent in the normal kidney and no new glomeruli or tubules can be formed. All renal growth from this point onward is the result of the enlargement of existing structures. The path of ascent of the kidney as it moves from the caudal region of the embryo toward its eventual

Figure 1-3

DIAGRAM OF NEPHRON DEVELOPMENT IN THE METANEPHRIC KIDNEY

a: Nephrogenic tissue capping the ampulla of the collecting tubule.

b: Enlarged blind end of the ampulla.

c: Primordium of the uriniferous tubule just formed from nephrogenic tissue.

d: Vessel which forms the glomerulus.

e: Bowman's capsule cut open.

f: Uriniferous tubule at a later stage of development.

g: Collecting tubule formed from ureteric bud of the mesonephric duct.

h: Ampulla of the collecting tubule cut open. (Fig. 28-22 from Bloom W, Fawcett DW. A textbook of histology. 8th ed. New York: Chapman & Hall, 1962 [Modified from Corning].)

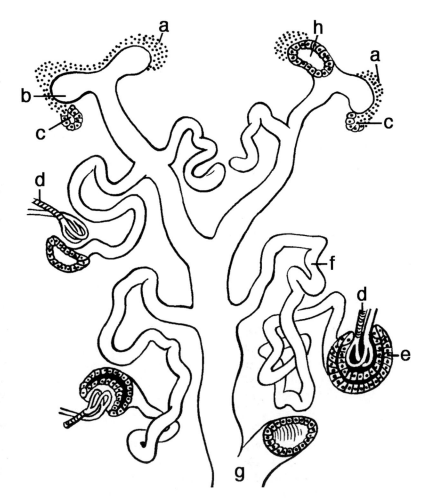

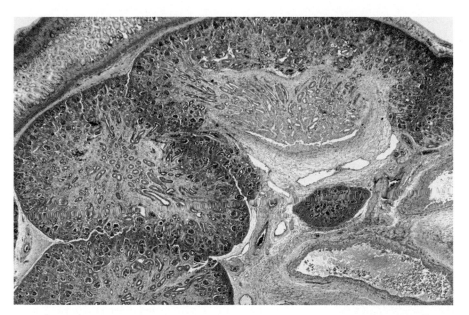

Figure 1-4

DEVELOPING KIDNEY IN A 21-WEEK FETUS

The lobar pattern is well established, with blastemal cells concentrated at the cortical periphery. The first generations of cortical nephrons are situated at the corticomedullary junction.

position in the abdomen determines the position of the future ureter.

The mature human kidney is a bean-shaped organ located in the lumbar retroperitoneal space opposite vertebrae T-12 to L-3 (4,11,14). On average, each adult kidney is 12 cm in length, 6 cm in width, and 2.5 cm in thickness. In men, the average weight varies from 125 to 170 g, whereas in women it is 115 to 155 g. The kidney consists of independently functional units fused together to form eight renal lobes, each composed of a medullary pyramid and the adjacent cortical mantle. This lobar structure is usually prominent on the external surface of the kidney in newborns as "fetal lobations." Fetal lobations are usually absent in adults, where the differential growth of nephrons has obliterated them.

The convex outer surface of the kidney is invested with a capsule composed of a thin fibroblastic layer that is difficult to dissect from the underlying nephrons, and an outer, thicker, collagenous layer easily stripped by blunt dissection (fig. 1-6). The renal capsule is covered by fat, which is in turn surrounded by a condensation of retroperitoneal connective tissue, the perirenal fascia of Gerota. Gerota's fascia may be in direct contact with the renal capsule anteriorly, where perirenal fat is scant.

An important but rarely emphasized component of the kidney is the renal sinus (figs. 1-7–1-9). Located on the medial aspect of the kidney, this concave structure is a major pathway of

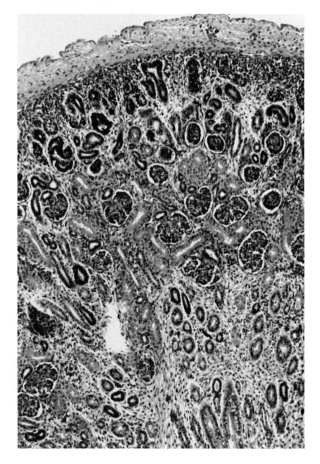

Figure 1-5

DEVELOPING KIDNEY AT 16 WEEKS

Blastemal cells and early glomerular development are confined to the periphery of the lobe.

tumor dissemination and an important landmark for evaluating tumor extension (2). The renal sinus contains the renal calices, variable portions of the pelvis, and the major vascular and neural structures that supply the kidney. These structures are surrounded by richly vascularized connective tissue contiguous with the perirenal fat. The most distinguishing feature of the renal sinus in histologic sections is the lack of a capsule separating the kidney from the perirenal fat (figs. 1-7–1-9). This contrasts with the thick fibrous capsule that covers the convex portion of the renal cortex and the pelvicaliceal system within the sinus.

The vascular supply of the normal kidney is variable, although most kidneys have a single renal artery and vein. These vessels arborize in the renal sinus and supply the parenchyma in such a way that each nephron is a self-contained functioning unit with its own blood supply and filtration system. Lymphatics are numerous in the renal cortex but are absent in the medulla. They drain via the renal sinus into hilar and regional lymph nodes adjacent to the aorta and vena cava. The kidney is supplied with adrenergic nerve fibers from the celiac plexus (13). Most nerves reach the renal parenchyma via the renal sinus and arborize with the vascular system.

The gross appearance of the cut surface of the human kidney is distinctive. The cortex is 0.7 to 1.0 cm in thickness and is easily distinguished from the medulla by its configuration, position, and color. The extensions of cortical tissue between the medullary pyramids of each lobe are usually referred to as the columns of Bertin. Closer inspection reveals radially arranged medullary rays extending from the cortex into the medulla (fig. 1-7). These rays are composed of collecting ducts, the straight segments of proximal and distal tubules, and straight blood vessels. Each kidney contains 1 to 2 million nephrons, the glomerular portions of which can often be seen with the unaided eye.

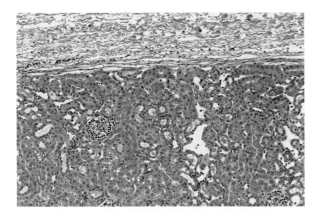

Figure 1-6

RENAL CAPSULE

A discrete layer of fibroblasts is seen adjacent to the cortex, with a condensed collagenous layer above.

Figure 1-7

KIDNEY IN CROSS SECTION

The renal sinus in this adult specimen is filled with fat, which surrounds the major renal vessels and pelvicaliceal system. (Fig. 4 from Beckwith JB. Renal neoplasms in childhood. In: Sternberg SS, ed. Diagnostic surgical pathology. New York: Raven Press; 1994:1741–66.)

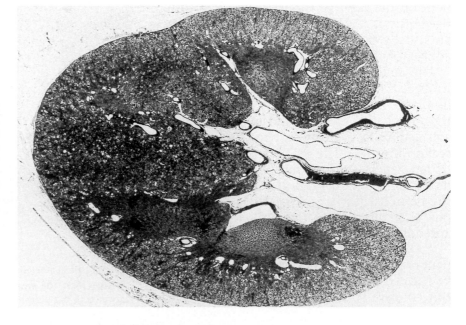

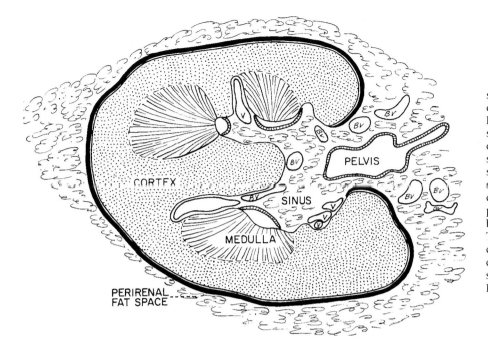

Figure 1-8

KIDNEY IN CROSS SECTION

Drawing of specimen shown in figure 1-7. The renal capsule, shown as a thick black line, surrounds the convex surface of the kidney but disappears from the cortical surface as it enters the renal sinus. Cortical surfaces of the sinus lack a capsule. The capsule surrounding the pelvicaliceal system is shown by crosshatched markings. This may extend over adjacent medullary pyramids but does not cover cortical structures. (Fig. 1-8 from Fascicle 11, 3rd Series.)

Histologically, the normal renal parenchyma consists of four parts: blood vessels, glomeruli, tubules, and interstitium. Excellent reviews of the microscopic anatomy are available (4,11,15) and only the most pertinent features are described here. The renal blood vessels are structurally similar to those in other body sites. Glomeruli are complex structures composed of specialized endothelial, epithelial, and mesangial cells arranged around a relatively thick basement membrane (1,9). The juxtaglomerular apparatus is a structure composed of vascular smooth muscle cells, cells of the extraglomerular mesangium, and the macula densa of the distal tubule. It occupies a portion of the vascular pole of the glomerulus (fig. 1-10).

A complex tubular system begins at the urinary pole and extends to the renal papilla. This system is traditionally divided into the proximal tubule, loop of Henle, distal tubule, and collecting duct, although each consists of distinctive subunits (fig. 1-11). The proximal tubule is composed of convoluted and straight portions; it is lined by tall columnar cells with acidophilic cytoplasm rich in structures necessary for active fluid transport, including densely packed microvilli, endocytic vacuoles, and mitochondria (fig. 1-12). The loop of Henle has thin

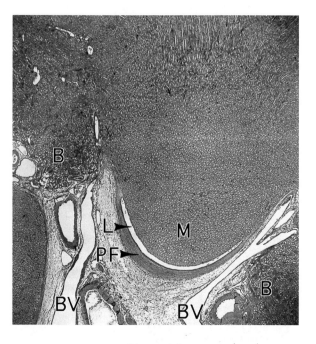

Figure 1-9

RENAL SINUS

This low-power photomicrograph shows the capsular tissue surrounding the pelvicaliceal system and the lack of capsule over cortical tissues of the sinus. B: Cortex adjacent to renal sinus; BV: branches of renal vein; PF: fascial layer surrounding pelvicaliceal system; M: medullary pyramid; L: caliceal lumen. (Fig. 1-9 from Fascicle 11, 3rd Series.)

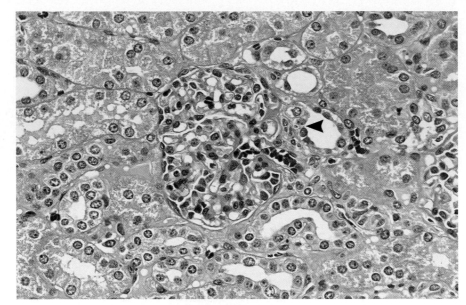

Figure 1-10

JUXTAGLOMERULAR APPARATUS

The juxtaglomerular apparatus can be identified at the vascular pole of this glomerulus. The specialized cells of the extraglomerular mesangium are seen in the small space of connective tissue located between the macula densa of the distal tubule (arrowhead) and the afferent arteriole.

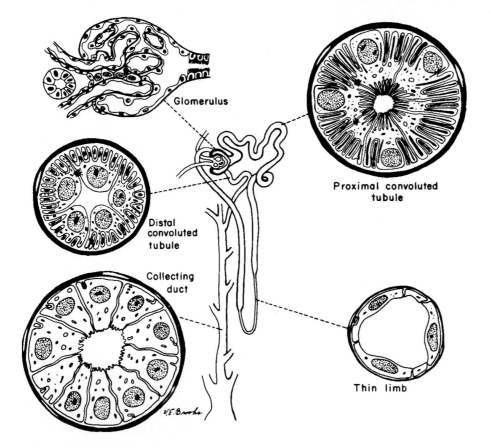

Figure 1-11

GENERAL HISTOLOGIC FEATURES OF THE NEPHRON

Cross sections of the various segments of the tubule roughly indicate the cellular morphologic features, and the relative size of cells and tubules at these sites. (Fig. 1-5 from Bennington JL, Kradjian R. Renal carcinoma. Philadelphia: WB Saunders; 1967:11.)

descending and thick ascending portions that are lined by cuboidal and columnar cells with variable quantities of microvilli and cytoplasmic organelles (fig. 1-13). Tamm-Horsfall protein is an antigenic substance produced by these cells (17). The distal tubule is narrower and shorter than the proximal tubule, and has fewer microvilli and organelles. It contains the specialized

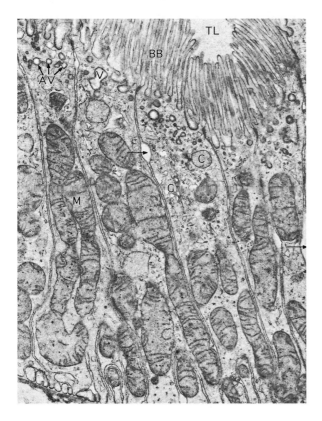

Figure 1-12

PROXIMAL CONVOLUTED TUBULAR CELL

In proximal convoluted tubular cells, the mitochondria (M) are often elongated and tortuous. The apical part of the proximal convoluted tubular cell is covered by tightly packed microvilli that form the brush border (BB). Deep invaginations of the apical cell membrane form apical tubules, vesicles (AV), and vacuoles (V). Note the dense homogenous material in some apical vacuoles and similar dense bodies in the apical cytosomes (C). The golgi (G), brush border (BB), and tubular lumen (TL) are also indicated. (Fig. 7 from Tisher CC. Human renal ultrastructure. I. Proximal tubule of healthy individuals. Lab Invest 1966;15:1357–94.)

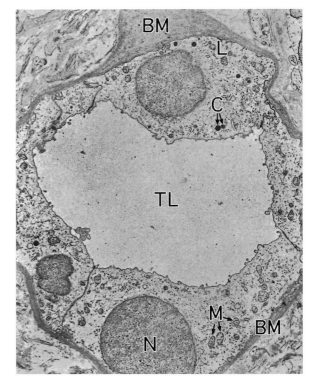

Figure 1-13

LOOP OF HENLE

In the thin limb of the loop of Henle, the cells assume a more squamoid configuration, with nuclei (N) that often display infolding. Basal and lateral cell interdigitations are infrequent. The basement membrane (BM) is often quite variable in thickness. Occasional small mitochondria (M), cytosomes (C), and droplets of lipid (L) are present. The tubular lumen (TL) is also indicated. (Fig. 1-13 from Fascicle 11, 3rd Series.)

cells of the macula densa of the juxtaglomerular apparatus. Collecting ducts consist of cuboidal cells with pale acidophilic cytoplasm and centrally placed nuclei (fig. 1-14). Cytoplasmic lipofuscin granules may be prominent. Collecting ducts coalesce to form the terminal ducts of Bellini; 10 to 25 terminal ducts open into the area cribrosa at the tip of a medullary papilla. The interstitium is more easily conceptualized as a space than a structure, it is usually visualized only when abnormal. It contains specialized interstitial cells and connective tissue elements.

Immunohistochemical observations indicate that the antigenic composition of the nephron varies considerably within different regions (1,5,7). The expression of high molecular weight cytokeratins, such as 34ßE12, is confined to the urothelium. In contrast, cytokeratins like AE1/3, cytokeratin 19, and cytokeratin 8, and epithelial membrane antigen are reliably expressed by the collecting ducts, the distal tubules, and the urothelium. The proximal tubules are ordinarily nonreactive or only focally reactive, and the glomeruli are negative for these markers (fig. 1-15). Cytokeratin 18 immunoreactivity is present in all the epithelial components of the nephron except the glomerulus and cytokeratin 20 is not expressed in the nephron. Cytokeratin 7 expression within the kidney is distinctive. It is

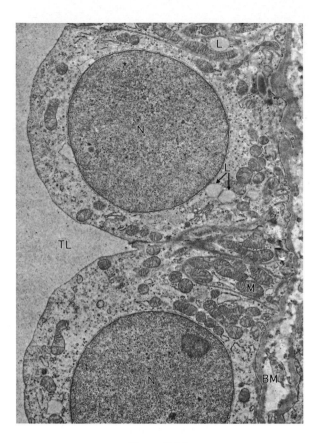

Figure 1-14

CORTICAL COLLECTING TUBULE CELLS

Note the paucity of organelles as compared to proximal tubular cells. Cortical collecting ducts often have a relatively smooth apical surface, although short plicae may be seen, and are more prominent in medullary collecting duct cells along with microvilli on some cells. A single cilium is usually present in the apex of the collecting duct cell, best shown with scanning electron microscopy. Membrane-bound lipid (L) is present in the basal cytoplasm. The tubular lumen (TL), nucleus (N), and basal lamina (BM) are also indicated. (Fig. 1-14 from Fascicle 11, 3rd Series.)

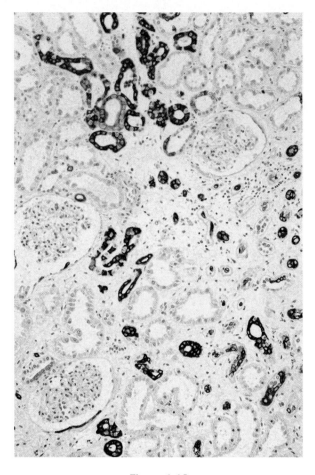

Figure 1-15

EPITHELIAL MARKERS IN THE NORMAL KIDNEY

Immunohistochemical expression of epithelial markers, including epithelial membrane antigen, cytokeratin cocktail AE1/AE3, cytokeratin 19, and cytokeratin 8, is present in the distal tubule and collecting duct, but is absent in the glomerulus and only focally identified in the proximal tubule (AE1/AE3 shown).

strongly expressed by the collecting ducts and to a lesser extent by isolated and small clusters of cells within the distal tubules; cytokeratin 7 is only focally expressed in the proximal tubules (fig. 1-16). Within the developing kidney, WT1 expression is restricted to the condensing metanephric blastema, renal vesicles, and glomerular epithelium, in keeping with its presumed role in the cessation of proliferation of blastemal cells and the initiation of epithelial differentiation at the tip of the ureteric bud (fig. 1-17) (3,8). WT1 expression persists in the glomerular podocytes into adulthood (3).

TUMORS OF INFANCY AND CHILDHOOD

It has long been recognized that the types of renal tumors that characteristically arise in children are different from those occurring in adults. These differences are apparent when observing the pathologic features of pediatric renal tumors as well as when assessing patient therapy and clinical outcome. As is the case with most pediatric tumors, neoplasms arising in the kidneys often have distinctive and characteristic molecular features, some of which have become diagnostically important.

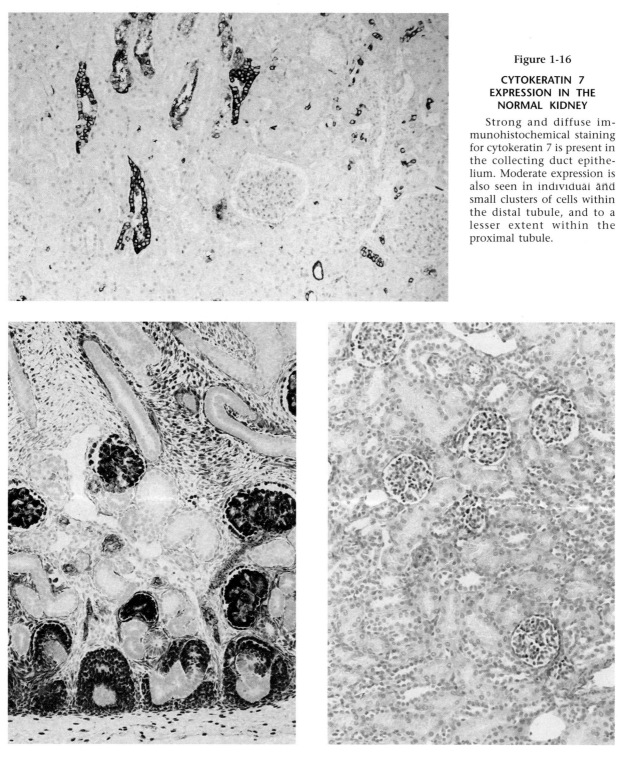

Figure 1-16

CYTOKERATIN 7 EXPRESSION IN THE NORMAL KIDNEY

Strong and diffuse immunohistochemical staining for cytokeratin 7 is present in the collecting duct epithelium. Moderate expression is also seen in individual and small clusters of cells within the distal tubule, and to a lesser extent within the proximal tubule.

Figure 1-17

WT1 EXPRESSION IN FETAL AND ADULT KIDNEY

Left: Strong nuclear immunohistochemical expression for WT1 is seen in the blastemal cells of the nephrogenic zone of the fetal kidney as well as in the differentiating glomeruli.

Right: Within the adult kidney, WT1 expression is limited to the parietal and visceral glomerular epithelium.

Table 1-1
CLASSIFICATION OF KIDNEY TUMORS IN INFANTS AND CHILDREN

Nephroblastic Tumors
  Nephroblastoma
    Favorable histology
    Anaplasia (diffuse and focal)
  Nephrogenic rests and nephroblastomatosis
  Cystic nephroma and cystic, partially differentiated
    nephroblastoma
  Metanephric tumors and related entities
    Metanephric adenoma
    Metanephric adenofibroma
    Metanephric stromal tumor

Mesoblastic Nephroma
  Cellular
  Classic
  Mixed

Clear Cell Sarcoma

Rhabdoid Tumor

Renal Epithelial Tumors of Childhood
  Papillary renal cell carcinoma
  Renal medullary carcinoma
  Renal tumors associated with Xp11.2 translocations

Rare Tumors
  Ossifying renal tumor of infancy
  Angiomyolipoma

Table 1-2
CONDITIONS ASSOCIATED WITH NEPHROBLASTOMA

Syndromes Associated with Highest Risk of Nephroblastoma
  Wilms-aniridia-genital anomaly-retardation
    (WAGR) syndrome (*WT1*, 11p13)
  Beckwith-Wiedemann syndrome (*WT2*, 11p15)
  Hemihypertrophy
  Denys-Drash syndrome (*WT1*, 11p13)
  Familial nephroblastoma (*FWT1*, 17q12-21;
    FWT2, 19q13.3-13.4)

Conditions Also Associated with Nephroblastoma
  Frasier's syndrome (*WT1*, 11p13)
  Simpson-Golabi-Behmel syndrome (*GPC3*, Xq26)
  Renal or genital malformations
  Cutaneous nevi, angiomas
  Trisomy 18
  Klippel-Trenaunay syndrome
  Neurofibromatosis
  Bloom's syndrome
  Perlman's syndrome
  Sotos' syndrome
  Cerebral gigantism

CLASSIFICATION

Kidney tumors arising in infants and children are described according to the classification shown in Table 1-1.

NEPHROBLASTOMA (WILMS' TUMOR)

Definition. Nephroblastoma is a malignant embryonal neoplasm derived from nephrogenic blastemal cells (25,27,28,111). Several lines of differentiation are commonly expressed in individual tumors and many nephroblastomas replicate the histology of the developing kidney. Although not preferred, the eponymic designation, Wilms' tumor, is commonly used, despite the fact that Wilms was not the first to describe this entity (117).

General Features. Nephroblastoma is the most common genitourinary cancer in children, affecting about 1 in every 8,000 children and accounting for approximately 400 new cases each year in the United States (38,111). There is a slight increase in frequency in girls, with a male to female ratio for patients with unilateral tumors of 0.9 to 1.0, and a ratio for those with bilateral tumors of 0.6 to 1.0 (34). Nephroblastomas occur with equal frequency in both kidneys. The mean age at diagnosis is approximately 36 and 42 months for males and females, respectively, and 98 percent of cases occur in individuals under 10 years of age (fig. 1-18) (37,38). Nephroblastomas rarely occur in adults (70,72). The relatively stable incidence of nephroblastoma in all geographic regions suggests that environmental factors do not play a major role in their etiology (38,105). The variation in incidence among different racial groups, however, indicates a genetic predisposition. The general risk among Caucasians is approximately 1 in 10,000 live births, the incidence among African-Americans is higher, and the frequency among Asians is lower (58). These incidences are not affected by immigration patterns (38,105).

Approximately 10 percent of nephroblastomas develop in association with one of several well-characterized dysmorphic syndromes (Table 1-2) (48,64). The first of these is the WAGR syndrome (Wilms' tumor, aniridia, genitourinary malformation, mental retardation), which carries a 30 percent risk of developing a nephroblastoma. Patients with this syndrome have a consistent deletion of chromosome 11p13 in their somatic cells. The observation

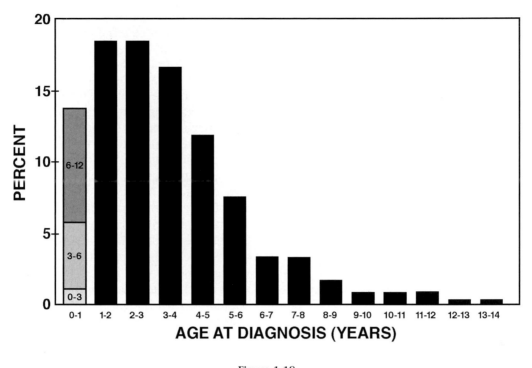

Figure 1-18

NEPHROBLASTOMA

Age distribution, based on 2,500 cases registered with the National Wilms Tumor Study Group protocols. (Fig. 1-15 from Fascicle 11, 3rd Series.)

that a similar deletion is confined to nephroblastoma cells in some patients without constitutional 11p13 abnormalities prompted intense research. In 1990, the gene on 11p13 was cloned and designated *WT1* (41,60). *WT1* encodes a zinc finger transcription factor that plays a major role in renal and gonadal development (67). Its normal expression is limited to the developing kidney, gonadal sex cord cells, and mesothelium. Abnormalities involving *WT1* are consistently found in the tumors of patients with WAGR as well as in patients with Denys-Drash syndrome (a syndrome characterized by mesangial sclerosis, pseudohermaphroditism, and a 90 percent risk of nephroblastoma). Different *WT1* abnormalities are associated with these different syndromes. Patients with WAGR have deletions of *WT1* whereas patients with Denys-Drash syndrome have constitutional inactivating point mutations in one copy of *WT1* and their nephroblastomas show loss of the remaining normal *WT1* allele (91). *WT1* alterations are strongly linked to the development of nephroblastoma

in syndromic cases, but their role in sporadic nephroblastoma appears to be limited, with only one third of all nephroblastomas showing loss of heterozygosity at this locus and only 10 percent harboring *WT1* mutations. Identical *WT1* mutations and loss of heterozygosity patterns have been reported in both nephroblastomas and their associated nephrogenic rests (42,90). This suggests that *WT1* inactivation may result in the formation of a nephrogenic rest and that at least some nephroblastomas are the result of subsequent genetic events occurring in a nephrogenic rest.

The low prevalence of *WT1* abnormalities in sporadic nephroblastomas led to the recognition that genes other than *WT1* must be involved in the pathogenesis of these tumors. Evidence supporting this was provided by the linkage of the familial Beckwith-Wiedemann syndrome (characterized by hemihypertrophy, macroglossia, omphalocele, and visceromegaly) to a locus at chromosome 11p15, designated *WT2* (55,77,93). The preferential loss of the maternal allele at this locus and duplication of the paternal allele in cases of sporadic nephroblastoma suggest that genomic imprinting is involved in the pathogenesis of some tumors (87). Attempts to determine the precise genetic event at this locus have revealed the presence of a cluster of imprinted genes, including *IGF2, H19,* and *LIT1,* among others. In particular, *IGF2* loss of imprinting occurs in 33 to 50 percent of nephroblastomas (84). Additional evidence suggesting an important role of *IGF2* in nephroblastoma tumorigenesis includes an association between *IGF2* loss of imprinting and the presence of perilobar nephrogenic rests, as well as the decreased incidence of both *IGF2* loss of imprinting and perilobar nephrogenic rests in nephroblastomas arising in Asian children (58,96). Whether a single gene at the 11p15 locus is responsible for the increased risk of nephroblastoma among patients with Beckwith-Wiedemann syndrome remains unclear (50).

Despite the success in defining *WT1* and *WT2,* it is clear that additional genetic loci are responsible for the pathogenesis of most nephroblastomas. This genetic heterogeneity is supported by the existence of familial nephroblastoma in patients with normal *WT1* and *WT2* genes (65,69,95). Among individuals registered in the National Wilms Tumor Study Group (NWTSG), approximately 1 percent have a positive family history of nephroblastoma. Most pedigrees suggest autosomal dominant transmission with variable penetrance and expressivity. Specific chromosomal loci identified and presumed responsible for familial nephroblastoma include 17q12-21 (*FWT1*), and 19q13.3-13.4 (*FWT2*) (69). It is apparent that nephroblastoma can be initiated by more than one factor and that a single hypothesis cannot account for all cases of this complex neoplasm.

The majority of nephroblastomas are unicentric, however, synchronous multicentric masses in a single kidney and bilateral primary lesions are observed in 7 and 5 percent of cases, respectively (34,47,101,115). Nephrogenic rests, most commonly of the perilobar type, are seen in the surrounding kidney in the majority of such cases. Patients with multiple nephroblastomas are more likely than those with single tumors to have an increased association with genetic syndromes. Patients with synchronous or metachronous bilateral nephroblastomas have a younger age of onset (27 months) and are more likely to have renal failure even with successful therapy than those with unicentric nephroblastomas (97,101).

Patients initially treated for unilateral nephroblastoma may develop a second tumor in the contralateral kidney at a later point in time. Studies analyzing the clinicopathologic risk factors associated with the development of a metachronous nephroblastoma show that children younger than 12 months of age who also have nephrogenic rests have a markedly increased risk of developing contralateral disease. This risk declines with increasing age at diagnosis, with the relative risk stabilizing at 5 years of age. Children whose nephroblastoma is diagnosed at birth in the presence of a nephrogenic rest have 15 times the chance of developing a metachronous bilateral nephroblastoma compared with those who do not have nephrogenic rests. This relative risk falls to 6 times by 4 years of age (47).

Nephroblastomas may arise adjacent to the kidney, possibly by exophytic growth from a narrow renal pedicle or from neoplastic transformation of an afferent branch of the ureteric bud (20,110). Inguinal, gonadal, or juxtagonadal nephroblastomas, while rare, are recorded and are thought to be derived from displaced mesonephric remnants (86). The immature masses of nephrogenic tissue occasionally found in proximity to a neural tube defect in the lumbosacral region may be related to nephrogenic mesenchyme displaced as part of the dysraphic process (18). Clear documentation of a pure testicular triphasic nephroblastoma arising from a germ cell origin, and confirmed by cytogenetic analysis, has been reported (61).

Clinical Features. Patients with nephroblastoma most commonly come to clinical attention due to the presence of an abdominal mass. Abdominal pain, hematuria, hypertension, and symptoms related to traumatic rupture are also common. Imaging usually reveals one or more intrarenal masses that are usually sharply demarcated and heterogeneous; however, radiographic studies are not ordinarily helpful for distinguishing nephroblastoma from other pediatric renal neoplasms (fig. 1-19). Ultrasonography is especially effective for evaluating cystic components and for demonstrating extension of the tumor into the venous system. Computed tomography

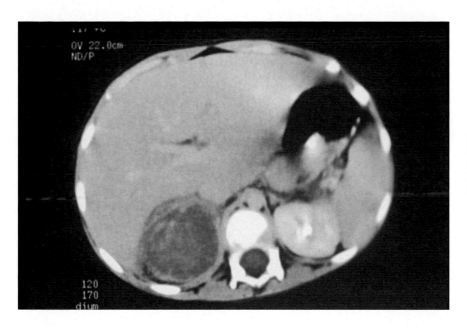

Figure 1-19

NEPHROBLASTOMA

Computerized tomography illustrates a circumscribed lesion with a heterogeneous appearance compressing the adjacent kidney. (Courtesy of Dr. David Kelly, Birmingham, AL.)

(CT) is useful for detecting small lesions and metastases. The demonstration of bilateral or multicentric tumors, features not observed in most other renal tumors of childhood, helps in the differential diagnosis.

Several potential serum tumor markers are associated with nephroblastoma, but no marker has been shown to be consistently present (46). Some patients have circulating serum mucin, which stains as blue granular material on conventionally prepared blood smears. An increased level of hyaluronic acid, apparently resulting from increased activity of hyaluronic acid–stimulating factor, is frequently present in the blood (79,104). Serum levels of erythropoietin may be increased, but the prevalence of this finding is probably no higher in patients with renal neoplasms than in other individuals. Urinary cytology and aspiration cytology are of limited value in the primary diagnosis of pediatric renal tumors because of the high error rate when tumors are classified using these methods.

Pathologic Findings. Grossly, nephroblastoma is usually a solitary, rounded mass sharply demarcated from the adjacent renal parenchyma by a peritumoral fibrous capsule. Tumor size is extremely variable. The combined weight of tumor and kidney ranges from 60 to 6,350 g, with a median of 550 g. The lesion tends to bulge from the sectioned surface and usually has a uniform, pale gray or tan appearance and a soft consistency (fig. 1-20). The sectioned surface may appear firm and whorled if a large fraction of the lesion is composed of mature stromal elements (fig. 1-21). The extremely soft consistency and friable texture of most nephroblastomas make them difficult to section without extensive displacement of tumor cells, an artifact that often complicates pathologic staging of the lesion. Nephroblastomas are often subdivided by prominent septa, imparting a lobulated appearance (figs. 1-20, 1-21). Multicentric tumors are identified in approximately 5 percent of nephrectomy specimens (fig. 1-22). Polypoid protrusions of tumor into the pelvicaliceal system may occur, resulting in a "botryoid" gross appearance (fig. 1-21) (81). Cystic spaces may be a prominent feature (fig. 1-23). Hemorrhage and necrosis are often present but are rarely prominent in the absence of abdominal trauma prior to nephrectomy. Local extension into the renal vein and metastases to regional lymph nodes are common. Extensive permeation of intrarenal blood and lymphatic vessels may produce a false impression of multicentricity during gross evaluation of the kidney.

Histologically, nephroblastoma rivals teratoma in the diversity of the histologic patterns. A variety of cell types including blastema, epithelium, and stroma are present in most lesions (fig. 1-24). The relative proportions of each cell or tissue type vary from specimen to specimen, and the diverse cell types may express variable degrees of differentiation, resulting in an almost

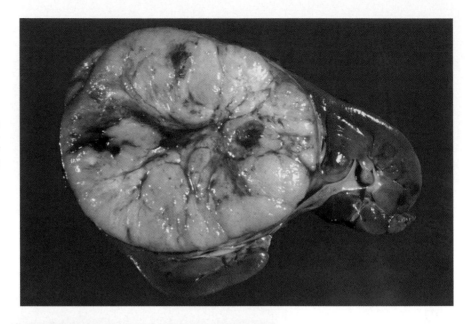

Figure 1-20

NEPHROBLASTOMA

Grossly, nephroblastomas commonly have a mucoid, gray-white appearance; a sharply demarcated, spherical shape; and a pushing growth pattern.

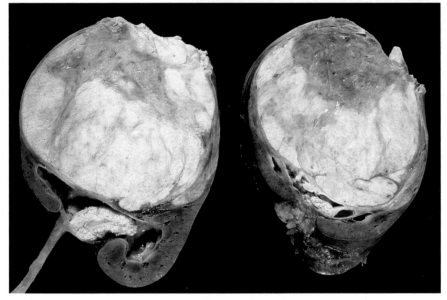

Figure 1-21

NEPHROBLASTOMA

Nephroblastomas are often lobulated and heterogeneous. Prominent septa subdivide the sectioned surface and the protrusion of tumor into the renal pelvis, resembling botryoid rhabdomyosarcoma. The irregular crescentic region between the mass and the renal capsule at the right of the section represents a nephrogenic rest. (Fig. 1-18, Fascicle 11, 3rd Series.)

infinite variety of potential patterns. Triphasic patterns, containing blastemal, stromal, and epithelial cell types, are the most characteristic, but biphasic and monophasic lesions are often observed. For the sake of clarity, the various histologic components are described individually. Most of these components represent various stages in normal or abnormal nephrogenesis. Some, such as skeletal muscle and cartilage, represent the differentiating potential of the nephrogenic precursor cells and are often referred to collectively as heterologous elements.

Blastemal Component. The blastemal cells of nephroblastoma resemble the condensed mesenchyme from which the kidney develops. Blastemal cells are small, closely packed, and mitotically active, with minimal evidence of differentiation. Blastema is present in most nephroblastomas and it may be the only element in the tumor. Cytologically, blastemal cells are usually rounded or polygonal but may be slightly elongated (fig. 1-25). Their nuclei are relatively small and regular, with evenly distributed, slightly coarse chromatin and small nucleoli.

It should be noted that details of nuclear structure may vary markedly under differing conditions of fixation. Delayed fixation often produces coarse clumping, and cross-linking fixatives can make the chromatin appear quite delicate. Cytoplasm is scanty and usually does not stain well with hematoxylin and eosin (H&E) although granular, brightly acidophilic cytoplasmic staining may be observed in some regions. Cytoplasmic acidophilia is a degenerative phenomenon that is usually accompanied by nuclear pyknosis. Cell borders are often indistinct especially when phosphate-buffered formalin fixation is used. A reliable feature of the blastema of nephroblastoma is the prominent

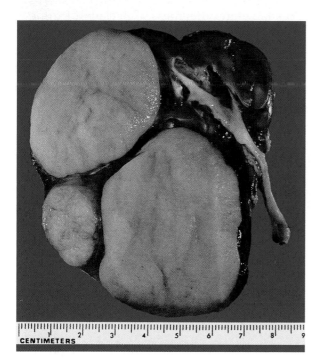

Figure 1-22

MULTICENTRIC NEPHROBLASTOMA

Three spherical tumor nodules are separated by renal parenchyma. (Fig. 1-20, Fascicle 11, 3rd Series.)

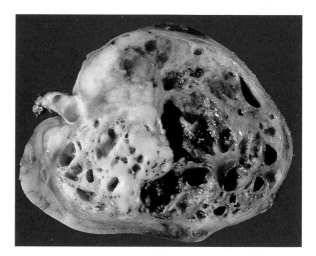

Figure 1-23

NEPHROBLASTOMA

Prominent cysts are seen, although solid areas differentiate this lesion from a cystic, partially differentiated nephroblastoma. (Fig. 1-19, Fascicle 11, 3rd Series.)

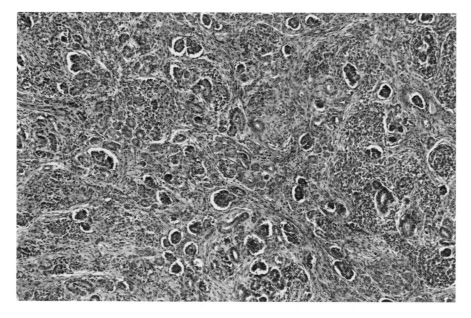

Figure 1-24

NEPHROBLASTOMA

Triphasic pattern, with blastemal, differentiated stromal, and tubular elements.

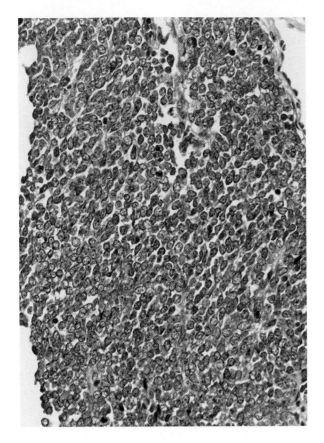

Figure 1-25

NEPHROBLASTOMA

Blastemal-predominant nephroblastomas may be confused with other small cell tumors of childhood. The cytologic features that are characteristic of nephroblastoma include finely dispersed chromatin and overlapping nuclei.

overlapping of adjacent nuclei. Mitotic figures are numerous in most specimens (fig. 1-25).

Blastemal cells occur in several distinctive patterns including serpentine, nodular, and basaloid. More than one pattern is often found in the same tumor. Recognition of these patterns facilitates diagnosis, especially of tumors at metastatic sites. Other embryonal tumors of childhood that arise in the kidney seldom demonstrate these distinctive patterns.

The *diffuse blastemal pattern* is characterized by a general lack of cellular cohesiveness and an aggressive pattern of invasion into adjacent connective tissues and vessels. This is in contrast to the typical circumscribed, encapsulated, and pushing border characteristic of most nephroblastomas. Despite its name, the diffuseness of the blastema is not the characteristic histologic feature, rather it is the invasive growth pattern. Tumors with this histologic pattern usually extend beyond the kidney and are diffusely infiltrative rather than sharply circumscribed (fig. 1-26). Nevertheless, such lesions generally respond to current therapeutic regimens and are not classified among those with unfavorable histology in the pre-therapy specimen. The presence of extensive blastemal cells in nephrectomy specimens following therapy, however, is associated with a poor response to therapy and a reduced survival rate (30,35). Diffuse blastemal nephroblastomas are histologically reminiscent of soft tissue embryonal tumors of childhood

Figure 1-26

NEPHROBLASTOMA

Invasive diffuse blastemal pattern shows discohesive cells extensively invading the soft tissue of the renal sinus.

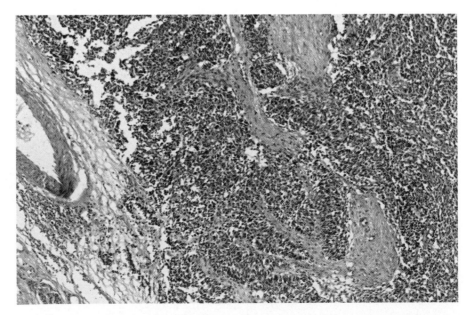

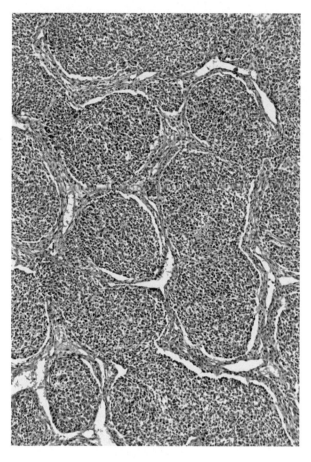

Figure 1-27

NEPHROBLASTOMA

This distinctive packaging of blastemal cells, seen in the nodular blastemal pattern, is seldom observed in other small blue cell tumors of childhood.

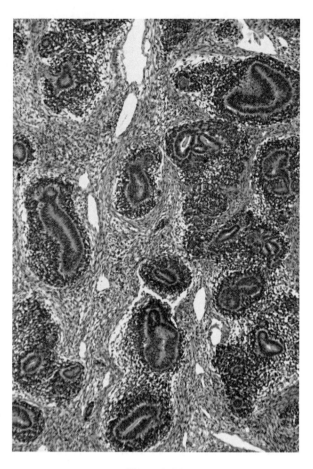

Figure 1-28

NEPHROBLASTOMA

The central epithelial pattern is characterized by a central tubule surrounded by blastemal cells.

such as primitive neuroectodermal tumor, neuroblastoma, synovial sarcoma, and lymphoma.

Other blastemal patterns tend to be cohesive and lack the aggressive invasiveness characterized by the diffuse blastemal type. The *nodular* and *serpentine blastemal patterns* are the most frequently encountered in nephroblastomas (fig. 1-27). These are characterized by round or undulating, sharply defined cords or nests of blastemal cells set in a loose, myxoid or fibromyxoid stroma. These growth patterns are rarely seen in other primitive neoplasms of childhood and are virtually diagnostic of a nephroblastoma. Well-defined tubules may be present centrally in some nodules, a configuration reminiscent of the condensations of blastema around the ampullary ends of the branching ureteric buds in the developing kidney (fig. 1-28). A *basaloid blastemal pattern* results when the serpentine or nodular patterns are outlined by a distinctive epithelial layer (fig. 1-29).

Epithelial Component. An epithelial component of differentiation is present in most nephroblastomas. In some lesions, this pattern is manifested by primitive rosette-like structures that are barely recognizable as early tubular forms. These are indistinguishable from similar structures seen in neuroblastomas and may result in diagnostic difficulty. Other nephroblastomas are composed predominantly or exclusively of easily recognizable tubular or papillary elements that recapitulate various stages of normal nephrogenesis (figs. 1-30, 1-31). Glomerular structures may closely resemble

17

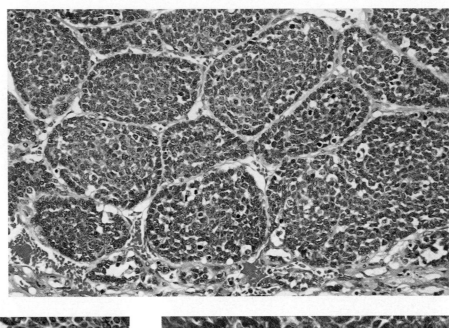

Figure 1-29

NEPHROBLASTOMA

The basaloid blastemal pattern contains an epithelial layer that outlines distinct nodules.

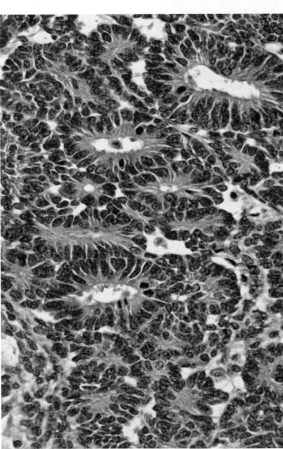

Figure 1-30

NEPHROBLASTOMA

Tall columnar cells and small lumens are seen in the embryonal tubular pattern.

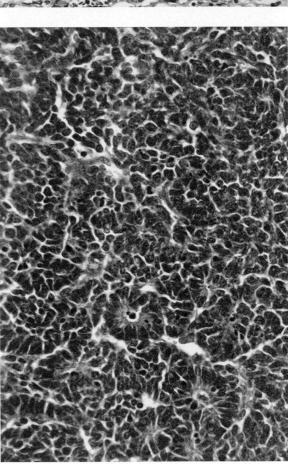

Figure 1-31

NEPHROBLASTOMA

Primitive tubular structures merge with undifferentiated areas.

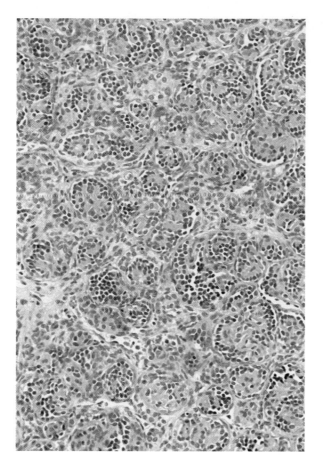

Figure 1-32

NEPHROBLASTOMA

Relatively mature glomeruloid differentiation predominates in this field.

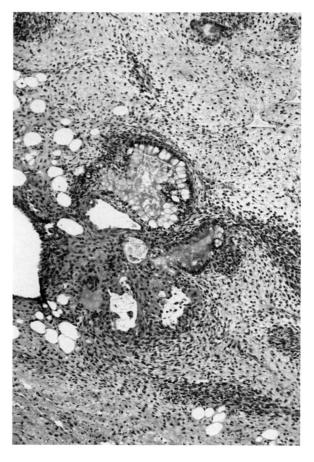

Figure 1-33

NEPHROBLASTOMA

A focus of mucinous epithelium is surrounded by myxoid stroma.

those of normal kidneys; they usually lack capillaries but many exceptions exist (fig. 1-32). Foci of mature cell types with low mitotic rates and increasing cytoplasmic content may represent differentiation toward a more mature state, particularly following therapy. Heterologous epithelial differentiation may occur; the most common elements are mucinous and squamous epithelia (fig. 1-33). Occasionally, ciliated epithelium is present.

Stromal Component. A variety of stromal patterns may cause diagnostic difficulty when blastemal or epithelial differentiation is absent. Myxoid and spindle cells resembling embryonic mesenchyme are found in nearly all specimens, and form the matrix for most of the blastemal and epithelial foci. Smooth muscle and fibroblasts may be present and may show varying degrees of differentiation (figs. 1-34, 1-35). Skeletal muscle is the most common heterologous stromal cell type and large fields of the tumor often contain this pattern (fig. 1-36). More primitive myoblastic elements can also be found, including the condensed mesenchyme characteristic of the cambium layer of botryoid embryonal rhabdomyosarcoma (fig. 1-37).

Almost any type of stromal differentiation, including adipose tissue, cartilage, osteoid, mature ganglion cells, and neuroglial tissue, may be observed in nephroblastomas (figs. 1-38–1-40) (78,80). This heterogeneity may be so prominent as to suggest a teratoma, and most pediatric renal tumors reported in the literature as renal teratoma are probably nephroblastomas. A useful distinguishing feature is the presence of organoid differentiation composed of more than one

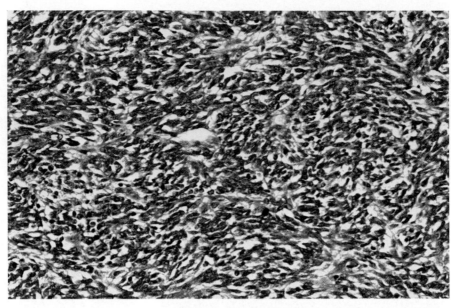

Figure 1-34

NEPHROBLASTOMA

A poorly differentiated spindle cell component may cause diagnostic difficulty if unaccompanied by epithelial elements.

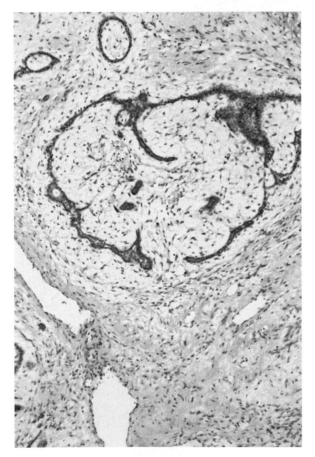

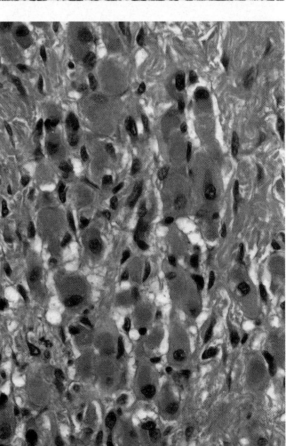

Figure 1-35

NEPHROBLASTOMA

Differentiated, myxoid stroma and branching trabeculae of epithelium form an adamantine pattern.

Figure 1-36

NEPHROBLASTOMA

Skeletal muscle is a commonly encountered element within nephroblastoma.

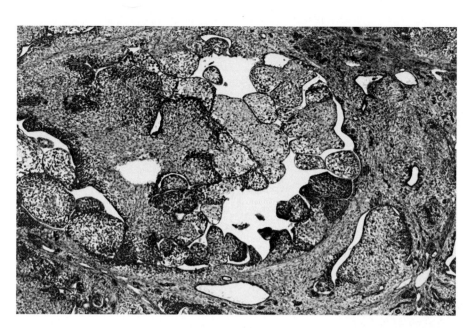

Figure 1-37

NEPHROBLASTOMA

Botryoid protrusions of tumor cells into the lumen of the pelvicaliceal system. (See figure 1-21 for the gross appearance.)

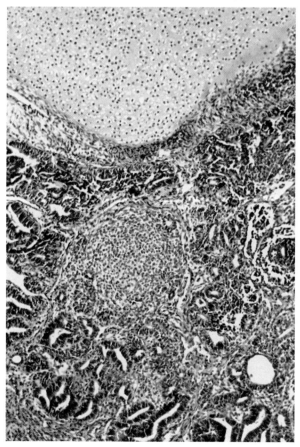

Figure 1-38

NEPHROBLASTOMA

Heterologous cartilage formation is evident.

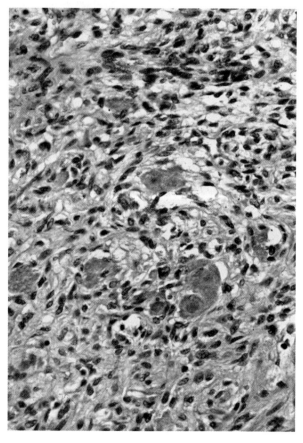

Figure 1-39

NEPHROBLASTOMA

Six mature ganglion cells are clustered near the center of this teratoid nephroblastoma, along with other mature tubular and stromal elements.

21

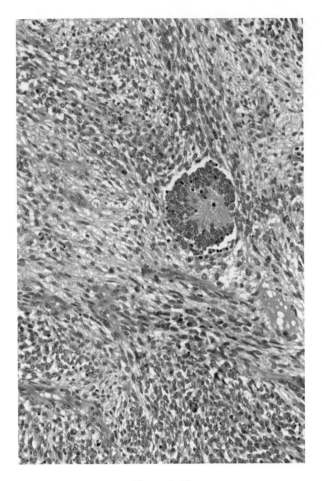

Figure 1-40

NEPHROBLASTOMA

Rosette-like structures are commonly seen in nephroblastoma.

Table 1-3

CRITERIA FOR FOCAL AND DIFFUSE ANAPLASIA

Histologic Criteria for Anaplasia
Presence of polyploid multipolar mitotic figures
Presence of nuclear enlargement with hyperchromasia

Histologic Criteria for Focal Anaplasia
Anaplastic regions that are circumscribed and the perimeter completely examined (may require mapping of anaplastic foci that extend to the edge of tissue sections)
Anaplasia confined to the renal parenchyma (presence in vascular spaces precludes the diagnosis)
Absence of severe nuclear pleomorphism and hyperchromasia (severe "nuclear unrest") in nonanaplastic tumor

tomas is important primarily in achieving the correct diagnosis. The effect of current therapy is such that the majority of tumors, regardless of their heterogeneity, can be considered to reside in the "favorable" histology group. Most tumors in this group are highly responsive to chemotherapy.

Unfavorable Histology. The majority of nephroblastomas associated with an adverse outcome are recognized by their unfavorable histology. Unfavorable histology is defined as the presence of nuclear anaplasia (39,119). Rarely, the development of a high-grade malignancy within a nephroblastoma also results in a poor prognosis. Such tumors include sarcomas as well as epithelial malignancies, and are recognized by an independent growth pattern that outstrips the growth of the underlying nephroblastoma (19,43).

Nuclear Anaplasia. As currently defined, anaplasia within a nephroblastoma refers to extreme nuclear atypia and hyperchromasia rather than to a lack of cellular differentiation. The overall frequency of anaplasia in nephroblastoma is 5 percent, but is age dependent. Anaplasia is rare in neoplasms diagnosed during the first 2 years of life, increases in prevalence to approximately 13 percent by 5 years of age, and remains at this level in tumors detected throughout the remainder of childhood and adolescence (63). Limited experience with adult nephroblastomas suggests that anaplasia has the same prognostic significance as in children. The rate of anaplasia is 2 to 3 times greater in black

cell type. Such organoid differentiation is characteristic of teratoma and is absent in teratoid nephroblastoma. Terms such as *fetal rhabdomyomatous nephroblastoma* and *teratoid nephroblastoma* have been suggested for lesions with prominent heterologous differentiation (56,81,116). The structural diversity inherent in nephroblastomas could engender an endless proliferation of similar descriptive terms and therefore the use of subdesignations based upon morphology alone is discouraged. Only those subtypes with important and consistent clinical implications should be considered in categories with separate names.

Favorable Histology. Recognition of the histologic diversity that may be seen in nephroblas-

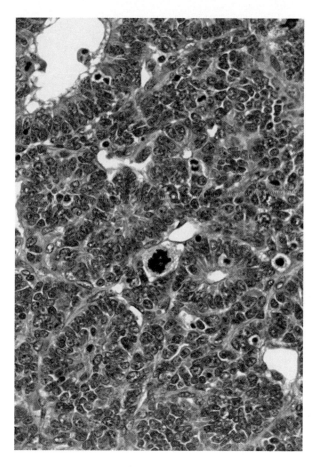

Figure 1-41

ANAPLASTIC NEPHROBLASTOMA

The polyploid multipolar mitotic figure contrasts with the numerous smaller normal mitotic figures in the field.

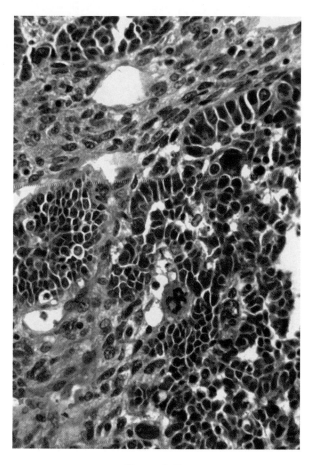

Figure 1-42

ANAPLASTIC NEPHROBLASTOMA

This field shows the enlarged, pleomorphic and hyperchromatic nuclei that are major criteria for recognition of anaplasia.

than in white patients. The histologic requirements to confirm anaplasia follow (Table 1-3).

The Presence of Multipolar Polyploid Mitotic Figures. The mitotic abnormalities must reflect an unequivocal increase in the total amount of DNA (fig. 1-41). In a true multipolar polyploid mitotic figure, each component must be as large or larger than a normal metaphase (fig. 1-42). Simple lagging of chromosomes on an anaphase spindle, although constituting an "abnormal mitosis," is not considered nuclear anaplasia. Uneven separation of a diploid metaphase plate can produce an X- or Y-shaped mitotic figure that might mimic a tripolar or tetrapolar mitosis, but these structures cannot be considered nuclear anaplasia if the total length of the X or

Y figure approximates that of a normal metaphase. Multipolar polyploid mitotic figures are required for the diagnosis of anaplasia, although in a limited sample, marked nucleomegaly with hyperchromasia alone may be sufficient to suggest this change.

Marked Nuclear Enlargement and Hyperchromasia. The major dimensions of affected nuclei meeting the criteria of nuclear anaplasia must be at least three times that of apparently nonanaplastic nuclei in other areas of the specimen (fig. 1-43) (119). Nuclear enlargement should involve all dimensions of the nuclei; simple elongation is insufficient. The enlarged nuclei must also be hyperchromatic, again indicating an unequivocal increase in DNA content.

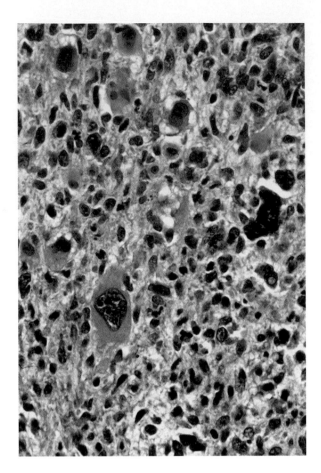

Figure 1-43

ANAPLASTIC NEPHROBLASTOMA

Stromal nephroblastoma with skeletal muscle differentiation shows the marked nuclear hyperchromasia and enlargement characteristic of anaplasia. The nuclear to cytoplasmic ratio is increased. Multipolar mitotic figures were present in other fields.

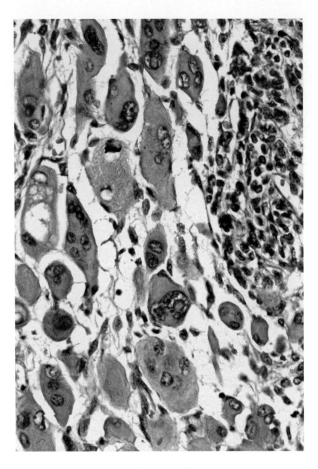

Figure 1-44

NEPHROBLASTOMA

Tumors cells with skeletal muscle differentiation may show striking nuclear hyperchromasia and pleomorphism, mimicking anaplasia. Note the parallel increase in cytoplasmic volume. No multipolar mitotic figures were present.

Areas of skeletal muscle differentiation within a nephroblastoma may have cells with dramatic nuclear enlargement, pleomorphism, and hyperchromasia (fig. 1-44). However, the nuclear enlargement is accompanied by increased cytoplasmic volume, and atypical mitotic figures are not seen. These findings are reminiscent of the regenerative features seen in normal skeletal muscle cells following surgery, and should not be mistaken for anaplasia.

The primary importance of nuclear anaplasia is its correlation with the responsiveness of the tumor to therapy rather than with any prediction of tumor aggressiveness (119). Accordingly, the presence of nuclear anaplasia is most consistently associated with a poor prognosis when it is diffusely distributed and when it appears in tumors of advanced stages (54). For this reason, pathologic and therapeutic distinctions have been made between *focal anaplasia* and *diffuse anaplasia*. Focal anaplasia is defined as the presence of one or a few sharply localized regions of anaplasia within a primary tumor, the majority of which contain no significant nuclear atypia (figs. 1-45, 1-46). To qualify as focal, the areas of anaplasia must be confined to the renal parenchyma. Under this definition, patients with focal anaplasia have a prognosis approximating that for patients with lesions of favorable histology (54). Focal anaplasia has restrictive

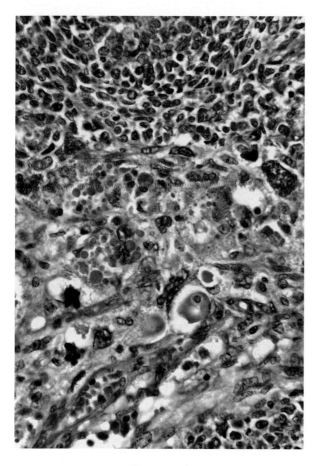

Figure 1-45

NEPHROBLASTOMA WITH FOCAL ANAPLASIA

A sharply demarcated nodular region is the only site of anaplasia in this tumor. The size discrepancy between nuclei in the two halves of this field is apparent even under low magnification.

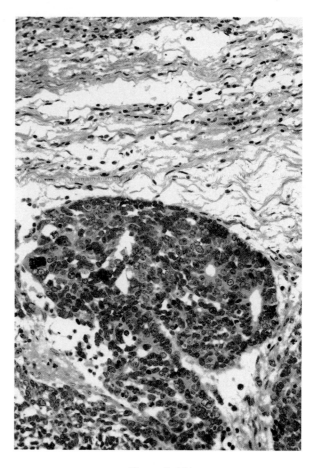

Figure 1-46

NEPHROBLASTOMA WITH FOCAL ANAPLASIA

Post-therapy nephrectomy specimens may show demarcated clusters of anaplastic cells due to the positive selection for these unresponsive cells by chemotherapy.

criteria, however, as indicated in Table 1-3. Anaplasia not meeting these requirements becomes classified as diffuse anaplasia.

Post-therapy nephrectomy specimens may contain circumscribed areas of anaplasia although the original biopsies were of favorable histology (fig. 1-46). This is because anaplastic foci do not respond to therapy whereas tumors of favorable histology do, resulting in the "selection" of anaplastic cells following therapy and the greater likelihood that these cells are both sampled for histology and detected microscopically. There is no evidence to suggest that therapy itself produces nuclear anaplasia.

The therapeutic and prognostic significance of nuclear anaplasia is profound, particularly in patients with high-stage tumors. A few tumors contain cells with features that straddle the imaginary line between favorable and unfavorable histology. These tumors have enlarged, hyperchromatic nuclei ("nuclear unrest") that do not meet the strict criteria for anaplasia. Such changes are particularly worrisome when identified in a small biopsy taken from a large mass. However, it has been the experience of the NWTSG pathology center and of others that many of these tumors respond quite well to treatment (68). Therefore, in the absence of a therapeutic regimen that successfully treats patients with anaplastic tumors, and considering the significant side effects of the aggressive therapy provided to such patients, tumors that

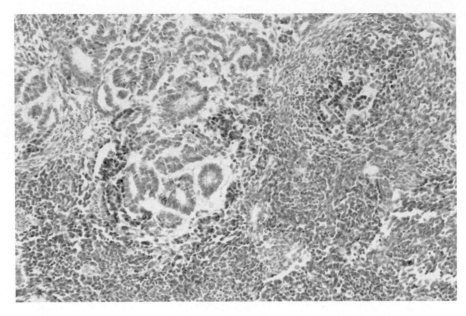

Figure 1-47

NEPHROBLASTOMA

Primitive blastemal and epithelial elements show WT1 expression, whereas differentiated epithelial and stromal components are commonly negative.

do not unequivocally meet the criteria for anaplasia are treated using the same protocols applied to neoplasms of favorable histology.

Immunohistochemical Findings. Immunohistochemical studies have a limited role in the pathologic evaluation of nephroblastomas. The results reflect the cell types and levels of differentiation present in the lesion: skeletal muscle fibers, neural elements, and tubular formations have the immunohistochemical characteristics of these cell types (52); structures in nephroblastomas that resemble components of the developing kidney have the same immunohistochemical features as their normal counterparts. The blastemal cells of nephroblastomas regularly express vimentin but other differentiation markers are usually absent (114). As in many other tumors, expression of neuron-specific enolase may be seen in the blastemal cells of nephroblastomas (53). Desmin may be both useful and misinterpreted when applied to blastemal patterns; a majority of tumors with blastemal patterns are at least focally positive for desmin yet usually negative for other primitive muscle markers such as myogenin and MyoD1 (57).

Immunohistochemical reactions for WT1 protein, confined to the nucleus, are variable and correlate with tumor histology. Areas of stromal differentiation have very low levels or no expression of WT1; areas of blastemal and early epithelial differentiation have consistently diffuse expression; areas of differentiated epithelium have patchy and variable reactions, with a positive reaction correlating best with glomerular differentiation (fig. 1-47) (42a,64a, 94). Whereas WT1 immunoreactivity may be useful in the distinction between blastemal nephroblastoma and other primitive tumors, it is not useful in tumors with only stromal differentiation. The presence of WT1 positivity in a primitive tumor supports the diagnosis of nephroblastoma. The rare exception is desmoplastic small round cell tumor, which likewise expresses high levels of WT1 (24). No single immunohistochemical reaction is universally diagnostic for nephroblastoma and the panel used must be determined on a case-by-case basis.

Ultrastructural Findings. Ultrastructural studies are usually not required for the diagnosis of nephroblastoma but can be helpful when a predominantly blastemal tumor must be distinguished from other "undifferentiated" neoplasms. Ultrastructurally, nephroblastoma cells closely resemble those of the developing metanephros (83). The findings are dependent upon the cell types present and their degree of differentiation (fig. 1-48). Primitive blastemal cells have sparse, poorly developed organelles, numerous free ribosomes, and a moderate number of mitochondria. Many cells interpreted as blastemal with the light microscope exhibit well-developed cell junctions and numerous organelles ultrastructurally. A layer of thick, flocculent, electron-dense material frequently

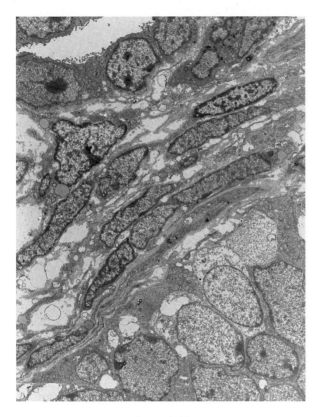

Figure 1-48

NEPHROBLASTOMA

Ultrastructural appearance of a triphasic specimen, with epithelial differentiation near the top of the field, stromal cells near the center, and blastemal cells near the bottom. (Fig. 1-50, Fascicle 11, 3rd Series.)

adheres to the cell surface. Microvilli vary in number and prominence. Phagolysosomes and lipid droplets may occur. The ultrastructural features that help confirm the diagnosis of a monophasic, poorly differentiated nephroblastoma include well-developed desmosomes and the characteristic flocculent coating. Cilia are more numerous than in other childhood tumors. The presence of paired, confronting cisternae in mitotically active blastemal cells is usually a more prominent feature than in most other pediatric renal neoplasms (83).

Prognosis. Nephroblastomas generally have a restricted pattern of local growth and metastasis (40). Locally, they may involve the renal vein and extend into the inferior vena cava, resulting in inoperability prior to therapy. The most common sites of metastasis are to the regional lymph nodes, lungs, and liver; unusual sites include the spinal epidural space, central nervous system, and mediastinal lymph nodes following pulmonary metastasis (33). Metastatic sites other than these are unusual and should always suggest alternative diagnoses. Bony metastases, for example, occur in less than 1 percent of nephroblastomas. Tumors that rupture before or during nephrectomy may become implanted widely in the flank or peritoneum.

A favorable outcome can be expected even among most patients having neoplasms with focal nuclear anaplasia. The prognosis is apparently not affected by tumor size or weight. The overall 4-year survival rate for patients with favorable histology nephroblastomas of all stages now approaches 90 percent. Specifically, patients with stages I, II, III, and IV tumors of favorable histology have 4-year overall survival rates of 96 percent, 91 percent, 90 percent, and 81 percent, respectively (49). The most significant unfavorable prognostic factors are age at detection, high stage, and unfavorable histology. Patients with diffuse anaplasia who received vincristine, dactinomycin, doxorubicin, cyclophosphamide, and radiation therapy, had a 4-year survival rate of 70 percent (for those with stage II tumor), 56 percent (stage III), and 17 percent (stage IV) (63).

Long-term follow-up of patients with nephroblastoma has shown that serious renal dysfunction is uncommon. When seen, the most frequent causes are renal failure associated with the Denys-Drash syndrome and renal failure caused by radiation nephritis (97). Sequelae that may be seen secondary to radiation therapy include decreased pulmonary function, infertility, and scoliosis. As many as 25 percent of nephroblastoma patients treated with doxorubicin develop some cardiac abnormality, depending on the cumulative dose and dose intensity (103). Survivors of nephroblastoma are at risk for second malignant neoplasms, which rarely are due to an inherited predisposition, but more commonly are the result of radiation and/or chemotherapy. The NWTSG experience suggests a cumulative incidence of second malignancies of 1.6 percent at 15 years after the initial diagnosis of nephroblastoma (40).

Differential Diagnosis. Nephroblastomas must be distinguished from other primary pediatric renal tumors, such as clear cell sarcoma,

Table 1-4

RELATIVE FREQUENCY OF
PEDIATRIC RENAL MALIGNANCIES

Neoplasm	Estimated Relative Frequency (%)
Nephroblastoma (nonanaplastic)	80
Nephroblastoma (anaplastic)	5
Mesoblastic nephroma	5
Clear cell sarcoma	4
Rhabdoid tumor	2

Miscellaneous
  Neuroblastoma
  Peripheral neuroectodermal tumor
  Synovial sarcoma
  Renal cell carcinoma
  Angiomyolipoma
  Lymphoma
  Other rare neoplasms
	4

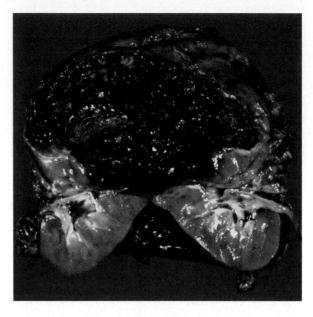

Figure 1-49

NEUROBLASTOMA

Neuroblastomas may be grossly indistinguishable from nephroblastomas. However, many cases, such as the one illustrated, have a hemorrhagic appearance and lack the sharp circumscription usually seen in nephroblastoma.

congenital mesoblastic nephroma, and rhabdoid tumor, as well as from pediatric embryonal soft tissue neoplasms that infrequently arise in the kidney. Table 1-4 presents an estimate of the likelihood of each tumor in childhood as a whole; the likelihood of each neoplasm during various periods of childhood is quite different. For example, congenital mesoblastic nephroma is far less common than nephroblastoma for all ages, but is the most common renal tumor in children less than 3 months of age. The diagnosis of congenital mesoblastic nephroma is highly suspect in a patient older than 2 years of age. Conversely, anaplastic nephroblastoma is virtually never encountered in infants. The differential diagnosis between nephroblastoma and the other primary renal neoplasms of childhood is considered in detail in the sections describing those lesions.

Tumors other than those detailed in this chapter are rare in children and young adults. Nearly all can be included among the so-called small, round, blue cell neoplasms. Since the accurate interpretation of these tumors ordinarily involves their distinction from nephroblastoma, and the differential diagnosis may depend on the clinical circumstances as well as the pathologic features, it seems appropriate to deal with these neoplasms in an expanded discussion in this section rather than by describing them in a separate section of rare renal tumors.

Neuroblastoma. Perhaps the most frequently encountered diagnostic problem is distinguishing nephroblastoma from undifferentiated or poorly differentiated neuroblastoma. Each year 2 to 3 tumors are registered by the NWTSG as blastemal nephroblastoma and are identified after central review as poorly differentiated or undifferentiated stroma-poor neuroblastoma (66). Surprisingly, the majority of these masses are clinically confined to the kidney, their epicenter is within the kidney, and the correct diagnosis is documented only following nephrectomy.

Clinical features that should raise the suspicion of neuroblastoma include elevated levels of catecholamine metabolites, stippled calcification on imaging studies, lack of circumscription, and widespread metastases to organs other than lung, liver, and lymph nodes. Grossly, neuroblastomas are often much more hemorrhagic than nephroblastomas (fig. 1-49). Histologically, the rosettes of some neuroblastomas or primitive neuroepithelial tumors closely resemble the nascent tubular formations of epithelial nephroblastoma (fig. 1-50). Epithelial differentiation in a nephroblastoma is usually

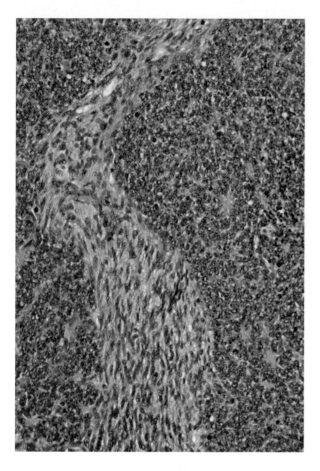

Figure 1-50

NEPHROBLASTOMA

Primitive tubules within a field of a nephroblastoma mimic the rosettes seen in neuroblastoma.

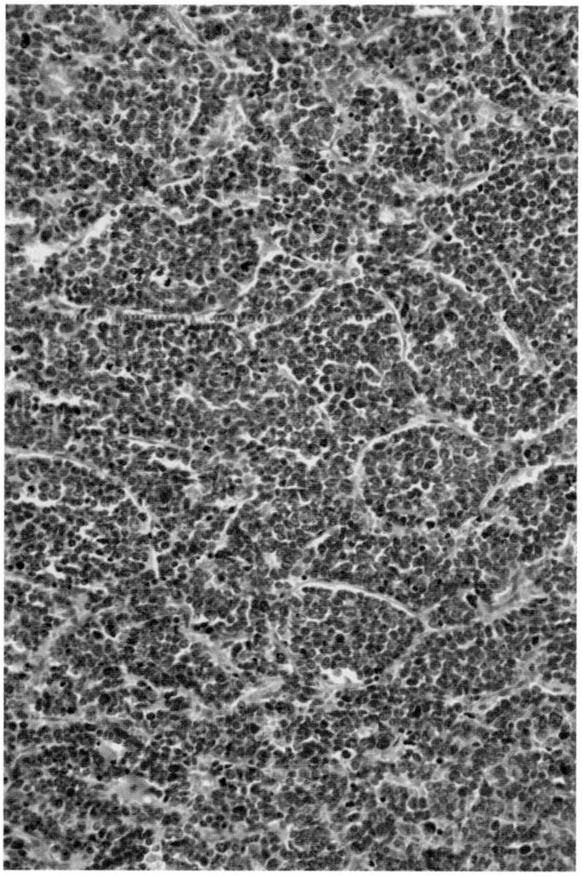

Figure 1-51

NEUROBLASTOMA

An organoid pattern of growth of undifferentiated cells with a "salt and pepper" nuclear chromatin pattern is characteristic of neuroblastoma.

characterized by a single layer of nuclei arranged in parallel, while the classic Homer-Wright rosette of a neuroblastoma tends to have a zone of nuclear concentration around a central fibrillary core, without the formation of a distinct layer of parallel nuclei. The absence of a well-developed peritumoral fibrous capsule, and the presence of an invasive growth pattern, prominent nesting of tumor cells, prominent hemorrhage, and nonoverlapping nuclei with coarse "salt and pepper" chromatin are histologic features that should raise the probability of a correct diagnosis of neuroblastoma (figs. 1-50, 1-51).

Immunohistochemical studies for markers such as WT1 and NB84 may be required to resolve difficult cases. Nephroblastoma and neuroblastoma may both show positivity for neuron-specific enolase and CD56, and variable expression for vimentin. A high proportion of intrarenal neuroblastomas are of unfavorable histology as defined by the International Neuroblastoma Pathology Classification and have a higher incidence of anaplasia (32 percent) when compared to both their adrenal counterparts and to nephroblastoma (66,102).

Synovial Sarcoma. These tumors rarely arise in the kidney, and are commonly misdiagnosed as nephroblastoma or another undifferentiated sarcoma (21,31,73,74). The 15 reported patients from the NWTSG pathology center range in age from 20 to 59 years (mean, 37 years). Grossly, these tumors are typically large, with a mean greatest dimension of 11 cm, and are usually at least focally cystic. Most renal synovial

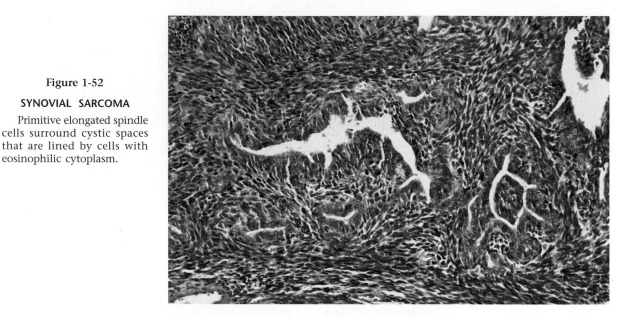

Figure 1-52

SYNOVIAL SARCOMA

Primitive elongated spindle cells surround cystic spaces that are lined by cells with eosinophilic cytoplasm.

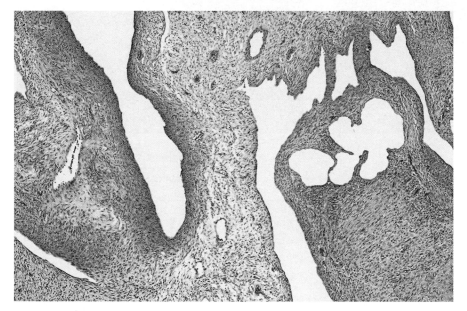

Figure 1-53

SYNOVIAL SARCOMA

Many synovial sarcomas contain a prominent cystic component; rare tumors are predominately cystic and mimic a cystic nephroma.

sarcomas are monophasic, although rare biphasic tumors have been reported (31). The tumor cells form short intersecting fascicles that readily dissect the native renal parenchyma (fig. 1-52). The serpentine and nodular patterns that are typical of blastemal nephroblastoma are not present in synovial sarcoma. The nuclei of synovial sarcoma cells are ovoid, with basophilic nuclei and indistinct cytoplasm. Similar to nephroblastoma, nuclear overlapping is present. Necrosis is a common feature, and often involves tumor cells distant from blood ves-

sels, resulting in the peritheliomatous pattern that is also often seen in primitive neuroectodermal tumors (PNETs). Cystic structures are common within synovial sarcomas, and are lined by cells having abundant acidophilic cytoplasm with luminal snouts and apically oriented nuclei, creating a hobnail appearance (figs. 1-52, 1-53). In the majority of cases, these cysts represent entrapped, dilated renal collecting ducts. A range of epithelial differentiation may be seen in the rare biphasic renal synovial sarcoma (fig. 1-54).

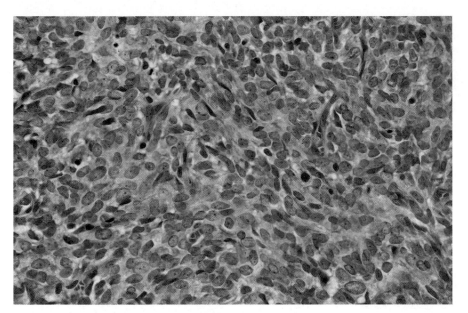

Figure 1-54

SYNOVIAL SARCOMA

Poorly differentiated sarcoma containing the t(X;18) translocation of monophasic synovial sarcoma.

Figure 1-55

GENETIC TRANSLOCATIONS CHARACTERISTIC OF SYNOVIAL SARCOMA AND PRIMITIVE NEUROECTODERMAL TUMOR

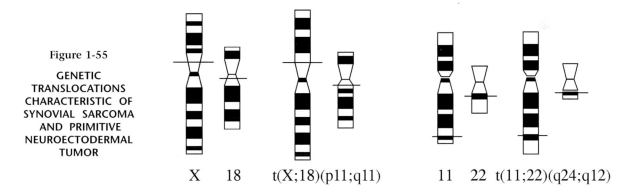

X   18   t(X;18)(p11;q11)   11   22   t(11;22)(q24;q12)

Immunohistochemical reactions are of some use in distinguishing synovial sarcoma from blastemal or primitive stromal-predominant nephroblastoma. If positive, epithelial markers are helpful. However, these are negative in the vast majority of synovial sarcomas and are positive in many nephroblastomas (21). WT1 is positive in the primitive elements of nephroblastoma and is negative in the histologically similar monophasic synovial sarcoma. While the combination of positivity for Bcl-2 and negativity for CD34 has been suggested to be relatively unique for synovial sarcoma and hence useful in its diagnosis, this feature is often shared by stromal-predominant nephroblastoma (106).

The ability to identify renal synovial sarcomas with confidence is the result of a variety of techniques to detect the t(X;18) translocation characteristic of this tumor (fig. 1-55). In addition to cytogenetic techniques, molecular analysis may document the presence of the *SYT/SSX* fusion transcripts resulting from this translocation (21,45,109).

The prognosis of patients with primary synovial sarcoma of the kidney is uncertain; of 20 reported patients, at least 7 had local or metastatic recurrence, and 2 died (21,73,74). It is doubtful that the majority of these patients received the currently recommended therapy for synovial sarcoma, which includes cyclophosphamide and etoposide.

Primitive Neuroectodermal Tumor. The history of primitive neuroectodermal tumors (PNETs) primary to the kidney is similar to that of synovial sarcoma. PNETs were largely unrecognized

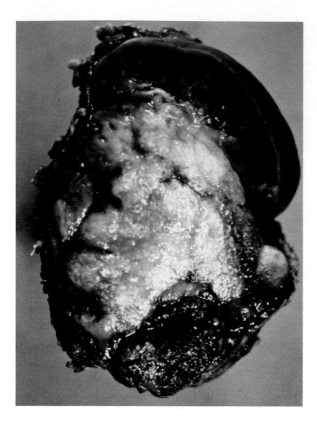

Figure 1-56

PRIMITIVE NEUROECTODERMAL TUMOR

The lack of circumscription is seen grossly.

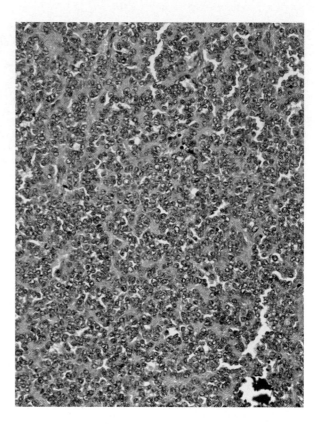

Figure 1-57

PRIMITIVE NEUROECTODERMAL TUMOR

This tumor contains numerous poorly formed pseudo-rosettes.

prior to the detection of the t(11;22) (q24;q12) and the other variant translocations characteristic for this tumor (fig. 1-55) (108). The development of immunohistochemical reactions for the MIC2 antigen (CD99), despite its lack of specificity, has likewise played an important role in the detection of PNETs, as blastemal nephroblastomas are negative for this marker. Primary renal PNETs are reported to affect patients from 1 month to 72 years of age, although most patients are adolescents or young adults (71,89,98). PNETs, unlike nephroblastomas, are grossly poorly circumscribed (fig. 1-56). Microscopically, PNETs of the kidney demonstrate primitive round cells with variable rosette formation (fig. 1-57). The cells are typically distributed in a nonoverlapping fashion, unlike those of nephroblastoma (fig. 1-58). Immunohistochemical studies demonstrate strong membranous positivity for CD99 and FLI1, and nega-

tivity for WT1, findings that would exclude the diagnosis of blastemal nephroblastoma (fig. 1-59). The outcome is poor, with metastasis and death in most patients (71,89,98).

Rhabdomyosarcoma. Rhabdomyosarcoma primary to the kidney is rare in the absence of a preceding nephroblastoma, with less than 10 cases seen in the 30-year history of the NWTSG pathology center. Equally rare are rhabdomyosarcomas that develop in the setting of a preexisting nephroblastoma. Such cases have included both embryonal and alveolar subtypes, complete with the cytogenetic translocation characteristic of the latter. In comparison, nephroblastomas composed of greater than two thirds skeletal muscle differentiation are common, with over 150 cases seen in the NWTSG pathology center. The distinction between a nephroblastoma predominantly composed of undifferentiated rhabdomyoblasts and a

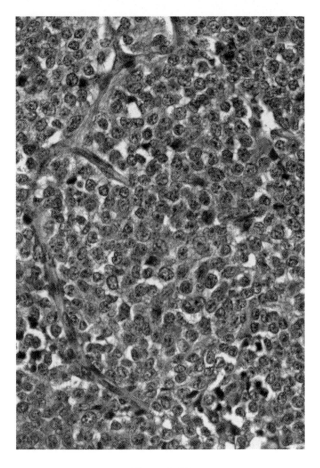

Figure 1-58

PRIMITIVE NEUROECTODERMAL TUMOR

The cells are often nonoverlapping, have fewer mitoses, and have a courser chromatin pattern than is seen in nephroblastomas.

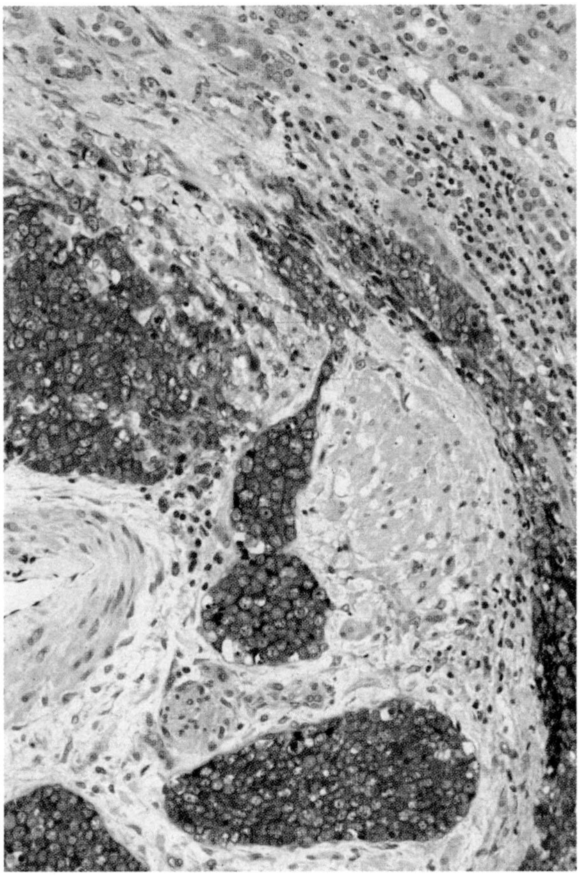

Figure 1-59

PRIMITIVE NEUROECTODERMAL TUMOR

Immunohistochemical staining for CD99 demonstrates the characteristic positivity of the cell membrane.

nephroblastoma with the secondary development of rhabdomyosarcoma may be difficult. It is based on clear evidence that the rhabdomyosarcomatous component is behaving in an independent fashion, outstripping the nephroblastoma component. A renal tumor composed only of rhabdomyoblasts on biopsy samples is presumed to represent a nephroblastoma until either: 1) confirmatory genetic evidence is available; 2) the tumor is refractory to nephroblastoma therapy; or 3) additional tissue provides information leading to an alternate diagnosis.

Other embryonal neoplasms that may present as primary renal lesions include desmoplastic small round cell tumor (which is often not desmoplastic), clear cell sarcoma of soft parts, and epithelioid sarcoma (59,99). The cells of a lymphoma occasionally resemble the diffuse blastemal pattern of a nephroblastoma; immunohistochemical phenotyping usually resolves this problem (fig. 1-60).

The above soft tissue lesions most commonly afflict adolescents or young adults. Most of the cases submitted to the NWTSG pathology center as "adult nephroblastomas" are in fact PNETs or synovial sarcomas. This may help explain the long-held view among oncologists that adult nephroblastomas are more aggressive than those in children. Recent evidence suggests that this is not the case, and that adult nephroblastomas are best treated using the same protocols provided to children (72).

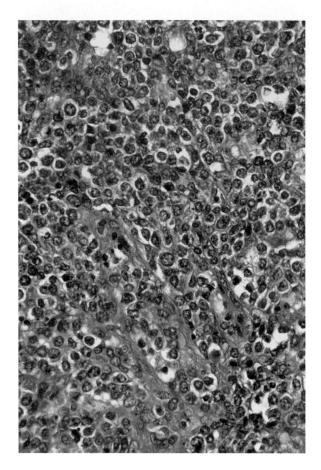

Figure 1-60

RENAL LYMPHOMA

This tumor with discohesive cells lacking particular architectural arrangements was diffusely positive for lymphoid markers.

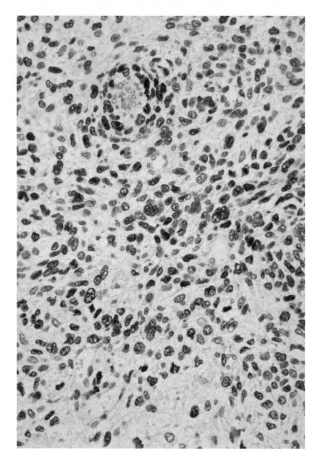

Figure 1-61

ANAPLASTIC NEPHROBLASTOMA

Immunohistochemical analysis for TP53 shows strong nuclear staining of the majority of cells within an anaplastic nephroblastoma.

Special Techniques. The histologic presence of anaplasia has long been associated with mutation of the *TP53* gene within nephroblastomas as well as other pediatric tumors (23,82, 107). Mutation of *TP53* often results in elevated protein levels due to the inability of the cell to degrade the abnormal protein. The resulting increase in TP53 protein levels may be detected by immunohistochemistry (fig. 1-61) (44,62, 75). While *TP53* gene mutation and anaplasia are closely linked, the association between TP53 protein overexpression and anaplasia is less clear, due in large part to the presence of occasional nonanaplastic nephroblastomas that have strong immunoreactivity for TP53 (greater than 20 percent nuclear staining). Patients whose tumors have increased levels of TP53 pro-

tein yet normal *TP53* gene sequences and no evidence histologically of anaplasia also seem to have a poor prognosis (75). Due to the variability of immunohistochemical reactions in the interpretation of TP53, this marker has not been used to date in cooperative group studies. Histologic evidence of anaplasia remains the most reliable indicator of poor prognosis in patients with nephroblastoma. Unfortunately, some patients whose tumors lack this feature, and are therefore classified as "favorable histology," are nonresponsive to current treatments and have a poor prognosis. Efforts to refine the definition of unfavorable histology in nephroblastomas using quantitative cytometric techniques have yielded conflicting results. With the currently available information, flow cytometry is

Table 1-5

STAGING OF PEDIATRIC RENAL TUMORS (NATIONAL WILMS TUMOR STUDY GROUP)[a]

Stage	Definition
I	**Limited to kidney and completely resected.** Renal capsule is intact. Renal sinus soft tissue may be minimally infiltrated.
II	**Tumor infiltrates beyond kidney, but is completely resected.** Tumor penetration of renal capsule or infiltration of vessels within the renal sinus (including the intrarenal extension of the sinus). Also includes tumors with prior open or large bore needle biopsies. May include tumors with local tumor spillage confined to flank.
III	**Residual nonhematogenous tumor confined to abdomen.** Includes cases with one of the following: Tumor in abdominal lymph nodes Diffuse peritoneal contamination by direct tumor growth, tumor implants, or spillage into peritoneum before or during surgery Involvement of specimen margins grossly or microscopically Residual tumor in abdomen Tumor removed noncontiguously (piece-meal resection)
IV	**Hematogenous metastases**
V	**Bilateral renal involvement at diagnosis.** The tumors in each kidney should be separately substaged in these cases.

[a]Data modified from reference 49.

less effective than conventional histology in identifying those tumors associated with a poor prognosis (51,76,85).

Staging. The most widely accepted staging system for nephroblastoma is that of the 5th protocol of the National Wilms Tumor Study Group (NWTSG-5) (Table 1-5) (49). This staging system relies on the identification of penetration of the renal capsule, and involvement of renal sinus vessels, surgical margins, and regional lymph nodes. The renal sinus is the most common site of extension of tumors beyond the renal parenchyma and it is essential that this region is generously sampled for histologic analysis. The renal sinus is identified histologically by the presence of adjacent renal pelvis, calyces, or medullary pyramids; the presence of unencapsulated renal cortex; and the presence of large vessels and nerves. The NWTSG-5 definition for stage I accepts minor degrees of infiltration of the soft tissues of the renal sinus, however, it does not allow the involvement of vessels within the renal sinus. The interpretation of vascular involvement of the renal sinus is hindered by the lack of recognition of the presence of tongue-like extensions of the renal sinus into the contour of the kidney itself (see fig. 1-7). Tumor involvement of the vessels within these extensions increases the stage to II (fig. 1-62). Bulky masses of apparent soft tissue invasion in the sinus are usually assumed to represent intravascular tumor that has effaced vessel walls.

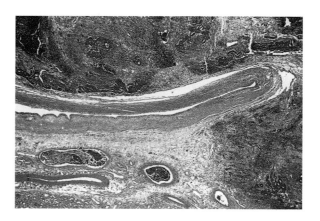

Figure 1-62

NEPHROBLASTOMA

Involvement of sinus vessels by tumor is one of the criteria for stage II.

Another major source of difficulty in differentiating stage I from stage II lesions is the microscopic distinction between the peritumoral fibrous pseudocapsule, the renal capsule, and an inflammatory pseudocapsule composed of active granulation tissue and scarring. An inflammatory pseudocapsule is usually caused by perirenal hemorrhage, extensive necrosis of the peripheral regions of the neoplasm, prior rupture of the tumor, or invasion of the renal capsule. It is possible for a tumor to grow until its capsule merges with the renal capsule, and then to continue to grow into the perirenal fat. It

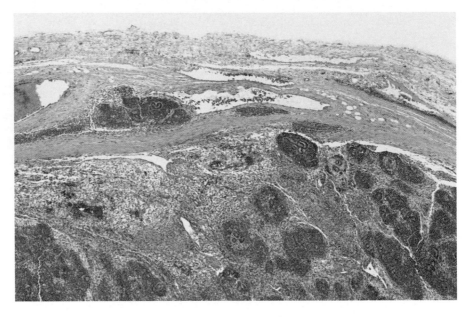

Figure 1-63

"HORIZONTAL ANALYSIS" OF RENAL TUMOR CAPSULE

The outermost tumor cells are in the same layer as perirenal fat, despite being overlain by a fibrous capsule. This appearance is consistent with a stage II designation.

may then form an inflammatory pseudocapsule that merges with the tumor capsule and renal capsule when the invaded fat disappears (112). In such cases, the seemingly simple criterion of "capsular penetration" can be difficult to assess since the "capsule" is a composite of the tumor capsule, the renal capsule, and an inflammatory pseudocapsule. This progression can sometimes be detected by sampling the tumor capsule at its intersection with the renal capsule (fig. 1-63). In this region, the capsule is best analyzed "horizontally," tracking laterally from the deepest level of tumor penetration, and demonstrating that tumor cells are in the same plane as perirenal fat.

Artifactual displacement of tumor cells within the lumens of vessels can likewise pose significant difficulties for pathologic staging. The presence of abundant artifactual tumor displacement elsewhere in the slide set should provide an important clue to the correct interpretation in most cases. Similarly, the presence of ink within the intravascular tumor points to its artifactual nature. Finally, the interpretation of true vascular involvement does not depend on the actual infiltration of the vascular wall by tumor. True vascular involvement is often seen as smooth aggregates of tumor cells floating within venous or lymphatic structures, accompanied by red blood cells or fibrin (fig. 1-64).

A tumor thrombus at the margin of the renal vein is another potential source of staging confusion. It is a relatively common occurrence for the surgeon to identify a renal vein thrombus and to transect the vein, completely excising the vessel proximal to the thrombus in this act. However, once transected, the vein margin usually retracts, leaving tumor protruding from the lumen, appearing to the pathologist to represent marginal involvement. The surgeon's observations are of great importance in the determination of stage in such cases. The most useful histologic section is a shave of the renal vein margin. In the absence of tumor invading the vascular wall in this section, and with the appropriate surgical opinion, the tumor may be safely classified as stage II.

The presence of lymph node metastases does not usually present difficulties. However, nephroblastomas are often difficult to recognize within lymph nodes due to similar staining properties and cellularity as lymphoid tissue. Particularly difficult are the small aggregates of tumor cells within the subcapsular lymph node sinus; these are a common cause of upstaging on central review. Another feature occasionally seen within regional lymph nodes accompanying a nephrectomy specimen is the presence of abundant Tamm-Horsfall protein within the subcapsular sinus. This is often accompanied by displaced renal tubular epithelial cells trapped within the protein. In some cases, these epithelial cells are quite prominent, even forming tubular structures, and result in the erroneous

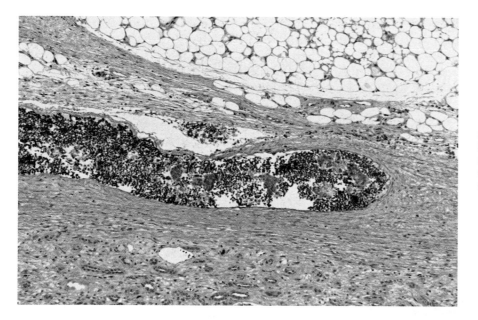

Figure 1-64

NEPHROBLASTOMA

Intravascular aggregates of tumor are intermixed with blood and fibrin, indicating that this intravascular tumor is unlikely to be due to artifactual displacement.

Figure 1-65

NEPHROBLASTOMA

The subcapsular sinus is distended with pink Tamm-Horsfall protein that contains many aggregates of displaced renal tubular epithelial cells (arrowheads), as well as a large cluster of tumor cells (arrow).

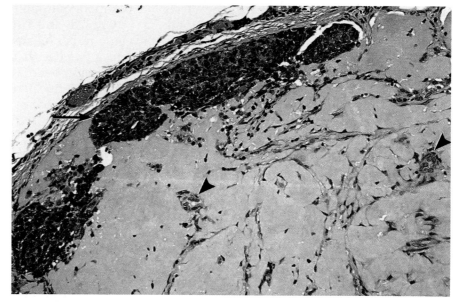

diagnosis of metastatic tumor (113). On the other hand, true tumor metastases may also be entrapped in Tamm-Horsfall protein (fig. 1-65).

Tumors that are not removed intact are considered, by definition, to represent stage III lesions. Therefore, if a surgeon removes the kidney separately from the adrenal gland and the adrenal gland resection has tumor cells in any part of the specimen, this tumor is stage III even if the surgical margins are clear. Similarly, if separately excised lymph nodes have perinodal soft tissue containing tumor, a stage of III is given even if the lymph nodes themselves are negative.

Few staging factors raise as much controversy, consternation, and confusion as that of tumor "spillage." The NWTSG-5 staging criteria indicate that a tumor that "spills" intraoperatively in a region confined to the pelvis or flank should be designated as stage II, while a tumor that "spills" intraperitoneally is designated as stage III, resulting in radiation therapy and more aggressive chemotherapy. This determination of spillage can only be made by the surgeon, and is by its very nature highly subjective. Candid communications with the oncologist and surgeon are essential.

Bilateral nephroblastomas occur in approximately 5 percent of patients and are designated as stage V. This designation has several disadvantages. Since the staging scheme represents a numerical progression that relates to an increasing likelihood for tumor relapse and death, the stage V designation can falsely suggest that the prognosis is even worse than that for stage IV. However, the prognosis in patients with bilateral tumors is determined by the stage of the most advanced tumor as well as by the presence or absence of other prognostic determinants, such as anaplasia. A patient with stage I nephroblastomas of favorable histology in both kidneys generally has a very favorable outcome, even though the bilateral situation is classified as stage V (39). Such cases can be assigned a designation using the stage of the most advanced lesion as the substage determinate (e.g., stage V, substage I).

Pathologic Effects of Treatment. The effects of therapy on the histology of nephroblastoma has been studied by the NWTSG as well as by the European cooperative group investigators (35, 120). Actively proliferating embryonal cell types rich in blastemal cells usually undergo a dramatic response to therapy, resulting in tumor necrosis. Mature tubular and skeletal muscle cells tend to remain unaltered by therapy. Anaplastic cells are also unaffected, although they may appear to be increased in number and frequency because of this unresponsiveness, the "selection factor." Infiltrating populations of histologically viable-appearing embryonal elements with easily identifiable mitoses that appear after recent therapy are a sign of unresponsiveness.

Treatment. Current protocols for favorable histology nephroblastomas are based on tumor stage, patient age, tumor size, and biologic indicators of poor prognosis. An example of the latter is loss of heterozygosity (LOH) for specific loci. Low- and intermediate-risk favorable histology tumors are those that are stage I or II and lack biologic indicators of poor prognosis. High-risk favorable histology tumors are all stages III and IV tumors, and tumors of all stages that have biologic indicators of poor prognosis.

Therapy for nephroblastoma is one of the great success stories in modern oncology. Dactinomycin and vincristine are the most effective drugs for most patients with favorable histology tumors and are now in standard use around the world. These drugs are used in conjunction with surgery, without radiotherapy, for all patients with stage I and II lesions with favorable histology. Radiotherapy and more toxic chemotherapeutic agents are reserved for patients with stage III and IV disease.

NEPHROGENIC RESTS AND NEPHROBLASTOMATOSIS

Definition. The term nephrogenic rest has been proposed for abnormally persistent foci of embryonal cells that are capable of developing into nephroblastomas (29). The term nephroblastomatosis is defined as the presence of diffuse or multifocal nephrogenic rests. These precursors of nephroblastoma are encountered in 25 to 40 percent of patients with nephroblastoma (25,26,29,36). Similar lesions have been observed in approximately 1 percent of routine postmortem examinations in infants (36).

Clinical and Pathologic Findings. Nephrogenic rests are classified into *perilobar (PLNR)* and *intralobar (ILNR)* types. These categories have a number of distinguishing structural features, as delineated in Table 1-6 and discussed below. Nephroblastomatosis can likewise be categorized according to the type of rests present. When only PLNRs or ILNRs are present and they are multiple, the designations *perilobar* or *intralobar nephroblastomatosis* is used; *combined nephroblastomatosis* refers to the presence of both PLNR and ILNR.

PLNR and ILNR have different epidemiologic features. PLNR is found in approximately 1 percent of infant autopsies whereas ILNR is found in only 0.1 percent. Not surprisingly, the prevalence of both types of rests is substantially higher in association with nephroblastoma than in the general infant population (Table 1-7). The association with metachronous bilateral nephroblastoma is especially relevant. Patients with any type of nephrogenic rest in a kidney removed for nephroblastoma should be considered at increased risk for tumor formation in the remaining kidney; the risk is the greatest with ILNRs and in patients less than 12 months of age (29,47). In contrast, when nephrogenic rests are not found in a generous sampling of renal parenchyma of patients with nephroblastoma, the risk for contralateral nephroblastoma is negligible. Both types of nephrogenic rests

Table 1-6		
FEATURES DISTINGUISHING PERILOBAR FROM INTRALOBAR RESTS		
	Perilobar Rests	Intralobar Rests
Position in lobe	Peripheral	Random
Margins	Sharply demarcated	Irregular and intermingling
Composition	Blastema, tubules	Stroma, blastema, tubules
	Stroma scant or sclerotic	Stroma often predominates
Distribution	Usually multifocal	Often unifocal

Table 1-7		
APPROXIMATE PREVALENCE OF NEPHROGENIC RESTS IN SELECTED PATIENT POPULATIONS		
Patient Category	Perilobar Rests	Intralobar Rests
Infant autopsies	0.01	0.001
Dysplastic kidneys	0.04	Unknown
Nephroblastoma cases		
Unilateral	0.25	0.15
Synchronous bilateral	0.80	0.40
Metachronous bilateral	0.40	0.75

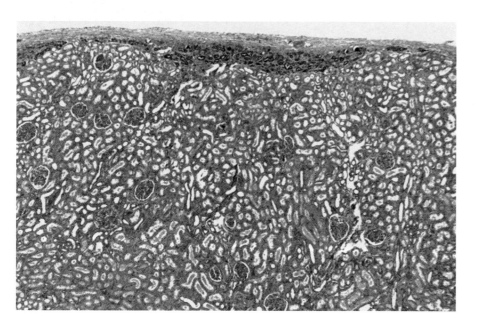

Figure 1-66

PERILOBAR NEPHROGENIC REST

Perilobar nephrogenic rests are located at the periphery of the renal lobule, and hence are commonly located on the surface of the kidney. Perilobar rests that are of microscopic size, quiescent, and composed of blastemal cells are termed "incipient" in a neonate and "dormant" in an older infant or child.

are associated with certain syndromes that carry a high risk for nephroblastoma (see Table 1-2).

PLNRs are characterized by sharp circumscription and a location at the periphery of the lobule. They are, therefore, most commonly located on the surface of the kidney, but may also be seen deep within the renal parenchyma along the edges of the lobule where the cortex follows the columns of Bertin. PLNRs may be seen at different stages of their development, resulting in different morphologies (26,29). *Dormant* or *incipient rests* are microscopic lesions with no evidence of proliferation, maturation, or involution. These rests usually contain well-formed tubular structures that are lined by a single layer of low cuboidal basophilic epithelium containing few or no mitotic figures (fig. 1-66). When PLNRs begin proliferating, they become larger and oval (fig. 1-67). A proliferating nephrogenic rest may then have one of several fates (fig. 1-68). Most commonly, the rest will regress, resulting in peritubular scarring and decreased proliferation. Following regression, islands of cells within the rest may continue to proliferate, waxing and waning over time (fig. 1-69). The end stage of a sclerosing rest is termed an *obsolescent rest*. These lesions are composed entirely of collagenous stroma and may be difficult to identify with certainty in the absence of other rests (fig. 1-70).

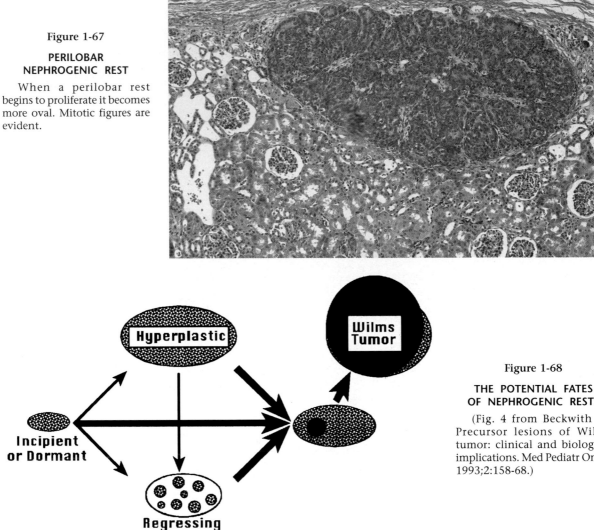

Figure 1-67

PERILOBAR NEPHROGENIC REST

When a perilobar rest begins to proliferate it becomes more oval. Mitotic figures are evident.

Figure 1-68

THE POTENTIAL FATES OF NEPHROGENIC RESTS

(Fig. 4 from Beckwith JB. Precursor lesions of Wilms tumor: clinical and biological implications. Med Pediatr Oncol 1993;2:158-68.)

PLNRs may also undergo diffuse or focal proliferative overgrowth, resulting in *hyperplastic nephrogenic rests*. Hyperplastic PLNRs are composed of blastemal and poorly differentiated tubular components that are actively proliferating. Hyperplastic PLNRs cannot be reliably distinguished from nephroblastoma by cytologic features alone. The most distinctive features of hyperplastic PLNRs are a tendency to preserve the original shape of the rest and a direct interface with the adjacent renal parenchyma (fig. 1-71).

In rare instances, the original PLNR forms a more or less continuous band around the surface of the kidney in a condition classified as *diffuse perilobar nephroblastomatosis* (DHPLN). Hyperplastic overgrowth of DHPLN results in massive renal enlargement (fig. 1-72). Children with DHPLN commonly present at 1 to 3 years of age with unilateral or bilateral renal masses (22). The renal enlargement may be massive, with weights up to 1,500 g. Histologically, DHPLN is composed of primitive epithelial and blastemal components, and demonstrates the

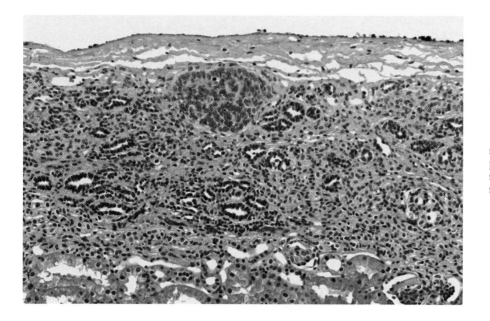

Figure 1-69

MULTIFOCAL HYPERPLASIA IN PERILOBAR NEPHROGENIC REST

Proliferating foci of various shapes and sizes within a perilobar nephrogenic rest are separated by regressing and sclerosing areas.

Figure 1-70

OBSOLESCENT PERILOBAR NEPHROGENIC REST

This lesion was distinguished from other causes of focal scarring only by the presence of other perilobar rests in the adjacent cortical surface.

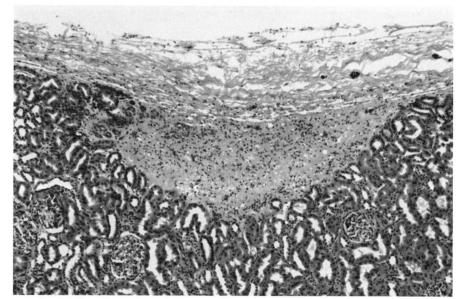

irregular contour and direct interface with the kidney that characterizes PLNRs (fig. 1-73). The distinctiveness of this lesion compared to nephroblastoma is evident radiographically by the diffuseness and homogeneity of the process (fig. 1-74). The diagnosis of nephroblastoma is often erroneously made unless the distinctive radiographic appearance is noted. As with all hyperplastic PLNRs, the fate of DHPLN is either regression or the development of nephroblastoma. However, in the waxing and waning course that is characteristic of DHPLN, it is not uncommon for small nests of cells to undergo epithelial differentiation, consisting of a trabecular growth of cells containing pale to acidophilic cytoplasm, somewhat resembling papillary renal cell carcinoma. These regions may also be associated with prominent sclerosis, particularly if chemotherapy has been provided. Such regions have been called *adenomatous nephrogenic rests* in the past, although it is doubtful that they represent the acquisition of a clonal genetic event that carries them further down the pathway toward neoplasia (fig. 1-75).

Figure 1-71

HYPERPLASTIC PERILOBAR NEPHROBLASTOMATOSIS

When composed of blastemal and other embryonal cells, a hyperplastic rest is distinguished from a small nephroblastoma by its shape, which preserves the original rest shape, and by the lack of a fibrous capsule separating it from the adjacent kidney. Note the adjacent dormant rest tissue.

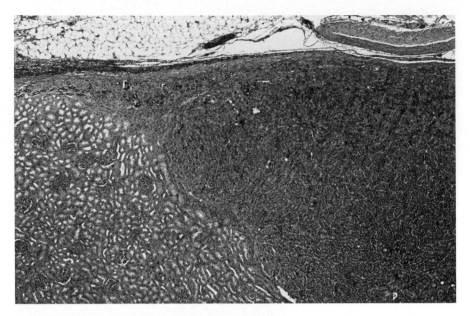

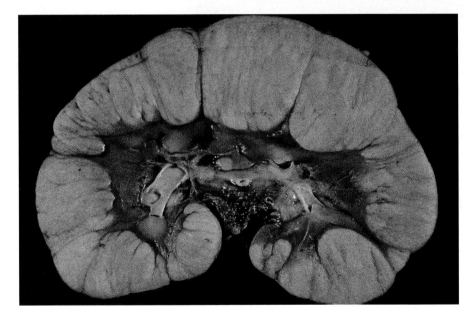

Figure 1-72

DIFFUSELY HYPERPLASTIC PERILOBAR NEPHROBLASTOMATOSIS

The kidney is enlarged but preserves its reniform shape due to relatively uniform overgrowth of a peripheral rim of nephroblastic tissue. (Fig. 1-64, Fascicle 11, 3rd Series.)

When clonal expansion develops within a PLNR, the resulting nephroblastoma is recognized by its propensity for spherical expansile growth and a peritumoral fibrous capsule that separates the neoplasm from the adjacent rest and normal kidney (figs. 1-76, 1-77). Nephrogenic rest tissue can often be seen at the periphery of the neuroblastoma, separated by the fibrous capsule (fig. 1-78). The cytology of the nephroblastoma is often indistinguishable from hyperplastic PLNR, and is characterized by blastemal and poorly differentiated epithelial or stromal components.

The distinction between nephrogenic rest and nephroblastoma can be made with confidence pathologically only when the shape of the lesion is known and the interface between the lesion and the surrounding kidney is included in the surgical excision. Therefore, a diagnosis by needle biopsy or fine needle aspiration is usually not possible. As knowledge of hyperplastic and neoplastic rests has increased, it has become apparent that many of the individual tumors previously diagnosed as one of multiple nephroblastomas actually represent hyperplastic rests.

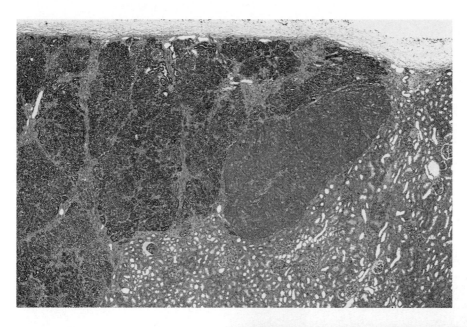

Figure 1-73

**DIFFUSELY
HYPERPLASTIC
PERILOBAR
NEPHROBLASTOMATOSIS**

A nearly confluent rind of hyperplastic perilobar rest tissue is evident in this enlarged kidney.

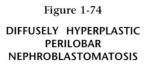

Figure 1-74

**DIFFUSELY HYPERPLASTIC
PERILOBAR
NEPHROBLASTOMATOSIS**

The rind-like proliferation of tissue with homogeneous signal results in a markedly enlarged left kidney. A small, subcapsular oval lesion of the same density is seen in the right kidney, consistent with a perilobar nephrogenic rest.

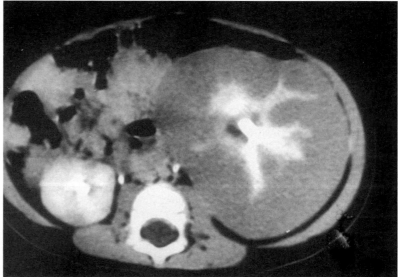

In contrast to PLNRs, ILNRs are typically located in the central areas of the lobule. In contrast to the sharply circumscribed PLNRs, ILNRs are characteristically poorly circumscribed, and intermingle with the normal renal parenchyma, particularly at their periphery. The cellular composition of ILNRs differs from that of PLNRs by often containing stromal elements as well as epithelial tubules (fig. 1-79). Like PLNRs, ILNRs may undergo hyperplasia, and this hyperplasia may involve stromal, epithelial, and/or blastemal elements (fig. 1-80). For these reasons, it may be difficult to distinguish a large

hyperplastic ILNR from a nephroblastoma. Clues to the correct diagnosis include the intermingling interface with the normal kidney characteristic of ILNR, and the histologic components of the lesion itself. For example, with few exceptions, fat is commonly found in ILNR but is uncommon in nephroblastoma; conversely, skeletal muscle differentiation is uncommon in ILNR but common in nephroblastoma. ILNRs are commonly found in the soft tissue of the renal sinus, and as suburothelial pads in the renal pelvis. These may result in a botryoid appearance similar to that seen in nephroblastoma. Rare

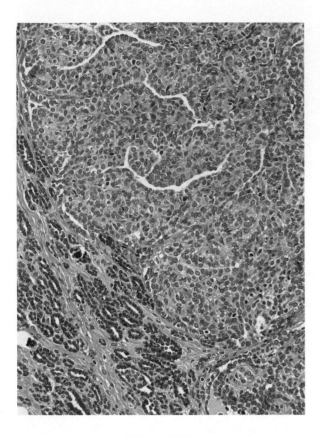

Figure 1-75

"ADENOMATOUS" CHANGE WITHIN HYPERPLASTIC PERILOBAR NEPHROBLASTOMATOSIS

Frequently identified in patients with perilobar nephroblastomatosis are nodules that show increased pale eosinophilic cytoplasm, often with a papillary architecture. These changes are referred to as "adenomatous."

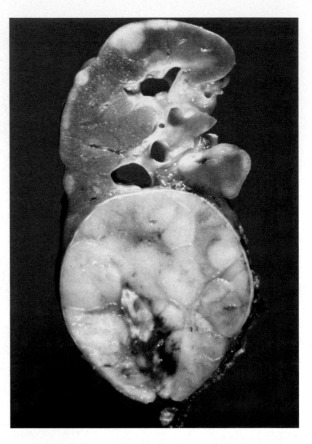

Figure 1-76

NEPHROBLASTOMA ARISING IN A PERILOBAR NEPHROGENIC REST

The large, rounded nephroblastoma occupies the lower pole. The smaller subcortical lesions are hyperplastic rests, as indicated by their irregular shape.

Figure 1-77

NEPHROBLASTOMA ARISING IN A PERILOBAR NEPHROGENIC REST

The spherical shape and presence of a peritumoral fibrous pseudocapsule indicate that this small lesion is a nephroblastoma. The primitive tubules outside the fibrous pseudocapsule provide a hint of the nephrogenic rest in which this nephroblastoma arose.

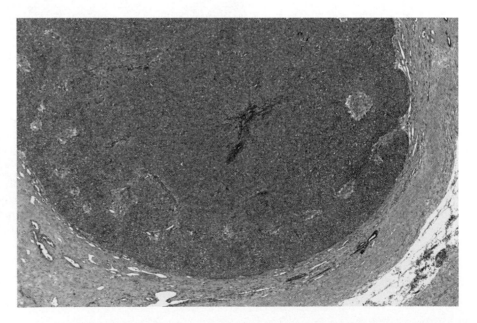

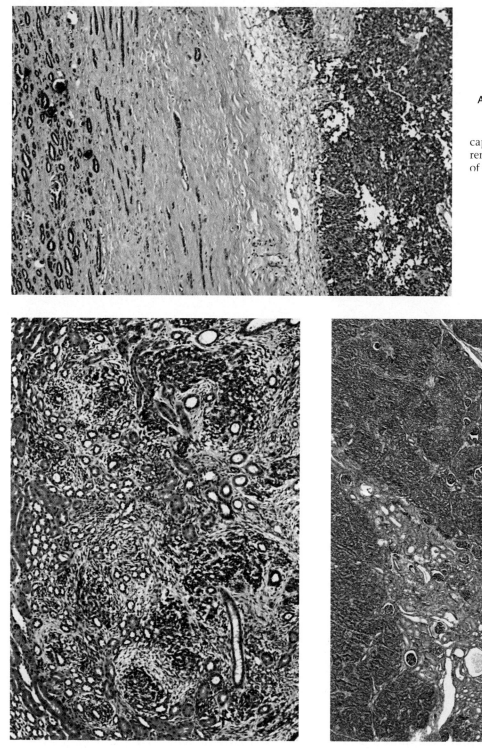

Figure 1-78

NEPHROBLASTOMA ARISING IN A PERILOBAR NEPHROGENIC REST

A prominent peritumoral capsule and compressed rest remnants are at the periphery of the expanding tumor.

Figure 1-79

INTRALOBAR NEPHROGENIC REST

This relatively small, blastemal lesion demonstrates the characteristic interstitial location and intermingling with normal nephronic elements.

Figure 1-80

HYPERPLASTIC INTRALOBAR NEPHROGENIC REST

When intralobar nephrogenic rests become hyperplastic, the interface of the tumor continues to be irregular in contour and lacks a fibrous pseudocapsule.

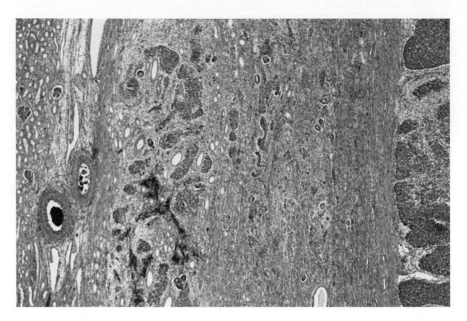

Figure 1-81

NEPHROBLASTOMA ARISING IN AN INTRALOBAR REST

The edge of the nephroblastoma at the right has a sharply defined border and dense cellularity. Most of the remainder of the field is occupied by intralobar nephrogenic rest tissue mingled with normal cortical and medullary structures. This appearance can easily be mistaken for tumor infiltrating the renal parenchyma.

examples have presented to the NWTSG pathology center as cystic abdominal masses which on review are ILNRs that have developed within a duplicated ureter.

Nephroblastoma commonly develops within ILNRs, and when this occurs the nephroblastoma is often separated from the underlying rest by a peritumoral fibrous capsule (fig. 1-81). Nephroblastomas associated with ILNRs have a greater degree of heterogeneity that those arising in PLNRs, and often contain abundant stromal and heterologous elements, such as differentiated skeletal muscle cells and cartilage. Such nephroblastomas are classified as "central" in contrast to the "peripheral" nephroblastomas associated with PLNRs that demonstrate predominantly epithelial and blastemal elements. ILNR-associated nephroblastomas are most common in young infants, and such patients have a high risk of developing contralateral lesions in the future (47).

Prognosis. The majority of PLNRs undergo regression and sclerosis without the development of a nephroblastoma. The risk of developing a nephroblastoma is considerably higher within an ILNR, and the frequency of uneventful regression is thought to be low. However, the relative risk of tumor development within patients with either PLNR or ILNR may not differ greatly because PLNRs are almost invariably multiple and ILNRs are usually single.

The prognosis for patients with DHPLN merits separate discussion. Because of the tremendous burden of proliferating nephroblastic cells, the risk for the development of a nephroblastoma is extraordinarily high in this group. For this reason, the chemotherapeutic regimen recommended for low stage, favorable histology nephroblastoma is commonly utilized in the treatment of patients with DHPLN, particularly when the lesions are bilateral (22). Chemotherapy is thought to be beneficial because it reduces the number of proliferating cells that may develop a clonal transformation into nephroblastoma, and it also reduces the burden of large quantities of nephroblastic tissue. Approximately half of patients with DHPLN who receive chemotherapy have complete resolution of the process and never develop tumors subsequently. The remaining patients have a waxing and waning course, both in the development and size of their rests and in the development of nephroblastoma, over a period of 5 to 10 years. The most critical determinant of long-term survival is the utilization of a treatment regimen that preserves the renal parenchyma. Patients with DHPLN have a 32 percent risk of developing anaplastic nephroblastoma, likely due to the increased number of tumors per patient. Therefore, their tumors must be carefully watched and monitored for responsiveness to therapy.

Differential Diagnosis. Rare entities that may be mistaken for nephrogenic rests include the dysplastic medullary ray nodules that are most commonly seen in association with Beckwith-Wiedemann syndrome (fig. 1-82). These are larger and more disorganized than the medullary ray nodules that may be seen in normal infant kidneys (32). Foci of embryonal hyperplasia found in end-stage kidneys and in patients with dysplastic kidneys may also be mistaken for nephrogenic rests (fig. 1-83).

CYSTIC NEPHROMA AND CYSTIC, PARTIALLY DIFFERENTIATED NEPHROBLASTOMA

Definition. Cystic nephroma (CN) and cystic, partially differentiated nephroblastoma (CPDN) are benign neoplasms currently considered to be a part of the spectrum of nephroblastoma (121,122,126). Current evidence supports a spectrum of morphologic changes from pure multicystic tumors without nephroblastic elements to obvious nephroblastoma with cysts. This nomenclature is most accurately applied to lesions in the kidneys of children; it is probable that many of the tumors classified as CNs in adults represent distinct entities unrelated to nephroblastoma.

General and Clinical Features. CN and CPDN have a 2 to 1 male predominance and are seen in children less than 4 years of age (124). Most patients are asymptomatic; tumors present as palpable masses, although hematuria

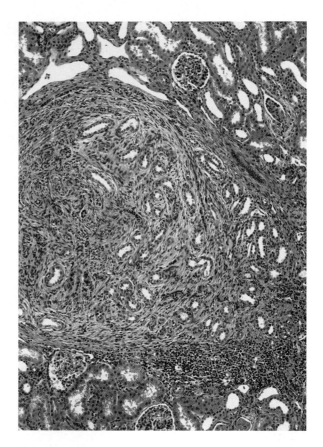

Figure 1-82

DYSPLASTIC MEDULLARY RAY NODULE

Unencapsulated nodules composed of several tubular cross-sections are surrounded by increased interstitial connective tissue, displacing and compressing the adjacent collecting ducts.

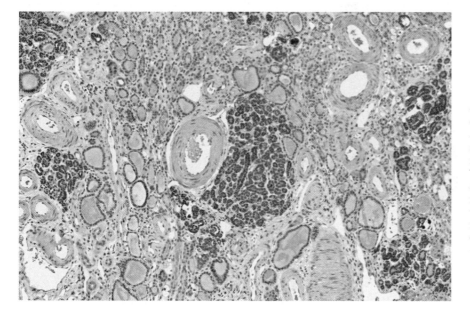

Figure 1-83

EMBRYONAL HYPERPLASIA

Embryonal hyperplasia is characterized by nodular proliferation of basophilic, embryonal-appearing tubular or papillary structures that differ from nephrogenic rests by their location. They are limited to the cortex, but are not usually seen in the immediate subcapsular region, the typical location of perilobar nephrogenic rests, which embryonal hyperplasia resembles.

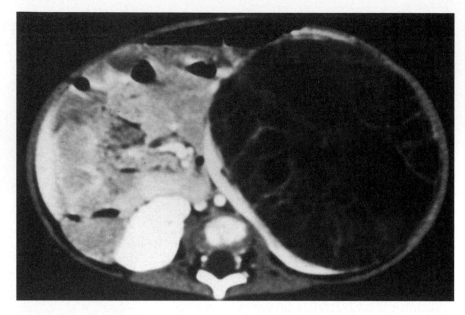

Figure 1-84

CYSTIC NEPHROMA

Computed tomographic image. (Fig. 1-74 from Fascicle 11, 3rd Series.)

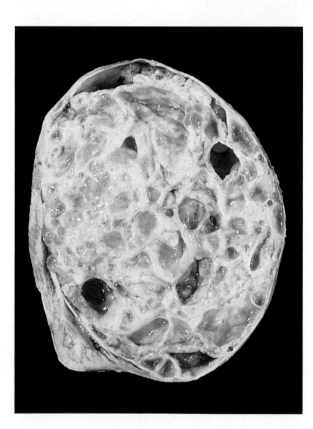

Figure 1-85

CYSTIC, PARTIALLY DIFFERENTIATED NEPHROBLASTOMA

Gross appearance of section surface. (Fig. 1-75 [top] from Fascicle 11, 3rd Series.)

is occasionally a presenting symptom. The cystic nature of the lesion is easily recognized by ultrasonography or CT (fig. 1-84). Nephroblastomas, clear cell sarcomas, and mesoblastic nephromas may also be predominantly cystic. An intriguing familial association between CN and the often cystic pleuropulmonary blastoma has recently been documented (123,127,128).

Pathologic Findings. CN and CPDN are solitary, multilocular lesions that are sharply demarcated from an otherwise normal remaining kidney (121,125,126). Tumors measure 5 to 10 cm in greatest dimension and appear as bulging masses, often with a bosselated surface. Cysts range from a few millimeters to several centimeters in diameter and are filled with colorless fluid. The intervening septa must conform to the contours of the cyst and do not contain grossly identifiable nodular masses (fig. 1-85). The microscopic distinction between cystic nephroblastoma, CPDN, and CN is usually straightforward. However, as with all entities that comprise a histologic spectrum, there are cases that lie in the diagnostic gray zone. CN, by definition, is composed of cysts with septa containing only mature elements (fig. 1-86). No nodular masses of mature or immature nephroblastic tissue should alter the contour of the cysts. CPDN differs from CN only in that the septa of CN contains blastemal or other poorly differentiated cell types (fig. 1-87). Any solid,

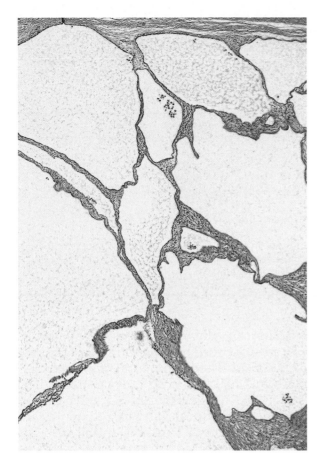

Figure 1-86

CYSTIC NEPHROMA

By definition, cystic nephroma contains no solid nodules and has only mature elements within septa.

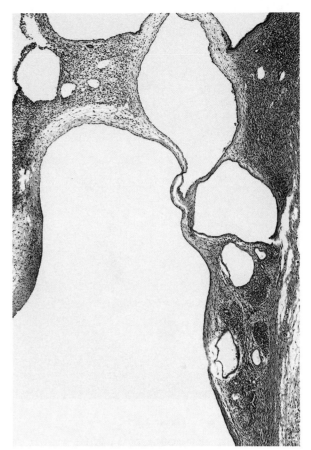

Figure 1-87

CYSTIC, PARTIALLY DIFFERENTIATED NEPHROBLASTOMA

Embryonal elements are present, but conform to septa between cysts; no solid nodules are present.

expansile, nodular proliferations indicate a diagnosis of cystic nephroblastoma (fig. 1-88). Extension of CN and CPDN beyond the renal capsule may occur and does not negate the diagnosis. Rarely, CN and CPDN protrude into the collecting system. The diagnosis of CN or CPDN should not be applied to tumors containing anaplasia or to tumors following chemotherapy. CNs can be distinguished from polycystic kidneys by their sharp circumscription and by a lack of mature renal parenchymal elements in the fibrous septa of the lesions.

Prognosis. As defined here, CN and CPDN are benign neoplasms adequately treated by complete resection (122). Some potential for recurrence exists if CPDN is incompletely excised, but metastases have not been documented. Some cystic carcinomas and sarcomas of adult kidneys

have been reported to arise within CN and CPDN, but it has not been conclusively proven that these lesions arose in preexistent cystic lesions rather than representing cystic change in a malignant neoplasm.

METANEPHRIC TUMORS

Definition. Metanephric tumors comprise a pathologic spectrum of lesions that are derived from the metanephric blastema. The individual components of these lesions distinguish them pathologically from nephroblastoma, and clinically they are distinguished by their benignity. At one end of the pathologic spectrum are tumors that are composed exclusively of epithelial nephroblastic cells, the *metanephric adenomas,* and at the other end are tumors that are

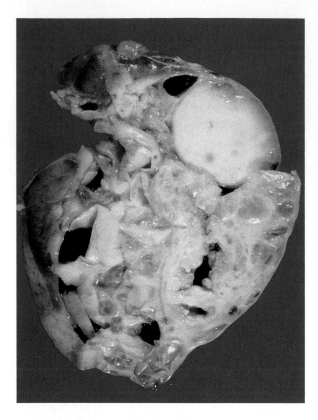

Figure 1-88

CYSTIC NEPHROBLASTOMA WITH A DISTINCT SOLID REGION

The solid region excludes the diagnosis of cystic, partially differentiated nephroblastoma or cystic nephroma. (Fig. 1-76 from Fascicle 11, 3rd Series.)

Table 1-8

FEATURES OF THE EPITHELIAL AND STROMAL COMPONENTS OF METANEPHRIC TUMORS (METANEPHRIC ADENOMA, METANEPHRIC ADENOFIBROMA, AND METANEPHRIC STROMAL TUMOR)

Epithelial Component
 Tubular, glomeruloid, or papillary architecture
 Virtual absence of mitoses
 Virtual absence of nucleoli
 No vascular involvement
 Negativity for epithelial membrane antigen and cytokeratin 7

Stromal Component
 Nodular low-power appearance
 Concentric collarettes around renal tubules and/or blood vessels
 Angiodysplasia
 Heterologous elements (glial, cartilage, fat)

composed exclusively of stromal elements, the *metanephric stromal tumors*. Tumors that include a composite of both are termed *metanephric adenofibromas*. The epithelial and stromal components identified in these lesions have characteristic histologic features (Table 1-8).

Clinical and Pathologic Findings. *Metanephric Adenoma.* The most commonly occurring member of the metanephric tumor family is the metanephric adenoma. These neoplasms occur most commonly in women; the mean age at presentation is 41 years, with a range of 5 to 83 years. Recorded lesions have varied from 0.3 to 15.0 cm in greatest dimension (132). Approximately 10 percent of patients with metanephric adenomas present with polycythemia, a higher frequency than has been recorded in patients with other pediatric renal tumors.

Microscopically, metanephric adenomas are well circumscribed but unencapsulated tumors. They consist of small, uniform, epithelial cells that form small acini in an acellular stroma (figs. 1-89, 1-90). Tubular, glomeruloid, and papillary formations may occur and calcospherites are common (fig. 1-91). Occasionally, the epithelial structures coalesce to form more solid sheets. Importantly, blastema is absent. Cytologically, the oval cells appear bland, with smooth nuclear contours, scant pale-staining cytoplasm, dark-staining nuclei, and inconspicuous to absent nucleoli. Mitoses are absent or quite rare. Vascular invasion is not a feature of metanephric adenoma and the presence of vascular invasion precludes this diagnosis (132,134).

There is considerable histologic overlap between metanephric adenoma, papillary renal cell carcinoma, and differentiated epithelial nephroblastoma. In order to assure a benign outcome, strict criteria are necessary for the diagnosis of metanephric adenoma. These criteria include: absence of a peritumoral fibrous capsule with a direct interface between the lesion and normal kidney; absent nucleoli; and virtually absent mitoses. For tumors meeting these criteria, no recurrences have been recorded (137).

Immunohistochemistry can help distinguish metanephric adenomas from other lesions. As in most maturing epithelial nephroblastomas, metanephric adenoma is negative for epithelial membrane antigen, compared with the positive results for this marker in papillary renal cell carcinoma. AE1/AE3 likewise shows predominant negativity within metanephric adenomas, although rare cells may be positive. The pattern of CD56, CD57, and WT1 staining identified in metanephric adenomas is similar to that seen in comparably differentiated nephroblastomas and nephrogenic rests (135). Cytokeratin 7, a useful positive immunohistochemical marker for papillary renal cell carcinoma, is only positive in rare cells in both metanephric adenoma and epithelial nephroblastoma (fig. 1-92) (137).

Metanephric Stromal Tumors. Metanephric stromal tumors (MSTs) are unencapsulated, benign tumors most commonly presenting in infancy, with a mean age at presentation of 2 years, although a 15-year-old patient has been reported (88,129). Within the NWTSG pathology center, 31 such cases have been identified. The majority of these were reclassified as MST during a retrospective review of cases previously considered to represent congenital mesoblastic

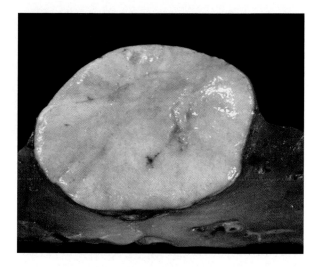

Figure 1-89

METANEPHRIC ADENOMA

The gross appearance demonstrates the sharp circumscription that characterizes metanephric adenoma.

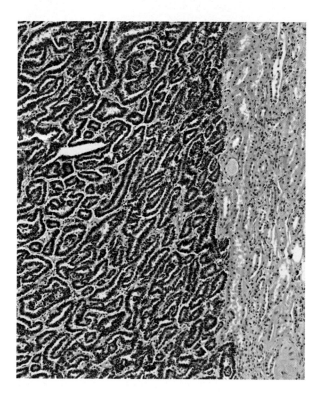

Figure 1-90

METANEPHRIC ADENOMA

The border of the lesion is sharply circumscribed but unencapsulated. The presence of a fibrous capsule precludes the diagnosis of metanephric adenoma.

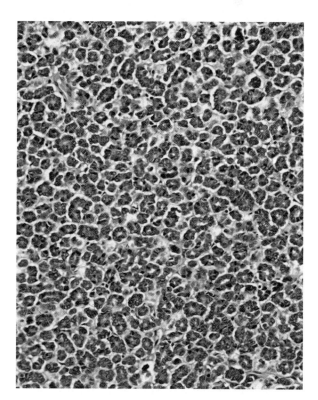

Figure 1-91

METANEPHRIC ADENOMA

Small tubules, papillary structures, or glomeruloid structures may be seen within a metanephric adenoma. Bland, overlapping, oval nuclei without nucleoli or mitotic figures are seen.

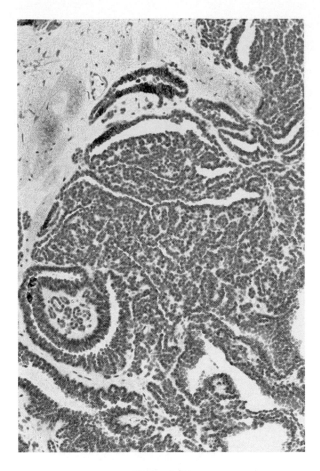

Figure 1-92

METANEPHRIC ADENOMA

Immunohistochemistry for cytokeratin 7 in metanephric adenoma shows rare or focal positivity, in contrast with the diffuse positivity characteristic of papillary renal cell carcinoma.

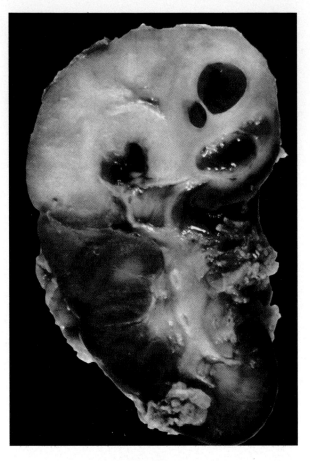

Figure 1-93

METANEPHRIC STROMAL TUMOR

There is a lack of circumscription and presence of cyst formation.

nephroma. The most common presentation of MST is that of a centrally located cystic or solid mass ranging from 3 to 10 cm in greatest dimension (fig. 1-93). Hematuria and hypertension are present in a minority of patients. No patients with bilateral tumors have been identified.

Microscopically, MSTs are composed of spindle to stellate cells with indistinct cytoplasmic processes. The degree of stromal cellularity in MST ranges from extreme hypocellularity with sclerosis, to extreme hypercellularity reminiscent of a cellular mesoblastic nephroma. The spindle cell stroma may have a number of architectural patterns, including a palisading pattern simulating the Verocay bodies of a schwannoma, a storiform pattern, and a hemangiopericytomatous pattern.

Mitoses are usually inapparent, but may be as numerous as 7 per 20 high-power fields. The distinctive characteristics of MST follow.

Alternating regions of myxoid or sclerotic hypocellularity and fibroblastic hypercellularity result in a distinctive nodular appearance on low-power microscopy that provides an important clue to the diagnosis (figs. 1-94–1-96). The cellular zones are commonly composed of spindle cells reminiscent of those identified in congenital mesoblastic nephroma. A striking epithelioid appearance is seen in a minority of cases; these regions are negative for epithelial markers (fig. 1-96).

Concentric collarettes of stromal cells around renal tubules or blood vessels is the feature that most commonly prompts the consideration of

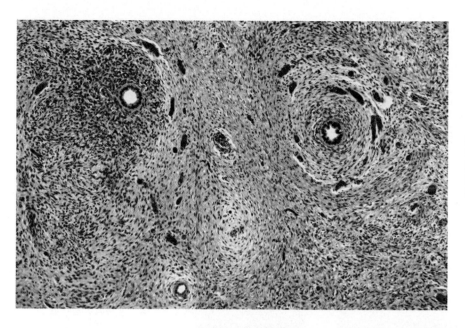

Figure 1-94

METANEPHRIC STROMAL TUMOR

Collars of stromal cells surround entrapped tubules and vessels. These collars may be hypercellular or hypocellular relative to the background stromal process.

Figure 1-95

METANEPHRIC STROMAL TUMOR

The collars of condensed stromal cells surrounding tubules are one component that results in the characteristic alternation of cellularity characteristic of this tumor.

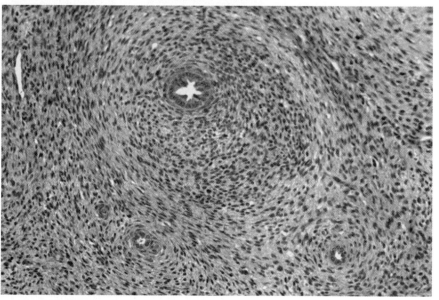

MST. It is quite similar to the cuffing that is characteristic of renal dysplasia, a feature also seen in ILNRs (figs. 1-94, 1-95). The collarette may be either hypercellular or hypocellular when compared to the surrounding stromal component.

Angiodysplasia of intratumoral arterioles with expansion and disorganization of vascular medial smooth muscle cells due to epithelioid transformation is seen in the majority of cases of MST (fig. 1-97). Desmin is nonimmunoreactive in tumoral spindle cells in most cases, but often highlights the epithelioid cells in dys-

plastic arterioles. Angiodysplasia may rarely involve extrarenal vessels, resulting in significant morbidity and mortality.

Nodules of heterologous tissue, such as glia, cartilage, or fat, are present in a minority of cases, with glial elements being the most common (fig. 1-98). When present, glial tissue is often in direct contact with epithelium, forming glial-epithelial complexes. Skeletal muscle differentiation has not been encountered in MSTs, although rare tumors may react for desmin within the stromal elements.

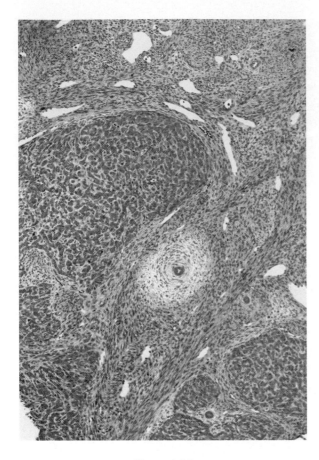

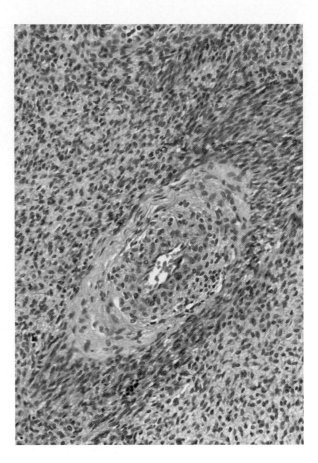

Figure 1-96

METANEPHRIC STROMAL TUMOR

Occasionally the stromal element contains nodules with a striking epithelioid appearance. These regions do not show epithelial differentiation by immunohistochemistry.

Figure 1-97

METANEPHRIC STROMAL TUMOR

Angiodysplasia is the most diagnostic feature of this tumor, although it is not seen in all cases.

Figure 1-98

METANEPHRIC STROMAL TUMOR

The heterologous elements most frequently seen are nodules of maturing glial tissue. These are commonly associated with epithelial elements.

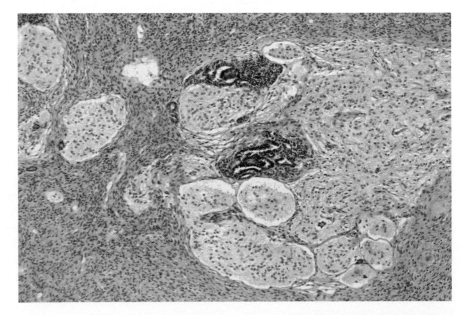

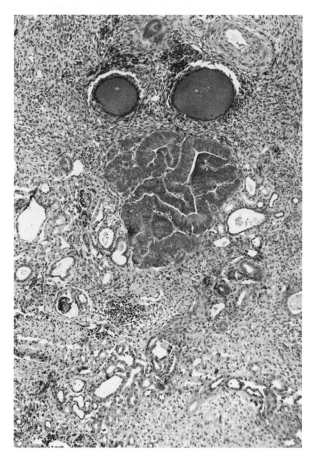

Figure 1-99

METANEPHRIC STROMAL TUMOR

Entrapped native renal epithelial structures may show a striking degree of embryonal hyperplasia.

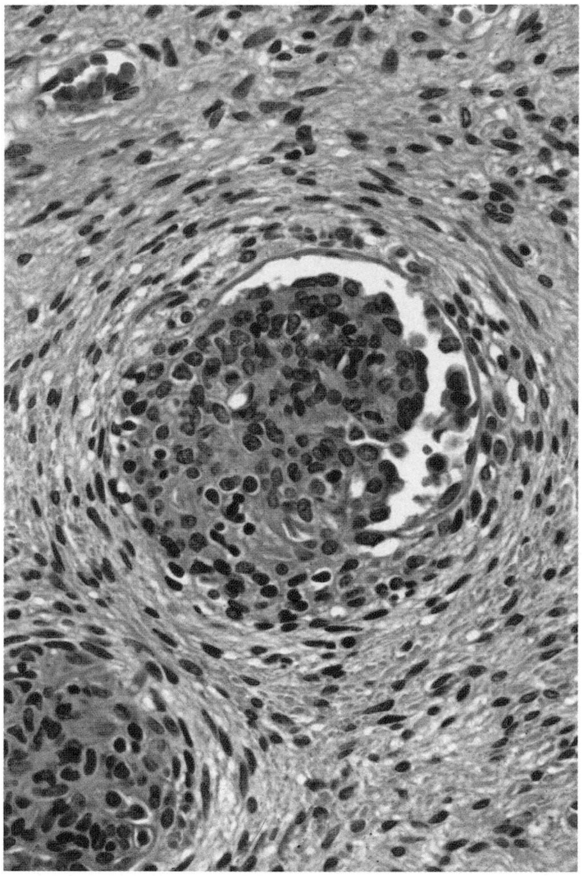

Figure 1-100

METANEPHRIC STROMAL TUMOR

Juxtaglomerular hyperplasia may be striking.

MSTs are unencapsulated and may extend as tongues of stromal tissue into the surrounding renal parenchyma, often entrapping normal renal elements and causing dilatation and cyst formation. The entrapped epithelium, particularly native glomeruli, may undergo embryonal hyperplasia, simulating the appearance of papillary renal cell carcinoma (fig. 1-99). Juxtaglomerular cell hyperplasia has also been commonly recorded, resulting in nodules of polygonal cells with minimal clear cytoplasm at the vascular pole (fig. 1-100). Many patients with juxtaglomerular cell hyperplasia have increased renin levels and hypertension.

Metanephric Adenofibroma. Metanephric adenofibroma is a lesion that contains both the epithelial and stromal components of meta-nephric adenoma and MST, respectively (130, 131,133,138). In the files of the NWTSG pathology center, 25 patients are described, ranging in age from 5 months to 36 years, with a mean age of 82.2 months and a male to female ratio of 2 to 1 (130). All recorded tumors are unilateral. Clinical features include polycythemia, hematuria, and hypertension. These tumors range in size from 1.8 to 11 cm in greatest dimension. They have indistinct borders and are commonly centered in the renal medulla. Microscopically, some tumors are predominantly stromal, whereas others are almost entirely composed of metanephric adenoma except for a peripheral band of stroma. The stromal component typically infiltrates the native kidney in a pattern similar to that of ILNRs (fig 1-101).

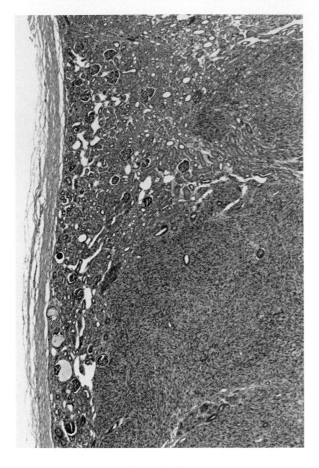

Figure 1-101

METANEPHRIC STROMAL TUMOR

The interface between the stromal component and the kidney is irregular and unencapsulated.

The epithelial component may be present as a single nodule or multiple nodules (fig. 1-102).

Prognosis. To date, the majority of MSTs have been completely excised, usually by nephrectomy. No recurrences or metastases have been documented. This includes one case in which a MST had a microscopically positive medial margin and a second case in which the tumor ruptured into the abdomen but was treated by nephrectomy alone. Three patients with MSTs had life-threatening sequelae due to extrarenal angiodysplasia associated with their tumors (129).

The lesions within the metanephric tumor family behave in a benign fashion, but either the epithelial or the stromal component may be associated with the development of malignancy. This is most commonly seen in the epithelial component. Of the 25 cases of metanephric adenofibroma identified within the NWTSG pathology center files, 7 tumors contained an epithelial nodule with features characteristic of epithelial-predominant nephroblastoma, including tall columnar cells with embryonal-appearing nuclei, a high mitotic rate, and epithelial membrane antigen immunoreactivity. These cases were classified as nephroblastoma arising in a metanephric adenofibroma. In five additional cases, the metanephric adenofibroma contained nodules of epithelial proliferation with architectural and cytologic features similar to those described for papillary renal cell carcinoma, including the presence of

Figure 1-102

METANEPHRIC ADENOFIBROMA

The epithelial component of a metanephric adenofibroma is typically circumscribed.

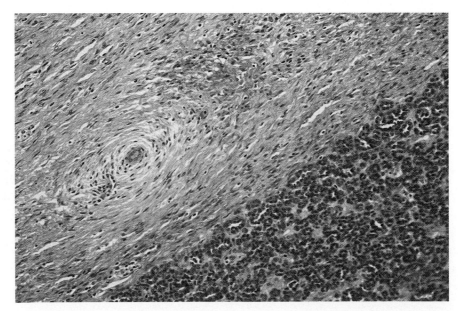

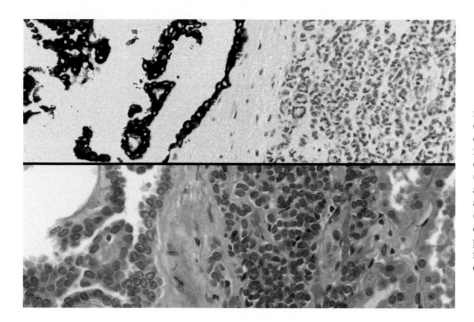

Figure 1-103

PAPILLARY RENAL CELL CARCINOMA ARISING IN A METANEPHRIC ADENOMA

A nodule of cells with a papillary architecture, increased nuclear size, mitotic activity, and occasional nucleoli (left) was identified within this otherwise diagnostic metanephric adenoma (lower middle). Note the lack of a fibrous capsule separating the adenoma from the normal kidney (lower right). Immunohistochemistry demonstrates diffuse positivity for cytokeratin 7 confined to the papillary renal cell carcinoma (top).

foamy macrophages within papillary stalks and immunoreactivity for both cytokeratin 7 and epithelial membrane antigen (fig. 1-103). The cytologic grade of these areas ranged from low-grade with rare mitotic figures and only mild to moderate pleomorphism, to high-grade with marked nuclear atypia and lymph node metastases. Such tumors merit the diagnosis of papillary renal cell carcinoma arising in a metanephric adenofibroma. The occurrence of both nephroblastoma and papillary renal cell carcinoma has been documented within metanephric adenomas at similar frequencies to that in metanephric adenofibromas. Patients with a malignancy arising within a metanephric adenofibroma or metanephric adenoma tend to be older than other patients with metanephric tumors, suggesting that malignant differentiation represents a late event in tumorigenesis.

The malignant potential of the stromal component within benign metanephric tumors remains unresolved. While no MST in the NWTSG pathology center has behaved aggressively, the theoretic potential for sarcomatous transformation associated with an adverse outcome remains. There are unclassified sarcomas and stromal tumors of the pediatric kidney that could represent malignant counterparts of MST or possibly even malignant transformation of MST. However, at this time no such sarcoma has been associated with a definite benign MST component. A tumor has been reported that contained both epithelial and stromal components in which the stromal component was widely metastatic (136). It was suggested that this might represent a metanephric adenosarcoma, but the spindle cell component lacked the distinctive features of a MST.

Most tumors within this family are classified as stage I, using the NWTSG-5 staging criteria. They may infiltrate the fibroadipose tissue of the renal sinus and entrap nerves, however, vascular invasion has not been identified. Stromal proliferation may focally undermine the caliceal or pelvic urothelium and form a suburothelial "pad."

CONGENITAL MESOBLASTIC NEPHROMA

Definition. Congenital mesoblastic nephroma (CMN) is a stromal neoplasm of infancy. These tumors have been described under other names, most notably *leiomyomatous hamartoma*, but the term initially suggested by Bolande is preferred (143,144).

General and Clinical Features. CMN is virtually confined to infancy. The median age at diagnosis is 2 months and over 90 percent of cases appear within the first year of life (fig. 1-104). The diagnosis should be questioned when applied to individuals over 2 years of age. Rare cases have been reported in older children and adults, but these tumors have been reclassified in current schemes, most commonly as cystic hamartoma or MST (152). With the widespread application

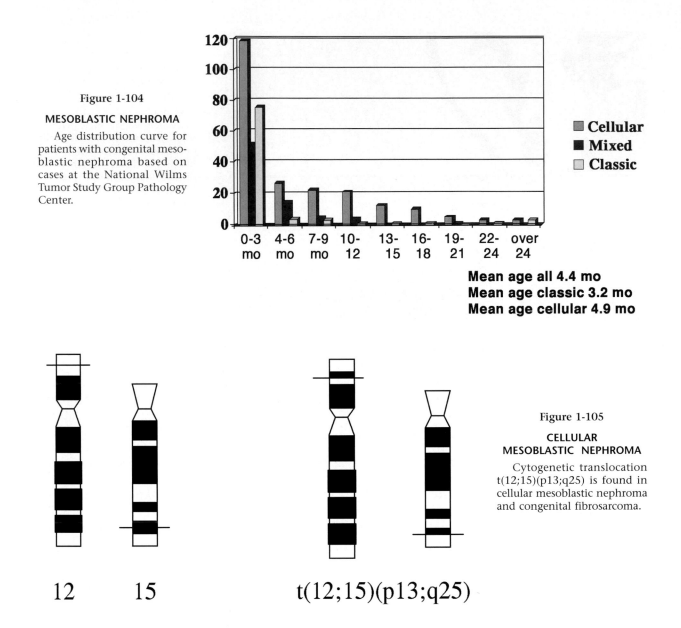

Figure 1-104

MESOBLASTIC NEPHROMA

Age distribution curve for patients with congenital mesoblastic nephroma based on cases at the National Wilms Tumor Study Group Pathology Center.

Mean age all 4.4 mo
Mean age classic 3.2 mo
Mean age cellular 4.9 mo

Figure 1-105

CELLULAR MESOBLASTIC NEPHROMA

Cytogenetic translocation t(12;15)(p13;q25) is found in cellular mesoblastic nephroma and congenital fibrosarcoma.

of ultrasound imaging, many CMNs are recognized prior to birth. The tumor has been reported on rare occasion in children with Beckwith-Wiedemann syndrome but has not been reported in other syndromes associated with nephroblastoma (168).

The molecular pathogenesis of CMN is gradually becoming clarified. Chromosomal and genetic abnormalities have been identified only in the cellular type. Initially, the most consistent genetic change in cellular CMN was trisomy for chromosome 11, which has also been reported in infantile fibrosarcoma (146,158,164,166). The potential linkage between infantile fibrosarcoma

and cellular CMN was then established when both were shown to contain the same t(12;15) (p13;q25) chromosomal translocation (154, 156,162). The cloning of the genes involved in this translocation has allowed more reliable molecular detection assays to be applied to formalin-fixed and paraffin-embedded sections (140). The *ETV6* gene on 12p13, which belongs to the *ETS* transcription factor family, is fused to the neurotrophin-3 receptor (*NTRK3*) gene on 15q25, a membrane-bound protein with tyrosine kinase activity (fig. 1-105). The consensus is that cellular CMN represents infantile fibrosarcoma arising within the kidney. In contrast, no consistent

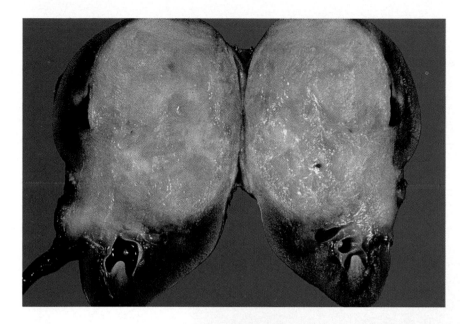

Figure 1-106

MESOBLASTIC NEPHROMA

Gross appearance of the classic pattern. Features include the whorled, myomatous appearance of the sectioned surface, the extensive involvement of the medial aspect of the kidney, and the lack of a sharply demarcated tumor-kidney junction. (Fig. 1-80 from Fascicle 11, 3rd Series.)

Figure 1-107

MESOBLASTIC NEPHROMA

Gross appearance often associated with the cellular pattern, with foci of hemorrhage, necrosis, and scattered cysts. (Fig. 1-81 from Fascicle 11, 3rd Series.)

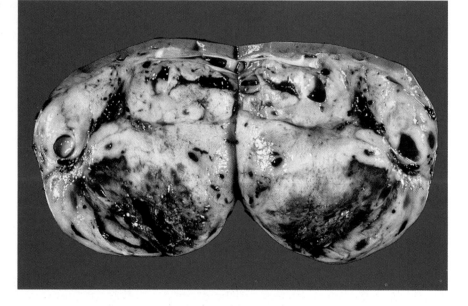

genetic abnormalities have been identified in the classic type of CMN. It has been suggested that classic CMN may represent infantile fibromatosis, rather than fibrosarcoma, involving the kidney. This is supported by the strong histologic similarity between these two entities.

Most CMNs are detected because of an abdominal mass; polyhydramnios, hydrops, and premature delivery often occur in affected fetuses (139,147,151). Hypercalcemia is identified in some patients and is attributed to excessive production of prostaglandin E by the tumor (165,

167). Hyperreninism, due to the production of the hormone by entrapped renal elements rather than by tumor cells, is common (145,157,169).

Pathologic Findings. Grossly, CMNs vary from 0.8 to 14 cm in greatest dimension (mean, 6.2 cm). They appear as solitary, unilateral masses with soft or firm, bulging cut surfaces often indistinguishable from a nephroblastoma (figs. 1-106, 1-107). Cysts, hemorrhage, and necrosis are common features, although some lesions are quite firm (149). Most CMNs are centered near the hilus of the kidney and nearly all involve

Table 1-9

DISTINGUISHING FEATURES OF CELLULAR AND CLASSIC CONGENITAL MESOBLASTIC NEPHROMA

	Cellular	Classic
Interface with kidney	Circumscribed, unencapsulated	Highly irregular, interdigitating
Genetic features	t(12;15)(p13;q25), trisomy chromosome 11	None known
Cytology	Plump, slightly spindled cells	Markedly elongated
Extrarenal equivalent	Infantile fibrosarcoma	Infantile fibromatosis

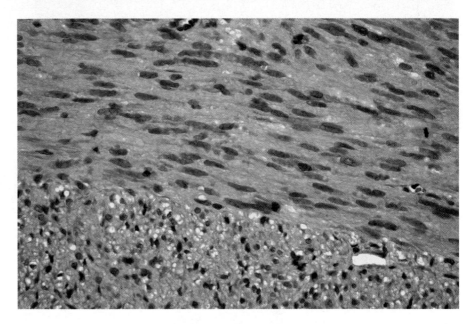

Figure 1-108

MESOBLASTIC NEPHROMA

The spindle cells forming the lesion are not densely aggregated. A prominent interlacing bundle pattern is characteristic of the classic pattern.

the renal sinus (141a). Recognizing this, both surgeon and pathologist should take particular care to establish that the medial aspect of the nephrectomy specimen is free of tumor.

Histologically, CMNs are predominantly monomorphic neoplasms composed of spindled mesenchymal cells of fibroblastic or myofibroblastic lineage. They can be divided into two major types: classic and cellular. The classic subtype is that originally described by Bolande, although fewer than one third of CMNs have this histology (144). The cellular pattern is most common. The distinguishing features of these two histologic subtypes are listed in Table 1-9.

CMN, classic type, closely resembles infantile fibromatosis in its pathologic features. It is characterized by intersecting fascicles of spindle cells, resembling fibroblasts or myofibroblasts, interspersed with scant collagen fibers (figs. 1-108, 1-109). Dilated, thin-walled vascular spaces are

often prominent. Mitotic activity is variable but generally less conspicuous than in the cellular pattern. The tumor margins are highly irregular, with radiating bands of cells extending into the renal parenchyma and often into the perirenal soft tissue (fig. 1-109). There is usually little compression of adjacent renal structures, suggesting that the tumor and fetal kidney grow as an integrated unit. Entrapped renal elements are common and can be misinterpreted as components of the neoplasm, especially since they are often not completely mature in these infants. Extensions of tumor tissue characteristically consist of long, narrow "tongues" of spindle cells that may continue for some distance beyond the gross margins of the tumor, especially at the hilus of the kidney. It is for this reason that wide surgical margins and careful pathologic documentation are important. Abnormal metaplastic changes in tubules or glomeruli adjacent to or entrapped by the lesion are present

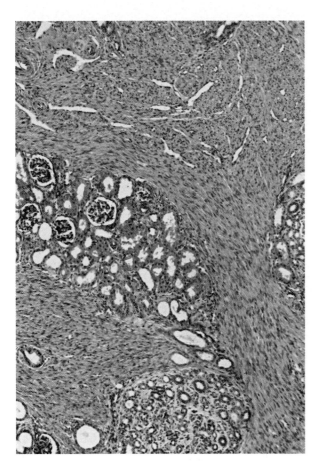

Figure 1-109

MESOBLASTIC NEPHROMA

In this classic pattern, the tumor interdigitates with renal parenchyma without compression or distortion of renal structures.

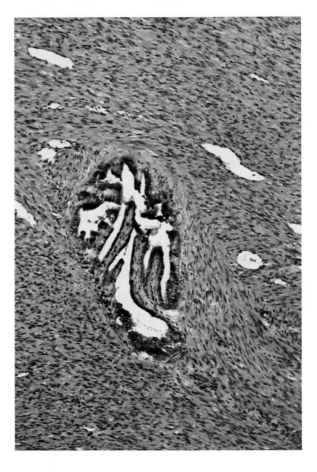

Figure 1-110

MESOBLASTIC NEPHROMA

Embryonal metaplasia of entrapped tubules is sometimes accompanied by epithelial hyperplasia.

in many specimens (fig. 1-110). These meta-plastic cells have an embryonal appearance and may exhibit papillary hyperplasia, a feature that can be mistaken for evidence of mixed stromal and epithelial nephroblastoma. Small nodules of hyaline cartilage are often encountered and are likely a reflection of dysplastic changes within the surrounding kidney secondary to the effect of tumor on normal renal development. Ex-tramedullary hematopoiesis is common. Skeletal muscle differentiation is not a feature of CMN.

CMN, cellular type, is characterized by in-creased cellular density and a high proliferative rate, imparting a sarcomatous appearance to the tumor. Cellular CMNs most commonly consist of plump cells with vesicular nuclei and a small

to moderate amount of cytoplasm (figs. 1-111, 1-112). Lesions are sharply circumscribed grossly, without the interdigitating margins of classic le-sions. Nevertheless, a peritumoral fibrous cap-sule is seldom present and the tumor subtly in-filtrates the adjacent normal renal parenchyma (fig. 1-111). Slight to moderate nuclear pleo-morphism may be present and the cells often grow in sheets of somewhat elongated cells remi-niscent of fibroblast cell cultures (fig. 1-113). Rare tumors contain cells with prominent nucleoli as well as areas of necrosis, closely resembling the features of a rhabdoid tumor (153). In some cellular CMNs, a prominent capillary vascula-ture that mimics the vasculature of a clear cell sarcoma of the kidney (CCSK) is present.

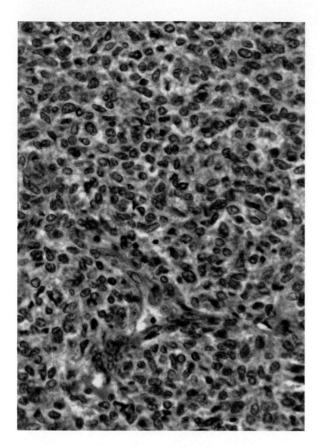

Figure 1-111

MESOBLASTIC NEPHROMA

The cellular variant is composed of monomorphous sheets of closely packed cells imparting a small blue cell appearance. Note the prominent irregular vascular spaces, which are a feature of many cellular mesoblastic nephromas.

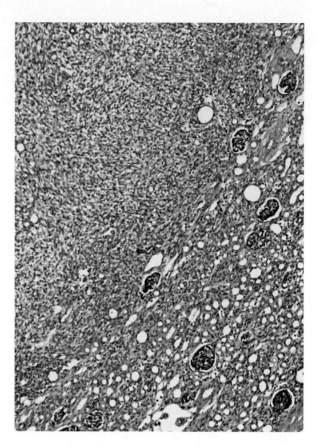

Figure 1-112

MESOBLASTIC NEPHROMA

The most common variant is cellular, composed of plump spindle cells growing in a diffuse pattern. The tumor is frequently circumscribed yet unencapsulated.

Figure 1-113

MESOBLASTIC NEPHROMA

"Plump" cell mesoblastic nephroma, cellular type, shows elongation of the cells, resembling fibroblast cultures.

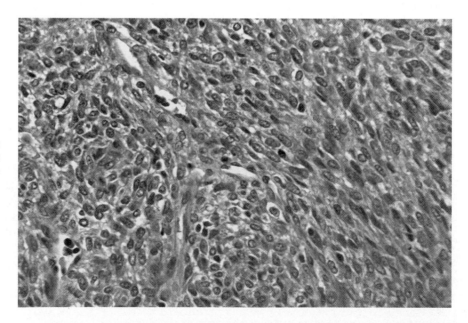

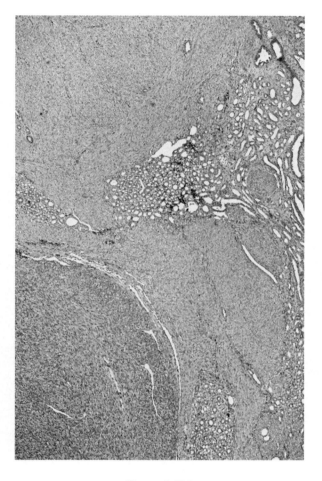

Figure 1-114

MESOBLASTIC NEPHROMA

A nodule of cellular mesoblastic nephroma can be seen within a background of classic mesoblastic nephroma.

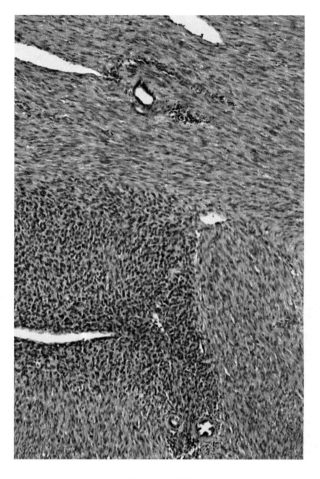

Figure 1-115

MESOBLASTIC NEPHROMA

A microscopic focus of increased cellularity is evident within this otherwise classic mesoblastic nephroma.

Cellular and classic patterns coexist in approximately 20 percent of CMNs, and such cases have been classified as *mixed mesoblastic nephroma* (figs. 1-114, 1-115). The majority of mixed CMNs have multiple foci of cellular histology in a background of classic histology, suggesting a "field effect." In some cases, a rim of cells consistent with classic CMN are associated with a single nodule of cellular CMN. There are two hypotheses to explain the occurrence of mixed CMNs. At least some cellular CMNs may arise within regions of classic morphology. Alternatively, the morphologic spectrum of both classic and cellular CMN may significantly overlap one another, resulting in tumors that appear to be mixed yet are biologically either classic or cellular.

Immunohistochemical Findings. Immunohistochemical reactions in both types of CMN are consistently positive using antibodies directed toward myofibroblasts (160,161,167a). Epithelial markers are positive only for entrapped epithelium. In addition to vimentin, desmin, and actin, reactions for fibronectin are positive. Negative reactions occur with antibodies to laminin, cytokeratins, and S-100 protein (155). WT1 positivity has been reported in CMNs, but this has not been the experience of all observers (163).

Ultrastructural Findings. Ultrastructural studies reveal elongated mesenchymal cells with prominent arrays of anastomosing rough endoplasmic reticulum (fig. 1-116) (159,161). Thin cytoplasmic filaments are often present. The basal

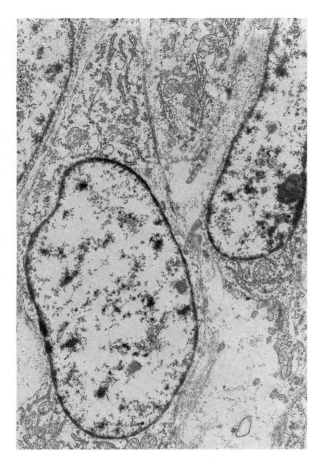

Figure 1-116

MESOBLASTIC NEPHROMA

Electron micrograph. (Fig. 1-92 from Fascicle 11, 3rd Series.)

Table 1-10

RECURRENCE AND/OR METASTASIS DOCUMENTED IN 415 MESOBLASTIC NEPHROMAS

Sites	No. of Cases
Abdominal recurrence only	18
Distant metastasis (lung, brain, bone)	9
Both local recurrence and distant metastasis	2
Total	29

lamina is absent and only sparse tight junctions of the macula adherens type have been observed.

Prognosis. CMNs are treated by complete surgical excision without adjuvant chemotherapy unless gross residual tumor remains. Almost all CMNs are predominantly localized to the kidney and perinephric or hilar soft tissue at the time of detection. Recurrences and metastases occur in approximately 5 to 10 percent of patients overall and are confined to tumors containing cellular histology (Table 1-10) (148). Of 415 CMNs evaluated by the NWTSG pathology center, 29 patients had documented recurrences (148). Local recurrence, usually to the flank, occurred in 18, and was associated with positive surgical margins at the time of original resection. This underscores the need for wide surgical resection and careful evaluation of the medial margin. Eleven patients developed distant metastases, most commonly involving the lung (161). The most significant factors associated with local recurrence and metastases are: 1) the presence of cellular histology; 2) tumors of stage III or greater (see Table 1-5); and 3) involvement of intrarenal or sinus vessels (fig. 1-117) (148). Virtually all recurrences develop during the 12 months following diagnosis, with several occurring within 1 month following negative ultrasound surveillance (148). As a result, it is recommended that patients with cellular CMN of either stage III or with vascular invasion should be screened via abdominal ultrasound monthly for 1 year. When gross residual tumor is left behind following surgery, adjuvant chemotherapy is indicated (142,150).

Differential Diagnosis. CMN must be differentiated from other pediatric renal neoplasms. Previously treated nephroblastomas may be especially rich in well-differentiated spindle cell stroma and one should be wary of the diagnosis of a CMN in such cases. The most commonly encountered and challenging problem is the differentiation of CMN from clear cell sarcoma. Both tumors occur in infancy and both are exclusively mesenchymal. Entrapped renal elements and embryonal metaplastic changes are often present in both. Helpful features in the differential diagnosis are listed in Table 1-11, however, no single criterion can be relied upon. Rhabdoid tumor is usually easily distinguished from CMN but the occasional CMN with unusually prominent nucleoli can lead to diagnostic difficulties. Immunohistochemistry is valuable in this situation.

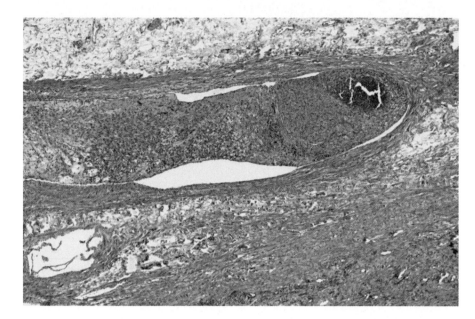

Figure 1-117

MESOBLASTIC NEPHROMA

Vascular invasion may be associated with a higher risk of recurrence or metastasis.

CLEAR CELL SARCOMA

Definition. Clear cell sarcoma of the kidney (CCSK) is a malignant mesenchymal neoplasm characterized by undifferentiated cells with abundant extracellular matrix that are separated into cords and nests by a fine vascular network (177,178,183,186). The tumor has a striking predilection to metastasize to bone, resulting in its historic classification as "bone metastasizing renal tumor of childhood."

General and Clinical Features. CCSK comprises 5 percent of primary pediatric renal tumors, with an incidence peaking during the second year of life and progressively falling thereafter (fig. 1-118). Patients as young as 2 months and as old as 54 years have been reported (171). Males are affected at least twice as frequently as females. The rare adult CCSK does not differ from childhood tumors in demographics, pathology, or clinical features. No racial or geographic predisposition has been observed, and CCSKs have not been associated with specific malformations, chromosomal defects, genetic abnormalities, or unusual syndromes.

Three patients have been reported with extrarenal masses histologically identical to CCSK, suggesting the possibility that CCSKs may present at extrarenal sites (171,181). However, these masses presented at sites where mesonephric remnants and nephrogenic rests are common, including the pelvic soft tissue, ovary, and retroperitoneum.

Only a few cases of CCSK have been examined by techniques other than light and electron microscopy. Almost all have had diploid DNA content with relatively low proliferation

Table 1-11

FEATURES DIFFERENTIATING MESOBLASTIC NEPHROMA FROM CLEAR CELL SARCOMA OF KIDNEY

Mesoblastic Nephroma	Clear Cell Sarcoma of Kidney
Clinical	
Age less than 6 months	Age more than 1 year
Increased renin, calcium	Metastases (except lung)
Light Microscopy	
Classic mesoblastic pattern[a]	**Classic CCSK pattern**[b]
Renal dysplasia (e.g., cartilage)	**Most variant CCSK patterns**
Coarse chromatin	Fine chromatin
High mitotic rate	Low mitotic rate
Extensively infiltrating margins	Extensive sclerosis
Staghorn vessels in tumor	Tumor entraps isolated nephrons
Tumor surrounds groups of nephrons	
Immunohistochemistry	
Positivity for desmin and/ or actin	Negativity for desmin and actin

[a]Features in boldface are diagnostic, others are supportive.
[b]CCSK = clear cell sarcoma of kidney.

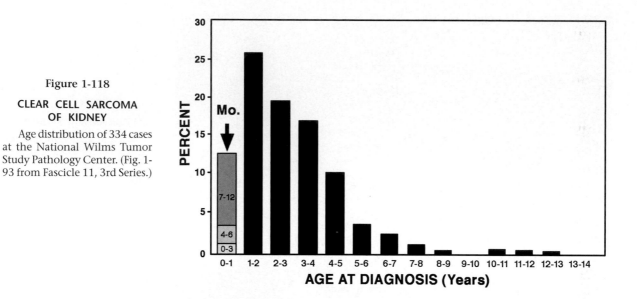

Figure 1-118

CLEAR CELL SARCOMA OF KIDNEY

Age distribution of 334 cases at the National Wilms Tumor Study Pathology Center. (Fig. 1-93 from Fascicle 11, 3rd Series.)

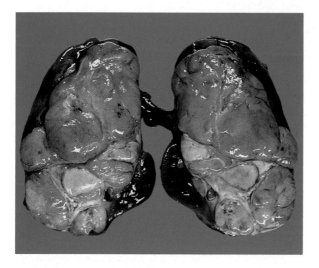

Figure 1-119

CLEAR CELL SARCOMA OF KIDNEY

Clear cell sarcomas of the kidney are homogenous, mucoid, and often irregular in contour. A tumor-kidney junction that is sharply defined is present. (Fig. 1-94 from Fascicle 11, 3rd Series.)

indices. Several tumors have been studied cytogenetically and have been interpreted as normal, but there is a single case report of a translocation involving chromosomes 10 and 17 (182). Studies using comparative genomic hybridization to analyze CCSKs for chromosomal gains and losses confirm that most tumors have no gains or losses, and no consistent changes have been identified (185).

Pathologic Findings. CCSKs vary in weight from 43 g to nearly 3,000 g, with both a mean and median weight of 500 to 600 g. The majority arise within the renal medulla, and almost all lesions are unilateral and unicentric (171). On sectioning, CCSKs are usually homogeneous and light brown or gray. Some tumors are soft and mucoid, but the majority have a dense, firm texture. The lesions are more often irregular in contour than spherical, and lack the multinodular appearance characteristic of nephroblastoma (fig. 1-119). The tumor-kidney junction appears sharply defined, although unencapsulated, and the tumor is usually confined within the renal capsule. Involvement of the renal vein has been recorded in approximately 5 percent of cases (171). Cysts are often present and may be the predominant feature in some specimens, resulting in a radiographic suspicion of multiloculated renal cyst or cystic nephroma.

Histologically, CCSKs are composed of undifferentiated plump cells arranged in nests or cords of 6 to 10 cells in width. These "cord" cells are separated by evenly dispersed, regularly branching small vessels, similar to the "chicken wire" vascular pattern seen in myxoid liposarcomas (fig. 1-120). These small vessels are accompanied by a variable component of spindle cells, often referred to as "septal" cells. The prominence of the vascular septa depends upon the number of septal cells accompanying the vessels. In well-fixed material, the cord cells are uniform in size,

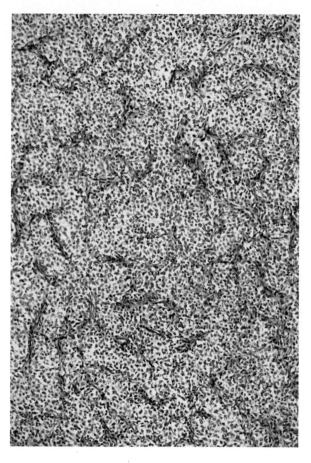

Figure 1-120

CLEAR CELL SARCOMA OF KIDNEY

Classic pattern, with cell cords demarcated by delicate, regularly spaced fibrovascular arcades.

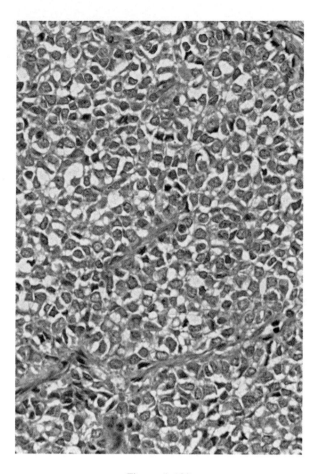

Figure 1-121

CLEAR CELL SARCOMA OF KIDNEY

The cells are separated by clear spaces and contain nuclei with finely dispersed chromatin. Often, the nuclei have a characteristic empty appearance.

loosely spaced, and have indistinct cell borders. They are separated from their neighbors by an extracellular, alcian blue–positive, mucopolysaccharide matrix that contributes to the pale, vesicular appearance of most specimens and provides the basis for the term clear cell sarcoma. The cord cells of CCSK are commonly separated from one another and are rarely as densely packed or overlapping as those of nephroblastoma. The nuclei of the cord cells contain finely dispersed chromatin without prominent nucleoli or chromatin condensation. "Empty"-appearing nuclei are frequent, and provide a valuable diagnostic clue for CCSK (fig. 1-121).

Most CCSKs are not composed entirely of clear cells but have at least some fields in which the cytoplasm is more condensed and acidophilic (fig. 1-122). When such cells predominate, the lesion may resemble a rhabdoid tumor. However, cells of CCSK lack the prominent nucleoli characteristic of a rhabdoid tumor. The mitotic rate is variable but considerably lower than that in other malignant pediatric renal neoplasms.

Cord cells are the predominant cell type in the majority of CCSKs, and septal cells are usually inconspicuous. However, in an occasional tumor, the septal cells may proliferate to varying degrees. These are recognized by their close apposition to the vascular septa, and by their elongated, spindled morphology (fig. 1-123). Their nuclear and cytoplasmic features are otherwise similar. The morphologic distinction between cord cells and septal cells recognizes their

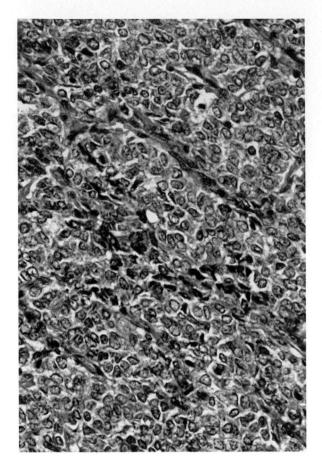

Figure 1-122

CLEAR CELL SARCOMA OF KIDNEY

In areas, the cells contain more condensed, eosinophilic cytoplasm, yet the regular vascular pattern is retained.

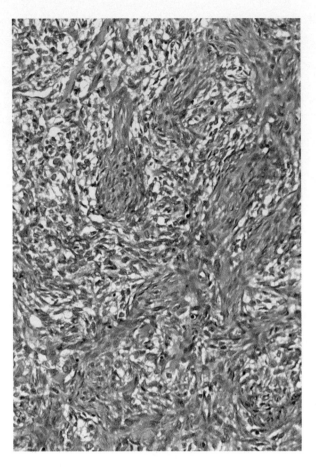

Figure 1-123

CLEAR CELL SARCOMA OF KIDNEY

The spindle cell pattern is caused by a proliferation of septal cells.

contribution to tumor architecture but does not necessarily imply that these cell types are biologically distinct from one another.

A distinctive and diagnostically useful feature of CCSK is the microscopic appearance of the kidney-tumor interface. Although the tumor margin is sharply demarcated grossly and under low magnification, higher magnification reveals tumor cells subtly infiltrating the normal renal parenchyma for short distances, nibbling into the adjacent renal parenchyma (fig. 1-124). This is in contrast to other malignant pediatric renal neoplasms, which usually have either a sharply defined, pushing border or an aggressively invasive, widely infiltrating margin. The slowly infiltrative nature of CCSK characteristically results in entrapment and separation of individual nephrons, tubules, or collecting ducts at the periph-

ery of the tumor, a feature virtually never seen in nephroblastomas (fig. 1-125). The cells of these entrapped tubules often assume a reactive, "embryonal" appearance that may be easily mistaken for the tubules of nephroblastoma, especially when they undergo reactive hyperplasia known as embryonal metaplasia (fig. 1-126). Similar features may be seen in mesoblastic nephromas and rhabdoid tumors, however, larger groups of nephrons tend to be entrapped by these neoplasms rather than the individually entrapped elements of CCSK. Entrapped tubules may dilate, forming cysts that are evident grossly or microscopically.

The histologic features of the *classic pattern* of CCSK are present at least focally in over 90 percent of cases. These features are distinctive, but the diagnosis of CCSK is often made difficult by the presence of a large number of variant

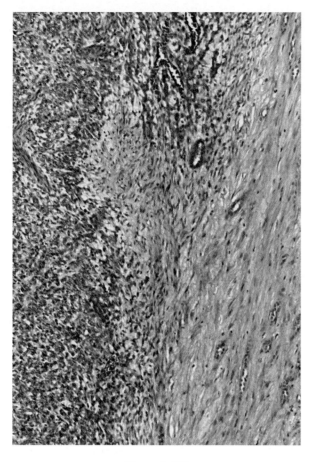

Figure 1-124

CLEAR CELL SARCOMA OF KIDNEY

The tumor-kidney interface shows the slowly infiltrative pattern, with entrapment of individual tubules.

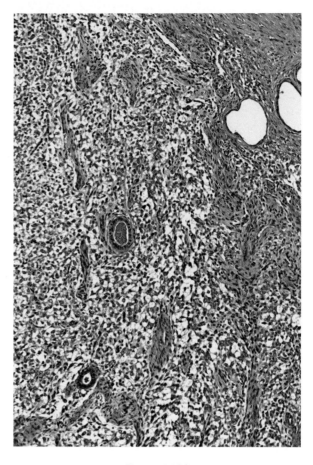

Figure 1-125

CLEAR CELL SARCOMA OF KIDNEY

Entrapped single renal tubules are commonly seen, particularly at the edge of the lesion.

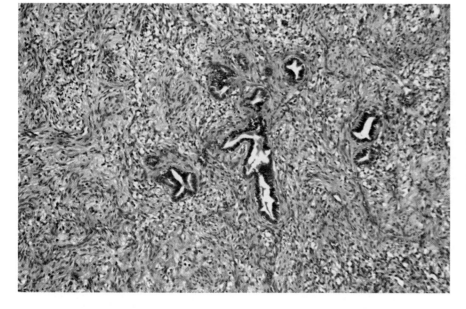

Figure 1-126

CLEAR CELL SARCOMA OF KIDNEY

Entrapped tubules and nephrons commonly have a reactive, embryonal, and metaplastic appearance that can lead to an erroneous diagnosis of nephroblastoma.

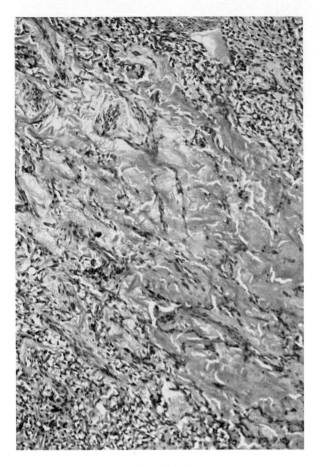

Figure 1-127

CLEAR CELL SARCOMA OF KIDNEY

The myxoid pattern shows focal accumulation of mucopolysaccharides, often associated with cyst formation.

patterns which may differ dramatically in histology and mimic almost any other pediatric renal tumor. Such variant patterns are common and in most cases, more than one variant pattern appears in the same lesion.

The most common variant pattern, seen in at least half of CCSKs, is the *myxoid pattern*, which results from the diffuse accumulation of mucopolysaccharide matrix between cord and septal cells, often obscuring the original classic histology (fig. 1-127). Coalescent pools of mucopolysaccharide may result in a cystic appearance.

In the *sclerosing pattern* (seen in 35 percent of CCSKs), abundant acellular collagen develops, often limited to the region of cord cells (fig. 1-128). These collagen bundles often isolate single cells or small groups of cells in a dense matrix that may become hyalinized, mimicking osteoid.

The *cellular pattern* is seen in approximately 25 percent of CCSKs, and is characterized by decreased intercellular material with close spacing and overlapping of nuclei. Mitotic activity is often increased in this variant, providing the appearance of an undifferentiated small blue cell tumor (fig. 1-129). This pattern may closely mimic primitive neuroectodermal tumor as well as blastemal nephroblastoma and cellular mesoblastic nephroma. Careful attention to the presence of the regularly spaced vascular network characteristic of CCSK is important.

The *epithelioid pattern* (identified in 13 percent) is the pattern that most often results in a

Figure 1-128

CLEAR CELL SARCOMA OF KIDNEY

The sclerosing pattern shows extensive sclerosis of the cord cells with persistence of the vascular septa.

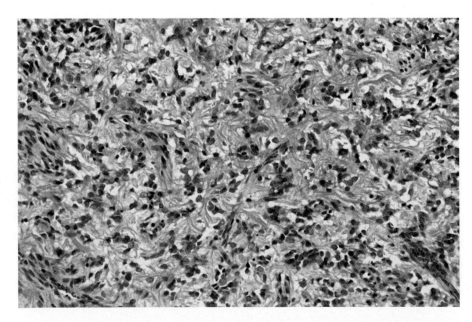

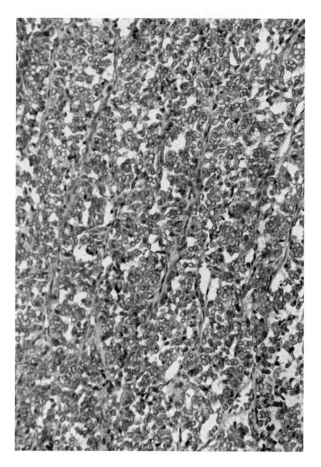

Figure 1-129

CLEAR CELL SARCOMA OF KIDNEY

The cellular pattern shows closely spaced, overlapping, embryonal-appearing cells, with persistence of the vascular pattern.

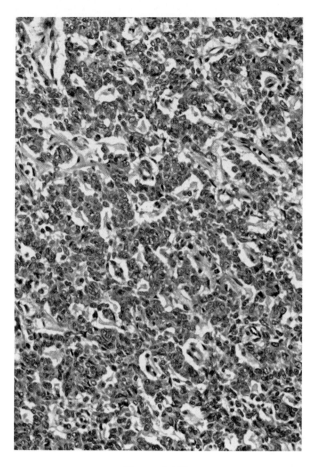

Figure 1-130

CLEAR CELL SARCOMA OF KIDNEY

In the epithelioid pattern, the cord cells have become condensed, creating cohesive epithelioid ribbons of cells.

mistaken diagnosis of nephroblastoma. Condensation of the cord cells may result in ribbons, tubules, rosettes, and trabeculae (fig. 1-130) (184). The intervening vascular septa are usually retained between the condensed cell cords but are not always conspicuous. A characteristic variation is the formation of undulating, elongated ribbons of single cell thickness, producing a sharply defined filigree pattern (fig. 1-131). Within the broader cords of the ribbon pattern, coalescent aggregates of interstitial mucin create a tubular or cystic appearance (180,184). Despite the strong resemblance of these changes to tubular differentiation, the cells participating in these structures do not react with antibodies to cytokeratins or epithelial membrane antigen. In contrast, entrapped renal tubules are strongly reactive for these antigens.

A *spindle cell pattern* may sometimes be prominent in CCSK, however, it is only seen in 7 percent of tumors. Both the septal and cord cells may have spindle cell features, resulting in a wide variety of histologic appearances reminiscent of other sarcomas and soft tissue lesions (figs. 1-132, 1-133). When the expansion of septal spindle cells is extreme, cord cells may be obliterated, resulting in a complex pattern of intersecting spindle cell bundles reminiscent of CMN.

One of the more distinctive variants of CCSK is the *palisading pattern*, which is observed in approximately 15 percent of specimens (fig. 1-133). This pattern is characterized by the alignment of spindle cell nuclei in parallel linear arrays, alternating with nuclear free zones. The resemblance to Verocay bodies of schwannomas is striking, however, these areas do not

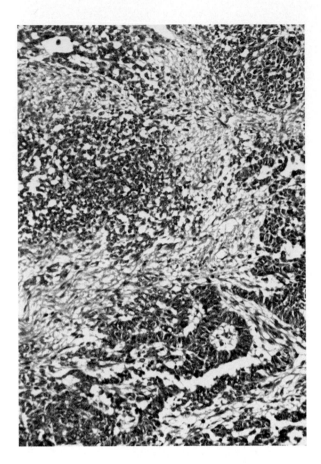

Figure 1-131

CLEAR CELL SARCOMA OF KIDNEY

The epithelioid pattern is composed of both trabecular condensations as well as condensations of cord cells that are 1 to 2 cells in thickness, forming a "filagree" pattern.

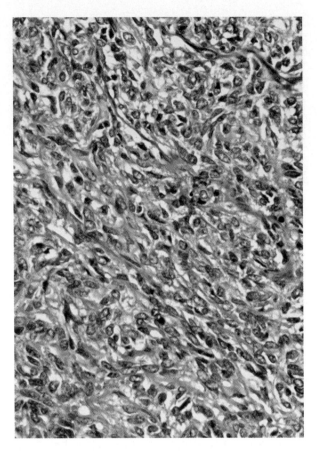

Figure 1-132

CLEAR CELL SARCOMA OF KIDNEY

The spindle cell pattern shows cord cells that have spindled, although the vascular septa are still recognizable.

Figure 1-133

CLEAR CELL SARCOMA OF KIDNEY

A palisading pattern reminiscent of nerve sheath tumors is common.

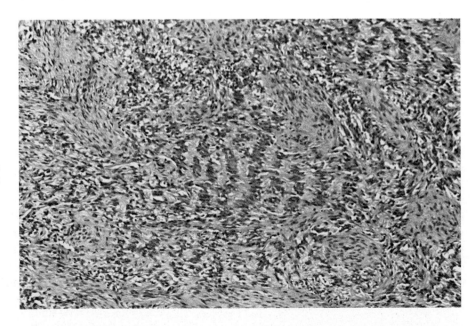

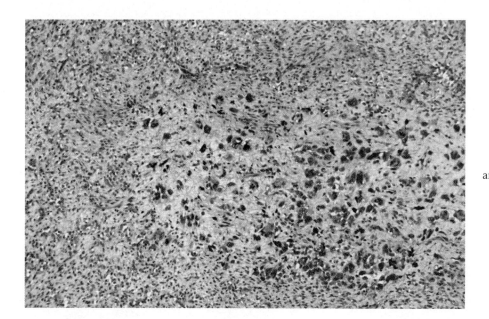

Figure 1-134

**CLEAR CELL
SARCOMA OF KIDNEY**

A circumscribed region of anaplasia is seen.

manifest S-100 protein expression or neural features ultrastructurally (186).

In the *sinusoidal (pericytomatous) pattern*, blood vessels comprising a part of the classic CCSK pattern become distended, resembling a hemangiopericytoma.

Anaplasia, characterized by the presence of markedly enlarged, polypoid nuclei with multipolar mitotic figures, is seen in approximately 3 percent of primary and recurrent CCSKs (fig. 1-134). In the majority of cases, anaplasia is evident in small, circumscribed foci within an otherwise nonanaplastic CCSK. Anaplasia has also been identified in metastases from a nonanaplastic primary tumor (171). Due to its rarity, the clinical significance of anaplasia in CCSK is unknown. The strong immunohistochemical positivity of anaplastic cells for TP53 protein suggests that, similar to other childhood tumors, such change is accompanied by a *TP53* gene mutation.

The histologic appearance of recurrent or metastatic CCSK following chemotherapy is usually similar to that of the primary tumor. However, such lesions may be hypocellular, sclerotic, and infiltrative, and may therefore resemble a wide spectrum of benign fibrous or myxomatous lesions, fibromatosis, or hamartomas (173). The correct identification of these lesions as recurrent or metastatic CCSK is made even more problematic by the tendency for CCSKs to recur very late, often decades after the initial diagnosis, and to

recur in unlikely sites (fig. 1-135). Therefore, recurrences are often present in situations where suspicion for metastasis has diminished. In general, a mass at any site in a patient with a previous history of CCSK should be considered a metastasis until proven otherwise.

Cytologic preparations of CCSK reveal cells with irregular nuclei containing evenly dispersed chromatin. The cytoplasm is often eccentric, with poorly defined cytoplasmic borders. Fine nuclear grooves may be seen and may be more prominent in aspirated specimens, although their diagnostic usefulness has not been established (fig. 1-136) (172).

Immunohistochemical Findings. The primary contribution of immunohistochemistry to the diagnosis of CCSK is the exclusion of other pediatric renal neoplasms (170,171,179). Vimentin is demonstrated in most tumors and is useful to verify preservation of tumor antigenicity, since nearly all other markers are negative. Epithelial markers are negative in the tumor cells, even in epithelioid variants, but react strongly with entrapped non-neoplastic nephrons and tubules.

Ultrastructural Findings. Electron microscopy shows that the cells of CCSK generally contain abundant, pale, extracellular matrix with scant collagen fibers (fig. 1-137). Elongated cytoplasmic processes frequently partially enfold pools of matrix. Mitochondria and rough endoplasmic reticulum are the most conspicuous organelles, and rare cytoplasmic cilia and

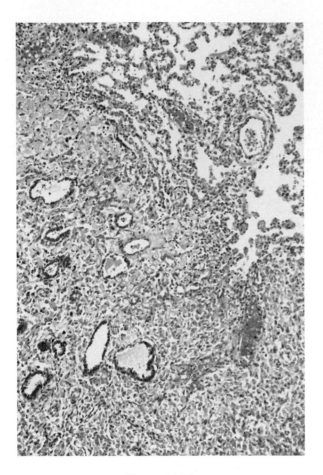

Figure 1-135

CLEAR CELL SARCOMA OF KIDNEY

Somewhat hypocellular, sclerotic, infiltrative metastasis within the lung.

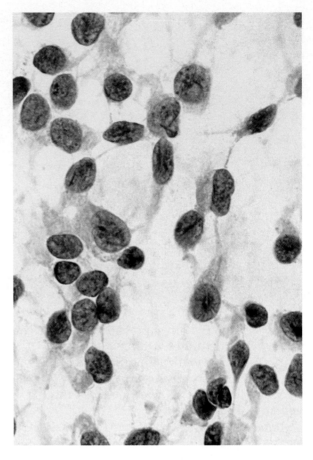

Figure 1-136

CLEAR CELL SARCOMA OF KIDNEY

Fine needle aspiration cytology shows nuclei with fine, evenly dispersed chromatin and nuclear grooves.

lipid droplets have been described. A basal lamina is not associated with the tumor cells. Cell junctions are infrequent and of the primitive type. Intermediate filaments are variable in their presence and amount (175,179,186).

Prognosis. Using the same staging criteria applied to nephroblastomas (see Table 1-5), 25 percent of CCSKs are localized stage I tumors, 37 percent are stage II, 34 percent are stage III, and 4 percent are stage IV. An unusual finding for a sarcoma, 29 percent of patients with CCSKs have regional lymph node involvement at diagnosis. Bone metastasis is the most common mode of relapse; other commonly observed metastatic sites are brain, lung, liver, and soft tissue. Unusual metastatic sites include testis and salivary gland, and the skeletal muscle of the distal extremities. Late onset of first relapse is a distinc-

tive feature of CCSK. Relapses after intervals as long as 8 and 10 years have been documented (171,176). Late relapses are especially prevalent among children treated with doxorubicin.

Patients with CCSKs are treated with nephrectomy followed by adjuvant therapy with regimens that include doxorubicin, actinomycin, and vincristine (171,174). The prognosis varies with stage at presentation: 97 percent 6-year survival for those with stage I; 75 percent for stage II; 77 percent for stage III; and 50 percent for stage IV (171).

Differential Diagnosis. The most difficult and frequent differential diagnostic considerations for CCSKs are nephroblastoma and CMN (Tables 1-11, 1-12). The presence of any element that is unambiguously nephroblastomatous excludes the diagnosis of CCSK. This includes the

Table 1-12

FEATURES DIFFERENTIATING NEPHROBLASTOMA FROM CLEAR CELL SARCOMA

Nephroblastoma	Clear Cell Sarcoma
Clinical	
Nephroblastoma syndromes[a]	Metastases to bone, brain, or other sites (except
Bilateral/multicentric tumors	lung, lymph nodes, liver)
Gross and Light Microscopy	
Heterologous cell types (skeletal muscle, etc.)	**Classic or variant CCSK patterns form entire tumor**[b]
Classic blastemal patterns (serpentine, etc.)	Homogeneous, pale H&E appearance
Nodular growth pattern	Tumor surrounds, isolates nephrons
Botryoid intrapelvic growth	Prominent collagen (except in treated or
Tumor in renal veins	infarcted tumor)
Nephrogenic rests	
Immunohistochemistry	
Positivity for WT1 or CD56	Negativity for immunohistochemical markers other
Positivity for epithelial, muscle, or neural differentiation	than vimentin

[a]Features in boldface are diagnostic, others are supportive.
[b]CCSK = clear cell sarcoma of kidney; H&E = hematoxylin and eosin.

presence of heterologous elements, and the presence of a botryoid-like growth pattern within the renal pelvis. Similarly, the presence of a nephrogenic rest within the same kidney should cast extreme doubt on the diagnosis of CCSK. The age of presentation must be considered when differentiating CCSK and CMN. While rare cases of CCSK in children less than 6 months have been reported, this is the most common age of presentation of those with CMN. Positivity of the tumor cells for desmin tends to confirm the diagnosis of CMN in such cases.

Rarely, other entities cause diagnostic difficulty, including primitive neuroectodermal tumor and synovial sarcoma, entities that have only relatively recently been recognized to involve the kidney. The presence of CD99 (MIC2) or epithelial membrane antigen positivity in such cases is useful. While not a frequent source of diagnostic confusion, occasional CCSKs may contain focal areas suggestive of a rhabdoid tumor. The inconspicuous nucleoli, clear cytoplasm, and less aggressive infiltrative marginal pattern of CCSKs are the most helpful diagnostic considerations. It is important to remember that CCSKs may both mimic, and be mimicked by, all other pediatric renal neoplasms. Therefore, a confident diagnosis of CCSK on a small biopsy specimen is virtually impossible. Furthermore, the performance of frozen section analysis for the purpose of diagnosis commonly results in an error.

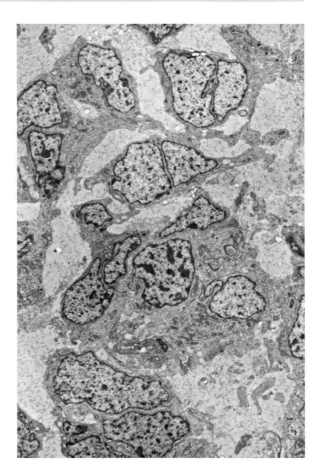

Figure 1-137

CLEAR CELL SARCOMA OF KIDNEY

Electron microscopy demonstrates that the "clear" cell appearance is due to extracellular matrix.

RHABDOID TUMOR

Definition. Rhabdoid tumor of the kidney (RTK) is a rare, highly malignant neoplasm of infancy characterized by a monomorphous population of large, relatively noncohesive cells with vesicular nuclei and large nucleoli (190,207). The misleading name was originally suggested by a perceived resemblance to other skeletal muscle tumors, but neither ultrastructural nor other features support a myogenic origin for rhabdoid tumors. Following the description of RTK, the lesion has become increasingly recognized at extrarenal sites, particularly in the central nervous system (CNS) (192,200,206,208). The unifying feature of infantile rhabdoid tumors at all sites is the presence of a mutation or deletion of the *INI1* gene located at chromosome 22q11.

General and Clinical Features. RTK is a neoplasm of unknown etiology that constitutes only 2.5 percent of pediatric renal tumors (207). The median age at diagnosis is 11 months and more than 95 percent of patients are under 3 years of age. This diagnosis should be considered suspect in patients over the age of 5 years. Males predominate over females in a ratio of 1.5 to 1. Extrarenal tumors with rhabdoid features have been reported in one pair of siblings (196). A few rhabdoid tumors have been associated with hypercalcemia and elevated levels of parathormone (197).

Cytogenetic analysis of RTK demonstrates a high frequency of abnormalities involving the long arm of chromosome 22, characterized by both deletions and translocations (188,193). These results are confirmed by the loss of chromosome 22q in 80 percent of rhabdoid tumors of the kidney, brain, and other soft tissue sites (187,189,201,209). The common area of deletion on chromosome 22q11.2 has been mapped to the *hSNF5/INI1* gene (189,203). Of tumors with documented *hSNF5/INI1* abnormalities, approximately half have shown homozygous deletions of *hSNF5/INI1* and half have contained mutations. In addition, germline mutations have been demonstrated in four children (189). Currently available data suggest that patients with both CNS and renal rhabdoid tumors have germline mutations involving one copy of the *hSNF5/INI1* gene, with different alterations involving the second copy confined to the separate tumors (199). The *hSNF5/INI1* gene product is thought to normally function by altering the conformation of the DNA-histone complex so that transcription factors have access to target genes (203).

While no syndromes are associated with RTK, CNS tumors are observed in approximately 15 percent of patients. Most of these CNS tumors are located in the midline cerebellum and morphologically resemble medulloblastoma or primitive neuroectodermal tumor (190–192,194). However, it has been well established that rhabdoid tumors of the CNS (also called atypical teratoid tumors) often have a small blue cell tumor appearance, yet contain the same genetic changes seen in RTKs (189,191). It has been suggested that most patients with both renal and CNS rhabdoid tumors have constitutional abnormalities in the *hSNF5/INI1* gene (189).

Pathologic Findings. Grossly, RTKs are bulky, soft, pale, and relatively uniform. They are moderately well demarcated from the adjacent kidney, although the tumor-kidney junction is often indistinct and the tumor usually lacks a capsule (fig. 1-138). Most recorded tumors weigh less than 500 g (207). Small tumors tend to arise in the renal medulla. These neoplasms are unicentric and unilateral, with multiple renal nodules considered to represent intrarenal or contralateral metastases.

Histologically, RTKs have a monotonous pattern composed of sheets of large, loosely cohesive cells with distinct cell borders. The cells often contain large whorls of intermediate filaments, resulting in the appearance of acidophilic cytoplasmic inclusions. Cells have large nuclei with prominent, centrally placed nucleoli, although the size of the nuclei and the nucleoli vary from field to field (fig. 1-139). The cells with characteristic cytoplasmic inclusions tend to be clustered rather than uniformly distributed, and not all cells of any given neoplasm contain these cytoplasmic inclusions (figs. 1-140–1-143). The growth pattern is infiltrative with frequent invasion of local blood vessels (fig 1-142). Sections taken from the tumor-kidney interface commonly have nephrons isolated by tumor cells, a pattern similar to that seen with CMN and CCSK.

Nearly all RTKs contain areas that are classic, but a number of pattern variations may be seen, including sclerosing, epithelioid,

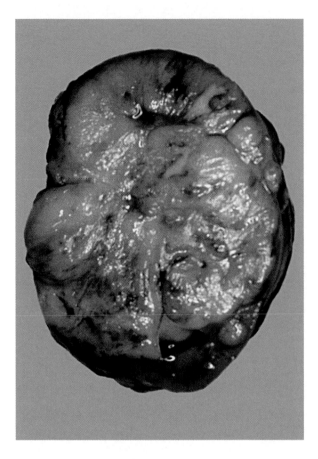

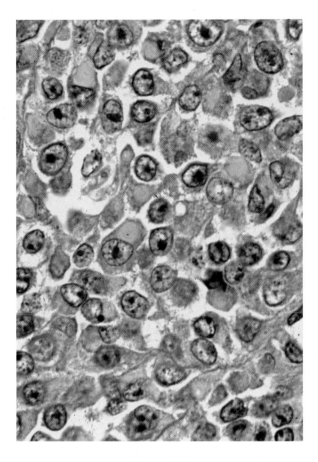

Figure 1-138

RHABDOID TUMOR

Rhabdoid tumors are often poorly circumscribed, with numerous satellite lesions present due to intrarenal metastases.

Figure 1-139

RHABDOID TUMOR

Characteristic appearance in well-fixed, routinely processed sections.

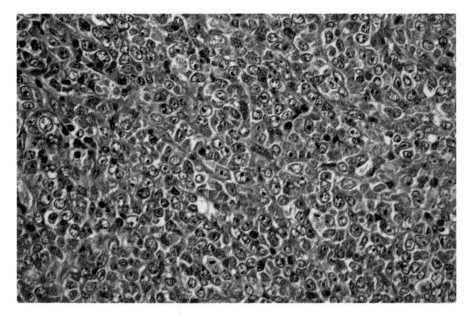

Figure 1-140

RHABDOID TUMOR

Characteristic vesicular nuclei, prominent nucleoli, and occasional pale cytoplasmic inclusions are seen in this diffuse growth pattern.

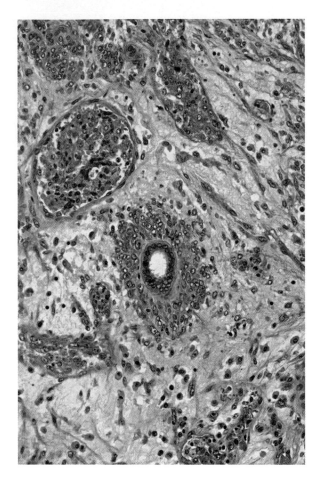

Figure 1-141

RHABDOID TUMOR

Tumor cells surround native structures, with alternating regions of increased and decreased cellularity.

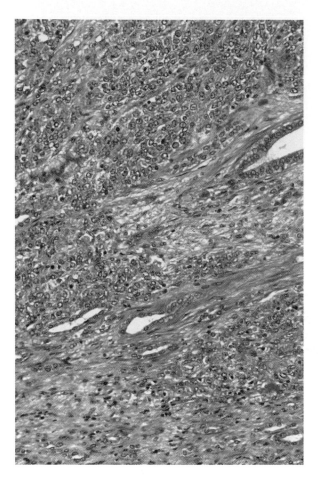

Figure 1-142

RHABDOID TUMOR

Aggressive infiltration of soft tissue and vessels in the renal parenchyma and sinus is characteristic of this neoplasm.

spindled, and lymphomatoid (207). In the *sclerosing variant,* the stroma of the rhabdoid tumor becomes densely collagenous, separating nests, cords, or single tumor cells (fig. 1-143). Basophilic ground substance may accumulate to such a degree as to suggest chondroid differentiation, and dense collagen may resemble osteoid. Cords of cohesive tumor cells that result in a trabecular arrangement are seen in the *epithelioid variant*, and may resemble nephroblastoma (fig. 1-144). The addition of mucoid substances or cyst formation may then result in the appearance of pseudoglandular or alveolar configurations. Occasional tumors show no differentiation and are composed of solid sheets of noncohesive cells with scant cytoplasm.

Such tumors may resemble large cell lymphomas and comprise the *lymphomatoid variant* (fig. 1-145). A *spindled variant* is also encountered and may cause great diagnostic difficulty, particularly in biopsy specimens and in the absence of the classic histology. This pattern includes tumors with fascicles of deceptively bland-appearing cells resembling mesoblastic nephroma as well as tumors with dispersed spindled cells within a loose matrix, resulting in a myxoid appearance (fig. 1-146). As with many other tumors, spindled RTKs may arrange themselves around prominent vessels, resulting in a hemangiopericytomatous appearance. Cystic dilatation of entrapped renal tubules may result in the formation of multiple cysts.

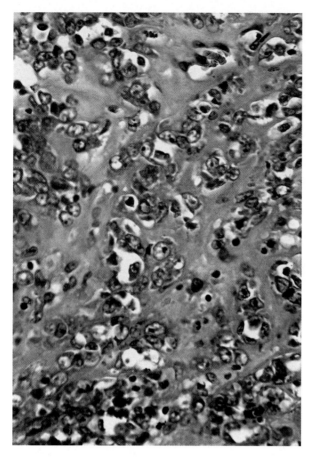

Figure 1-143

RHABDOID TUMOR

Dense sclerosis may be seen, resembling osteoid production.

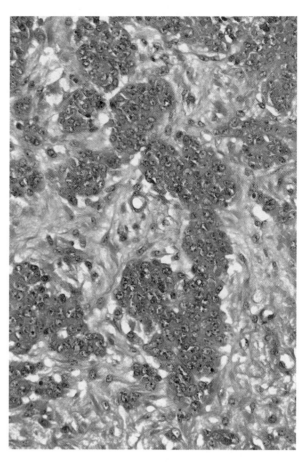

Figure 1-144

RHABDOID TUMOR

The epithelioid pattern consists of irregular nests and trabeculae of cells resembling a poorly differentiated carcinoma.

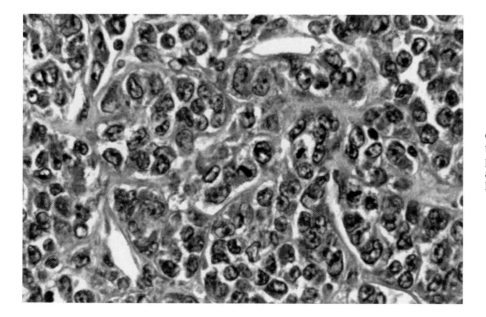

Figure 1-145

RHABDOID TUMOR

Rhabdoid tumors are often discohesive. In addition, rare tumors contain little cytoplasm, resulting in a histologic appearance resembling a hematopoietic lesion.

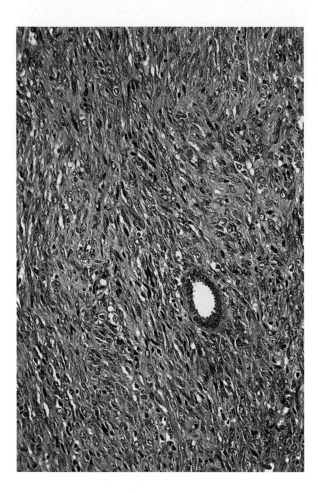

Figure 1-146

RHABDOID TUMOR

Spindling of the tumor cells is occasionally seen.

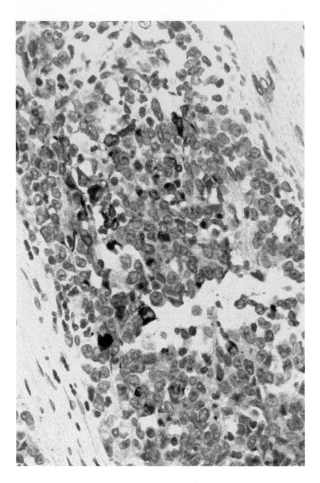

Figure 1-147

RHABDOID TUMOR

Polyphenotypic differentiation in a pattern characterized by very focal but intense staining is seen in rhabdoid tumors. Positivity for epithelial membrane antigen is shown.

Immunohistochemical Findings. RTKs are characterized by a polyphenotypic immunoreactive pattern (200,202,204,207,209a). Vimentin immunoreactivity is uniform and intense in all tumors. In addition, tumor cells may react simultaneously with a variety of markers including (but not limited to) cytokeratin, epithelial membrane antigen, desmin, and neurofilament. The reaction pattern for these is characteristically patchy and strong, with small clusters of cells having intense positivity. One particularly helpful pattern of reaction is the presence of scattered clusters of intensely epithelial membrane antigen- or cytokeratin-positive cells in a background of nonreactive tumor cells. This pattern is seen in over 90 percent of RTKs, and few other pediatric tumors react in this distinct fashion (fig. 1-147). For this reason, epithelial membrane antigen or pancytokeratins are commonly used as confirmatory markers for RTKs (Table 1-13). Rare RTKs with the characteristic *INI1* mutation may have either no epithelial immunoreactivity or diffusely positive immunoreactivity.

Ultrastructural Findings. Ultrastructurally, the prominent aggregates of filaments that characterize RTKs range in thickness from 6 to 10 nm and form tightly whorled structures adjacent to the nucleus (fig. 1-148). Rudimentary cell junctions, cytoplasmic organelles, and glycogen may be present, but they are not abundant. Dense core granules, alternating thick and thin filaments, and cell-associated basal laminae are

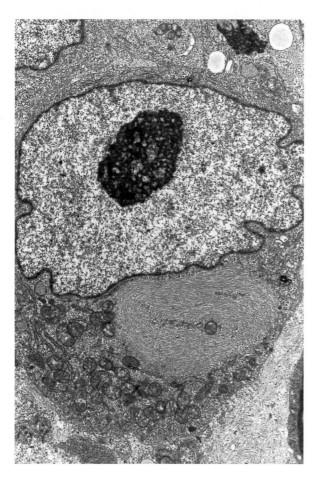

Figure 1-148

RHABDOID TUMOR

The characteristic electron microscopic appearance of a whorled aggregate of intermediate filaments can occur in many other neoplasms. (Fig. 1-123 from Fascicle 11, 3rd Series.)

Table 1-13

RENAL NEOPLASMS MIMICKING RHABDOID TUMOR OF KIDNEY

Nephroblastoma with cytoplasmic inclusions
Renal cell carcinoma with inclusions
Renal medullary carcinoma
Transitional cell carcinoma
Mesoblastic nephroma
Rhabdomyosarcoma
Leiomyosarcoma
Neuroepithelial tumors
Metastases from extrarenal "pseudorhabdoid" tumor

Table 1-14

EXTRARENAL NEOPLASMS MIMICKING RHABDOID TUMOR

Rhabdomyosarcoma
Leiomyosarcoma
Ganglioneuroblastoma
Carcinoid, other neuroendocrine tumors
Epithelioid schwannoma
Melanoma
Glioma
Epithelioid sarcoma
Synovial sarcoma
Histiocytic sarcoma
Large cell lymphoma
Yolk sac tumor
Hepatocellular carcinoma
Angiosarcoma

conspicuously absent, suggesting that these lesions are not differentiating toward neuroendocrine, skeletal muscle, or smooth muscle cells (195,200,207). It should be emphasized that whorled aggregates of filaments are not diagnostic of RTK and can be seen in a number of other neoplasms, and otherwise classic RTKs may contain few if any cells with filamentous inclusions.

Prognosis. RTK is one of the most lethal neoplasms of childhood: 80 percent of patients die of their cancers within 1 year of diagnosis (205, 207). The tumor is usually disseminated at diagnosis, with 80 percent of patients presenting with stage III or IV tumors (207). Chemotherapy has not altered the dismal prognosis associated with RTK. Combinations of etoposide and cisplatin or ifosfamide are employed, but the results have not been encouraging. Rare patients with documented negative lymph nodes at presentation have survived (207).

Differential Diagnosis. The diagnosis of rhabdoid tumor at any site is complicated by the fact that a wide variety of tumors may have rhabdoid features (Tables 1-13, 1-14) (198,208). Nonetheless, the establishment of a common genetic deletion on the long arm of chromosome 22 in both renal and extrarenal rhabdoid tumors in infants has allowed a unifying approach to the recognition of primary rhabdoid tumors of childhood. Differentiating rhabdoid tumor from other renal neoplasms of infancy and childhood is usually straightforward. Neuroblastoma may offer a challenge due to the common presence of nuclei with large nucleoli and cells with abundant cytoplasm and ganglionic differentiation. At times, foci in a nephroblastoma, neuroblastoma, CMN, or CCSK may resemble a RTK. However, the careful examination of the specimen in its entirety usually reveals the histologic appearance characteristic of the correct diagnosis. The prognosis for patients with CMN and nephroblastoma appears to be unaffected by the presence of rhabdoid features, and aggressive therapy triggered by the diagnosis of RTK is contraindicated in these patients (208). Renal medullary carcinoma accounts for many of the cases previously reported as RTK in patients over the age of 5 years. This highly lethal tumor is virtually restricted to adolescent patients with sickle cell hemoglobinopathy.

Occasional RTKs lack the typical cytoplasmic inclusions and resemble other small blue cell tumors of childhood. Immunohistochemistry is quite useful in this setting. A panel of immunohistochemical markers that includes epithelial membrane antigen, a cytokeratin cocktail, and vimentin as well as other positive markers for differentiating small blue cell tumors of childhood will usually point to the correct diagnosis.

More troubling are tumors that contain cells with the characteristic nuclear features of rhabdoid tumor, but a moderate amount of cytoplasm that lacks prominent inclusions and is negative for both specific positive markers and epithelial markers. It is known that such tumors may contain the *hSNF5/INI1* mutation. Conversely, it is amply recognized that a number of tumors mimic rhabdoid tumor. This places the pathologist in the distinctly uncomfortable situation of suggesting the diagnosis of RTK, implying an abysmal prognosis, without the ability to confirm the diagnosis. It is hoped that a clinically useful method for documenting *hSNF5/INI1* mutation or deletion will be available in the near future.

PEDIATRIC RENAL CELL CARCINOMA

Malignant epithelial tumors arising in the kidneys of children are rare, accounting for less than 0.1 percent of new pediatric malignancies (214,220,225,229). The mean age at presentation in children is 9 to 10 years (214). Unlike renal cell carcinomas (RCC) in adults, environmental factors have not been shown to play a role. Furthermore, pediatric RCCs often differ in their histologic appearance from those of adulthood. Clear cell RCC is quite rare in patients under the age of 25 in the absence of a predisposing genetic condition such as von Hippel-Lindau syndrome. These factors strongly suggest that RCCs in children do not simply represent the lower range of the age distribution curve of adult-type renal tumors, but instead are intrinsically different, at least in part. This is supported by genetic changes that have been reported in pediatric RCCs in recent years. Given the currently available information, RCCs in children most commonly fall into three categories: papillary RCC; renal medullary carcinoma; and RCCs with an Xp11.2 translocation.

Papillary Renal Cell Carcinoma

Papillary RCC is the most common histologic subtype of RCC occurring in children, and represents the pediatric counterpart of the papillary RCC found in adults (211,219,228). The pathologic appearance and genetic changes are those described in chapter 2 for adults. The differential diagnosis includes differentiated epithelial nephroblastoma and metanephric adenoma. The most valuable histologic clues for distinguishing these similar lesions follow.

Peritumoral Pseudocapsule. Most epithelial nephroblastomas and papillary RCCs have a prominent peritumoral pseudocapsule composed of compressed kidney and collagen. Papillary RCCs also characteristically have an abundant lymphocytic infiltrate around the periphery of their pseudocapsule (227). Metanephric adenomas, by definition, lack a peritumoral pseudocapsule, although this assessment may be difficult when the metanephric adenoma approaches normal renal architectural barriers such as the renal capsule or the edge of the renal lobule (see fig. 1-90).

Cytology. Nephroblastomas are proliferative lesions that contain at least occasional mitotic figures, whereas mitotic figures are absent in metanephric adenoma, and are often rare in papillary RCC. The cells of nephroblastoma are generally columnar with large, overlapping nuclei and finely dispersed chromatin (see figs. 1-30, 1-31). The cells of metanephric adenoma are oval with

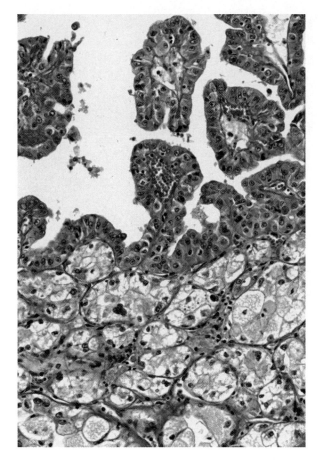

Figure 1-149

PAPILLARY RENAL CELL CARCINOMA

Typical papillary architecture with foam cells. Pale cytoplasm and prominent nucleoli are seen.

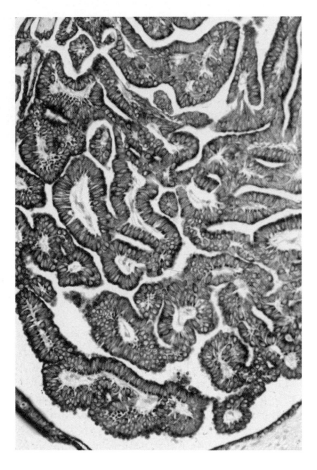

Figure 1-150

PAPILLARY RENAL CELL CARCINOMA

Cytokeratin 7 staining of papillary renal cell carcinoma. Compare to figure 1-92.

bland nuclei that lack prominent nucleoli (see figs. 1-90, 1-91). Papillary RCCs may contain cells with prominent nucleoli (fig. 1-149). Aggregates of foamy macrophages are seen in over 80 percent of papillary RCCs, but these may also be seen focally in epithelial-predominant nephroblastomas as well as in metanephric adenomas. Calcospherites may be a prominent feature in each of these tumors.

Immunohistochemical Findings. Papillary RCCs are characteristically strongly and homogeneously positive for cytokeratin 7, a marker that is at most only focally positive in nephroblastomas and metanephric adenomas (fig. 1-150) (227). Metanephric adenomas are negative for epithelial membrane antigen, a marker that is strongly positive in papillary RCC.

Despite these helpful features, basophilic papillary renal tumors in children are frequently difficult to categorize definitively as metanephric adenoma, differentiated epithelial nephroblastoma, or papillary RCC. It is useful to remember that all of these tumors typically are low stage at presentation. In addition, any residual tumor is commonly unresponsive to chemotherapy, and surgery remains the cornerstone of treatment for patients with these entities.

Renal Medullary Carcinoma

Renal medullary carcinoma is a rare tumor that afflicts young individuals with sickle cell hemoglobinopathy (210,217,224,230,233,236). While nearly all reported patients have sickle cell trait, a single case of an individual with sickle cell

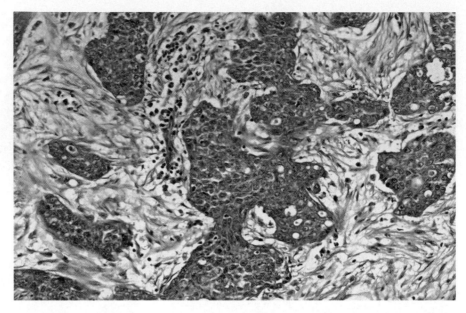

Figure 1-151

RENAL MEDULLARY CARCINOMA

Prominent sclerosis is present in most tumors and often surrounds irregular clusters of cells that show variable degrees of gland formation.

disease is recorded (233). The relative frequency of sickle cell trait and sickle cell disease appears to be the same in the population at large as it is in patients with renal medullary carcinoma (233). Most reported patients are African-Americans, but patients with Caucasian European and Brazilian backgrounds have also been reported; these populations have a high prevalence of the sickle cell gene (221,222). The age at presentation has ranged from 5 to 32 years, with a mean of 14.8 years (233). Clinical symptoms at presentation include the classic triad of flank pain, hematuria, and a palpable abdominal mass. A surprisingly high number of patients are suspected of having abdominal infection and treated with antibiotics for variable lengths of time prior to the discovery of a renal mass.

Pathologically, most renal medullary carcinomas are poorly circumscribed and involve the medulla. Intrarenal hematogenous spread is common. Microscopically, a cribriform architecture is most often present, but other growth patterns are identified, including microcystic, solid, and sarcomatoid (figs. 1-151, 1-152). Stromal desmoplasia is commonly identified and is usually a prominent feature. Another characteristic feature is the presence of a striking acute and chronic inflammatory infiltrate. These tumors have infiltrative margins and single cell infiltration is commonly observed. The nuclei are large and vesicular, with prominent nucleoli in most cases. Aci-

dophilic cytoplasm is abundant, with striking cytoplasmic lumens in some cases. Cytoplasmic inclusions resembling rhabdoid tumor are noted in most cases (fig. 1-153).

Renal medullary carcinomas have homogeneous expression for low molecular weight cytokeratins such as Cam 5.2 and epithelial membrane antigen, and demonstrate co-expression with vimentin. The high molecular weight cytokeratin 34ßE12 is negative in all cases. Drepanocytes (sickled cells) can be identified in most cases, although sometimes a diligent search of the tissue is required (fig. 1-154).

Renal medullary carcinoma is characterized clinically by a high stage at the time of detection, widespread metastases, and lack of response to both chemotherapy and radiotherapy. Survival ranges from 2 weeks to 15 months, with a mean of 4 months.

Renal Tumors with Xp11.2 Translocations

Renal neoplasms have been traditionally defined according to their histologic characteristics, but certain renal tumors in children and young adults merit recognition by their genetic features. The majority of these lesions have histologic features that overlap those of other RCCs, yet have genetic translocations involving the *TFE3* gene located at Xp11.2 and a number of variant partner genes (Table 1-15) (212, 215,216,218,223,226,231,234,235,237). These tumors tend to have a nested or tubulopapillary

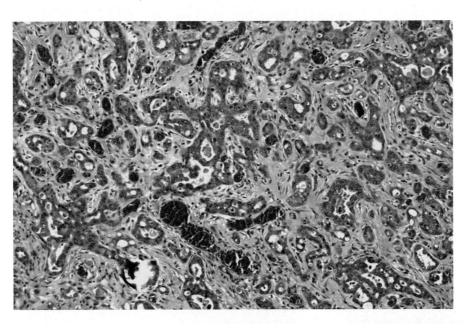

Figure 1-152

RENAL MEDULLARY CARCINOMA

In some tumors, glandular formation is well-developed and contains eosinophilic contents.

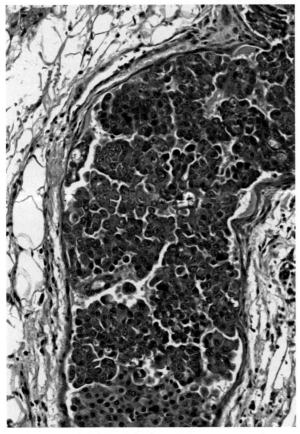

Figure 1-153

RENAL MEDULLARY CARCINOMA

Vascular involvement is common. Eosinophilic cytoplasmic inclusions and prominent nucleoli, often indistinguishable from rhabdoid tumor, are present in most tumors.

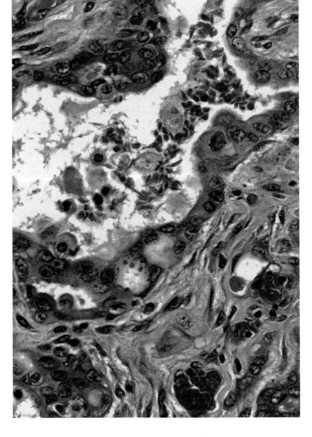

Figure 1-154

RENAL MEDULLARY CARCINOMA

Drepanocytes (sickled cells) can be found in most cases as a result of formalin fixation. Some specimens may require a diligent search.

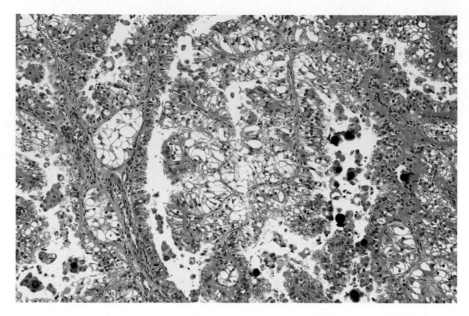

Figure 1-155

RENAL CELL CARCINOMA WITH Xp11.2 TRANSLOCATION

The tumor cells commonly show voluminous cytoplasm and form a papillary architecture.

Table 1-15			
RENAL CELL CARCINOMAS WITH THE XP11 TRANSLOCATION			
Variant	Frequency	Fusion Product	Reference
t(X;1)(p11.2;q21)	~78%	*PRCC-TFE3*	(231,237)
t(X;1)(p11.2;p34)	~20%	*PSF-TFE3*	(215)
t(X;17)(p11.2;q25)	rare	*ASPL-TFE3*	(212,223,234)

Table 1-16
PEDIATRIC RENAL TUMORS MIMICKING CLEAR CELL RENAL CELL CARCINOMA
Epithelioid angiomyolipoma
t(Xp11) renal carcinomas
Alveolar soft part sarcoma
t(6;11) renal tumors
Chromophobe or oncocytic renal tumors

morphology composed of cells with voluminous clear to acidophilic cytoplasm and distinct cell borders separated by thin fibrovascular septa (figs. 1-155, 1-156). The Xp11.2 translocation is not specific for RCC and may also be seen in alveolar soft part sarcoma. The full histologic spectrum of tumors with this group of genetic abnormalities is not known.

The immunohistochemical reaction pattern of tumors with an Xp11.2 translocation differs from that of most other categories of RCC. These tumors have no or only focal immunoreactivity for epithelial membrane antigen, cytokeratin Cam 5.2, and vimentin. This is in sharp contrast to other RCCs, which have a more diffuse reaction pattern for these antibodies. More recently, aberrant nuclear immunoreactivity for antibodies to the TFE3 protein has been reported in patients with TFE3 fusions (213a).There is insufficient long-term follow-up to provide meaningful prognostic information

for the Xp11.2 translocation group of tumors, although lymph node metastases are common and late metastases have been reported (216).

The primary differential diagnostic problem is epithelioid angiomyolipoma, which may likewise be composed of nests of polygonal oncocytic cells with well-defined borders (Table 1-16; fig. 1-157). Immunohistochemistry may be helpful as angiomyolipomas are positive for melanocytic markers such as HMB-45 and Melan A.

A small number of renal tumors in children are also composed of polygonal cells with well-defined cell borders, and are arranged in a strikingly nested and focally acinar growth pattern (213). Subpopulations of smaller cells are often seen surrounding hyaline material which by electron microscopy represents basement membrane material (fig. 1-158). These tumors do not react for epithelial markers and do not have desmosomes. They may react focally with HMB-45

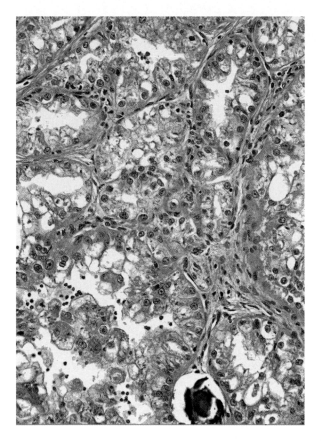

Figure 1-156

**RENAL CELL CARCINOMA
WITH Xp11.2 TRANSLOCATION**

Some tumors have a tubular appearance and may mimic clear cell renal cell carcinoma. Psammomatous calcifications are commonly seen.

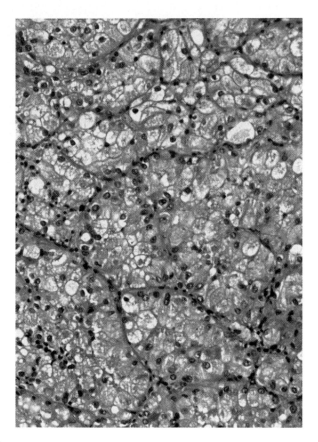

Figure 1-157

EPITHELIOID ANGIOMYOLIPOMA

A variant of angiomyolipoma that contains foamy epithelioid cells, which may mimic clear cell renal cell carcinoma.

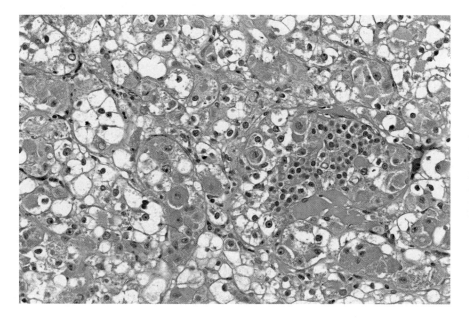

Figure 1-158

**RENAL TUMOR WITH
t(6;11) TRANSLOCATION**

These rare tumors are predominately composed of clear cells with cytoplasmic granules. Characteristic of this tumor are rare clusters of cells with small nuclei, scant cytoplasm, and associated pink basement membrane-like material.

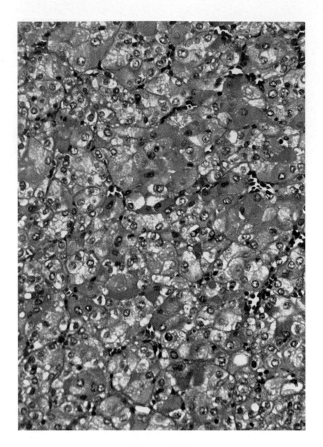

Figure 1-159

**POSTNEUROBLASTOMA ONCOCYTOID
RENAL CELL CARCINOMA**

Cells containing a spectrum of cytoplasmic appearances are present, some with a striking oncocytoid appearance. While this tumor is predominantly solid, papillary growth patterns are seen.

and Melan A. These tumors have a recurrent t(6;11)(p21;q13) cytogenetic translocation. Cloning of this translocation has shown TFEB to be involved. TFEB is a member of the same transcription factor family as TFE3 (217a).

A rare form of renal cell carcinoma has been seen in a handful of children previously treated for neuroblastoma (219a,225a). The majority of these tumors show unusual oncocytoid histologic features, with solid and papillary architecture, and do not fit into the spectrum of known renal tumors (fig. 1-159). Reported patients with tumors having these histologic features have come to clinical attention 5 to 13 years following their original neuroblastoma diagnosis. While secondary tumors are commonly attributed to the therapeutic agents necessary

for the treatment of the primary tumor, this is unlikely in these neuroblastoma-associated cases. There have been no agents utilized only for neuroblastoma, and this oncocytoid histology has not been associated as a second tumor with any other pediatric tumor. In addition, two of the reported tumors were identified in patients with stage 4S neuroblastoma disease who were never treated. Therefore, these tumors may have a closer association with neuroblastoma than is usual for a secondary malignancy.

In summary, RCCs in children sharing clear cell features may represent entities distinct from tumors of similar histology arising in adults. In the absence of a genetic syndrome, the diagnosis of the clear cell type of RCC should be highly suspect in a patient less than 25 years of age. Immunohistochemical evaluation for the Xp11.2 translocation-containing RCC and for angiomyolipoma should be performed. A useful panel of markers for this purpose includes HMB-45, Melan A, epithelial membrane antigen, vimentin, AE1/3, and Cam 5.2.

RARE RENAL TUMORS OF CHILDHOOD

Ossifying Renal Tumor of Kidney

This is a rare neoplasm that characteristically presents as a calcified mass in the renal pelvis (232). It may mimic a renal calculus both clinically and radiologically. The majority of patients are boys less than 1 year of age. Hematuria is the usual presenting symptom.

The lesion is relatively small and attached to the renal parenchyma at or near the papilla so that most of the mass lies free in the pelvic cavity. Grossly, the tumors resemble renal calculi except for their firm attachment to the parenchyma. Microscopically, ossifying renal tumors are composed of proliferating spindle cells admixed with partially calcified osteoid matrix (fig. 1-160). The prognosis is excellent; there are no known cases with recurrences or metastases.

PROCEDURE FOR
PATHOLOGIC EXAMINATION

The correct diagnosis and treatment of pediatric renal tumors depend on adequate sampling of tumors that are often large and friable. Adequate sampling is defined as one generous sample for every centimeter of greatest tumor

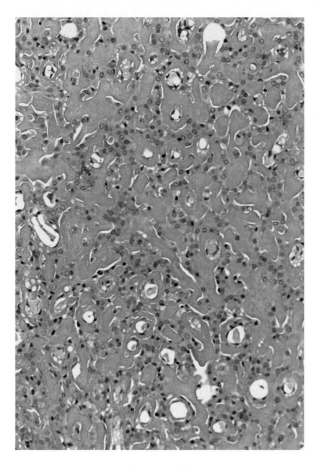

Figure 1-160

OSSIFYING RENAL TUMOR OF INFANCY

Spindle cells with focal osteoid matrix characterize this lesion.

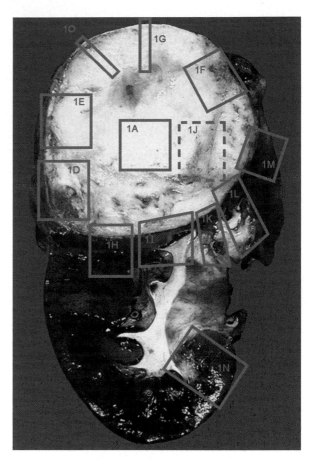

Figure 1-161

NEPHROBLASTOMA

The utilization of digital mapping can aid in the designation of sections submitted from a nephroblastoma. Most of the sections are taken from the periphery of the lesion, maximizing the pathologist's ability to detect renal sinus invasion and capsular penetration. (Courtesy of Dr. Paul Dickman, Pittsburgh, PA.)

dimension. In addition, the diagnosis of focal anaplasia can only be accurately made if the location of each section is precisely documented, preferably with a gross photograph or diagram (fig. 1-161) (238). In multicentric neoplasms, each individual tumor should be sampled using the above recommendations. Listed below are key points to aid in the correct evaluation, processing, and staging of pediatric renal tumors.

Avoid Intraoperative Frozen Sections Whenever Possible. Pediatric renal tumors pose a significant potential for diagnostic error even on permanent sections. Intraoperative frozen sections should be reserved for those instances when the operative procedure will be determined by the result. Intraoperative biopsies taken prior to the nephrectomy result in the upstaging of a stage I tumor.

Encourage Surgeons to Submit the Nephrectomy Specimen Intact. Bivalving the specimen in the operating room results in retraction of the tumor capsule and extravasation of tumor, precluding adequate staging in many cases.

Carefully Ink the Tumor Prior to Taking Any Sections. The distinction between stages I and II as well as stages II and III is complicated by the extreme friability of most nephroblastomas, often resulting in displacement of tumor during sectioning of the gross specimen. This may make interpretation of both vascular involvement and margin involvement difficult. If the specimen has been carefully inked first, displaced tumor will be located outside the ink.

Do not remove the perirenal fat or strip the renal capsule at any time during the evaluation.

Submit Shave Margins of the Renal Vein, the Renal Artery, and the Ureter. If a tumor thrombus is protruding from the lumen of the renal vein, evaluate the gross appearance of the surface of the thrombus. Submit a shave of the actual renal vein margin. A thrombus that has not been transected is not considered to be a positive margin unless the vascular wall is involved by tumor at its margin.

Carefully Search the Hilar Adipose Tissue for Lymph Nodes. One of the most important determinants of therapy is the presence or absence of lymph node metastasis. Unfortunately, it is not the practice of many surgeons to conduct a formal lymph node search when performing a nephrectomy. A lymph node search is also made difficult by the fact that these lymph nodes are often quite small in infants. A marker of poor prognosis within tumors that are stage II is the absence of lymph nodes available for histologic evaluation. This is presumably due to the failure to detect some lymph node metastases due to lack of lymph node sampling. The surgeon relies on the pathologist for the careful examination of the hilar adipose tissue for lymph nodes.

Carefully Examine the External Surfaces of the Kidney. Look for nodules that protrude from the contours of the kidney, areas in which the serosal surface is irregular, and any other signs that the tumor has penetrated the renal capsule or is approaching the surgical margin of resection.

Bivalve the Kidney and Submit Sections for Clinical Protocols and Ancillary Studies. Samples of the tumor and adjacent normal kidney should be frozen or placed in tissue culture medium for clinical protocols. Samples of the tumor should be placed in glutaraldehyde or tissue culture medium for electron microscopy and cytogenetic analysis when indicated. Renal tumors of patients older than 10 years of age should be submitted for cytogenetic analysis whenever possible and feasible.

Submit Routine Sections, Obtaining the Majority of Sections from the Periphery of the Tumor. The single most important practice for the adequate staging of pediatric renal tumors is to take the majority of sections along the periphery of the tumor. This maximizes the number of sections that demonstrate the relationship of the tumor to the capsule and the tumor to the renal sinus, including the intrarenal extension of the sinus (fig 1-161). It also allows the pathologist to evaluate the pattern of invasion of the tumor, which is an important clue to the correct diagnosis of many renal tumors. Any grossly distinctive internal foci should be sampled (92).

Carefully Evaluate the Normal Kidney for Nephrogenic Rests. Grossly evaluate the renal parenchyma bordering the dominant neoplasm for any differences in color or texture, which may indicate the presence of a nephrogenic rest (see figs. 1-21, 1-76). Submit at least two random sections of non-neoplastic kidney.

REFERENCES

Normal Anatomy

1. Bander NH, Cordon-Cardo C, Finstad CL, et al. Immunohistologic dissection of the human kidney using monoclonal antibodies. J Urol 1985;133:502–5.
2. Bonsib SM, Gibson D, Mhoon M, Greene GF. Renal sinus involvement in renal cell carcinomas. Am J Surg Pathol 2000;24:451–8.
3. Charles AK, Mall S, Watson J, Berry PJ. Expression of the Wilms' tumour gene WT1 in the developing human and in paediatric renal tumours: an immunohistochemical study. Mol Pathol 1997;50:138–44.
4. Clapp WL. Adult kidney. In: Sternberg S, ed. Histology for pathologists. New York: Raven Press; 1992:677–707.
5. Cohen C, McCue PA, Derose PB. Histogenesis of renal cell carcinoma and renal oncocytoma. An immunohistochemical study. Cancer 1988;62:1946–51.
6. Dressler GR. Development of the excretory system. In: Rossant J, Tam PP, eds. Mouse development: patterning, morphogenesis, and organogenesis. Academic Press; 2002:395–420.
7. Fleming S, Lindop GB, Gibson AA. The distribution of epithelial membrane antigen in the kidney and its tumours. Histopathology 1985;9:729–39.

8. Grubb GR, Yun K, Williams BR, Eccles MR, Reeve AE. Expression of WT1 protein in fetal kidneys and Wilms tumors. Lab Invest 1994;71:472–9.

9. Hennigar RA, Spicer SA, Sens DA, Othersen HB Jr, Garvin AJ. Histochemical evidence for tubule segmentation in a case of Wilms' tumor. Am J Clin Pathol 1986;85:724–31.

10. Inke G. The protolobar structure of the kidney. Its biologic and clinical significance. New York: Alan R. Liss; 1988.

11. Kissane JM. Development and structure of the urogenital system. In: Murphy WM, ed. Urological pathology. Philadelphia: WB Saunders; 1989:1–12.

12. Kuure S, Vuolteenaho R, Vainio S. Kidney morphogenesis: cellular and molecular regulation. Mech Dev 2000;92:31–45.

13. Mitchell GA. The nerve supply of the kidneys. Acta Anat 1950;10:1–37.

14. Pirani CL. Evaluation of kidney biopsy specimens. In: Tisher CC, Brenner BM, eds. Renal pathology with clinical and functional correlation. Philadelphia: J.B. Lippincott; 1989:11–42.

15. Potter EL. Normal and abnormal development of the kidney. Chicago: Year Book Medical Publishers; 1972.

16. Schedl A, Hastie ND. Cross-talk in kidney development. Curr Opin Genet Dev 2000;10:543–9.

17. Schenk EA, Schwartz RH, Lewis RA. Tamm-Horsfall mucoprotein. I. Localization in the kidney. Lab Invest 1971;25:92–5.

Nephroblastoma and Nephroblastomatosis

18. Abrahams JM, Pawel BR, Duhaime AC, Sutton LN, Schut L. Extrarenal nephroblastic proliferation in spinal dysraphism. A report of 4 cases. Pediatr Neurosurg 1999;31:40–4.

19. Allsbrook WC Jr, Boswell WC Jr, Takahashi H, et al. Recurrent renal cell carcinoma arising in Wilms' tumor. Cancer 1991;67:690–5.

20. Andrews PE, Kelalis PP, Haase GM. Extrarenal Wilms' tumor results of the National Wilms Tumor Study Group. J Pediatr Surg 1992;27:118–4.

21. Argani P, Faria PA, Epstein JI, et al. Primary renal synovial sarcoma: molecular and morphologic delineation of an entity previously included among embryonal sarcomas of the kidney. Am J Surg Pathol 2000;24:1087–96.

22. Barbosa AS, Faria PA, Beckwith JB. Diffuse hyperplastic perilobar nephroblastomatosis (DHPLN): pathology and clinical biology. Lab Invest 1998;78:1P.

23. Bardeesy N, Falkoff D, Petruzzi MJ, et al. Anaplastic Wilms' tumour, a subtype displaying poor prognosis, harbours p53 gene mutations. Nat Genet 1994;7:91–7.

24. Barnoud R, Sabourin JC, Pasquier D, et al. Immunohistochemical expression of WT1 by desmoplastic small round cell tumor: a comparative study with other small round cell tumors. Am J Surg Pathol 2000;24:830–6.

25. Beckwith JB. Nephrogenic rests and the pathogenesis of Wilms tumor: developmental and clinical considerations. Am J Med Genet 1998;79:268–73.

26. Beckwith JB. Precursor lesions of Wilms tumor: clinical and biological implications. Med Pediatr Oncol 1993;21:158–68.

27. Beckwith JB. Renal tumors. In: Stocker JT, Askin FB, eds. Pathology of solid tumors in children. New York: Chapman & Hall Medical; 1998:1–23.

28. Beckwith JB. Wilms' tumor and other renal tumors of childhood: a selective review from the National Wilms' Tumor Study Pathology Center. Hum Pathol 1983;14:481–92.

29. Beckwith JB, Kiviat NB, Bonadio JF. Nephrogenic rests, nephroblastomatosis, and the pathogenesis of Wilms' tumor. Pediatr Pathol 1990;10:1–36.

30. Beckwith JB, Zuppan CE, Browning NG, Moksness J, Breslow NE. Histological analysis of aggressiveness and responsiveness in Wilms' tumor. Med Pediatr Oncol 1996;27:422–8.

31. Bella AJ, Winquist EW, Perlman EJ. Primary synovial sarcoma of the kidney diagnosed by molecular detection of SYT-SSX fusion transcripts. J Urol 2002;168:1092–3.

32. Benjamin DR, Beckwith JB. Medullary ray nodules in infancy and childhood. Arch Pathol 1973;96:33–5.

33. Bever CT Jr, Koenigsberger MR, Antunes JL, Wolff JA. Epidural metastasis by Wilms' tumor. Am J Dis Child 1981;135:644–6.

34. Blute ML, Kelalis PP, Offord KP, Breslow N, Beckwith JB, D'Angio GJ. Bilateral Wilms tumor. J Urol 1987;138(Pt 2):968–73.

35. Boccon-Gibod L, Rey A, Sandstedt B, et al. Complete necrosis induced by preoperative chemotherapy in Wilms tumor as an indicator of low risk: report of the International Society of Pediatric Oncology (SIOP) nephroblastoma trial and study 9. Med Pediatr Oncol 2000;34:183–90.

36. Bove KE, McAdams AJ. The nephroblastomatosis complex and its relationship to Wilms' tumor: a clinicopathologic treatise. Perspect Pediatr Pathol 1976;3:185–223.

37. Breslow N, Beckwith JB, Ciol M, Sharples K. Age distribution of Wilms' tumor: report from the National Wilms' Tumor Study. Cancer Res 1988;48:1653–7.

38. Breslow N, Olshan A, Beckwith JB, Green DM. Epidemiology of Wilms tumor. Med Pediatr Oncol 1993;21:172–81.

39. Breslow NE, Churchill G, Nesmith B, et al. Clinicopathologic features and prognosis for Wilms' tumor patients with metastases at diagnosis. Cancer 1986;58:2501–11.

40. Breslow NE, Takashima JR, Whitton JA, Moksness J, D'Angio GJ, Green DM. Second malignant neoplasms following treatment for Wilm's tumor: a report from the National Wilms' Tumor Study Group. J Clin Oncol 1995;13:1851–9.

41. Call KM, Glaser T, Ito CY, et al. Isolation and characterization of a zinc finger polypeptide gene at the human chromosome 11 Wilms' tumor locus. Cell 1990;60:509–20.

42. Charles AK, Brown KW, Berry PJ. Microdissecting the genetic events in nephrogenic rests and Wilms' tumor development. Am J Pathol 1998;153:991–1000.

42a. Charles AK, Mall S, Watson J, Berry PJ. Expression of the Wilms' tumour gene WT1 in the developing human and in paediatric renal tumours: an immunohistochemical study. Mol Pathol 1997;50:138–44.

43. Chatten J. Epithelial differentiation in Wilms' tumor: a clinicopathologic appraisal. Perspect Pediatr Pathol 1976;3:225–54.

44. Cheah PL, Looi LM, Chan LL. Immunohistochemical expression of p53 proteins in Wilms' tumour: a possible association with the histological prognostic parameter of anaplasia. Histopathology 1996;28:49–54.

45. Clark J, Rocques PJ, Crew AJ, et al. Identification of novel genes, SYT and SSX, involved in the t(X;18)(p11.2;q11.2) translocation found in human synovial sarcoma. Nat Genet 1994;7:502–8.

46. Coppes MJ. Serum biological markers and paraneoplastic syndromes in Wilms tumor. Med Pediatr Oncol 1993;21:213–21.

47. Coppes MJ, Arnold M, Beckwith JB, et al. Factors affecting the risk of contralateral Wilms tumor development: a report from the National Wilms Tumor Study Group. Cancer 1999;85:1616–25.

48. Coppes MJ, Haber DA, Grundy PE. Genetic events in the development of Wilms' tumor. N Engl J Med 1994;331:586–90.

49. D'Angio GJ, Breslow N, Beckwith JB, et al. Treatment of Wilms' tumor. Results of the Third National Wilms' Tumor Study. Cancer 1989;64:349–60.

50. DeBaun MR, Niemitz EL, McNeil DE, Brandenburg SA, Lee MP, Feinberg AP. Epigenetic alterations of H19 and LIT1 distinguish patients with Beckwith-Wiedemann syndrome with cancer and birth defects. Am J Hum Genet 2002;70:604–11.

51. Douglass EC, Look AT, Webber B, et al. Hyperdiploidy and chromosomal rearrangements define the anaplastic variant of Wilms' tumor. J Clin Oncol 1986;4:975–81.

52. Droz D, Rousseau-Merck MF, Jaubert F, et al. Cell differentiation in Wilms' tumor (nephroblastoma): an immunohistochemical study. Hum Pathol 1990;21:536–44.

53. Ellison DA, Silverman JF, Strausbauch PH, Wakely PE, Holbrook CT, Joshi VV. Role of immunocytochemistry, electron microscopy, and DNA analysis in fine-needle aspiration biopsy diagnosis of Wilms tumor. Diagn Cytopathol 1996;14:101–7.

54. Faria P, Beckwith JB, Mishra K, et al. Focal versus diffuse anaplasia in Wilms tumor—new definitions with prognostic significance: a report from the National Wilms Tumor Study Group. Am J Surg Pathol 1996;20:909–20.

55. Feinberg AP. Multiple genetic abnormalities of 11p15 in Wilms' tumor. Med Pediatr Oncol 1996;27:484–9.

56. Fernandes ET, Parham DM, Ribeiro RC, Douglass EC, Kumar AP, Wilimas J. Teratoid Wilms' tumor: the St Jude experience. J Pediatr Surg 1988;23:1131–4.

57. Folpe AL, Patterson K, Gown AM. Antibodies to desmin identify the blastemal component of nephroblastomas. Mod Pathol 1997;10:895–900.

58. Fukuzawa R, Breslow NE, Morison IM, et al. Epigenetic differences between Wilms tumor in Caucasian and Asian children. Lancet (In press)

59. Gerald WL, Miller HK, Battifora H, Miettinen M, Silva EG, Rosai J. Intra-abdominal desmoplastic small round-cell tumor. Report of 19 cases of a distinctive type of high-grade polyphenotypic malignancy affecting young individuals. Am J Surg Pathol 1991;15:499–513.

60. Gessler M, Poustka A, Cavenee W, Neve RL, Orkin SH, Bruns GA. Homozygous deletion in Wilms tumours of a zinc-finger gene identified by chromosome jumping. Nature 1990;343:774–8.

61. Gillis AJ, Osterhuis JW, Schipper ME, et al. Origin and biology of a testicular Wilms' tumor. Genes Chromosomes Cancer 1994;11:126–35.

62. Govender D, Harilal P, Hadley GP, Chetty R. p53 protein expression in nephroblastomas: a predictor of poor prognosis. Br J Cancer 1998;77:314–8.

63. Green DM, Beckwith JB, Breslow NE, et al. Treatment of children with stages II to IV anaplastic Wilms' tumor: a report from the National Wilms' Tumor Study Group. J Clin Oncol 1994;12:2126–31.

64. Green DM, Breslow NE, Beckwith JB, Norkool P. Screening of children with hemihypertrophy, aniridia, and Beckwith-Wiedemann syndrome in patients with Wilms tumor: a report from the National Wilms Tumor Study. Med Pediatr Oncol 1993;21:188–92.

64a. Grubb GR, Yun K, Williams BR, Eccles MR, Reeve AE. Expression of WT1 protein in fetal kidneys and Wilms tumors. Lab Invest 1994;71:472–9.

65. Grundy P, Koufos A, Morgan K, Li FP, Meadows AT, Cavenee WK. Familial predisposition to Wilms' tumour docs not map to the short arm of chromosome 11. Nature 1988;336:374–6.

66. Gupta A, Perlman EJ. Neuroblastoma arising in the kidney: 90 cases from the National Wilms Tumor Study Group Pathology Center. Lab Invest 2003;83:4P.

67. Haber DA, Englert C, Maheswaran S. Functional properties of WT1. Med Pediatr Oncol 1996;27:453–5.

68. Hill DA, Sheer TD, Liu T, et al. Clinical and biologic significance of nuclear unrest in Wilms tumor. Cancer 2003;97:2318–26.

69. Huff V, Amos CI, Douglass EC, et al. Evidence for genetic heterogeneity in familial Wilms' tumor. Cancer Res 1997;57:1859–62.

70. Huser J, Grignon DJ, Ro JY, Ayala AG, Shannon RL, Papadopoulos NJ. Adult Wilms' tumor: a clinicopathologic study of 11 cases. Mod Pathol 1990;3:321–6.

71. Jimenez RE, Folpe AL, Lapham RL, et al. Primary Ewing's sarcoma/primitive neuroectodermal tumor of the kidney: a clinicopathologic and immunohistochemical analysis of 11 cases. Am J Surg Pathol 2002;26:320–7.

72. Kalapurakal JA, Norkool P, Nan B, et al. Clinical characteristics and treatment outcomes in adult favorable histology Wilms tumor. A report from the National Wilms Tumor Study Group. Med Pediatr Oncol 2001;37:187.

73. Kim DH, Sohn JH, Lee MC, et al. Primary synovial sarcoma of the kidney. Am J Surg Pathol 2000;24:1097–104.

74. Koyama S, Morimitsu Y, Morokuma F, Hashimoto H. Primary synovial sarcoma of the kidney: report of a case confirmed by molecular detection of the SYT-SSX2 fusion transcripts. Pathol Int 2001;51:385–91.

75. Lahoti C, Thorner P, Malkin D, Yeger H. Immunohistochemical detection of p53 in Wilms' tumors correlates with unfavorable outcome. Am J Pathol 1996;148:1577–89.

76. Layfield LJ, Ritchie AW, Ehrlich R. The relationship of deoxyribonucleic acid content to conventional prognostic factors in Wilms tumor. J Urol 1989;142:1040–3.

77. Li M, Squire JA, Weksberg R. Molecular genetics of Wiedemann-Beckwith syndrome. Am J Med Genet 1998;79:253–9.

78. Llombart-Bosch A, Peydro-Olaya A, Cerda-Nicolas M. Presence of ganglion cells in Wilm's tumours: a review of the possible neuroepithelial origin of nephroblastoma. Histopathology 1980;4:321–30.

79. Longaker MT, Adzick NS, Sadigh D, et al. Hyaluronic acid-stimulating activity in the pathophysiology of Wilms' tumors. J Natl Cancer Inst 1990;82:135–9.

80. Magee F, Mah RG, Taylor GP, Dimmick JE. Neural differentiation in Wilms' tumor. Hum Pathol 1987;18:33–7.

81. Mahoney JP, Saffos RO. Fetal rhabdomyomatous nephroblastoma with a renal pelvic mass simulating sarcoma botryoides. Am J Surg Pathol 1981;5:297–306.

82. Malkin D, Sexsmith E, Yeger H, Williams BR, Coppes MJ. Mutations of the p53 tumor suppressor gene occur infrequently in Wilms' tumor. Cancer Res 1994;54:2077–9.

83. Mierau GW, Beckwith JB, Weeks DA. Ultrastructure and histogenesis of the renal tumors of childhood: an overview. Ultrastruct Pathol 1987;11:313–33.

84. Ogawa O, Eccles MR, Szeto J, et al. Relaxation of insulin-like growth factor II gene imprinting implicated in Wilms' tumour. Nature 1993;362:749–51.

85. Oppedal BR, Glomstein A, Zetterberg A. Feulgen DNA values in Wilms' tumour in relation to prognosis. Pathol Res Pract 1988;183:756–60.

86. Orlowski JP, Levin HS, Dyment PG. Intrascrotal Wilms' tumor developing in a heterotopic renal anlage of probable mesonephric origin. J Pediatr Surg 1980;15:679–82.

87. Pal N, Wadey RB, Buckle B, Yeomans E, Pritchard J, Cowell JK. Preferential loss of maternal alleles in sporadic Wilms' tumour. Oncogene 1990;5:1665–8.

88. Palese MA, Ferrer F, Perlman E, Gearhart JP. Metanephric stromal tumor: a rare benign pediatric renal mass. Urology 2001:58:462.

89. Parham DM, Roloson GJ, Feely M, Green DM, Bridge JA, Beckwith JB. Primary malignant neuroepithelial tumors of the kidney: a clinicopathologic analysis of 146 adult and pediatric cases from the National Wilms' Tumor Study Group Pathology Center. Am J Surg Pathol 2001;25:133–46.

90. Park S, Bernard A, Bove KE, et al. Inactivation of WT1 in nephrogenic rests, genetic precursors to Wilms' tumour. Nat Genet 1993;5:363–7.

91. Pelletier J, Bruening W, Kashtan CE, et al. Germline mutations in the Wilms' tumor suppressor gene are associated with abnormal urogenital development in Denys-Drash syndrome. Cell 1991;67:437–47.

92. Perlman EJ. Pediatric tumors. In: Westra WH, ed. Surgical pathology dissection: an illustrated guide, 2nd ed. New York: Springer; 2003:212–5.

93. Ping AJ, Reeve AE, Law DJ, Young MR, Boehnke M, Feinberg AP. Genetic linkage of Beckwith-Wiedemann syndrome to 11p15. Am J Hum Genet 1989;44:720–3.

94. Pritchard-Jones K, Fleming S. Cell types expressing the Wilms' tumour gene (WT1) in Wilms' tumours: implications for tumour histogenesis. Oncogene 1991;6:2211–20.

95. Rahman N, Abidi F, Ford D, et al. Confirmation of FWT1 as a Wilms' tumour susceptibility gene and phenotypic characteristics of Wilms' tumour attributable to FWT1. Hum Genet 1998;103:547–56.

96. Ravenel JD, Broman KW, Perlman EJ, et al. Loss of imprinting of insulin-like growth factor-II (IGF2) gene in distinguishing specific biological subtypes of Wilms tumor. J Natl Cancer Inst 2001;93:1698–703.

97. Ritchey ML, Green DM, Thomas PR, et al. Renal failure in Wilms' tumor patients: a report from the National Wilms' Tumor Study Group. Med Pediatr Oncol 1996;26:75–80.

98. Rodriguez-Galindo C, Marina NM, Fletcher BD, Parham DM, Bodner SM, Meyer WH. Is primitive neuroectodermal tumor of the kidney a distinct entity? Cancer 1997;79:2243–50.

99. Rubin BP, Fletcher JA, Renshaw AA. Clear cell sarcoma of soft parts: report of a case primary in the kidney with cytogenetic confirmation. Am J Surg Pathol 1999;23:589–94.

100. Shao L, Hill DA, Perlman EJ. Expression of WT-1, Bcl-2, and CD34 by primary renal spindle cell tumors in children. Pediatr Dev Pathol 2002;5:101.

101. Shearer P, Parham DM, Fontanesi J, et al. Bilateral Wilms tumor. Review of outcome, associated abnormalities, and late effects in 36 pediatric patients treated at a single institution. Cancer 1993;72:1422–6.

102. Shimada H, Ambros IM, Dehner LP, et al. The International Neuroblastoma Pathology Classification (the Shimada system). Cancer 1999;86:364–72.

103. Sorensen K, Levitt G, Seba-Montefiore D, Bull C, Sullivan I. Cardiac function in Wilms' tumor survivors. J Clin Oncol 1995;13:1546–56.

104. Stern M, Longaker MT, Adzick NS, Harrison MR, Stern R. Hyaluronidase levels in urine from Wilms' tumor patients. J Natl Cancer Inst 1991;83:1569–74.

105. Stiller CA, Parkin DM. International variations in the incidence of childhood renal tumours. Br J Cancer 1990;62:1026–30.

106. Suster S, Fisher C, Moran CA. Expression of bcl-2 oncoprotein in benign and malignant spindle cell tumors of soft tissue, skin, serosal surfaces, and gastrointestinal tract. Am J Surg Pathol 1998;22:863–72.

107. Takeuchi S, Bartram CR, Ludwig R, et al. Mutations of p53 in Wilms' tumors. Mod Pathol 1995;8:483–7.

108. Thorner PS, Squire JA. Molecular genetics in the diagnosis and prognosis of solid pediatric tumors. Pediatr Dev Pathol 1998;1:337–65.

109. Turc-Carel C, Dal Cin P, Limon J, et al. Involvement of chromosome X in primary cytogenetic change in human neoplasia: nonrandom translocation in synovial sarcoma. Proc Natl Acad Sci U S A 1987;84:1981–5.

110. Wakely PE Jr, Sprague RI, Kornstein MJ. Extrarenal Wilms' tumor: an analysis of four cases. Hum Pathol 1989;20:691–5.

111. Webber BL, Parham DM, Drake LG, Wilimas JA. Renal tumors in childhood. Pathol Annu 1992;27(Pt 1):191–232.

112. Weeks DA, Beckwith JB, Luckey DW. Relapse-associated variables in stage I favorable histology Wilms' tumor. A report of the National Wilms' Tumor Study. Cancer 1987;60:1204–12.

113. Weeks DA, Beckwith JB, Mierau GW. Benign nodal lesional mimicking metastases from pediatric renal neoplasms: a report of the National Wilms' Tumor Study Pathology Center. Hum Pathol 1990;21:1239–44.

114. Wick MR, Cherwitz DL, Manivel JC, Sibley R. Immunohistochemical finding in tumors of the kidney. In: Eble JN, ed. Tumors and tumor-like conditions of the kidneys and ureters. New York: Churchill Livingstone; 1990:207–47.

115. Wiener JS, Coppes MJ, Ritchey ML. Current concepts in the biology and management of Wilms tumor. J Urol 1998;159:1316–25.

116. Wigger HJ. Fetal rhabdomyomatous nephroblastoma—a variant of Wilms' tumor. Hum Pathol 1976;7:613–23.

117. Wilms M. Mischgeschwulste der Niere. Die Mischgeschwulste. Leipzig: A. Georgi; 1899:5–90.

118. Zuppan CW. Handling and evaluation of pediatric renal tumors. Am J Clin Pathol 1998;109 (Suppl 1):S31–7.

119. Zuppan CW, Beckwith JB, Luckey DW. Anaplasia in unilateral Wilms' tumor: a report from the National Wilms' Tumor Study Pathology Center. Hum Pathol 1988;19:1199–209.

120. Zuppan CW, Beckwith JB, Weeks DA, Luckey DW, Pringle KC. The effect of preoperative therapy on the histologic features of Wilms' tumor. An analysis of cases from the Third National Wilms' Tumor Study. Cancer 1991;68:385–94.

Cystic Nephroma and Cystic, Partially Differentiated Nephroblastoma

121. Beckwith JB, Kiviat NB. Multilocular renal cysts and cystic renal tumors. AJR Am J Roentgenol 1981;136:435–6.
122. Blackely ML, Shamberger RC, Norkool P, Beckwith JB, Greene DM, Ritchey ML. Outcome of children with cystic partially differentiated nephroblastoma treated with or without chemotherapy. J Pediatr Surg 2003;38:897–900.
123. Delahunt B, Thomson KJ, Ferguson AF, Neale TJ, Meffan PJ, Nacey JN. Familial cystic nephroma and pleuropulmonary blastoma. Cancer 1993;71:1338–42.
124. Eble JN, Bonsib SM. Extensively cystic renal neoplasms: cystic nephroma, cystic partially differentiated nephroblastoma, multilocular cystic renal cell carcinoma, and cystic hamartoma of renal pelvis. Semin Diagn Pathol 1998;15:2–20.
125. Joshi VV. Cystic partially differentiated nephroblastoma: an entity in the spectrum of infantile renal neoplasia. Perspect Pediatr Pathol 1979;5:217–35.
126. Joshi VV, Beckwith JB. Multilocular cyst of the kidney (cystic nephroma) and cystic, partially differentiated nephroblastoma. Terminology and criteria for diagnosis. Cancer 1989;64:466–79.
127. Priest JR, McDermott MB, Bhatia S, Watterson J, Manivel JC, Dehner LP. Pleuropulmonary blastoma: a clinicopathologic study of 50 cases. Cancer 1997;80:147–61.
128. Priest JR, Watterson J, Strong L, et al. Pleuropulmonary blastoma: a marker for familial disease. J Pediatr 1996;128:220–4.

Benign Metanephric Tumors

129. Argani P, Beckwith JB. Metanephric stromal tumor: report of 31 cases of a distinctive pediatric renal neoplasm. Am J Surg Pathol 2000;24:917–26.
130. Arroyo MR, Green DM, Perlman EJ, Beckwith JB, Argani P. The spectrum of metanephric adenofibroma and related lesions: clinicopathologic study of 25 cases from the National Wilms Tumor Study Group Pathology Center. Am J Surg Pathol 2001;25:433–44.
131. Bigg SW, Bari WA. Nephrogenic adenofibroma: an unusual renal tumor. J Urol 1997;157:1835–6.
132. Davis CJ Jr, Barton JH, Sesterhenn IA, Mostofi FK. Metanephric adenoma. Clinicopathological study of fifty patients. Am J Surg Pathol 1995;19:1101–14.
133. Hennigar RA, Beckwith JB. Nephrogenic adenofibroma. A novel kidney tumor of young people. Am J Surg Pathol 1992;16:325–34.
134. Jones EC, Pins M, Dickersin GR, Young RH. Metanephric adenoma of the kidney. A clinicopathological, immunohistochemical, flow cytometric, cytogenetic, and electron microscopic study of seven cases. Am J Surg Pathol 1995;19:615–26.
135. Muir TE, Cheville JC, Lager DJ. Metanephric adenoma, nephrogenic rests, and Wilms' tumor: a histologic and immunophenotypic comparison. Am J Surg Pathol 2001;25:1290–6.
136. Picken MM, Curry JL, Lindgren V, Clark J, Eble JN. Metanephric adenosarcoma in a young adult: morphologic, immunophenotypic, ultrastructural, and fluorescence in situ hybridization analyses: a case report and review of the literature. Am J Surg Pathol 2001;25:1451–7.
137. Pins MR, Jones EC, Martul EV, Kamat BR, Umlas J, Renshaw AA. Metanephric adenoma-like tumors of the kidney: report of 3 malignancies with emphasis on discriminating features. Arch Pathol Lab Med 1999;123:415–20.
138. Shek TW, Luk IS, Peh WC, Chan KL, Chan GC. Metanephric adenofibroma: report of a case and review of the literature. Am J Surg Pathol 1999;23:727–33.

Mesoblastic Nephroma

139. Angulo JC, Lopez JI, Ereno C, Unda M, Flores N. Hydrops fetalis and congenital mesoblastic nephroma. Child Nephrol Urol 1991;11:115–6.
140. Argani P, Fritsch M, Kadkol SS, Schuster A, Beckwith JB, Perlman EJ. Detection of the ETV6-NTRK3 chimeric RNA of infantile fibrosarcoma/cellular congenital mesoblastic nephroma in paraffin-embedded tissue: application to challenging pediatric renal stromal tumors. Mod Pathol 2000;13:29–36.
141. Beckwith JB. National Wilms Tumor Study: an update for pathologists. Pediatr Dev Pathol 1998;1:79–84.
141a. Beckwith JB. Wilms' tumor and other renal tumors of childhood: a selective review from the National Wilms' Tumor Study Pathology Center. Hum Pathol 1983;14:481–92.
142. Beckwith JB, Weeks DA. Congenital mesoblastic nephroma. When should we worry? Arch Pathol Lab Med 1986;110:98–9.
143. Bolande RP. Congenital mesoblastic nephroma of infancy. Perspect Pediatr Pathol 1973;1:227–50.
144. Bolande RP, Brough AJ, Izant RJ. Congenital mesoblastic nephroma of infancy. A report of eight cases and the relationship to Wilms' tumor. Pediatrics 1967;40:272–8.

145. Cook HT, Taylor GM, Malone P, Risdon RA. Renin in mesoblastic nephroma: an immunohistochemical study. Hum Pathol 1988;19:1347–51.

146. Dal Cin P, Lipcsei G, Hermand G, Boniver J, Van den Berghe H. Congenital mesoblastic nephroma and trisomy 11. Cancer Genet Cytogenet 1998;103:68–70.

147. Favara BE, Johnson W, Ito J. Renal tumors in the neonatal period. Cancer 1968;22:845– 55.

148. Fitchev P, Beckwith JB, Perlman EJ. Congenital mesoblastic nephroma: prognosis and outcome. Lab Invest 2003;83:2P.

149. Ganick DJ, Gilbert EF, Beckwith JB, Kiviat N. Congenital cystic mesoblastic nephroma. Hum Pathol 1981;12:1039–43.

150. Gormley TS, Skoog SJ, Jones RV, Maybee D. Cellular congenital mesoblastic nephroma: what are the options. J Urol 1989;142(Pt 2):479–83.

151. Gray ES. Mesoblastic nephroma and non-immunological hydrops fetalis. Pediatr Pathol 1989;9:607–9.

152. Howell CG, Othersen HB, Kiviat NE, Norkool P, Beckwith JB, D'Angio GJ. Therapy and outcome in 51 children with mesoblastic nephroma: a report of the National Wilms' Tumor Study. J Pediatr Surg 1982;17:826–31.

153. Joshi VV, Kasznica J, Walters TR. Atypical mesoblastic nephroma. Pathologic characterization of a potentially aggressive variant of conventional congenital mesoblastic nephroma. Arch Pathol Lab Med 1986;110:100–6.

154. Knezevich SR, Garnett MJ, Pysher TJ, Beckwith JB, Grundy PE, Sorensen PH. ETV6-NTRK3 gene fusions and trisomy 11 establish a histogenetic link between mesoblastic nephroma and congenital fibrosarcoma. Cancer Res 1998;58: 5046–8.

155. Kumar S, Marsden HB, Carr T, Kodet R. Mesoblastic nephroma contains fibronectin but lacks laminin. J Clin Pathol 1985;38:507–11.

156. Lowery M, Issa B, Pysher T, Brothman A. Cytogenetic findings in a case of congenital mesoblastic nephroma. Cancer Genet Cytogenet 1995;84:113–5.

157. Malone PS, Duffy PG, Ransley PG, Risdon RA, Cook T, Taylor M. Congenital mesoblastic nephroma, renin production, and hypertension. J Pediatr Surg 1989;24:599–600.

158. Mascarello JT, Cajulis TR, Krous HF, Carpenter PM. Presence or absence of trisomy 11 is correlated with histologic subtype in congenital mesoblastic nephroma. Cancer Genet Cytogenet 1994;77:50–4.

159. Mierau GW, Beckwith JB, Weeks DA. Ultrastructure and histogenesis of the renal tumors of childhood: an overview. Ultrastruct Pathol 1987;11:313–33.

160. Nadasdy T, Roth J, Johnson DL, et al. Congenital mesoblastic nephroma: an immunohistochemical and lectin study. Hum Pathol 1993;24:413–9.

161. Pettinato G, Manivel JC, Wick MR, Dehner LP. Classical and cellular (atypical) congenital mesoblastic nephroma: a clinicopathologic, ultrastructural, immunohistochemical, and flow cytometric study. Hum Pathol 1989;20:682–90.

162. Rubin BP, Chen CJ, Morgan TW, et al. Congenital mesoblastic nephroma t(12;15) is associated with ETV6-NTRK3 gene fusion: cytogenetic and molecular relationship to congenital (infantile) fibrosarcoma. Am J Pathol 1998;153:1451–8.

163. Satoh F, Tsutsumi Y, Yokoyama S, Osamura RY. Comparative immunohistochemical analysis of developing kidneys, nephroblastomas, and related tumors: considerations on their histogenesis. Pathol Int 2000;50:458–71.

164. Schofield DE, Yunis EJ, Fletcher JA. Chromosome aberrations in mesoblastic nephroma. Am J Pathol 1993;143:714–24.

165. Shanbhogue LK, Gray E, Miller SS. Congenital mesoblastic nephroma of infancy associated with hypercalcemia. J Urol 1986;135:771–2.

166. Varsa EW, McConnell TS, Dressler LG, Duncan M. Atypical congenital mesoblastic nephroma. Report of a case with karyotypic and flow cytometric analysis. Arch Pathol Lab Med 1989;113:1078–80.

167. Vido L, Carli M, Rizzoni G, et al. Congenital mesoblastic nephroma with hypercalcemia. Pathogenetic role of prostaglandins. Am J Pediatr Hematol Oncol 1986;8:149–52.

167a. Wick MR, Cherwitz DL, Manivel JC, Sibley R. Immunohistochemical finding in tumors of the kidney. In: Eble JN, ed. Tumors and tumor-like conditions of the kidneys and ureters. New York: Churchill Livingstone; 1990:207–47.

168. Wockel W, Scheibner K, Lageman A. A variant of the Wiedemann-Beckwith syndrome. Eur J Pediatr 1981;135:319–24.

169. Yokomori K, Hori T, Takemura T, Tsuchida Y. Demonstration of both primary and secondary reninism in renal tumors in children. J Pediatr Surg 1988;23:403–9.

Clear Cell Sarcoma of Kidney

170. Altmannsberger M, Osborn M, Schafer H, Schauer A, Weber K. Distinction of nephroblastomas from other childhood tumors using antibodies to intermediate filaments. Virchows Arch B Cell Pathol Incl Mol Pathol 1984;45:113–24.

171. Argani P, Perlman EJ, Breslow NE, et al. Clear cell sarcoma of the kidney: a review of 351 cases from the National Wilms Tumor Study Group Pathology Center. Am J Surg Pathol 2000;24:4–18.

172. Drut R, Pomar M. Cytologic characteristics of clear-cell sarcoma of the kidney (CCSK) in fine–needle aspiration biopsy (FNAB): a report of 4 cases. Diagn Cytopathol 1991;7:611–4.

173. Florine BL, Simonton SC, Sane SM, Stickel FR, Singher LJ, Dehner LP. Clear cell sarcoma of the kidney: report of a case with mandibular metastasis simulating a benign myxomatous tumor. Oral Surg Oral Med Oral Pathol 1988;65:567–74.

174. Green DM, Breslow NE, Beckwith JB, Moksness J, Finklestein JZ, D'Angio GJ. Treatment of children with clear-cell sarcoma of the kidney: a report from the National Wilms' Tumor Study Group. J Clin Oncol 1994;12:2132–7.

175. Haas JE, Bonadio JF, Beckwith JB. Clear cell sarcoma of the kidney with emphasis on ultrastructural studies. Cancer 1984;54:2978–87.

176. Kusumakumary P, Chellam VG, Rojymon J, Hariharan S, Krishnan NM. Late recurrence of clear cell sarcoma of the kidney. Med Pediatr Oncol 1997;28:355–7.

177. Marsden HB, Lawler W. Bone metastasizing renal tumour of childhood. Histopathological and clinical review of 38 cases. Virchows Arch A Pathol Anat Histol 1980;387:341–51.

178. Marsden HB, Lawler W, Kumar PM. Bone metastasizing renal tumor of childhood: morphological and clinical features, and differences from Wilms' tumor. Cancer 1978;42:1922–8.

179. Mierau GW, Weeks DA, Beckwith JB. Anaplastic Wilms' tumor and other clinically aggressive childhood renal neoplasms: ultrastructural and immunocytochemical features. Ultrastruct Pathol 1989;13:225–48.

180. Morgan E, Kidd JM. Undifferentiated sarcoma of the kidney: a tumor of childhood with histopathologic and clinical characteristics distinct from Wilms' tumor. Cancer 1978;42:1916–21.

181. Patterson LS. Ovarian sarcoma with pathologic features of clear cell sarcoma of the kidney. Pediatr Dev Pathol 2000;3:487–91.

182. Punnett HH, Halligan GE, Zaeri N, Karmazin N. Translocation 10;17 in clear cell sarcoma of the kidney. A first report. Cancer Genet Cytogenet 1989;41:123–8.

183. Sandstedt BE, Delemarre JF, Harms D, Tournade MF. Sarcomatous Wilms' tumour with clear cells and hyalinization. A study of 38 tumours in children from the SIOP nephroblastoma file. Histopathology 1987;11:273–85.

184. Schmidt D, Harms D, Evers KG, Bliesener JA, Beckwith JB. Bone metastasizing renal tumor (clear cell sarcoma) of childhood with epithelioid elements. Cancer 1985;56:609–13.

185. Schuster AE, Schneider DT, Fritsch MK, Grundy P, Perlman EJ. Genetic and genetic expression analysis in clear cell carcinoma of the kidney. Lab Invest 2003;83:1293–9.

186. Sotelo-Avila C, Gonzalez-Crussi F, Sadowinski S, Gooch WM 3rd, Pena R. Clear cell sarcoma of the kidney: a clinicopathologic study of 21 patients with long-term follow-up evaluation. Hum Pathol 1985;16:1219–30.

Rhabdoid Tumor

187. Biegel JA, Allen CS, Kawasaki K, Shimizu N, Budarf ML, Bell CJ. Narrowing the critical region for a rhabdoid tumor locus in 22q11. Genes Chromosomes Cancer 1996;16:94–105.

188. Biegel JA, Rorke LB, Packer RJ, Emanuel BS. Monosomy 22 in rhabdoid or atypical tumors of the brain. J Neurosurg 1990;73:710–4.

189. Biegel JA, Zhou JY, Rorke LB, Stenstrom C, Wainwright LM, Fogelgren B. Germ-line and acquired mutations of INI1 in atypical teratoid and rhabdoid tumors. Cancer Res 1999;59:74–9.

190. Bonnin JM, Rubinstein LJ, Palmer NF, Beckwith JB. The association of embryonal tumors originating in the kidney and in the brain. A report of seven cases. Cancer 1984;54:2137–46.

191. Burger PC, Yu IT, Tihan T, et al. Atypical teratoid/rhabdoid tumor of the central nervous system: a highly malignant tumor of infancy and childhood frequently mistaken for medulloblastoma: a Pediatric Oncology Group study. Am J Surg Pathol 1998;22:1083–92.

192. Chang CH, Ramirez N, Sakr WA. Primitive neuroectodermal tumor of the brain associated with malignant rhabdoid tumor of the liver: a histologic, immunohistochemical, and electron microscopic study. Pediatr Pathol 1989;9:307–19.

193. Douglass EC, Valentine M, Rowe ST, et al. Malignant rhabdoid tumor: a highly malignant childhood tumor with minimal karyotypic changes. Genes Chromosomes Cancer 1990;2:210–6.

194. Fort DW, Tonk VS, Tomlinson GE, Timmons CF, Schneider NR. Rhabdoid tumor of the kidney with primitive neuroectodermal tumor of the central nervous system: associated tumors with different histologic, cytogenetic, and molecular findings. Genes Chromosomes Cancer 1994;11:146–52.

195. Haas JE, Palmer NF, Weinberg AG, Beckwith JB. Ultrastructure of malignant rhabdoid tumor of the kidney. A distinctive renal tumor of children. Hum Pathol 1981;12:646–57.

196. Lynch HT, Shurin SB, Dahms BB, Izant RJ Jr, Lynch J, Danes BS. Paravertebral malignant rhabdoid tumor in infancy. In vitro studies of a familial tumor. Cancer 1983;52:290–6.

197. Mayes LC, Kasselberg AG, Roloff JS, Lukens JN. Hypercalcemia associated with immunoreactive parathyroid hormone in a malignant rhabdoid tumor of the kidney (rhabdoid Wilms' tumor). Cancer 1984;54:882–4.

198. Parham DM, Weeks DA, Beckwith JB. The clinicopathologic spectrum of putative extrarenal rhabdoid tumors. An analysis of 42 cases studied with immunohistochemistry or electron microscopy. Am J Surg Pathol 1994;18:1010–29.

199. Savla J, Chen TT, Schneider NR, Timmons CF, Delattre O, Tomlinson GE. Mutations of the hSNF5/INI1 gene in renal rhabdoid tumors with second primary brain tumors. J Natl Cancer Inst 2000;92:648–50.

200. Schmidt D, Leuschner I, Harms D, Sprenger E, Schafer HJ. Malignant rhabdoid tumor. A morphological and flow cytometric study. Pathol Res Pract 1989;184:202–10.

201. Schofield DE, Beckwith JB, Sklar J. Loss of heterozygosity at chromosome regions 22q11-12 and 11p15.5 in renal rhabdoid tumors. Genes Chromosomes Cancer 1996;15:10–7.

202. Sotelo-Avila C, Gonzalez-Crussi F, deMello D, et al. Renal and extrarenal rhabdoid tumors in children: a clinicopathologic study of 14 patients. Semin Diagn Pathol 1986;3:151–63.

203. Versteege I, Sevenet N, Lange J, et al. Truncating mutations of hSNF5/INI1 in aggressive pediatric cancer. Nature 1998;394:203–6.

204. Vogel AM, Gown AM, Caughlan J, Haas JE, Beckwith JB. Rhabdoid tumors of the kidney contain mesenchymal specific and epithelial specific intermediate filament proteins. Lab Invest 1984;50:232–8.

205. Vujanic GM, Sandstedt B, Harms D, Boccon-Gibod L, Delemarre JF. Rhabdoid tumour of the kidney: a clinicopathological study of 22 patients from the International Society of Paediatric Oncology (SIOP) nephroblastoma file. Histopathology 1996;28:333–40.

206. Weeks DA, Beckwith JB, Mierau GW. Rhabdoid tumor. An entity or a phenotype? Arch Pathol Lab Med 1989;113:113–4.

207. Weeks DA, Beckwith JB, Mierau GW, Luckey DW. Rhabdoid tumor of kidney. A report of 111 cases from the National Wilms' Tumor Study Pathology Center. Am J Surg Pathol 1989;13:439–58.

208. Weeks DA, Beckwith JB, Mierau GW, Zuppan CW. Renal neoplasms mimicking rhabdoid tumor of kidney. A report from the National Wilms' Tumor Study Pathology Center. Am J Surg Pathol 1991;15:1042–54.

209. White FV, Dehner LP, Belchis DA, et al. Congenital disseminated malignant rhabdoid tumor: a distinct clinicopathologic entity demonstrating abnormalities of chromosome 22q11. Am J Surg Pathol 1999;23:249–56.

209a. Wick MR, Cherwitz DL, Manivel JC, Sibley R. Immunohistochemical finding in tumors of the kidney. In: Eble JN, ed. Tumors and tumor-like conditions of the kidneys and ureters. New York: Churchill Livingstone; 1990:207–47.

Pediatric Renal Cell Carcinoma and Rare Tumors

210. Adsay NV, deRoux SJ, Sakr W, Grignon D. Cancer as a marker of genetic medical disease: an unusual case of medullary carcinoma of the kidney. Am J Surg Pathol 1998;22:260–4.

211. Amin MB, Corless CL, Renshaw AA, Tickoo SK, Kubus J, Schultz DS. Papillary (chromophil) renal cell carcinoma: histomorphologic characteristics and evaluation of conventional pathologic prognostic parameters in 62 cases. Am J Surg Pathol 1997;21:621–35.

212. Argani P, Antonescu CR, Illei PB, et al. Primary renal neoplasms with the ASPL-TFE3 gene fusion of alveolar soft part sarcoma: a distinctive tumor entity previously included among renal cell carcinomas of children and adolescents. Am J Pathol 2001;159:179–92.

213. Argani P, Hawkins A, Griffin CA, et al. A distinctive pediatric renal neoplasm characterized by epithelioid morphology, basement membrane production, focal HMB45 immunoreactivity, and t(6;11)(p21.1;q12) chromosome translocation. Am J Pathol 2001;158:2089–96.

213a. Argani P, Lal P, Hutchinson B, Lui MY, Reuter VE, Ladanyi M. Aberrant nuclear immunoreactivity for TFE3 in neoplasms with TFE3 gene fusions: a sensitive and specific immunohistochemical assay. Am J Surg Pathol 2003;27:750–61.

214. Carcao MD, Taylor GP, Greenberg ML, et al. Renal-cell carcinoma in children: a different disorder from its adult counterpart? Med Pediatr Oncol 1998;31:153–8.

215. Clark J, Lu YJ, Sidhar SK, et al. Fusion of splicing factor genes PSF and NonO (p54nrb) to the TFE3 gene in papillary renal cell carcinoma. Oncogene 1997;15:2233–9.

216. Dal Cin P, Stas M, Sciot R, De Wever I, Van Damme B, Van den Berghe H. Translocation (X;1) reveals metastasis 31 years after renal cell carcinoma. Cancer Genet Cytogenet 1998;101:58–61.

217. Davis CJ Jr, Mostofi FK, Sesterhenn IA. Renal medullary carcinoma. The seventh sickle cell nephropathy. Am J Surg Pathol 1995;19:1–11.

217a. Davis IJ, Hsi BL, Arroyo JD, et al. Cloning of an alpha-TFEB fusion in renal tumors harboring the t(6;11)(p21;q13) chromosome translocation. Proc Natl Acad Sci 2003;100:6051–6.

218. de Jong B, Molenaar IM, Leeuw JA, Idenberg VJ, Oosterhuis JW. Cytogenetics of a renal adenocarcinoma in a 2-year-old child. Cancer Genet Cytogenet 1986;21:165–9.

219. Delahunt B, Eble JN. Papillary renal cell carcinoma: a clinicopathologic and immunohistochemical study of 105 tumors. Mod Pathol 1997;10:537–44.

219a. Eble JN. Mucinous tubular and spindle cell carcinoma and post-neuroblastoma carcinoma: newly recognized entities in the renal cell carcinoma family. Pathology 2003;35:499–504.

220. Eckschlager T, Kodet R. Renal cell carcinoma in children: a single institution's experience. Med Pediatr Oncol 1994;23:36–9.

221. Gelpi AP, Perrine RP. Sickle cell disease and trait in white populations. JAMA 1973;224:605–8.

222. Goncalves MS, Nechtman JF, Figueiredo MS, et al. Sickle cell disease in a Brazilian population from Sao Paulo: a study of the beta s haplotypes. Hum Hered 1994;44:322–7.

223. Hernandez-Marti MJ, Orellana-Alonso C, Badia-Garrabou L, Verdeguer Miralles A, Paradis-Alos A. Renal adenocarcinoma in an 8-year-old child, with a t(X;17)(p11.2;q25). Cancer Genet Cytogenet 1995;83:82–3.

224. Kalyanpur A, Schwartz DS, Fields JM, Rayes-Mugica M, Keller MS, Gosche J. Renal medulla carcinoma in a white adolescent. AJR Am J Roentgenol 1997;169:1037–8.

225. Leuschner I, Harms D, Schmidt D. Renal cell carcinoma in children: histology, immunohistochemistry, and follow-up of 10 cases. Med Pediatr Oncol 1991;19:33–41.

225a. Medeiros LJ, Palmedo G, Krigman HR, Kovacs G, Beckwith JB. Oncocytoid renal cell carcinoma after neuroblastoma: a report of four cases of a distinct clinicopathologic entity. Am J Surg Pathol 1999;23:772–80.

226. Meloni AM, Dobbs RM, Pontes JE, Sandberg AA. Translocation (X;1) in papillary renal cell carcinoma. A new cytogenetic subtype. Cancer Genet Cytogenet 1993;65:1–6.

227. Renshaw AA. Basophilic tumors of the kidney. J Urologic Pathol 1998;8:85–102.

228. Renshaw AA, Corless CL. Papillary renal cell carcinoma. Histology and immunohistochemistry. Am J Surg Pathol 1995;19:842–9.

229. Renshaw AA, Granter SR, Fletcher JA, Kozakewich HP, Corless CL, Perez-Atayde AR. Renal cell carcinomas in children and young adults: increased incidence of papillary architecture and unique subtypes. Am J Surg Pathol 1999;23:795–802.

230. Rodriguez-Jurado R, Gonzalez-Crussi F. Renal medullary carcinoma. J Urologic Pathol 1996;4:191–203.

231. Sidhar SK, Clark J, Gill S, et al. The t(X;1)(p11.2;q21.2) translocation in papillary renal cell carcinoma fuses a novel gene PRCC to the TFE3 transcription factor gene. Hum Mol Genet 1996;5:1333–8.

232. Sotelo-Avila C, Beckwith JB, Johnson JE. Ossifying renal tumor of infancy: a clinicopathologic study of nine cases. Pediatr Pathol Lab Med 1995;15:745–62.

233. Swartz MA, Karth J, Schneider DT, Rodriguez R, Beckwith JB, Perlman EJ. Renal medullary carcinoma: clinical, pathologic, immunohistochemical, and genetic analysis with pathogenetic implications. Urology 2002;60:1083–9.

234. Tomlinson GE, Nisen PD, Timmons CF, Schneider NR. Cytogenetics of a renal cell carcinoma in a 17-month-old child. Evidence for Xp11.2 as a recurring breakpoint. Cancer Genet Cytogenet 1991;57:11–7.

235. Tonk V, Wilson KS, Timmons CF, Schneider NR, Tomlinson GE. Renal cell carcinoma with translocation (X;1). Further evidence for a cytogenetically defined subtype. Cancer Genet Cytogenet 1995;81:72–5.

236. Wesche WA, Wilimas J, Khare V, Parham DM. Renal medullary carcinoma: a potential sickle cell nephropathy of children and adolescents. Pediatr Pathol Lab Med 1998;18:97–113.

237. Weterman MA, Wilbrink M, Geurts van Kessel A. Fusion of the transcription factor TFE3 gene to a novel gene, PRCC, in t(X;1)(p11;q21)-positive papillary renal cell carcinomas. Proc Natl Acad Sci U S A 1996;93:15294–8.

238. Zuppan CW. Handling and evaluation of pediatric renal tumors. Am J Clin Pathol 1998;109(Suppl 1):S31–7.

2 KIDNEY TUMORS IN ADULTS

The broad separation of renal tumors according to patient age rather than histology is an arbitrary but widely accepted practice whose usefulness has been validated by many years of experience. Exceptions to this method of classification are well known, however, and the reader should be aware that histologically similar renal neoplasms occur over a wide age range. Studies of the molecular biology of renal neoplasms promise to help answer the question of whether tumors arising in children are different entities from those arising in adults or simply lesions at the extreme end of the age distribution.

CLASSIFICATION

Significant advances in the appropriate classification of renal cell carcinomas (RCCs) have resulted from the application of immunohistochemistry, electron microscopy, cytogenetics, and molecular genetics. It now seems clear that a number of distinctive entities exist under this heading. In the future, molecular diagnostic studies to further categorize neoplasms that are grouped on the basis of their histologic features may help design appropriate therapeutic strategies and predict the likelihood of progression. Several classification schemes have been proposed. The renal neoplasms and non-neoplastic tumorous conditions included in this section are categorized in Table 2-1. Table 2-2 presents a classification of RCCs modified from that proposed at a consensus meeting in 1997 and followed in its essentials in the 2004 World Health Organization system (WHO) (77,289).

RENAL CELL NEOPLASMS

Definition. Renal cell neoplasms are tumors arising in the kidney that differentiate in whole or in part toward mature renal tubular structures.

General Features. RCC accounts for 3 percent of adult malignancies; all RCCs are malignant. In the United States, more than 35,000 new cases and approximately 12,480 deaths per year are expected, and the incidence is appar-

ently increasing (52,145). Tumors are found among all ethnic groups and geographic areas, with the highest incidence reported in northern Europe and North America and the lowest incidence in Asian countries and areas of Central and South America (218). There is a higher incidence among blacks than among whites in the United States (52). Men are more often affected than women in a ratio of approximately 1.5 to 1. The disease arises mainly in adult kidneys but histologically similar tumors have been observed in children and infants as young as 6 months of age (170,253). RCCs and oncocytomas have developed in the remaining kidneys of young adults previously treated by radical nephrectomy plus adjuvant therapy for nephroblastoma (46). The incidence of RCC increases with age, with a peak in the sixth decade of life and a median patient age of 55 years.

Renal cell neoplasms have been studied for more than 100 years, but the etiology and histogenesis remain obscure. The term "hypernephroma," for example, was introduced by Grawitz to describe the clear cell type of RCC in the belief that the tumor arose from heterotopic adrenal (hypernephroid) rests in the kidney (59,111). Modern studies strongly indicate differentiation toward mature renal tubular structures, but in most cases the exact portion of the nephron involved is difficult to confirm, and heterogeneous nephron differentiation is likely in most renal neoplasms (26,109,178,324).

A variety of agents, including viruses, estrogens, lead compounds, X rays, and over 100 chemicals including aromatic hydrocarbons, can induce RCCs in experimental animals (21). None of these agents has been proven to be an important etiologic factor for renal cancers in humans, however. A slightly increased frequency of kidney cancer has been documented in men exposed to cadmium and rare cases have been observed after exposure to thorotrast (163,317). The most important known etiologic factor for RCC in men involves constituents of tobacco,

Table 2-1
RENAL TUMORS AND TUMOR-LIKE CONDITIONS OF ADULTS

Renal Cell Carcinoma

Renal Cortical Adenoma

Metanephric Tumors
  Metanephric adenoma
  Metanephric adenofibroma
  Metanephric stromal tumor
  Metanephric adenosarcoma

Oncocytoma

Rare Tumors with Epithelial and/or Parenchymal
    Differentiation
  Carcinoid tumor
  Small cell carcinoma
  Primitive neuroectodermal tumor
  Juxtaglomerular cell tumor
  Teratoma
  Nephroblastoma and other "pediatric" renal tumors
  Multilocular cyst (cystic nephroma)
  Mixed epithelial and stromal tumor
  Spiradenocylindroma

Mesenchymal Tumors
  Angiomyolipoma
    Epithelioid angiomyolipoma
  Medullary fibroma
  Leiomyoma
  Lipoma
  Hemangioma
  Lymphangioma
  Other benign mesenchymal tumors
  Leiomyosarcoma
  Liposarcoma
  Solitary fibrous tumor
  Hemangiopericytoma
  Fibrosarcoma and malignant fibrous histiocytoma
  Rhabdomyosarcoma
  Angiosarcoma
  Osteosarcoma
  Synovial sarcoma
  Other malignant mesenchymal tumors

Lymphoid Tumors
  Plasmacytoma

Metastatic Tumors

Tumor-Like Lesions
  Xanthogranulomatous pyelonephritis
  Inflammatory myofibroblastic pseudotumor
  Perirenal and sinus cysts

Table 2-2
CLASSIFICATION OF RENAL CELL CARCINOMA

Clear cell
  Multilocular cystic

Papillary

Chromophobe cell

Collecting duct

Medullary

Mucinous tubular and spindle cell

Associated with Xp11.2 translocations/*TFE3* gene fusion

Unclassified

higher risk in those with the highest 5 percent body mass index compared to the lowest quartile (191,217,321). Dietary studies have generally found reduced risk with increased consumption of fruits and vegetables (218).

Cytogenetic studies of renal neoplasms have documented abnormalities in most types of tumors, the chromosomal and genetic aberrations tending to be associated with specific histopathologic patterns (247). Most RCCs have multiple chromosomal aberrations but the most commonly observed abnormality is a terminal deletion of the short arm of one of the two homologous chromosomes 3, beginning at 3p13 (166,323). Using restriction fragment length polymorphism (RFLP) analysis, DNA sequence deletions have been found consistently on chromosome 3 in RCCs, mainly of the clear cell type (326). These findings led to the identification of the von Hippel-Lindau (*VHL*) gene at chromosome 3p25 (165,175). This gene is mutated or lost in both *VHL*-related and sporadic clear cell RCC. Expression of a protein product of the *VHL* gene is widespread in human tissues but the chromosomal and genetic abnormalities associated with RCCs are almost always localized to the tumors themselves and do not appear in non-neoplastic cells.

Additional tumor suppressor genes associated with familial and nonfamilial clear cell RCC are also found on chromosome 3 (297). Most frequent is the region of 3p14, possibly involving the *FHIT* gene. In up to 96 percent of clear cell RCCs, a continuous deletion at 3p14.2-p25, including both the *FHIT* and *VHL* genes, can be identified (294). A minority of papillary and chromophobe RCCs also have

whether smoked or chewed (177,204,218); in general, heavy smokers are considered to have a 2- to 2.5-fold increased risk compared to nonsmokers. Hypertension has been identified as a significant risk factor in several studies (60). Obesity, particularly in women, has also been linked to an increased risk of RCC, with up to a 5-fold

loss of heterozygosity involving 3p, possibly involving *FHIT* in addition to different molecular targets (294,314).

The papillary type of RCC most commonly manifests trisomy of chromosomes 7 and 17, but additional trisomies of chromosomes 12, 16, and 20 are frequent (146,164,166,258). As with the clear cell type, numerous other abnormalities have been reported but with less consistency (19,273). Hereditary papillary RCC is characterized by a germline mutation of the *c-met* gene (270). This mutation can also be found in sporadic papillary RCC (271,272). In addition, a group of tumors previously considered to represent a subset of papillary RCC manifest translocations involving chromosomes X and 1, most often t (x;1) (p11.2;q 21) (10,56,278). This results in a fusion of the *TFE3* and *PRCC* genes (278). As a group, these tumors seem to have distinctive morphologic characteristics, such as a mixture of architectural patterns including nested, solid, alveolar, tubular, and papillary, and tumor cells with clear to acidophilic cytoplasm (see figs. 1-156, 1-157, chapter 1) (10).

A group of renal neoplasms occurring in the pediatric age group (range, 17 months to 17 years), having the der (17) t(x;17)(p11.2;q25) translocation typical of alveolar soft part sarcoma, has been described (11).

Cytogenetic studies of the chromophobe cell type of RCC have yielded a relatively consistent pattern of monosomies involving chromosomes 1, 2, 6, 10, 13, and 17 (124,213). This is reflected in the consistent finding of hypodiploidy by flow cytometry (4). Loss of heterozygosity analyses demonstrate a consistent abnormality at 10q23.3 involving the *PTEN/MMAC1* gene, an alteration not present in oncocytomas (293).

Chromosomal and genetic studies of collecting duct carcinomas are limited. The most characteristic changes are deletions involving chromosomes 1, 6, 8, 14, 15, 21, and 22 (94,242,288).

The recognition of chromosomal and genetic aberrations in RCCs, especially as they are associated with histologic subtypes, has been an important contribution to our understanding of neoplasia in the kidney, but the practical value of this information should not be overemphasized. These abnormalities are not confined to renal neoplasms, may occur in renal tumors of different histologic types, and have not been documented in every case. Until further refinements in knowledge occur, the temptation to rely entirely upon molecular diagnostic approaches for classification or for the determination of the primary site of a metastasis should be resisted.

RCCs are commonly associated with other renal diseases, malformations, and paraneoplastic syndromes. RCC has been reported in association with hemihypertrophy and situs inversus totalis (235,308). Authentic examples of RCC have been documented in supernumerary kidneys as well as in teratomas (37,42). It must be noted, however, that if rigid diagnostic criteria are applied, most cases of extrarenal RCC are poorly documented tumors attributed to a renal cell origin primarily because of their clear cell histology (196). A possible association with hairy cell leukemia has been reported (227).

RCCs are often associated with cysts (fig. 2-1). In most cases, the cyst is of the common variety generally considered a cortical retention cyst, but associations with both acquired and hereditary polycystic diseases have been well documented (figs. 2-2, 2-3) (34,54,97,114,148,168,224). There is an estimated 10- and 50-fold increase in the risk of RCC for patients with chronic renal failure and with acquired cystic kidney disease, respectively (141,197). The renal neoplasms associated with acquired cystic kidney disease in patients on chronic hemodialysis generally occur after dialysis for several years (mean, 3.5 years) and the frequency of RCC varies directly with both the duration of dialysis and the number of cysts (141,198). Patients are younger than the usual patients with RCC (136). RCC has been reported in a nonfunctioning transplanted kidney in a patient on hemodialysis after failure of the transplant (161). Tumors also occur in patients with chronic renal failure who have not been dialyzed. Although renal tumors are found in 25 percent of patients with acquired cystic disease, not all lesions are histologically malignant and only 4 to 7 percent metastasize. Kidneys are usually small, with scattered cysts localized to the cortex, but may be markedly enlarged (up to 700 g) with innumerable cysts. The number of cysts is important for establishing a diagnosis of RCC associated with acquired cystic disease: at least five cysts are necessary for diagnosis of acquired cystic disease.

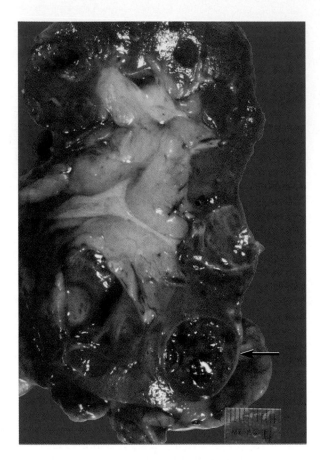

Figure 2-1

RENAL CELL CARCINOMA

This papillary renal cell carcinoma (arrow) is associated with two benign cortical cysts.

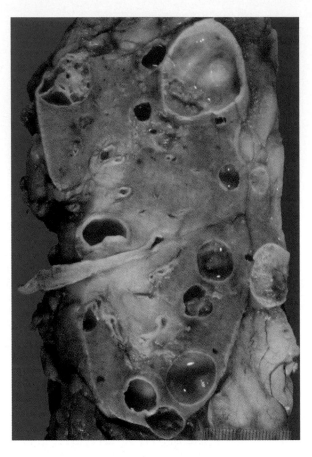

Figure 2-2

RENAL CELL CARCINOMA

Renal cell carcinoma arising in acquired cystic kidney disease. The tumor at the upper right is arising within a preexisting cyst.

Figure 2-3

RENAL CELL CARCINOMA

This clear cell renal cell carcinoma is arising in a background of adult polycystic kidney disease.

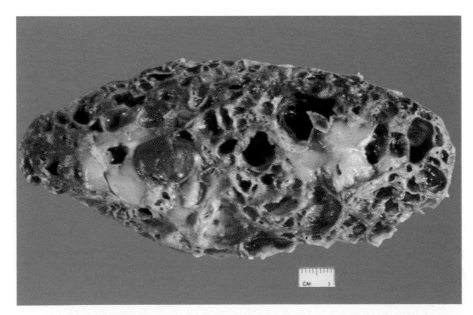

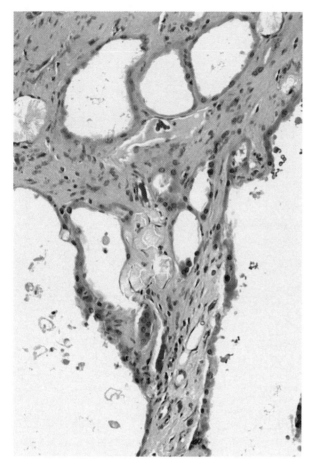

Figure 2-4

ACQUIRED CYSTIC KIDNEY DISEASE

The cysts are lined by flattened to cuboidal epithelium.

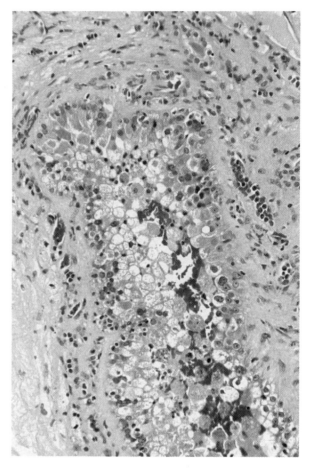

Figure 2-5

ACQUIRED CYSTIC KIDNEY DISEASE

The cyst lining is hyperplastic, and many cells have clear cytoplasm and enlarged nuclei with small nucleoli.

Cysts in this setting tend to be lined by a flat to cuboidal epithelium that may become focally columnar (fig. 2-4). The cytoplasm of the lining cells is clear, granular, or acidophilic. In most cases of RCC associated with acquired cystic disease, there is focal hyperplasia of the epithelium, with or without atypia (fig. 2-5). These atypical epithelial proliferations harbor cytogenetic abnormalities and are hypothesized to represent early neoplastic lesions (47). Histologically, small papillary lesions are most frequent (both adenomas and carcinomas) but the clear cell type of RCC has also been recorded (140). Intratumoral deposition of calcium oxalate crystals is seen in some cases (260). Clear cell RCC arising in this setting has been shown to have *VHL* gene mutations (322). Rare cases of oncocytoma have been described (187).

An association of RCC with autosomal dominant (adult) polycystic kidney disease has not been completely established (168,224). Intracystic epithelial hyperplasia occurs in up to 90 percent of polycystic kidneys and various tumors are identified in up to 25 percent of cases, but almost all are small and well differentiated, with the histologic features of cortical adenomas (114). RCCs are rare in adult polycystic kidneys and probably occur with no greater frequency than might be expected based on the prevalence of the two conditions.

RCC occurs in 38 to 55 percent of patients with von Hippel-Lindau syndrome (50,281). Lesions tend to be bilateral and multicentric, are often associated with cysts, and occur at an earlier age than sporadic RCC (figs. 2-6, 2-7). As

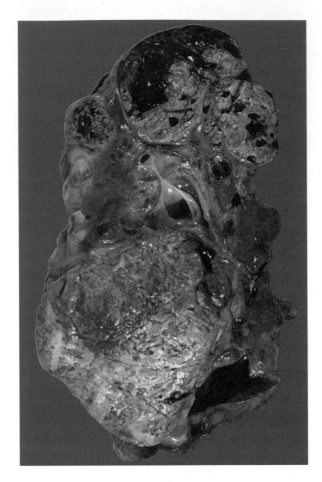

Figure 2-6

VON HIPPEL-LINDAU DISEASE

Multiple tumors and cysts are present in this kidney. The tumor in the lower left had a sarcomatoid clear cell carcinoma.

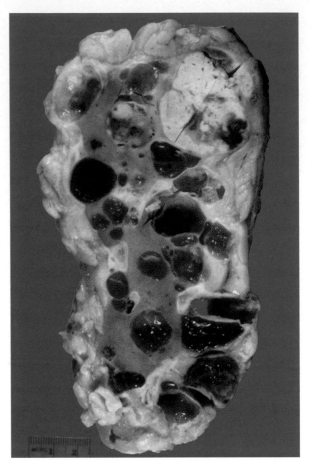

Figure 2-7

VON HIPPEL-LINDAU DISEASE

The kidney contains numerous clear cell carcinomas and cysts.

many as one third of patients with von Hippel-Lindau syndrome die of RCC. Pathologically, there is hyperplasia of the cyst epithelium with varying degrees of cytologic atypia (fig. 2-8). Papillary and solid tumor nodules are seen intracystically and typical clear cell RCCs may ultimately develop (fig. 2-9). The abnormal gene associated with this syndrome is linked to *RAF1*, a gene located on the distal portion of chromosome 3p25-26 (135,183,259). This gene is a recessive oncogene and patients with a germline mutation of this gene develop all the hallmarks of von Hippel-Lindau disease, including renal cysts and RCCs.

An increased risk of RCC is also seen in patients with tuberous sclerosis. On average, patients with tuberous sclerosis develop RCC in the fourth decade, with some cases occurring in childhood (6,28,181). Other renal lesions associated with this disorder include angiomyolipomas and cysts. The histologic types of RCC reported in these patients are clear cell, papillary, and chromophobe, with the former predominating (6,28,147).

Familial cases of RCC other than those detailed above are uncommon but well described (297). Familial non-*VHL* clear cell RCC occurs with and without associated translocations in chromosome 3 (3p14, 3q13.3, and 3q21) (101, 299). Clear cell, chromophobe, and papillary RCCs have been reported in patients with the Birt-Hogg-Dube syndrome (17p12-q11.2) (237,

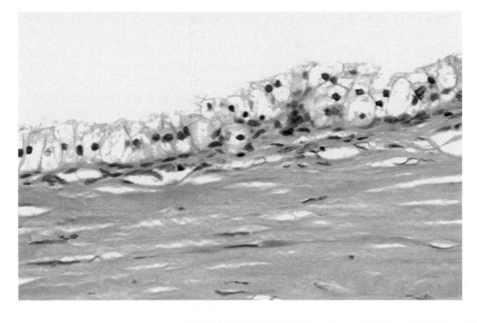

Figure 2-8

VON HIPPEL-LINDAU DISEASE

The lining of one of the cysts shows clear cells.

Figure 2-9

VON HIPPEL-LINDAU DISEASE

There is a proliferation of clear cells admixed with inflammatory cells within the wall of a cyst.

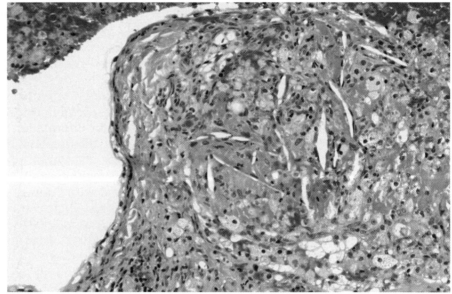

306). About half of the tumors in these patients have features of both chromophobe RCC and oncocytoma, and have been referred to as "hybrid oncocytic tumors" (237). Papillary RCC also occurs in association with hereditary leiomyomatosis related to a genetic abnormality at 1q42-44 (160,176). There have been isolated reports of familial papillary thyroid carcinoma and papillary RCC, and of RCC in a patient with the multiple hamartoma syndrome (Cowden's disease) (128,194). Patients with sickle cell trait (and rarely, hemoglobin SS) are at risk for the development of a highly aggressive RCC type—medullary carcinoma (17,67). These patients are younger than those with more usual RCC, and many cases have been recorded in the pediatric age group.

A peculiar hepatic disease unrelated to metastatic liver deposits has been reported in approximately 20 percent of patients with RCC (33). The liver is enlarged, but is not tender or nodular, and the patient is not icteric. Chemical studies have revealed some combination of increased alkaline phosphatase, increased indirect bilirubin, increased alpha-2 globulin, and decreased prothrombin time. Histologic changes in the liver include nonspecific triaditis, Kupffer's cell hyperplasia, and vascular dilatation (peliosis). Although the liver disease is reversible after nephrectomy, its presence is a poor prognostic sign and most patients with RCC and this type of liver disease do not survive 5 years (69).

Paraneoplastic syndromes occasionally occur in patients with renal tumors, particularly when the tumor is RCC (291). Some of these syndromes are nonspecific and common to patients with many forms of advanced cancer. Some accompany even small renal neoplasms and are thought to result from an elaboration of physiologically active substances by the tumor, such as renin, erythropoietin, prolactin, and gonadotropin (107,286,287,292). The substances may be normally produced in the kidney or ectopically produced by the tumor.

Clinical Features. RCCs may remain clinically occult for most of a patient's lifespan. In fact, most tumors are confined to the kidneys for substantial periods and may cause no changes in renal structure or function that would result in signs and symptoms. Patients manifesting the "classic triad" of hematuria, flank pain, and a flank mass generally have advanced disease. The importance of this often quoted symptom complex, present in less than 20 percent of patients, antedates modern diagnostic techniques (104). Hematuria is reported in 6 to 83 percent of patients and is usually gross rather than microscopic. Pain is documented in 20 to 45 percent of affected individuals and may represent distension of the renal capsule or traction on perinephric structures from the tumor itself. Flank masses are palpated in 6 to 48 percent of cases. They are usually nontender and indicative of a large tumor. An acquired scrotal mass due to a varicocele secondary to obstruction of the spermatic vein is observed in a few patients.

Many nonspecific symptoms, such as fever (10 to 20 percent), weight loss (15 to 30 percent), fatigue (30 to 40 percent), nausea and vomiting (8 to 14 percent), and neuropathy or muscle tenderness (4 percent), are more commonly observed than the classic triad. Approximately 30 percent of patients with RCC present with signs and symptoms of metastatic disease. Polycythemia, mostly in the form of erythro-

cytosis, is found in up to 6 percent of patients with RCC. Conversely, 2 to 4 percent of individuals with polycythemia have RCC. In most cases, erythropoietin production by the tumor can be documented. Normochromic, normocytic anemia unrelated to blood loss is seen in approximately 75 percent of patients; an increase in the erythrocyte sedimentation rate occurs in nearly 70 percent. Hypercalcemia, attributed to the production of parathormone-like substances by the tumor, may also occur.

Detection. Renal tumors are most accurately and consistently detected with some type of radiographic procedure (figs. 2-10, 2-11) (69). An increasing proportion of newly diagnosed cases can be considered incidental findings during some type of imaging examination (243). Calcification occurs in 10 to 15 percent of lesions and is usually localized to nonperipheral portions of the mass. Rarely, tumors are surrounded by a rim of calcification with ossification (125). Excretory urography may provide important information about the location and function of the contralateral kidney but is not particularly sensitive or specific in localizing small renal tumors. Computed tomography (CT) is much more useful in this regard (133,173). Important staging information regarding extension to perirenal tissues, including the renal vein, vena cava, and lymph nodes, is best obtained using this technique. CT functions such as enhancement with contrast may even provide clues to the histologic subtype.

Ultrasonography is particularly useful in the evaluation of cystic lesions detected by other modalities as well as for localizing needles in percutaneous procedures (90). The composition of the cyst and its fluid can be helpful in determining the nature of cystic tumors. In general, benign cysts appear radiologically as homogeneous spheres with regular, smooth internal borders whereas neoplasms may contain nodules protruding into the cysts. Benign cysts are typically filled with clear, straw-colored fluid, which is low in fat, protein, and lactic dehydrogenase, while cystic carcinomas may be bloody, contain necrotic tissue, and have an elevated fat, protein, or lactic dehydrogenase content (150).

Renal arteriography is no longer the procedure of choice in the evaluation of renal masses and is

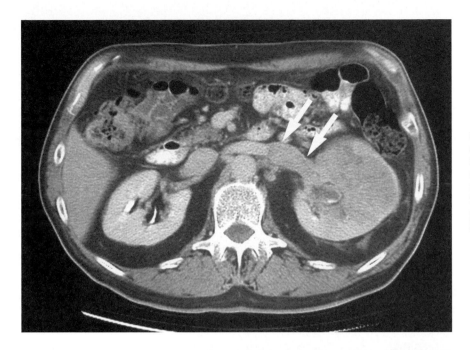

Figure 2-10

RENAL CELL CARCINOMA

As seen with computerized tomography, a large renal cell carcinoma in the kidney extends into the major renal vein (arrows). (Fig. 8-39 from Farrow GM. Diseases of the kidney. In: Murphy WM, ed. Urological pathology. Philadelphia: WB Saunders; 1989:409-82.)

Figure 2-11

RENAL CELL CARCINOMA

As seen with magnetic resonance imaging, there is massive extension of renal cell carcinoma into the inferior vena cava (arrows). (Fig. 1-132 from Fascicle 11, 3rd Series.)

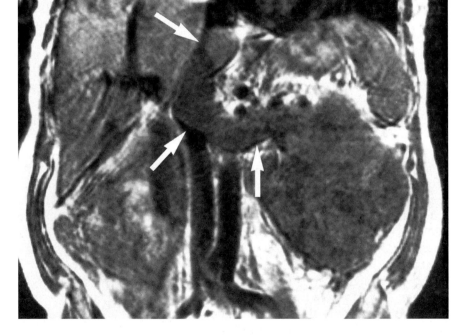

generally reserved for special situations. In RCC, the arteriogram often reveals neovascularity in the tumor, arteriovenous fistulas, and pooling of the contrast medium accentuating the capsular vessels (200). Magnetic resonance imaging (MRI) may provide accurate staging information as well as a three-dimensional representation of the tumor to help plan a surgical approach (152).

RENAL CELL CARCINOMAS

Renal Cell Carcinoma, Clear Cell Type

Definition. The clear cell type is the most common histologic variant of RCC, accounting for approximately 70 percent of cases. This type of RCC has been combined with a category of lesions labeled the "granular cell type" of RCC

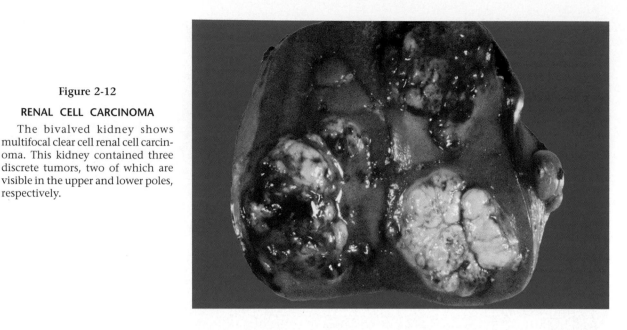

Figure 2-12

RENAL CELL CARCINOMA

The bivalved kidney shows multifocal clear cell renal cell carcinoma. This kidney contained three discrete tumors, two of which are visible in the upper and lower poles, respectively.

in previous schemes and, because the new category now includes neoplasms that may (rarely) be entirely composed of cells with granular, acidophilic cytoplasm, some authors advocate the term "conventional" as a substitute for "clear cell" in the classification (165,221,289).

Pathologic Findings. Grossly, most clear cell RCCs are solitary and randomly distributed in the renal cortex. They occur with equal frequency in either kidney. Multiple neoplasms may occur, and in such cases, coexistence of a carcinoma with a papillary adenoma is the rule. Multicentricity in the same kidney occurs in approximately 4 percent of patients, whereas bilaterality is seen in 0.5 to 3.0 percent (fig. 2-12) (142). The pathologic criteria for the distinction of multicentricity from intrarenal or contrarenal metastases have not been established but a significant difference in the morphology of various tumors in the same or opposite kidneys favors multifocality. Among multifocal cases, 75 percent of lesions are synchronous; the remainder are asynchronous (327). Multicentricity and bilaterality are often associated with familial and associated conditions such as von Hippel-Lindau disease (figs. 2-6, 2-7) (249). In one such case, as many as 15 discrete carcinomas were found (50).

RCC, clear cell type characteristically presents as a rounded, bosselated mass that may protrude from the renal cortex. The interface of the tumor and the adjacent kidney is usually non-encapsulated but well demarcated, with a "pushing" margin (fig. 2-13). Rarely, RCC is diffusely infiltrative (fig. 2-14). These neoplasms may be over 15 cm in greatest dimension, but the frequency of small lesions is rapidly increasing in countries where radiologic imaging is widely applied. Size itself is not a determinant of malignancy and all kidney tumors of the clear cell type are considered malignant. According to the classification used here, renal tumors with any element of nonpapillary, clear cell carcinoma are included among the clear cell variant.

On section, areas of necrosis, cystic degeneration, hemorrhage, and calcification are commonly present (fig. 2-15). Calcification and even ossification typically occur within necrotic zones and are demonstrated in 10 to 15 percent of RCCs (25,93). Variations in consistency tend to accompany tumor size, with small tumors being much more homogeneous than large lesions.

The clear cell type of RCC is typically golden due to the rich lipid content of its cells: cholesterol, neutral lipids, and phospholipids are abundant. These accumulate as droplets in the cytoplasm of tumor cells due to deficient glycogenolysis and lipolysis associated with an unresponsiveness of the tumor cell adenylate cyclase to glucagon and beta-catecholamines (157). The lipid content is similar to that of the proximal convoluted tubules (178).

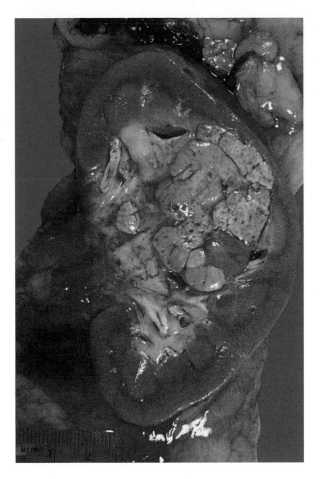

Figure 2-13

RENAL CELL CARCINOMA

This clear cell renal cell carcinoma has the typical golden yellow appearance. In this case there is extension of the tumor into the renal pelvis.

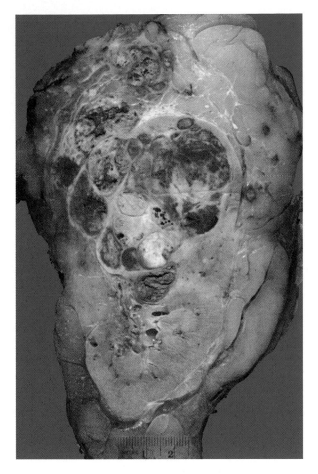

Figure 2-14

RENAL CELL CARCINOMA

This large clear cell renal cell carcinoma is infiltrating the surrounding perirenal adipose tissue.

Histologically, cells interspersed with abundant, thin-walled blood vessels that result in a sinusoidal vascular pattern characterize the clear cell type of RCC (figs. 2-16, 2-17). The cells are filled with lipids and cholesterol, which are ordinarily dissolved in usual histologic preparations, creating a clear cytoplasm surrounded by a distinct cell membrane (fig. 2-18). These neutral lipids can be identified in unfixed material using oil red O and Sudan IV reactions. The phospholipid components are the most resistant to solvents and may be identified with Sudan black B reactions. Glycogen can be identified by the periodic acid–Schiff (PAS) stain (fig. 2-19). Both types of cytoplasmic substances are readily observed in electron microscopic prepa-

rations. Other cytoplasmic components include hyaline intracytoplasmic globules and structures resembling Mallory bodies (64,143). The hyaline globules are 5 to 7 µm in greatest dimension and stain brightly acidophilic in usual preparations (figs. 2-20, 2-21), but also react with PAS, phosphotungstic acid, and Luxol fast blue reagents. The presence of a coarsely granular brown pigment, suggestive of neuromelanin, has also been described (151). A tumor with melanin-like pigment and HMB-45 positivity has been described as clear cell carcinoma with melanocytic differentiation (179). Basophilic inclusions that ultrastructurally have a myelinoid lamellated structure occur (138). The accumulation of altered red blood cells in tumor cell cytoplasm,

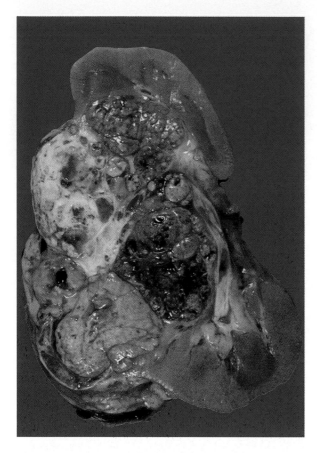

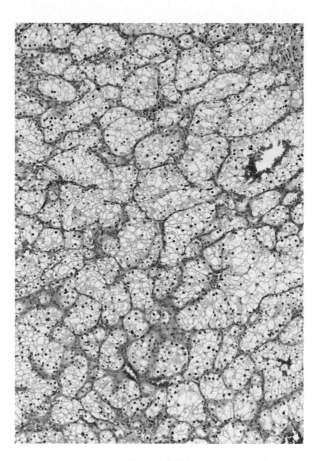

Figure 2-15

CLEAR CELL RENAL CELL CARCINOMA

Large renal cell carcinoma with a variegated appearance is bulging into perinephric adipose tissue. The tumor also involves the renal pelvis.

Figure 2-16

CLEAR CELL RENAL CELL CARCINOMA

Typical clear cell renal cell carcinoma contains solid nests of cells that are separated by a prominent sinusoidal vascular network.

Figure 2-17

**CLEAR CELL
RENAL CELL CARCINOMA**

Solid nests of clear cells are separated by a prominent sinusoidal vascular network. Many of the cells have fine granular acidophilic cytoplasm.

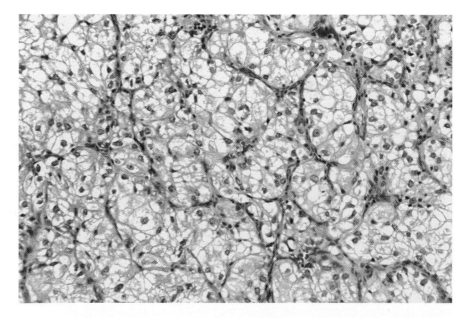

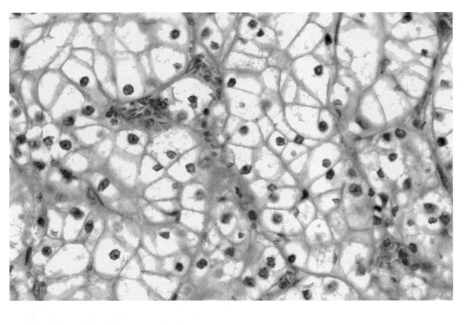

Figure 2-18

**CLEAR CELL
RENAL CELL CARCINOMA**

The clear cells are separated from one another by well-defined cell borders.

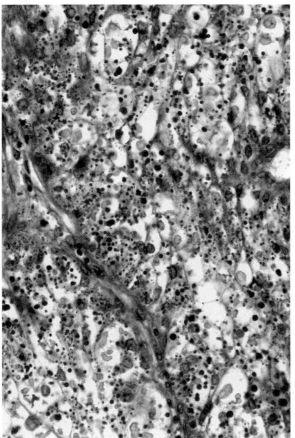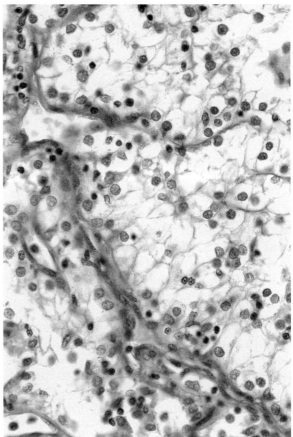

Figure 2-19

CLEAR CELL RENAL CELL CARCINOMA

Periodic acid–Schiff stain without (left) and with (right) diastase demonstrates the abundant glycogen in the cytoplasm.

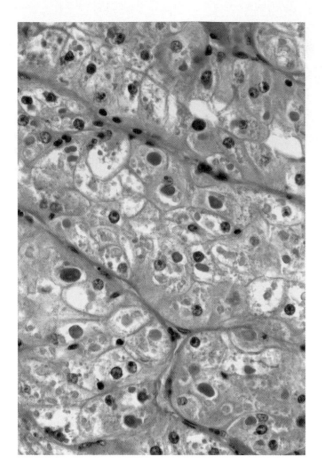

Figure 2-20

CLEAR CELL RENAL CELL CARCINOMA

Intracytoplasmic and extracytoplasmic hyaline globules are present.

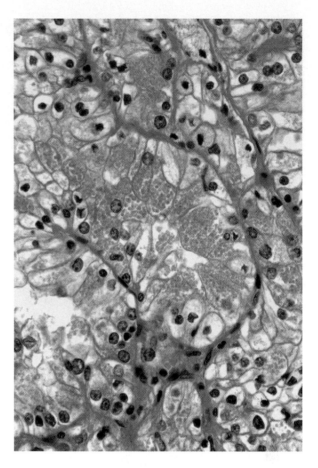

Figure 2-21

CLEAR CELL RENAL CELL CARCINOMA

Numerous intracytoplasmic acidophilic inclusions are present.

so-called myospherulosis, has been reported in clear cell carcinomas (45). This feature is rare in other types of RCC. Granular cytoplasmic acidophilia is a prominent feature of some clear cell RCCs (fig. 2-22). Cells with such cytoplasm have a higher nuclear grade.

In 4 to 5 percent of clear cell RCCs, there are focal or extensive areas of cells with a distinctive rhabdoid morphology (106). This can lead to confusion with rhabdoid tumor of the kidney (316). Less often this histology is present in papillary and chromophobe RCCs (106,277a). The rhabdoid cells are uniform, with large eccentric nuclei, prominent nucleoli, and abundant cytoplasm containing globular acidophilic inclusions (fig. 2-23). Multinucleated cells are common (fig. 2-24). The cells are most often arranged in a solid organoid or sheet-like pat-

tern. Spindle cell and pseudoglandular architecture can be seen. Approximately 25 percent of tumors with a rhabdoid morphology have a sarcomatoid component. The rhabdoid cells coexpress cytokeratin and vimentin, and are epithelial membrane antigen (EMA) positive.

RCC, clear cell type may grow in various architectural patterns, and knowledge of these is important only to avoid errors in classification. In addition to sinusoidal and sheet-like patterns, tumors may have a predominantly alveolar, tubular, or acinar appearance (figs. 2-25, 2-26). In these patterns, rounded collections of cells are peripherally demarcated by a network of delicate, interconnecting capillary or sinusoidal structures and supported by a network of thin reticulin fibers. No luminal differentiation is apparent in the alveolar pattern but a central,

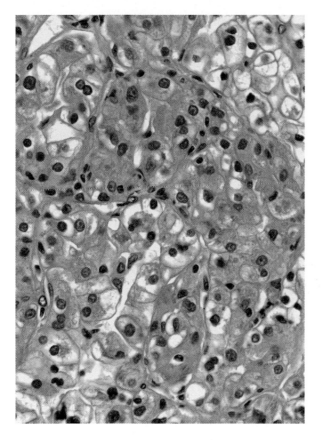

Figure 2-22

CLEAR CELL RENAL CELL CARCINOMA

Higher-grade clear cell renal cell carcinoma (nuclear grade 3) with granular acidophilic cytoplasm.

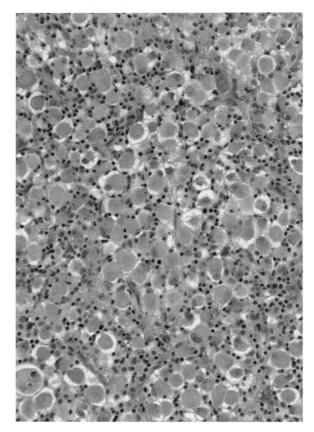

Figure 2-23

CLEAR CELL RENAL CELL CARCINOMA

Prominent rhabdoid cells have abundant acidophilic cytoplasm and eccentric nuclei with macronucleoli. Elsewhere, this tumor showed the typical appearance of clear cell renal cell carcinoma.

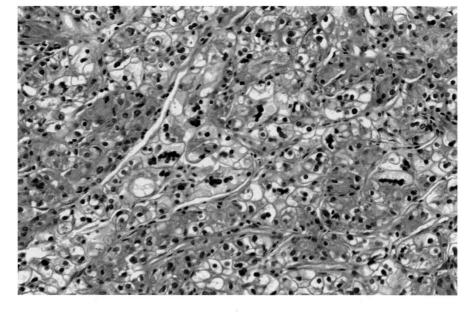

Figure 2-24

CLEAR CELL RENAL CELL CARCINOMA

Many of the tumor cells are multinucleated with small round uniform nuclei. The nuclear grade is based on the nuclear morphology and in this case the grade is 3; the nuclei in the multinucleated cells have grade 2 features.

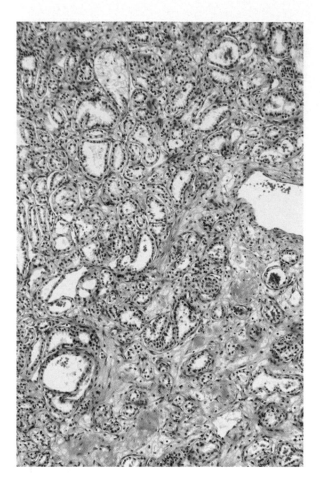

Figure 2-25

CLEAR CELL RENAL CELL CARCINOMA

This case illustrates prominent tubular differentiation.

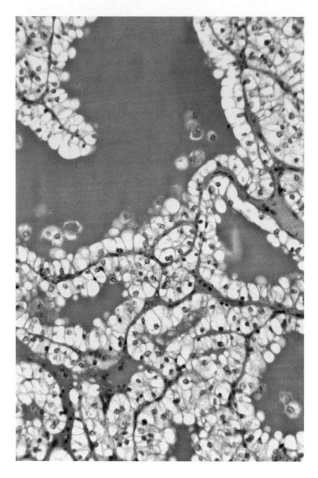

Figure 2-27

CLEAR CELL RENAL CELL CARCINOMA

There is tubule and microcyst formation. The lumens are filled with an amorphous proteinaceous material.

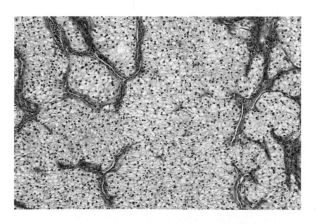

Figure 2-26

CLEAR CELL RENAL CELL CARCINOMA

The tumor is growing in wide solid trabeculae. The prominent sinusoidal vasculature remains evident.

rounded luminal space filled with lightly acidophilic serous fluid or erythrocytes occurs in the acinar pattern (figs. 2-27, 2-28). The alveolar and acinar structures may dilate, and produce microcystic and macrocystic patterns (fig. 2-29). Infrequently, clear cell RCC has a distinct tubular or tubulopapillary architecture (fig. 2-30) (95).

In well-preserved preparations, nuclei tend to be round and uniform, with finely granular, evenly distributed chromatin. Depending upon the degree of differentiation, nucleoli may be absent, sparse, large, or prominent. Occasionally, there are very large nuclei lacking nucleoli or bizarre nuclei. Intranuclear inclusions can be seen (122).

A host of unusual histologic findings have been described in the clear cell type of RCC.

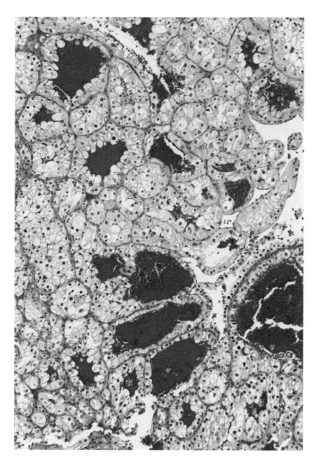

Figure 2-28

CLEAR CELL RENAL CELL CARCINOMA

The lumens of the tubules and microcystic spaces are filled with red blood cells.

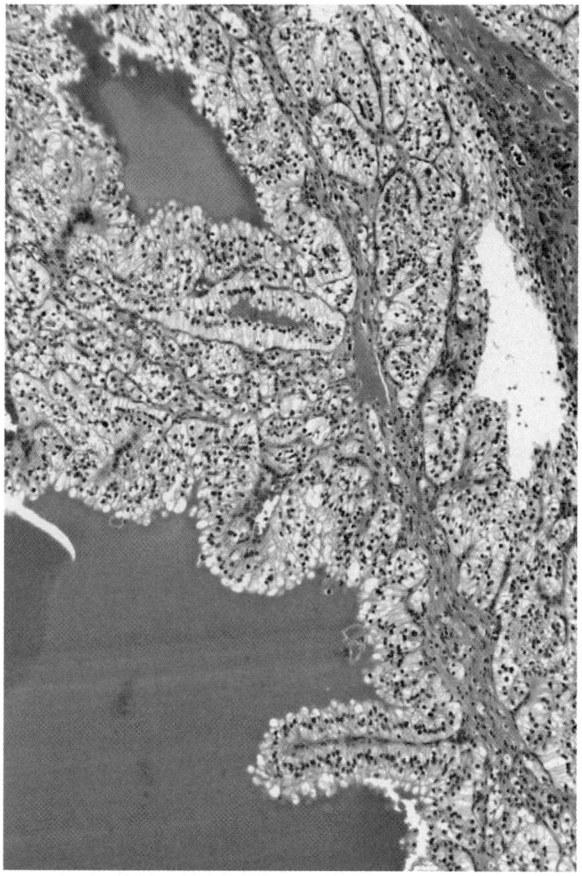

Figure 2-29

CLEAR CELL RENAL CELL CARCINOMA

There is microcyst and macrocyst formation. Papillae extend into the cystic area.

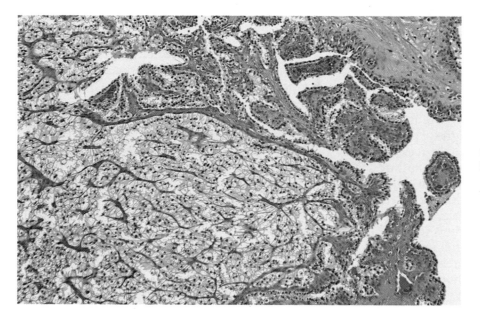

Figure 2-30

CLEAR CELL RENAL CELL CARCINOMA

This clear cell renal cell carcinoma has a prominent papillary architecture.

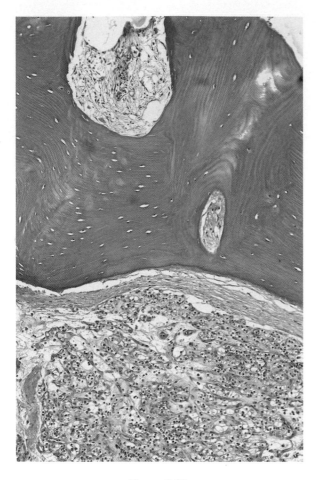

Figure 2-31

CLEAR CELL RENAL CELL CARCINOMA

There is prominent bone formation in association with a low-grade, clear cell renal cell carcinoma.

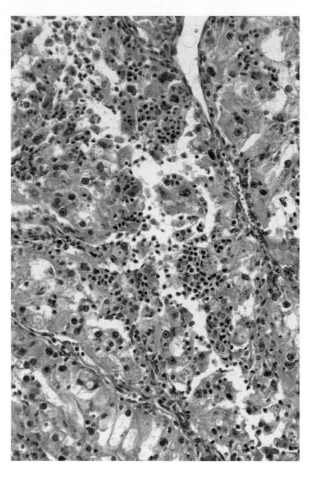

Figure 2-32

CLEAR CELL RENAL CELL CARCINOMA

There is a prominent neutrophilic infiltrate in this nuclear grade 3, clear cell renal cell carcinoma.

These include calcification, ossification, inflammation, and even sarcoid-like granulomas (figs. 2-31–2-33) (125,212). Most, if not all, probably represent nonspecific reactions to degeneration within the tumor.

Studies of the uninvolved parenchyma adjacent to RCCs have reported dysplasia of the tubular epithelium in over 20 percent of cases (216), although this is rare in the author's (DG) experience. Renal tubular dysplasia is defined by the presence of tubular cells that have nuclei that are at least two times the size of normal or reactive nuclei. It is most frequent in the collecting duct type of RCC, followed by the clear cell type. Similar changes rarely are observed in nontumor-bearing kidneys but are described in transplanted kidneys (210).

The cytologic changes observed in fine needle aspiration specimens are well described in the literature (121,256). Various histologic subtypes of RCC can be distinguished in aspirates but the identification of neoplastic cells is ordinarily sufficient for patient care. The cytologic interpretation is greatly facilitated in cases in which large groups of cohesive cells, associated with intact capillaries, are recognized by their endothelial cells and red and white blood cells.

Aspiration cytology is most often performed to document the presence of renal cancer when the tumor is clinically unresectable or to validate the radiologic impression of metastatic disease. In such cases, renal tumor cells tend to be large, with a moderate nuclear-cytoplasmic ratio. Nuclei are round or slightly irregular with finely

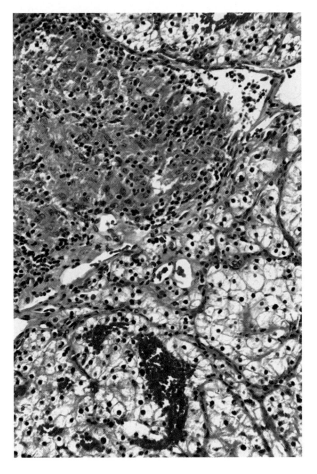

Figure 2-33

CLEAR CELL RENAL CELL CARCINOMA

This clear cell renal cell carcinoma contains numerous well-formed granulomata.

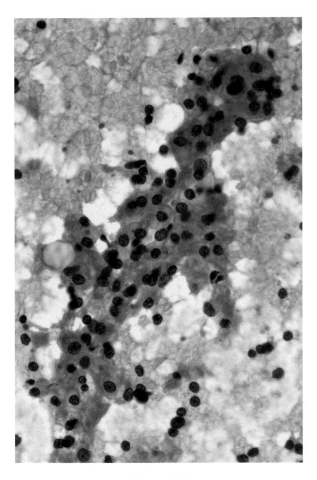

Figure 2-34

CLEAR CELL RENAL CELL CARCINOMA

Fine needle aspiration specimen shows cohesive nests of uniform cells with moderate amounts of pale-staining cytoplasm, well-defined cell borders, and uniform round nuclei with some small nucleoli.

granular, evenly distributed chromatin and a single, prominent nucleolus (fig. 2-34). Intranuclear pseudoinclusions may be present. The cytoplasm can be clear and foamy or have a granular acidophilic character. Cell borders may be ill-defined or sharp, often depending upon the shear artifact created during specimen extraction and preparation. In those few instances in which the tumor assessed by fine needle aspirate cytology is low grade, the nuclear changes are much less distinctive and more reliance must be placed on the presence of sheet-like patterns and lack of normal tubular structures.

Immunohistochemical Findings. Immunohistochemical studies confirm that the antigenic composition of RCC is variable, likely reflecting the heterogeneous differentiation of these tumors. A bewildering number of antigens have been documented in RCC, and it is common for antigens recognized in one study population to be absent from the tumors in another. In general, renal neoplasms manifest antigenic determinants common to renal tubules and the more the cells of any particular tumor are differentiating toward collecting tubules, the more likely they will react to certain cytokeratins (57).

Cells comprising the clear cell type of RCC tend to react with antibodies to brush border antigens, low molecular weight cytokeratins (8, 18, and 19), AE1, Cam 5.2, and vimentin (figs. 2-35, 2-36) (39,198,207,241,318,324). High molecular weight cytokeratins, including cytokeratin 14

119

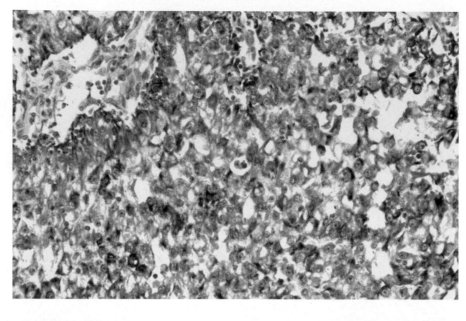

Figure 2-35

CLEAR CELL RENAL CELL CARCINOMA

Immunohistochemical stain with a pancytokeratin cocktail shows strong cytoplasmic reactivity.

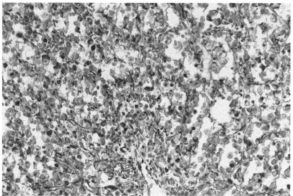

Figure 2-36

CLEAR CELL RENAL CELL CARCINOMA

Immunohistochemical stain demonstrates strong cytoplasmic reactivity for vimentin.

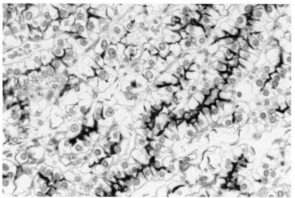

Figure 2-37

CLEAR CELL RENAL CELL CARCINOMA

Immunohistochemical stain for epithelial membrane antigen demonstrates a strong cytoplasmic membrane pattern.

and 34ßE12, are detected rarely (53). Many tumors express vimentin although the frequency varies widely in the literature. The majority of clear cell RCCs are positive for RCC marker and EMA (fig. 2-37) (84,203). MUC I is consistently expressed (39). Clear cell RCCs also express alpha-1–antichymotrypsin, alpha-1–antitrypsin, CD68, and CD10 (16,158,277). A significant number of tumors are reactive to placental alkaline phosphatase (PLAP). Rare lesions are reactive for carcinoembryonic antigens, alpha-fetoprotein, and S-100 protein (55,244,267). Clear cell RCCs do not react with antibodies to

Tamm-Horsfall protein (78). The majority of tumors do not express parvalbumin or beta-defensin-1 (325).

Antibodies to lectins reveal the variable antigenic composition in RCCs (311). Lectin-based studies indicate that even low-grade carcinomas may have lectin components in common with both proximal and distal tubules.

Ultrastructural Findings. Ultrastructurally, the cells of RCCs tend to have a tubular differentiation that is characterized by arrangement around microlumens, often with varying amounts of brush border, and demarcation of

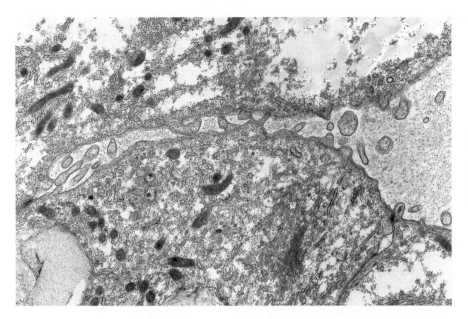

Figure 2-38

CLEAR CELL RENAL CELL CARCINOMA

There are microvilli on the luminal aspect of the cell membrane. (Fig. 8-31 from Farrow GM. Diseases of the kidney. In: Murphy WM, ed. Urological pathology. Philadelphia: WB Saunders; 1989:409–82.)

Figure 2-39

CLEAR CELL RENAL CELL CARCINOMA

The tumor cells feature cytoplasmic glycogen and lipid droplets (X2,500). (Fig. 8-30 from Farrow GM. Diseases of the kidney. In: Murphy WM, ed. Urological pathology. Philadelphia: WB Saunders; 1989:409–82).

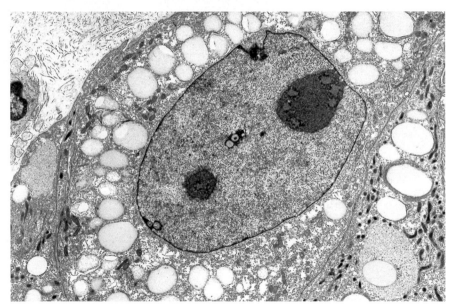

groups of cells by basal lamina (fig. 2-38). Abundant lipid vacuoles and glycogen are characteristically present when the cells have clear cytoplasm by light microscopy (fig. 2-39). In RCCs with granular acidophilic cytoplasm, large numbers of mitochondria may be present. These are haphazardly distributed and are large and pleomorphic (304). Other organelles, such as Golgi bodies and rough endoplasmic reticulum, are either absent or sparse.

Multilocular Cystic Renal Cell Carcinoma. In approximately 5 percent of clear cell RCCs, multiple cysts are the predominant pathologic finding (figs. 2-40, 2-41) (220). These so-called cystic or multilocular cystic RCCs are considered a subtype of the clear cell variety. The tumors are well circumscribed, with noncommunicating cysts separated by irregular, thick fibrous septa, reminiscent of a multilocular cyst. The correct interpretation is achieved by the recognition of the presence of small aggregates of low-grade clear cells in the walls of the cysts (figs. 2-42, 2-43). The lining epithelium of the cysts is often attenuated or even absent but the

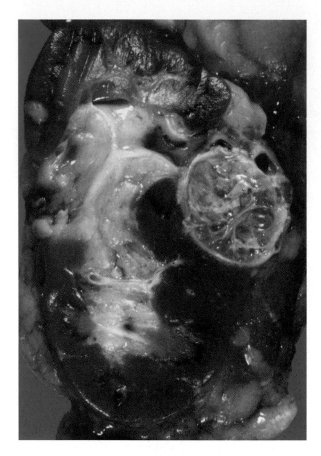

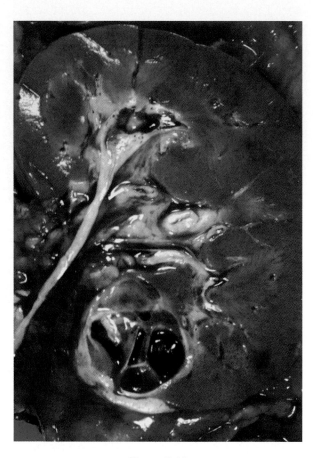

Figure 2-40

MULTILOCULAR CYSTIC RENAL CELL CARCINOMA

The tumor in the upper pole is well circumscribed and has a complex multicystic appearance, with thin fibrous septa and without expansile tumor nodules.

Figure 2-41

MULTILOCULAR CYSTIC RENAL CELL CARCINOMA

The tumor contains blood within one of the cystic spaces. Note the absence of any expansile component to the tumor.

Figure 2-42

MULTILOCULAR CYSTIC RENAL CELL CARCINOMA

The septa separating the cystic spaces are relatively thin and fibrous. Even at low magnification, a few clusters of clear cells are evident within the septal walls (arrow).

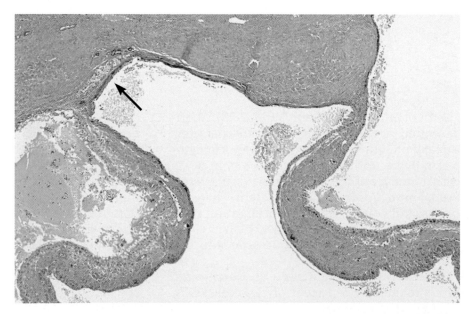

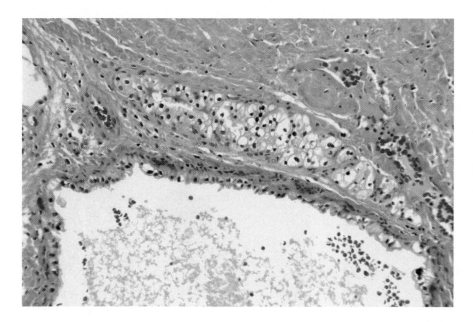

Figure 2-43

MULTILOCULAR CYSTIC RENAL CELL CARCINOMA

There are small nests of clear cells within the fibrous tissue. The tumor is of low nuclear grade (nuclear grade 1).

structures do not represent cystic degeneration of a clear cell RCC of the usual type. The septa are fibrotic or hyalinized and may be calcified, with or without ossification.

Multilocular cystic RCCs are distinguished from multilocular cysts by the presence of nodular aggregates of clear cells, in at least some portions of the cyst wall. The presence of clear cells lining the cystic spaces, a feature also found in multilocular cyst, is not sufficient for an interpretation of carcinoma. In some cases, immunohistochemical reactions for cytokeratins are necessary to confirm the epithelial nature of small groups of clear cells within the cystic septa. The criteria for diagnosis of multilocular cystic RCC include: 1) growth as an expansile mass surrounded by a fibrous pseudocapsule; 2) a tumor composed of cysts and septa without expansile solid nodules; and 3) septa containing aggregates of clear cells (76). If defined in this way, well-documented examples of malignant behavior of multilocular cystic RCCs have not come to our attention and there is considerable doubt as to whether or not these tumors are truly carcinomas (76,162,220,223,307).

Multilocular cystic RCCs must be distinguished from RCCs with cystic change. The latter may have expansile clear cell masses in their cyst walls or papillary excrescences covered by clear cells.

Renal Cell Carcinoma, Papillary Type

Definition. This histologically distinct type of RCC comprises 10 to 15 percent of RCCs (9,30, 49,71,137,171,172,195,229). Papillary RCCs are variable in size, and small tumors must be distinguished from true renal cortical adenomas. The classification of RCCs defines any papillary tumor larger then 0.5 cm as a carcinoma (289). In one large series, the mean size of papillary RCCs was 8 cm and a few tumors measured up to 23 cm in greatest dimension (195).

Pathologic Findings. Grossly, the papillary type of RCC is well circumscribed and eccentrically situated in the renal cortex. More than 80 percent of tumors are confined to the cortex within the renal capsule at the time of nephrectomy. In a high percentage of cases, a distinct fibrous capsule is evident (fig. 2-44). The cut surfaces of papillary RCC vary from light gray to red-brown to golden yellow, depending upon the number of lipid-laden macrophages in the stroma and the amount of hemosiderin in the tumor cells (figs. 2-45, 2-46). Intratumoral hemorrhage and necrosis are seen in two thirds of cases, a finding that correlates with the radiographic finding of reduced or absent tumor vascularity (22,29,246). Papillary RCCs can be found in the walls of cysts (148). Compared to other types of RCC, they are more often associated with cortical adenomas and are more often multiple (fig. 2-47) (51). In the

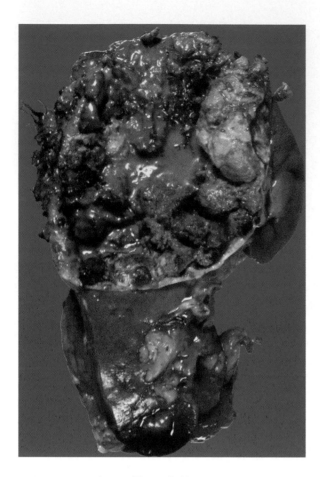

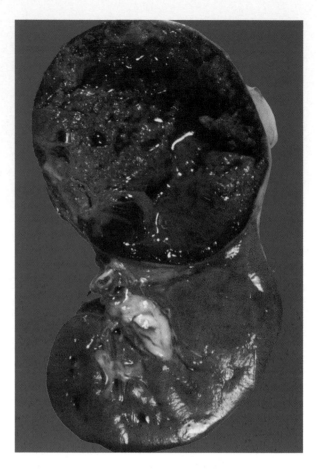

Figure 2-44

PAPILLARY RENAL CELL CARCINOMA

This large papillary renal cell carcinoma has a thick fibrous capsule that is evident on gross examination. The cut surface shows the friable, necrotic appearance that is often present in this tumor type.

Figure 2-45

PAPILLARY RENAL CELL CARCINOMA

This papillary renal cell carcinoma has a hemorrhagic friable cut surface. A thin capsule is present.

hereditary type of papillary RCC, numerous tumors may be grossly visible and many more found microscopically (232).

Histologically, papillary RCC is almost always surrounded by a fibrous capsule (fig. 2-48). The tumor is characterized by a single layer or pseudostratified layers of cells arranged on fibrovascular stalks (fig. 2-49). Most often, the entire tumor is papillary, but tubules may exist in some cases and can predominate (fig. 2-50). Collapse of the papillae and tubules may produce the impression of solid growth (fig. 2-51) (225). The accumulation of lipid-laden macrophages (xanthoma or foam cells) in the stalk is a characteristic feature (figs. 2-49, 2-52). These xanthoma cells may greatly expand the papil-

lary cores. The papillary cores can be thickened and hyalinized. Tumor necrosis may liberate large quantities of lipid, and cholesterol crystals are not rare. Psammomatous calcifications may be abundant (fig. 2-53). Sarcomatoid change is infrequent, but is well described and occurs in both basophilic and acidophilic variants (238,262). Mucin secretion occurs in a small percentage of cases (120,312). Staining with Hale's colloidal iron reveals coarse cytoplasmic droplets and can be intensely positive if there is abundant hemosiderin (73,303).

The cells of the papillary type of RCC can be basophilic, acidophilic, or clear. Most recently, papillary RCC has been separated into two subtypes, type 1 and type 2, based on morphologic

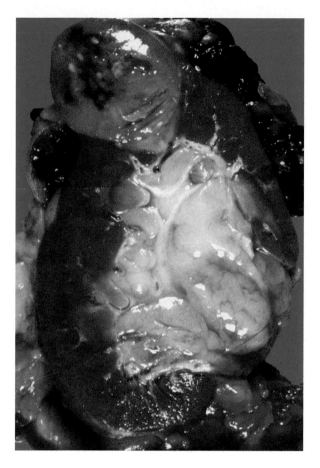

Figure 2-46

PAPILLARY RENAL CELL CARCINOMA

The tumor is homogenous tan brown, with small foci of necrosis.

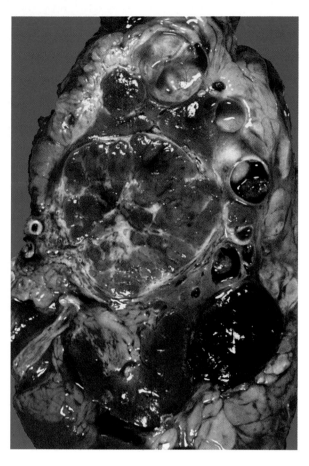

Figure 2-47

PAPILLARY RENAL CELL CARCINOMA

There are multiple papillary renal cell carcinomas.

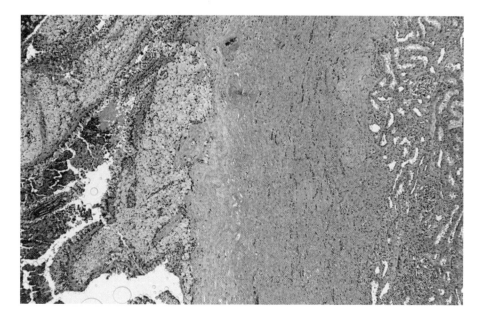

Figure 2-48

PAPILLARY RENAL CELL CARCINOMA

This low-power photomicrograph illustrates the thick fibrous capsule of the tumor. The abundant foamy macrophages in this particular case are evident even at this magnification.

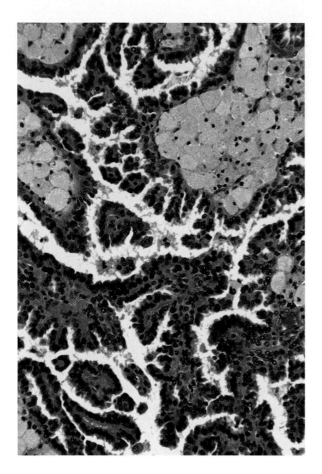

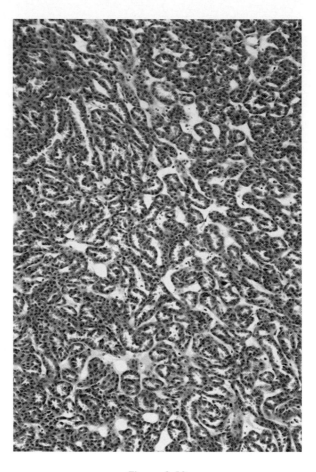

Figure 2-49

PAPILLARY RENAL CELL CARCINOMA

The papillary cores are filled and in some areas expanded by the presence of numerous foamy macrophages.

Figure 2-50

PAPILLARY RENAL CELL CARCINOMA

There is a prominent tubular architecture.

Figure 2-51

PAPILLARY RENAL CELL CARCINOMA

The papillae are collapsed, resulting in a "solid" appearance.

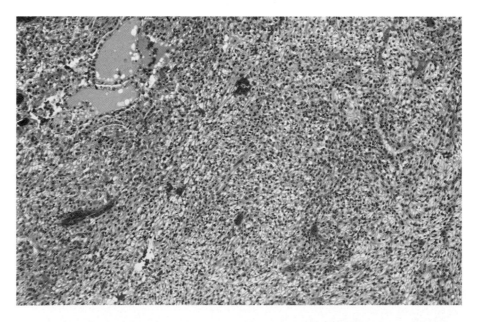

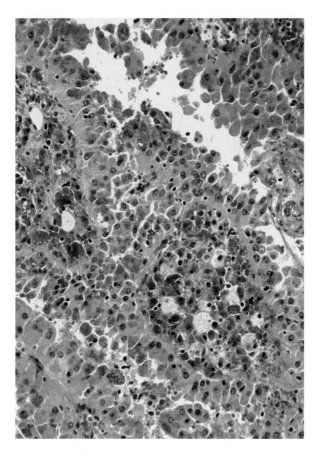

Figure 2-52

PAPILLARY RENAL CELL CARCINOMA

The papillary cores contain a mixture of foamy macrophages and hemosiderin-laden macrophages. The tumor cells also contain cytoplasmic hemosiderin. This tumor is a type with pseudostratified, tall columnar cells having nuclei with prominent nucleoli.

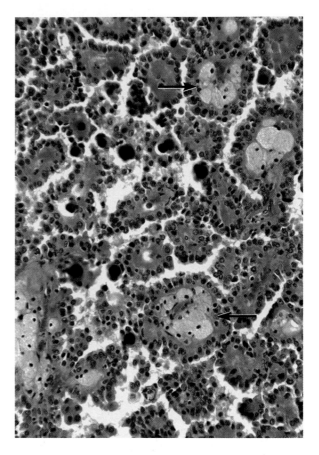

Figure 2-53

PAPILLARY RENAL CELL CARCINOMA

This papillary renal cell carcinoma contains numerous psammoma bodies. Note also the focal collections of macrophages (arrows).

features. This separation is included in the 2004 WHO classification of RCC (77). The distinction is reputed to have prognostic significance and there is data to suggest that molecular and genetic differences may exist as well (71,72,182,269).

Type 1 tumors comprise at least two thirds of reported cases. They are composed of small cells with scanty, pale, usually basophilic cytoplasm (figs. 2-54–2-56). The nuclei are small and ovoid with inconspicuous nucleoli (grades 1 and 2). Nuclear grooves may be present. The cells typically form a single layer on the papillae. Psammoma bodies and foamy macrophages are often abundant.

Type 2 tumors comprise less than one third of cases. They are composed of large cells with

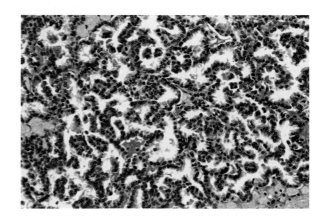

Figure 2-54

PAPILLARY RENAL CELL CARCINOMA

This papillary renal cell carcinoma is of low nuclear grade and would correspond to the type 1 category.

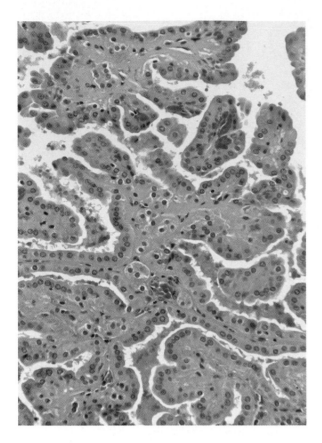

Figure 2-55

PAPILLARY RENAL CELL CARCINOMA

The cells have more abundant acidophilic cytoplasm than in figure 2-54, but still have small uniform nuclei with inconspicuous nucleoli and lack pseudostratification, corresponding to the type 1 category.

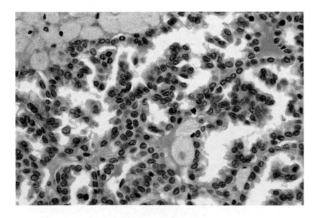

Figure 2-56

PAPILLARY RENAL CELL CARCINOMA

The nuclei in this papillary renal cell carcinoma are small and occasionally show the presence of nuclear grooves. This feature is often seen in the low-grade type 1 category.

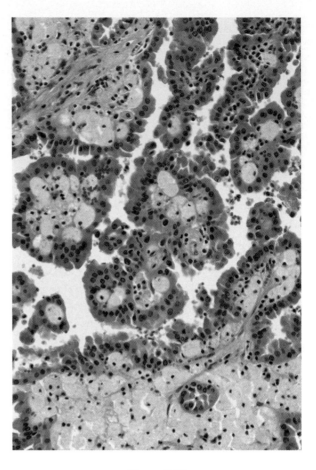

Figure 2-57

PAPILLARY RENAL CELL CARCINOMA

This papillary renal cell carcinoma is characterized by cells with abundant acidophilic cytoplasm and large nuclei with small nucleoli. This would correspond to the type 2 category.

voluminous cytoplasm that is usually acidophilic (figs. 2-57–2-59). Cytoplasmic clearing can be present and is characteristically apical. Nuclei are large and spherical with prominent nucleoli (grade 3). There is often focal pseudostratification of cells. The tumor cells may have intracytoplasmic lumens. Intracellular and extracellular PAS-positive hyaline globules are rare.

In those cases having an apparent mixture of the two types, classification is based on the predominant component. Whether or not distinguishing the subtypes of papillary RCC is important to patient care, considering that the poorer prognosis of type 2 lesions might well be conferred by their higher grade and stage, and that only one standard treatment is available for organ-confined RCC, remains to be determined.

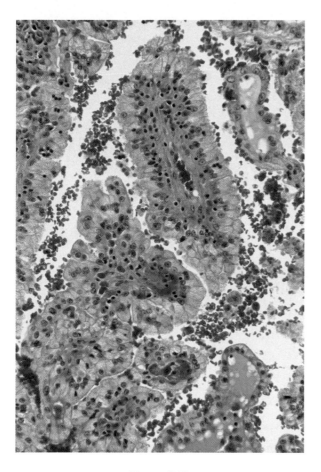

Figure 2-58

PAPILLARY RENAL CELL CARCINOMA

The tumor cells are tall and columnar, and show clearing of the cytoplasm. The cells contain enlarged nuclei with prominent nucleoli, corresponding to the type 2 category.

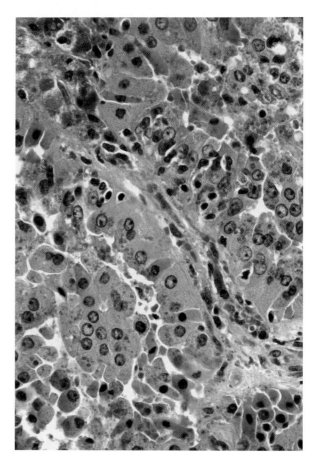

Figure 2-59

PAPILLARY RENAL CELL CARCINOMA

The papillary tumors with abundant acidophilic cytoplasm typically have higher-grade nuclei, as in this case.

Hereditary papillary RCCs are typically composed of small basophilic cells with scant cytoplasm and low-grade nuclei (188). Numerous foamy macrophages and psammoma bodies as well as extensive hemorrhage and necrosis are present. The tumors associated with the t(X;1) (p11.2;q21) translocation (so-called Xp11.2 tumors) are also usually, in part, papillary in type. The cells comprising these tumors are cuboidal to columnar, with clear to acidophilic cytoplasm and high-grade nuclei.

The cytologic changes in papillary RCCs include several characteristic features (86,110, 256). The presence of papillary clusters in a necrotic background is diagnostic but not uniformly present. Foamy macrophages and tumor cell intracytoplasmic hemosiderin are seen in most

papillary RCCs whereas they are found in less than 10 percent of other types of RCC (110,315). Not surprisingly, nuclear and cytoplasmic features depend on the subtype. In basophilic (type 1) papillary RCC, nuclei are small, with inconspicuous nucleoli and prominent nuclear grooves. Nuclei in the acidophilic (type 2) tumors are larger, often have prominent nucleoli, and infrequently exhibit nuclear grooves. Papillary RCC has been diagnosed from voided urine specimens (155). As with other types of RCC, the principal value of cytology is to document the presence of a neoplasm and to distinguish primary from metastatic lesions.

Immunohistochemical Findings. Immunohistochemical studies of papillary RCC have yielded variable results. The RCC marker is positive

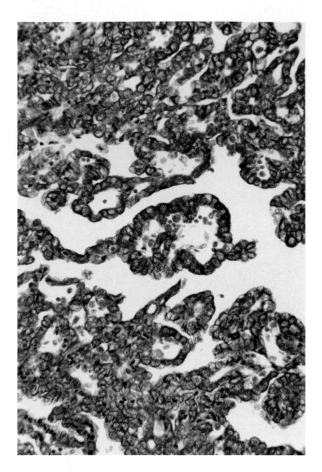

Figure 2-60

PAPILLARY RENAL CELL CARCINOMA

Immunohistochemical stain for cytokeratin 7 demonstrates strong immunoreactivity.

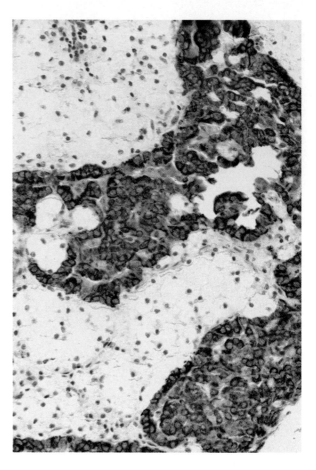

Figure 2-61

PAPILLARY RENAL CELL CARCINOMA

Immunohistochemical stain for vimentin shows immunoreactivity within the epithelial cells.

in over 90 percent of cases (203). Tumors react strongly with pancytokeratins and low molecular weight cytokeratin antibodies, but only rarely and focally for high molecular weight keratins (53,71,85,99,251). The basophilic (type 1) tumors are more intensely reactive for cytokeratin 7 than the acidophilic (type 2) neoplasms (fig. 2-60) (71). There is inconsistent reactivity for vimentin (fig. 2-61) (71); in one series, all hereditary papillary RCCs expressed vimentin (188). Reactivity for carcinoembryonic antigen is recorded in a small percentage of papillary RCCs (238). Papillary RCCs are positive for CD9 and CD10 (16,158,169). Many tumors express parvalbumin and beta-defensin-1 (325).

Ultrastructural Findings. Ultrastructurally, papillary RCC is characterized by cells with variably sized luminal microvilli resting on a basal lamina. The cytoplasm contains variable numbers of mitochondria (greater in cells with acidophilic cytoplasm as detected by light microscopy) with lamellar cristae. The microvesicles typical of the chromophobe cell type of RCC are absent and there is little or no glycogen (167).

Renal Cell Carcinoma, Chromophobe Cell Type

Definition. This is a variant with distinctive histologic and cytogenetic features. Tumors composed entirely of the distinctive "classic" (plant-like) cells are unusual, however, and the primary value of separating this lesion from other renal neoplasms is to distinguish it from benign oncocytoma (300). Chromophobe cell RCCs may contain foci of sarcomatoid carcinoma, in which case the tumor has been labeled *sarcomatoid*

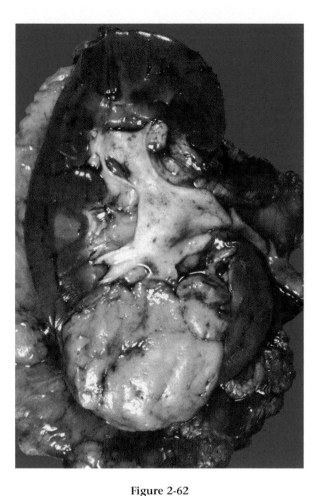

Figure 2-62

CHROMOPHOBE RENAL CELL CARCINOMA

The tumor is well circumscribed, nonencapsulated, and pale tan.

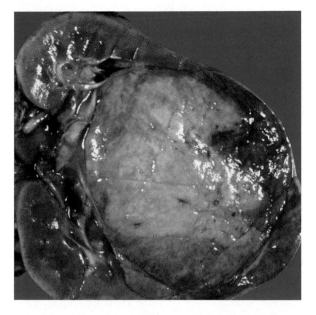

Figure 2-63

CHROMOPHOBE RENAL CELL CARCINOMA

This large chromophobe renal cell carcinoma has a homogeneous, pale yellow-tan color and small punctate areas of hemorrhage.

chromophobe RCC (5). Although initially recognized in men of Middle Eastern descent, it is unlikely that regional or ethnic factors are important in the etiology of these tumors.

As currently defined, chromophobe cell RCCs constitute approximately 5 percent of renal neoplasms (49). A similar neoplasm can be induced in rats, where it seems to differentiate toward the proximal nephron, but the presence of numerous cytoplasmic vesicles containing the enzyme carbonic anhydrase C in the tumors of humans suggests differentiation toward the intercalated cells of collecting ducts (20,290).

Pathologic Findings. Grossly, chromophobe cell RCCs range from 2 to 22 cm in greatest dimension (mean, 8 cm) (figs. 2-62–2-65). All recorded lesions have been well circumscribed and

solitary. The cut surfaces are typically pale yellow, tan, or brown and may closely mimic an oncocytoma. Small areas of hemorrhage, necrosis, or scarring may be seen, but are not typical. Calcification and ossification may be present (320).

Histologically, there are two major patterns of growth, referred to as the classic and the eosinophilic types. In most cases, mixtures of the two occur (figs. 2-66–2-70). The tumor cells are arranged in broad trabeculae and solid sheets. Tubule formation may be seen but rarely predominates. Psammoma bodies may be present. The cells of eosinophilic areas are essentially oncocytes and have many of the features expected in an oncocytoma. The cells of the classic type tend to be arranged along septa. They have well-defined borders and abundant, finely reticular, translucent to pale acidophilic cytoplasm. The pale acidophilic appearance is due to the presence of abundant microvesicles distending the cytoplasm. Any remaining organelles are pushed to the periphery, producing a more intense peripheral acidophilia, and giving the cell borders a distinctive thick "plant-like" appearance.

131

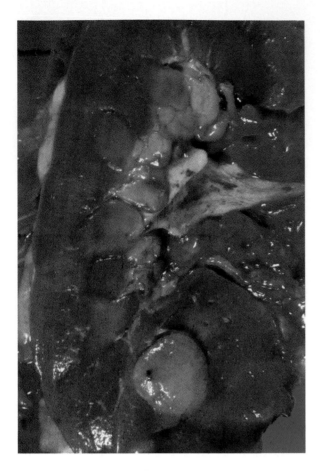

Figure 2-64

CHROMOPHOBE RENAL CELL CARCINOMA

A homogeneous, pale tan-brown tumor is seen.

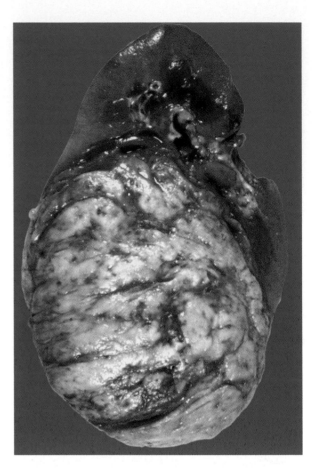

Figure 2-65

CHROMOPHOBE RENAL CELL CARCINOMA

The tumor is pale yellow with areas of hemorrhage and focal necrosis.

Figure 2-66

CHROMOPHOBE RENAL CELL CARCINOMA

This tumor shows a mixture of the classic plant-like cells and the eosinophilic-type cells. Note the "raisinoid" appearance of many of the nuclei in both cell types and the presence of a mitotic figure (arrow).

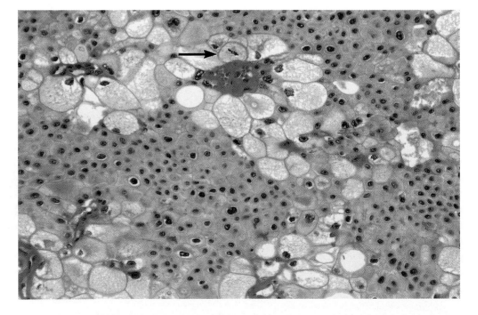

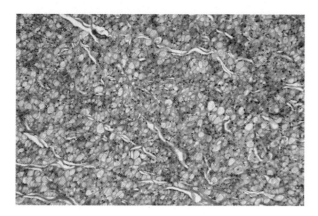

Figure 2-67

CHROMOPHOBE RENAL CELL CARCINOMA

In the classic type, the tumor cells are arranged in broad trabeculae with interspersed thin-walled blood vessels.

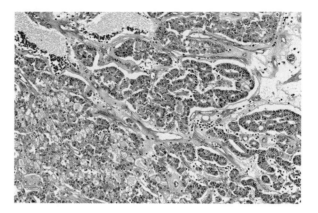

Figure 2-68

CHROMOPHOBE RENAL CELL CARCINOMA

Prominent tubule formation in association with classic chromophobe renal cell carcinoma.

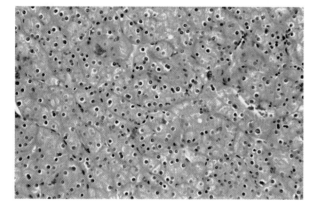

Figure 2-69

CHROMOPHOBE RENAL CELL CARCINOMA

In the eosinophilic variant, the tumor cells are arranged in small nests. The cells have granular eosinophilic cytoplasm with prominent perinuclear halos.

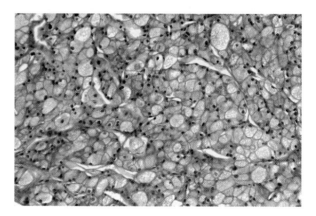

Figure 2-70

CHROMOPHOBE RENAL CELL CARCINOMA

In the classic type, the tumor cells have abundant vesicular cytoplasm. The cytoplasmic membranes appear prominent due to the concentration of cell organelles at the peripheral portion of the cytoplasm.

Many cells are of sufficient size that nuclei do not appear in the plane of section. In some cases, the predominant cell type contains numerous mitochondria, which are granular and strongly acidophilic, reminiscent of the old granular cell variant of RCC. Microvesicles may concentrate around the nucleus, producing a distinctive perinuclear halo (fig. 2-71). This is an important distinguishing feature from oncocytoma. The microvesicles of both types of chromophobe cells can be stained by the Hale colloidal iron technique, indicating a content of mu-

copolysaccharides unique to this type of RCC (figs. 2-72, 2-73) (300,301). If successful, staining is diffuse, intense, and reticular in character. The eosinophilic type often has weaker staining with greater intensity at the apical portion of the cells than the classic type (174,193,303). It should be noted that many laboratories have found Hale's colloidal iron technically challenging and a diagnostic interpretation based on this procedure should be approached with caution.

The nuclei of both classic and eosinophilic types of chromophobe RCC are similar. They

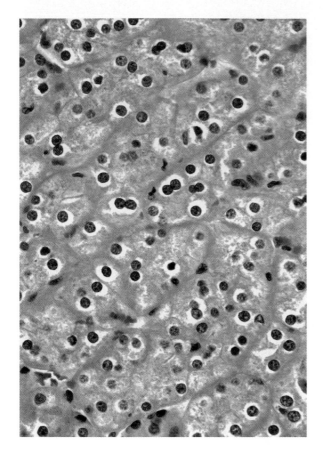

Figure 2-71

CHROMOPHOBE RENAL CELL CARCINOMA

Eosinophilic type of chromophobe renal cell carcinoma illustrates the granular eosinophilic cytoplasm with round uniform nuclei and perinuclear halos.

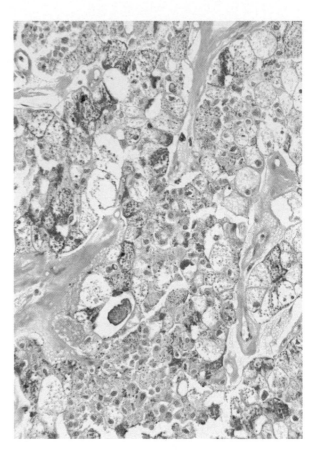

Figure 2-72

CHROMOPHOBE RENAL CELL CARCINOMA

Hale's colloidal iron stain of classic chromophobe renal cell carcinoma demonstrates strong cytoplasmic positivity.

Figure 2-73

CHROMOPHOBE RENAL CELL CARCINOMA

Hale's colloidal iron stain of the eosinophilic variant of chromophobe renal cell carcinoma shows diffuse cytoplasmic staining.

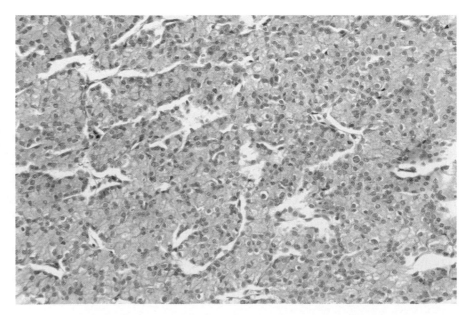

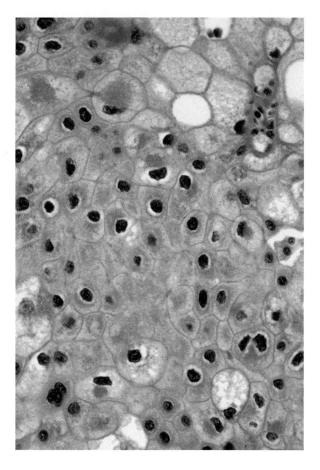

Figure 2-74

CHROMOPHOBE RENAL CELL CARCINOMA

Many of the nuclei in this mixed classic and eosinophilic chromophobe renal cell carcinoma have an irregular or raisinoid shape.

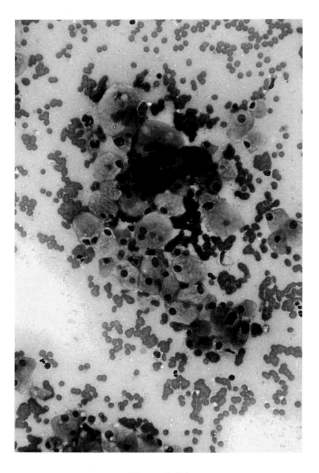

Figure 2-75

CHROMOPHOBE RENAL CELL CARCINOMA

Fine needle aspiration biopsy specimen shows cohesive groups of cells having abundant cytoplasm with a vesicular appearance. Binucleate cells are evident.

measure 10 to 15 µm in greatest dimension, are slightly pleomorphic, and contain granular chromatin and scattered nucleoli conforming to a nuclear grade 2/4 in the Fuhrman system; grade 3 and 4 tumors are distinctly unusual (91). In the classic cell type, the nuclear membrane is often irregular, resulting in a "raisinoid" appearance (fig. 2-74). Binucleate cells are often seen, a feature that is rare in oncocytomas.

The cytologic changes in chromophobe RCCs include the presence of small clusters and single cells having reticular, clear, or granular cytoplasm, with thick cell membranes (fig. 2-75) (254,256). The nuclei vary in size and have irregular outlines. Binucleate cells may be present. Most useful in distinguishing this tu-

mor from an oncocytoma is the variation in nuclear size and irregularity in nuclear outline. Hale's colloidal iron staining can also be diagnostically helpful (184).

Immunohistochemical Findings. Immunohistochemically, the tumor cells of chromophobe RCC react with antibodies to cytokeratins such as 7 and 14, EMA, soybean agglutinin, and carbonic anhydrase C. Cytokeratin reactivity is diffuse and strong when pancytokeratin antibodies are used (fig. 2-76) (53). High molecular weight cytokeratins are not expressed. Chromophobe RCCs do not react for vimentin (fig. 2-77). Approximately 50 percent of lesions are positive for the RCC marker and most express parvalbumin and beta-defensin-1 (203,325).

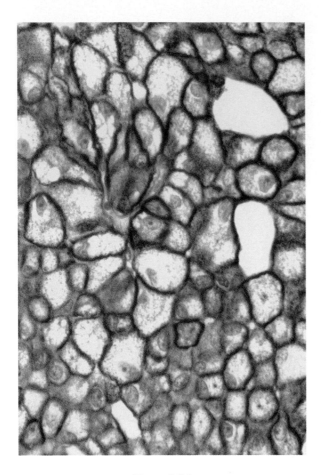

Figure 2-76

CHROMOPHOBE RENAL CELL CARCINOMA

Intense immunoreactivity for cytokeratin 7. The distinctive pseudomembrane-like pattern is due to compression of intermediate filaments towards the periphery of the cytoplasm.

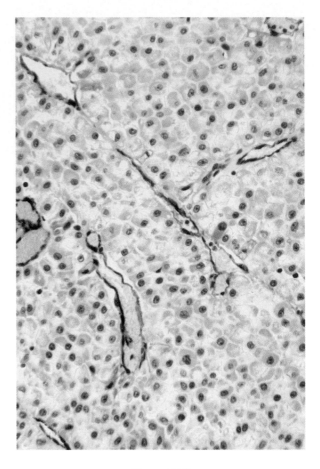

Figure 2-77

CHROMOPHOBE RENAL CELL CARCINOMA

Immunohistochemical stain for vimentin shows a complete absence of reactivity within the tumor cells.

Ultrastructural Findings. Ultrastructurally, the most characteristic feature of chromophobe RCCs is the presence of abundant cytoplasmic microvesicles, the feature that led to the initial separation of this lesion as a distinctive tumor (300). The cytoplasmic vesicles are round to oval and vary in size from 100 to 750 nm (figs. 2-78, 2-79) (304). Typically, they are complex, with vesicles inside vesicles, and they tend to be concentrated adjacent to and surrounding the nucleus. Mitochondria exist more peripherally in the classic form, concentrated adjacent to the cell membrane. Mitochondria are more diffusely distributed in the eosinophilic type, with intermingled microvesicles. The mitochondria are abnormal, with tubulovesicular cristae predominating, but also have circular or lamellar cristae (167,304). There is scant glycogen and lipid. Only a few short microvilli are present on the surface of the cells (167). Nuclei vary from round to highly convoluted with irregular nuclear membranes.

Renal Cell Carcinoma, Collecting Duct Type

Definition. This rare group of tumors constitutes less than 1 percent of malignant epithelial renal neoplasms in adults (8,43,61,83,127, 156,275,282). In the WHO classification, the tumor is grouped with RCC, but designated *carcinoma of the collecting ducts of Bellini* (77). An origin from the collecting ducts has been established, primarily from the medullary location of

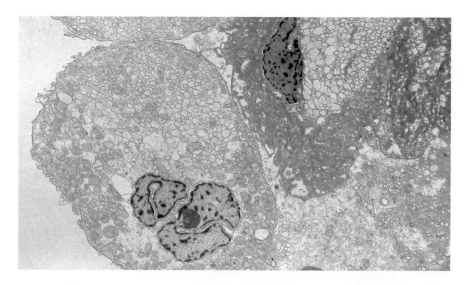

Figure 2-78

CHROMOPHOBE RENAL CELL CARCINOMA

Cytoplasmic vesicles of 150 to 300 nm are present in the cytoplasm along with scattered mitochondria. (Fig. 1-171 from Fascicle 11, 3rd Series.)

Figure 2-79

CHROMOPHOBE RENAL CELL CARCINOMA

The cytoplasmic vesicles are often paranuclear, with mitochondria present in the more peripheral cytoplasm. (Fig. 1-172 from Fascicle 11, 3rd Series.)

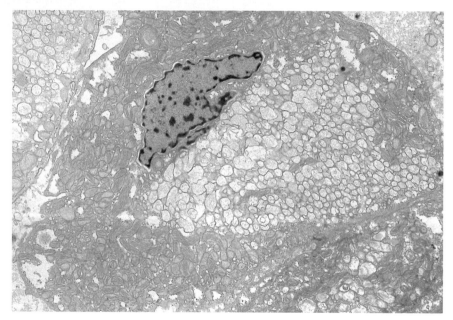

small tumors, but is supported by dysplasia of the collecting duct epithelium adjacent to the neoplasm in many instances, as well as by immunohistochemical and ultrastructural studies.

The category of collecting duct carcinoma includes at least three different clinicopathologic entities: 1) the classically described tubulopapillary type with stromal desmoplasia; 2) lower grade, often partially cystic tumors; and 3) a group of neoplasms with a possible derivation from the loop of Henle (discussed separately). Medullary tumors occurring in patients with sickle cell hemoglobinopathies could also be included, but they have been considered as a distinct entity in current classification schemes.

Pathologic Findings. Grossly, collecting duct carcinomas are predominantly localized to the medulla but may invade the cortex (figs. 2-80, 2-81). They tend to distort adjacent calyces and the renal pelvis. Hemorrhage, with or without necrosis, is typically present. The classic type is gray or very pale gray and has invasive borders. A multicystic appearance secondary to the dilated tubular structures often occurs, particularly in the low-grade variant. Other tumors have a glistening or gelatinous surface.

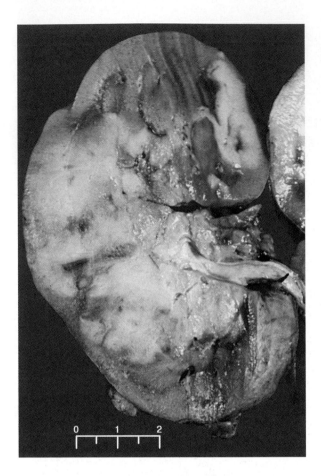

Figure 2-80

COLLECTING DUCT RENAL CELL CARCINOMA

The tumor is gray-white, with an infiltrative growth pattern extending outwards from the central portion of the kidney.

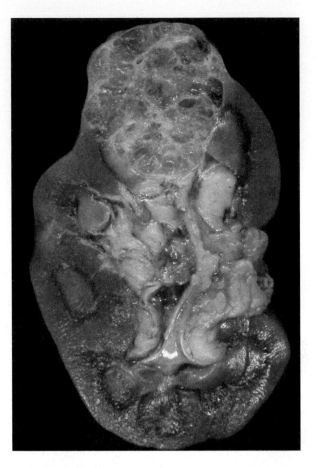

Figure 2-81

COLLECTING DUCT RENAL CELL CARCINOMA

This low-grade collecting duct carcinoma has a multicystic appearance and involves both the cortex and medulla. (Fig. 2-181 from Fascicle 11, 3rd Series.)

Histologically, the classic collecting duct type of RCC is composed of a mixture of dilated tubules and papillae (figs. 2-82–2-84). These tubules may be of varying dimensions and impart a sponge-like appearance to the tumor. In most cases, the predominant pattern is tubular. Both tubules and papillae are lined by a single layer of cuboidal to columnar cells that often have a hobnail pattern. The cytoplasm is amphophilic to acidophilic. Alcian blue-, mucicarmine-, and PAS-positive cytoplasmic mucins are present in some cases. Rarely, cytoplasmic mucins are associated with a signet ring morphology (239). There is marked nuclear pleomorphism, with vesicular to coarse chromatin and single or multiple nucleoli. Mitoses are frequent and abnormal forms may be present. Sar-

comatoid change can be seen (5,18,92). In more differentiated examples, a tubulocystic architecture often predominates, nuclear pleomorphism is minimal, and mitoses are infrequent (figs. 2-85, 2-86) (190). These tumors are considered by some to represent a distinct tumor type. Usually, collecting duct carcinomas infiltrate the adjacent renal parenchyma, producing a striking desmoplastic response (fig. 2-87). There may be dysplasia of the epithelium of the renal collecting ducts immediately adjacent to the tumor, a point of evidence for a collecting duct origin (fig. 2-88).

Collecting duct carcinomas are detected in urinary cytology specimens and diagnosed by fine needle aspiration biopsies (40,199,226, 231). Tumor cells occur singly or in cohesive

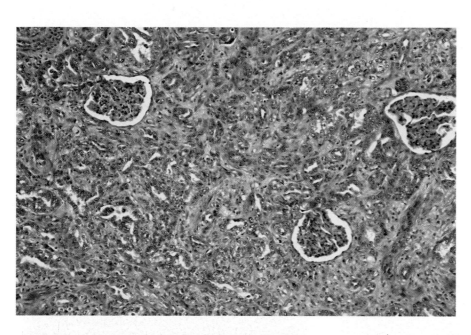

Figure 2-82

COLLECTING DUCT RENAL CELL CARCINOMA

This collecting duct carcinoma is made up of tubular or duct-like structures growing in an infiltrative pattern between residual glomeruli. The tumor is high grade and there is stromal desmoplasia.

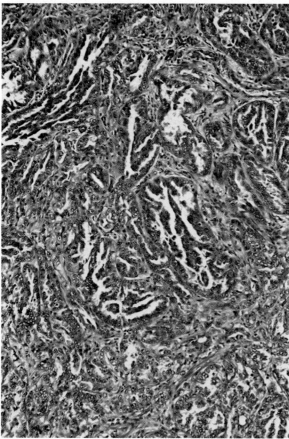

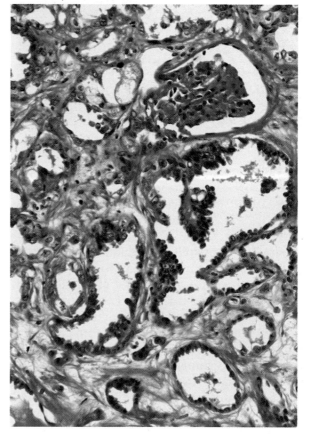

Figure 2-83

COLLECTING DUCT RENAL CELL CARCINOMA

The tumor has a combination of ductal and papillary architectures, and there is associated stromal desmoplasia.

Figure 2-84

COLLECTING DUCT RENAL CELL CARCINOMA

Collecting duct carcinoma with tubulopapillary architecture growing in an infiltrative fashion. Some cells are beginning to have a hobnail-like appearance.

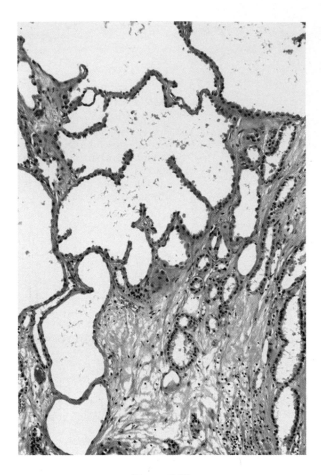

Figure 2-85

COLLECTING DUCT RENAL CELL CARCINOMA

This low-grade collecting duct carcinoma has a distinctive tubulocystic growth pattern, with the individual cells having a low cuboidal morphology and acidophilic cytoplasm.

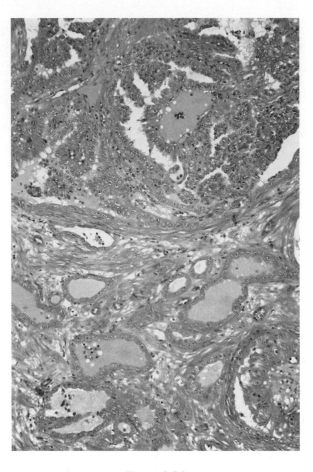

Figure 2-86

COLLECTING DUCT RENAL CELL CARCINOMA

This collecting duct carcinoma has a tubulopapillary architecture. The nuclei are of high grade and the acidophilic cytoplasm is abundant.

groups having papillary or glandular features. Individual cells have irregular, hyperchromatic nuclei with coarse or vesicular chromatin and single to multiple nucleoli. The cytoplasm is finely vacuolated and mucin may be present. The features are quite distinctive from clear cell, papillary, and chromophobe carcinomas, but the lesions cannot be reliably distinguished from metastatic lesions.

Immunohistochemical Findings. The recorded immunohistochemical features of collecting duct RCC are variable. Positive reactions for peanut agglutinin; EMA; cytokeratins 7, 8, 18; and high molecular weight cytokeratins have been observed in many cases (fig. 2-89) (85). The RCC marker is negative in the few lesions studied (203).

Ultrastructural Findings. The cells of collecting duct RCCs rest on a basal lamina and have short, irregular apical microvilli (266). There are well-formed cell junctions. The cytoplasm contains a mixture of organelles and may have small amounts of glycogen and lipid. Some tumors have features reminiscent of the loop of Henle (236,284).

Renal Cell Carcinoma, Medullary Type

Definition. Medullary RCC is a distinctive clinicopathologic entity that apparently occurs exclusively in patients with the sickle cell hemoglobinopathies, almost always the sickle cell trait (17,67,89,264,295). The tumor is believed to originate in the collecting ducts but is not considered a subtype of collecting duct carcinoma

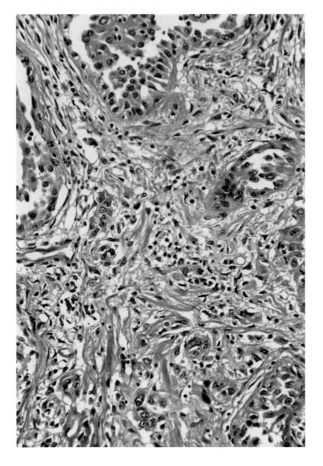

Figure 2-87

COLLECTING DUCT RENAL CELL CARCINOMA

There is striking stromal desmoplasia associated with the infiltrating carcinoma.

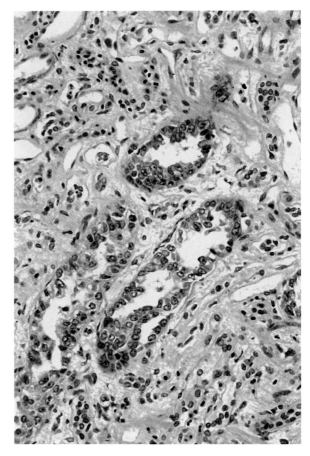

Figure 2-88

COLLECTING DUCT RENAL CELL CARCINOMA

There is dysplasia (carcinoma in situ) of collecting ducts away from the tumor.

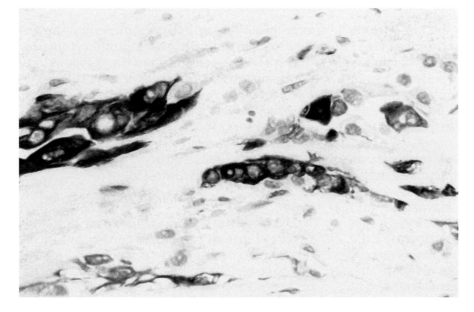

Figure 2-89

COLLECTING DUCT RENAL CELL CARCINOMA

Immunohistochemical stain for high molecular weight cytokeratin (clone 34ßE12) shows strong cytoplasmic reactivity.

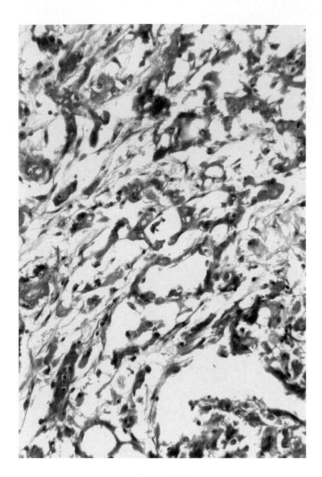

Figure 2-90

MEDULLARY RENAL CELL CARCINOMA

The yolk sac tumor-like appearance is present in many of these cases.

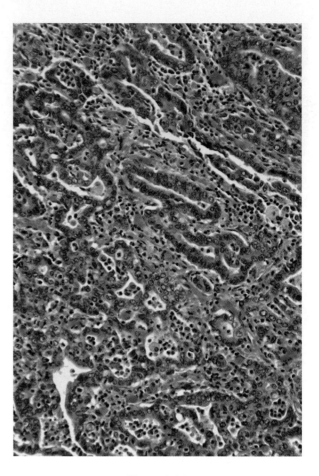

Figure 2-91

MEDULLARY RENAL CELL CARCINOMA

The tumor is forming tubules, some of which are fused. The neutrophils are abundant. (Courtesy of Dr. Volkan Adsay, Detroit, MI.)

in classification schemes (67,282). A *BRC/ABL* gene rearrangement has been described (285).

Pathologic Findings. Medullary carcinomas are typically located in the medullary region of the kidney. Recorded lesions are gray-white and infiltrative, often extending into the perihilar fat. Satellite nodules are often present in the adjacent cortex.

Histologically, the most characteristic feature is a reticular or yolk sac–like appearance (figs. 2-90–2-92). Other patterns include solid nests or tubules, or an adenoid cystic–like pattern. Infiltration by polymorphonuclear leukocytes is common. The stroma is typically desmoplastic. Mucin stains have revealed cytoplasmic mucins in approximately three quarters of lesions (67). Individual tumor cells are pleomorphic, with large nuclei containing macronucleoli and with moderate to abundant acidophilic cytoplasm (fig. 2-93). The cells may have a rhabdoid-like appearance that dominates the morphology. Cytologically, there are cohesive clusters of large epithelioid cells with abundant acidophilic cytoplasm. Nuclei have prominent nucleoli. The tumor cells are positive for cytokeratins, and variably reactive for carcinoembryonic antigens and EMA.

Cystic Changes in Renal Cell Carcinomas

Extensively cystic renal tumors are not classified as separate pathologic entities but must be discussed because they may present diagnostic challenges. Overall, cystic change occurs in up to 15 percent of RCCs (130). Radiologically,

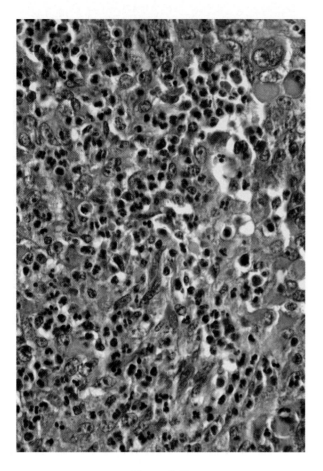

Figure 2-92

MEDULLARY RENAL CELL CARCINOMA

Solid area of a medullary carcinoma with diffuse infiltration by neutrophils. The cells in the upper left corner have a rhabdoid-like morphology.

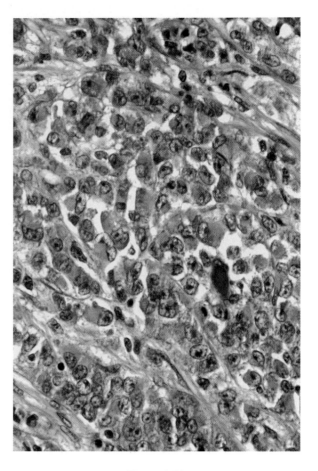

Figure 2-93

MEDULLARY RENAL CELL CARCINOMA

Many of the tumor cells in this solid area of medullary carcinoma have a distinctive rhabdoid appearance, with large acidophilic cytoplasmic inclusions and eccentric nuclei containing macronucleoli.

these tumors are classified into four categories: 1) cysts resulting from an intrinsic multilocular pattern of growth; 2) cysts resulting from an intrinsic unilocular pattern of growth; 3) cysts resulting from cystic degeneration of a previously solid tumor (fig. 2-94); and 4) cystic RCC originating in a preexisting, benign cyst (130). It is important to separate multilocular cystic RCC from this group, due to the distinctive clinicopathologic characteristics of these tumors.

In cases resulting from cystic necrosis of a previously solid tumor, the cysts may contain old and recent hemorrhage as well as necrotic tissue. The cyst wall may be thickened and irregular, reminiscent of the papillary type of RCC (fig. 2-95). Other tumors may be composed of cysts that mimic a multilocular cystic RCC or a multilocular cyst (fig. 2-96). These cases may be the most problematic because an epithelial lining is often absent in many if not all of the cysts. As a general rule, malignancy should be suspected when any cystic mass in the kidney contains hemorrhagic or necrotic material, and extensive sampling is warranted if necessary (figs. 2-97, 2-98). In such cases, identifiable tumor may be scant and the identification of any clear cell or papillary areas indicates the presence of a malignancy. RCCs may arise in preexisting, histologically benign cysts in the kidney (fig. 2-99) (185,268). The presence of extensive cystic necrosis has been reported to be associated with a poorer prognosis (35).

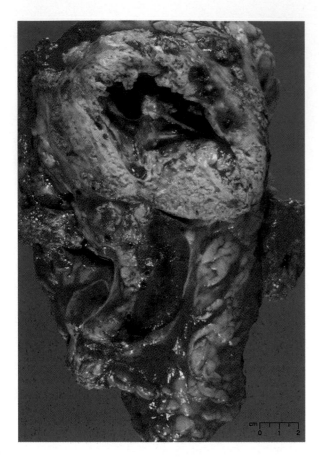

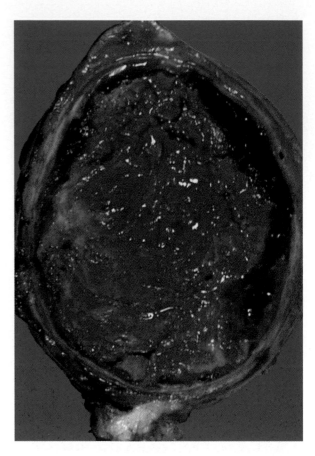

Figure 2-94

CYSTIC RENAL CELL CARCINOMA

There is cystic change in part of this large necrotic clear cell renal cell carcinoma. Diagnosis is not a problem.

Figure 2-95

CYSTIC RENAL CELL CARCINOMA

This papillary renal cell carcinoma has central necrosis and a residual thickened fibrotic wall. No viable tumor is present within the necrotic debris.

Figure 2-96

CYSTIC RENAL CELL CARCINOMA

This cystic variant has a thick wall that contains clear cell carcinoma.

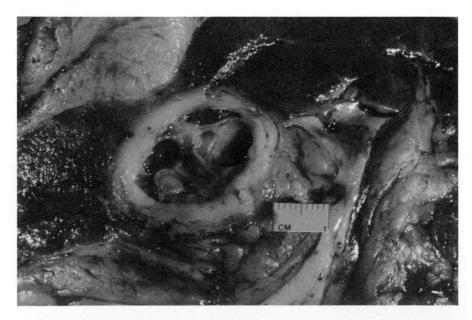

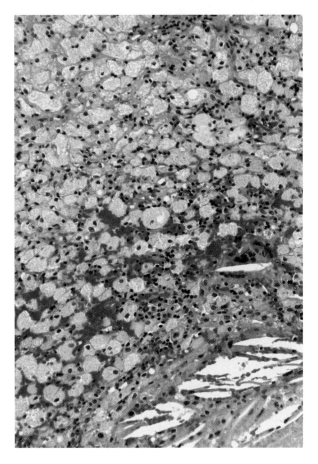

Figure 2-97

CYSTIC RENAL CELL CARCINOMA

The wall of this cystic renal cell carcinoma contains numerous foamy macrophages, inflammatory cells, and cholesterol clefts. (Figures 2-97 and 2-98 are from the same patient.)

Renal Cell Carcinoma, Sarcomatoid Type

Foci of high-grade spindle cells, often reminiscent of a malignant fibrous histiocytoma, can occur in all histologic subtypes of RCC and current classifications do not recognize tumors with these features as a distinctive subtype (77). Nevertheless, the presence of a sarcomatoid component in a RCC is widely considered to be a poor prognostic sign and has sufficient patient care implications to warrant inclusion in the diagnosis. The amount of sarcomatoid histology required for diagnosis has not been defined but the suggestion that the sarcomatoid area comprise at least one low-power (4X) field seems reasonable (238).

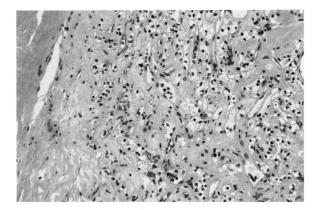

Figure 2-98

CYSTIC RENAL CELL CARCINOMA

Within the fibrous tissue of the wall are small clusters of clear cell renal cell carcinoma.

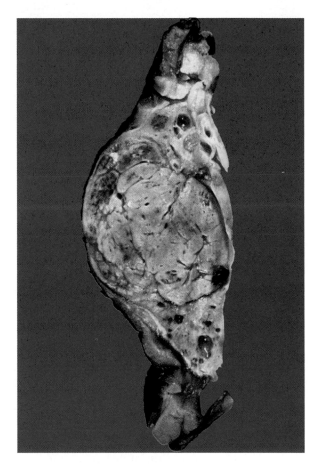

Figure 2-99

CLEAR CELL RENAL CELL CARCINOMA

This clear cell renal cell carcinoma is arising within a preexisting cyst. In this case the underlying disease is acquired cystic kidney disease.

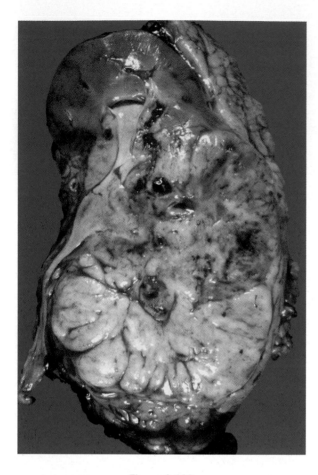

Figure 2-100

SARCOMATOID RENAL CELL CARCINOMA

This large renal cell carcinoma has a predominantly sarcomatoid growth pattern. This corresponds to the bulging, lobulated, gray-white areas seen grossly.

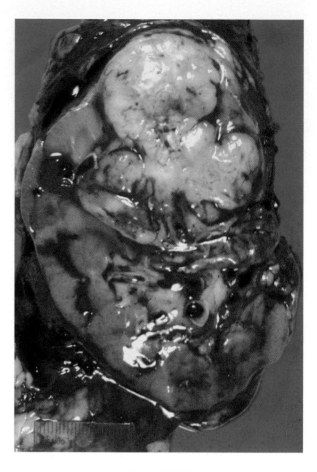

Figure 2-101

SARCOMATOID RENAL CELL CARCINOMA

This sarcomatoid renal cell carcinoma has a bulging, lobulated, pale gray-white cut surface.

Sarcomatoid areas are present in 1.0 to 6.5 percent of RCCs (27,79,154,238). The tumor may be almost entirely sarcomatoid but these neoplasms are classified among the carcinomas because of the invariable presence of histologic, immunohistochemical, or ultrastructural features of epithelial differentiation. The proportion of sarcomatous and carcinomatous differentiation in any particular tumor may vary but the greater the proportion of the sarcomatoid component, the worse the prognosis (192,262). The carcinomatous component in a sarcomatoid tumor is poorly differentiated in a significant number of cases and may be difficult to classify. In many cases, a sarcomatoid histology is associated with clear cell RCC, but it has also been documented in papillary, chro-

mophobe, collecting duct, and unclassified RCCs (5,18,58,92). A few reported tumors have manifested areas of chondrosarcoma and osteosarcoma. Such tumors could be designated carcinosarcoma (79,189,214) but there seems no compelling reason to consider them an entity other than sarcomatoid carcinoma with heterologous elements.

Pathologic Findings. Grossly, the sarcomatoid type of RCC is large and invasive; the inconspicuous lesions that present with large metastases are distinctly unusual (figs. 2-100, 2-101). Depending upon the relative proportions of sarcomatous and carcinomatous elements, the sarcomatoid type may present a bimorphic macroscopic appearance or may be firm and fibrous without hemorrhage and necrosis. The presence

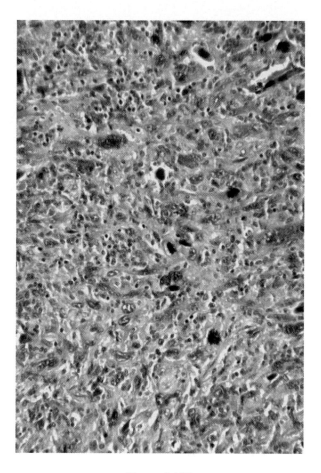

Figure 2-102

SARCOMATOID RENAL CELL CARCINOMA

The sarcomatoid component of this tumor has a poorly defined storiform architecture that results in a malignant fibrous histiocytoma-like appearance.

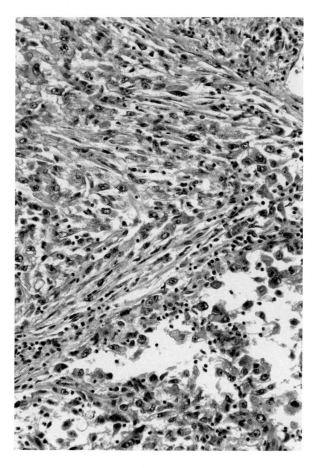

Figure 2-103

SARCOMATOID RENAL CELL CARCINOMA

Sarcomatoid clear cell renal cell carcinoma with high-grade spindle cells is adjacent to the epithelial component (bottom).

of a bulging, lobulated, soft, gray-white, fleshy component should alert the prosector to the possibility of a sarcomatoid element.

Histologically, the sarcomatoid component is characterized by interlacing or whorled bundles of spindle cells, sometimes in a storiform pattern (figs. 2-102–2-106) (262,305). Carcinomatous components may be distinctly separate from the spindled component and have a clear cell, chromophobe cell, and even papillary or collecting duct morphology. In some cases, there may be transition zones from carcinoma to sarcomatoid areas. Many tumors resemble malignant fibrous histiocytomas, but patterns mimicking leiomyosarcoma, fibrosarcoma, angiosarcoma, rhabdomyosarcoma, and hemangiopericytoma have also been recorded. Ultrastructural stud-

ies in some cases demonstrate desmosomal junctions among the spindle cells (68).

The most characteristic cytologic change in sarcomatoid RCC is the presence of cells of the malignant spindle cell component. These cells have marked nuclear pleomorphism and prominent nucleoli (15,256).

Immunohistochemical Findings. Not surprisingly, considerable heterogeneity is observed using histochemical and immunohistochemical techniques. Some tumors react with antibodies to cytokeratins in both the sarcomatous and carcinomatous components (fig. 2-107) (73). Immunoreactivity to desmin and smooth muscle myosin is rarely observed among the spindle cells. Plumper elements, which may represent transition forms between carcinoma and

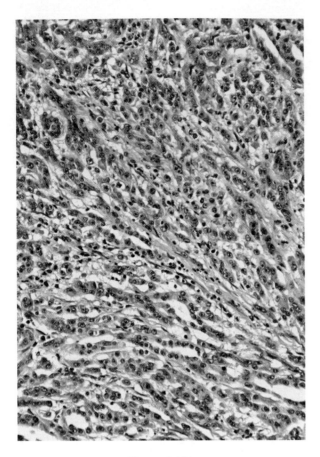

Figure 2-104

SARCOMATOID RENAL CELL CARCINOMA

Collecting duct carcinoma with an area of sarcomatoid differentiation indicated by poorly formed fascicles of spindle-shaped cells.

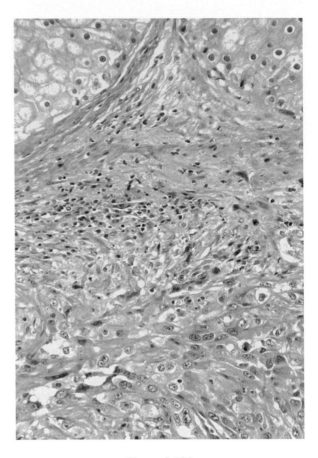

Figure 2-105

SARCOMATOID RENAL CELL CARCINOMA

Chromophobe renal cell carcinoma with sarcomatoid change. The classic chromophobe cell carcinoma element is present at the top of the figure. (Courtesy of Dr. John Eble, Indianapolis, IN.)

Figure 2-106

SARCOMATOID RENAL CELL CARCINOMA

This sarcomatoid clear cell renal cell carcinoma shows nests of clear cell carcinoma admixed with sarcomatoid elements.

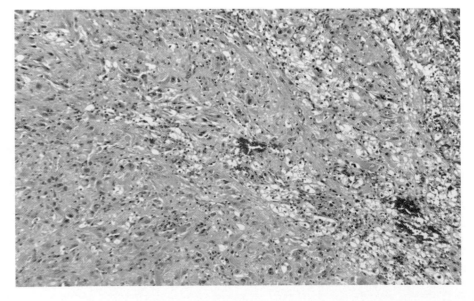

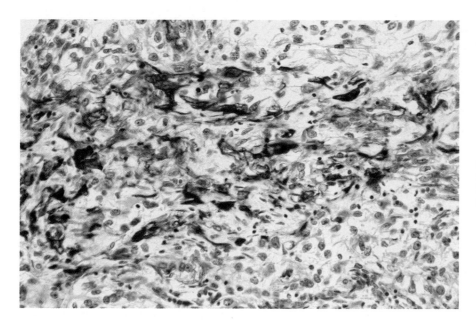

Figure 2-107

**SARCOMATOID RENAL
CELL CARCINOMA**

Sarcomatoid clear cell renal cell carcinoma shows focal immunohistochemical staining for cytokeratins within the spindle cell element.

sarcoma, react with antibodies to EMA. The RCC marker is positive in the epithelial component, but not in the sarcomatoid foci (203).

Mucinous Tubular and Spindle Cell Renal Carcinoma

Definition. A less common pattern of RCC that is postulated to be of collecting duct and possibly loop of Henle origin occurs predominantly in females (133a,236,248,284). Most tumors are single, although multifocality has been described. Despite the designation "carcinoma," these tumors are not associated with malignant behavior, although information is limited.

Pathologic Findings. Grossly, mucinous tubular and spindle cell tumors are solid, pale tan to yellow to gray-white lesions that may have slight focal areas of necrosis or hemorrhage (fig. 2-108). Histologically, they manifest elongated branching tubules in a bubbly myxoid stroma (figs. 2-109–2-111). The collapsed tubules result in a cord-like pattern and spindle cell areas are also present. The tubules are striking, with characteristic long profiles. The basal lamina, around the tubules, is highlighted with the PAS stain. The cells are cuboidal, with scant, clear to pale, acidophilic cytoplasm and low-grade nuclear features. The background is mucinous with basophilia and a characteristic bubbly appearance.

Immunohistochemical Findings. The results of immunohistochemical studies vary widely, but most tumors express cytokeratins 18 and 19, and EMA (248). Cytogenetic studies demonstrate consistent losses involving chromosomes 1, 4, 6, 8, 9, 13, 14, 15, and 22, supporting the view that this lesion is a distinctive entity.

Renal Cell Carcinoma, Unclassified

For approximately 6 to 7 percent of epithelial kidney tumors, classification into one of the categories defined above is extremely difficult (figs. 2-112, 2-113) (77,165,289). In most cases, the tumors are not undifferentiated but have features that would fit into more than one category of classification. This includes lesions with a well-defined differential diagnosis, but where a definitive conclusion cannot be reached. The most frequent problems in classification include: 1) separation of oncocytoma from chromophobe RCC; 2) distinction of papillary RCC from clear cell RCC with pseudopapillary areas; and 3) distinction of clear cell RCC from chromophobe RCC (257).

Another large group of difficult-to-classify tumors are high-grade carcinomas or sarcomatoid carcinomas in which the epithelial element cannot be recognized or classified (fig. 2-114). In sarcomatoid carcinomas, there may be no identifiable epithelial element, and the diagnosis is then based on immunohistochemical or ultrastructural evidence of epithelial derivation. Tumors in these groups are associated with an aggressive clinical course (8,328). Additionally,

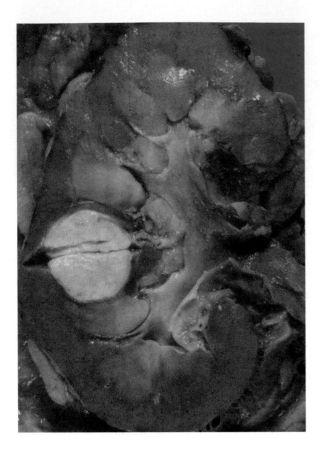

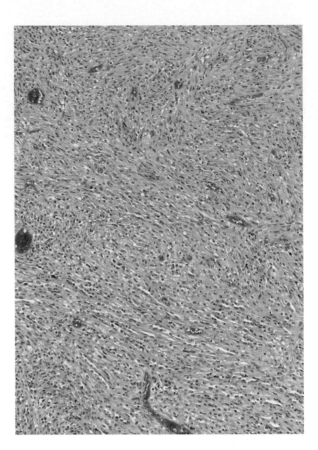

Figure 2-108

**MUCINOUS TUBULAR AND
SPINDLE CELL RENAL CARCINOMA**

The tumor is well circumscribed, gray-white, with a glistening cut surface and is located in the medullary region.

Figure 2-109

**MUCINOUS TUBULAR AND
SPINDLE CELL RENAL CARCINOMA**

In this example the tumor cells are forming collapsed tubules, resulting in a spindle-shaped appearance.

Figure 2-110

**MUCINOUS TUBULAR
AND SPINDLE
CELL RENAL CARCINOMA**

Higher-power magnification of the tumor in figure 2-109 shows the relative low-grade cytology. The basement membrane separating the collapsed tubules from each other can be appreciated as basophilic lines running between cords of cells.

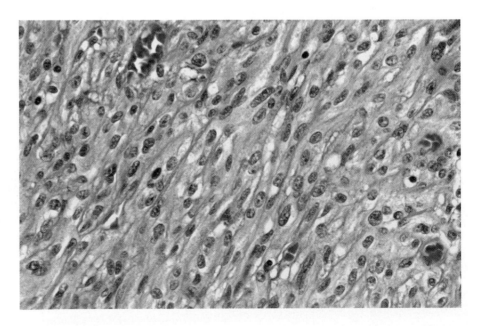

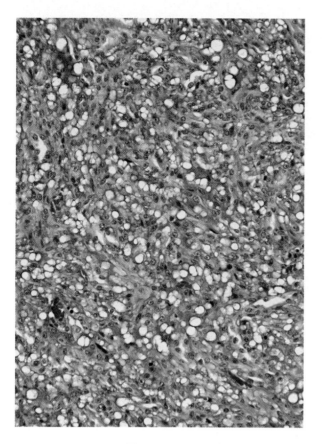

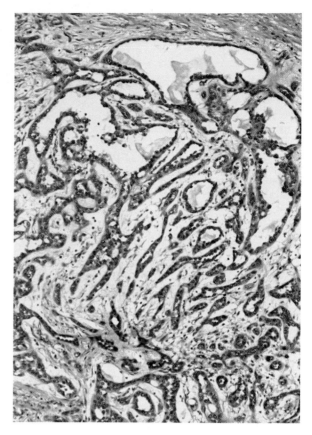

Figure 2-111

**MUCINOUS TUBULAR AND
SPINDLE CELL RENAL CARCINOMA**

This tumor is associated with abundant extracellular acidic mucin that has a bubbly basophilic appearance when stained with hematoxylin and eosin.

Figure 2-112

UNCLASSIFIED RENAL CELL CARCINOMA

In this unusual renal tumor, there is an adenoid cystic-like pattern, with infiltrating tubules and cords of cells in a basophilic stroma.

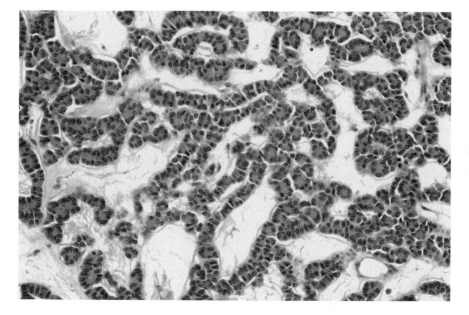

Figure 2-113

**UNCLASSIFIED RENAL
CELL CARCINOMA**

In this tumor, the neoplastic cells are arranged in narrow trabeculae growing in a serpiginous fashion.

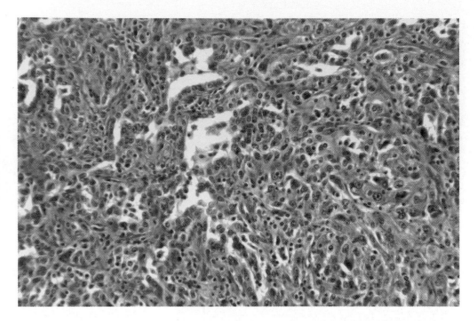

Figure 2-114

UNCLASSIFIED RENAL CELL CARCINOMA

In this high-grade epithelial neoplasm, there are some features that suggest the possibility of either collecting duct or papillary type, however, no characteristic features of either tumor type are present.

carcinomas that produce mucin, have mixtures of epithelial and stromal elements, or have unrecognizable cell types, not otherwise specified, are included here.

Patients with unclassifiable renal tumors may not necessarily have an uncertain prognosis. The poorly differentiated and sarcomatoid carcinomas are predictably aggressive, whether or not they are included in a category of sarcomatoid RCC. Localized tumors lacking significant nuclear atypia are best considered to be low-grade malignancies. For other unusual tumors, pathologic features such as size, stage, and nuclear grade, provide important clues to likely future events.

Grading of Renal Cell Carcinomas

With the exception of stage, nuclear grade is the most important prognostic feature of a RCC (41,48,80,91,112,117,129,132,186,280,283,330); its prognostic value has been validated in numerous studies over the past eight decades. Recent reports have supported its value for patients with papillary and chromophobe as well as clear cell RCCs (49,186). The preferred formulation is that of Fuhrman (91); the characteristics of the four groups of the Fuhrman system for classification by nuclear grade are detailed in Table 2-3. Mitotic activity is absent or rare in grades 1 and 2 tumors; mitoses are usually readily identified in grades 3 and 4 tumors. The majority of renal tumors are nuclear grades 2 and 3; grade 1

tumors are less common and grade 4 tumors account for only 5 to 10 percent of cases. The relatively small differences in nuclear size that separate nuclear grades in the Fuhrman system are often difficult to discern, and in practice most pathologists rely on the presence and relative size of nucleoli as well as the granularity of chromatin to assess grade. The quality of the specimen is important for accurate grading, since nucleoli and nuclear chromatin can be easily obscured in poorly preserved preparations.

Using the 10X objective, grade 1 nuclei are small and dense (like mature lymphocytes), with no nucleoli and little detail in the chromatin (fig. 2-115). Grade 2 nuclei have finely granular, "open" chromatin but inconspicuous nucleoli at this magnification. Nucleoli are often present, and may appear as small chromocenters at 10X. Importantly, nucleoli that can be confirmed only at the 40X magnification are not large enough to qualify for grade 3 (fig. 2-116). For nuclear grade 3, the nucleoli must be easily discerned and recognized as unequivocal at 10X (fig. 2-117). Grade 4 nuclei are characterized by nuclear pleomorphism, hyperchromasia, and single to multiple macronucleoli (fig. 2-118).

One issue in the application of the Fuhrman system concerns the heterogeneity of grade within a single tumor (fig. 2-119) (280). Most experts accept the worst grade approach: the worst grade is defined by the most abnormal

Table 2-3

FUHRMAN NUCLEAR GRADING SYSTEM

Grade	Nuclear Size	Nuclear Shape	Chromatin	Nucleoli
1	< 10 µm	Round	Dense	Inconspicuous
2	15 µm	Round	Finely granular	Small, not visible with 10X objective
3	20 µm	Round/oval	Coarsely granular	Prominent
4	> 20 µm	Pleomorphic, multilobated	Open, hyperchromatic	Macronucleoli

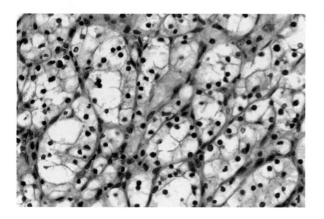

Figure 2-115

CLEAR CELL RENAL CELL CARCINOMA, FUHRMAN NUCLEAR GRADE 1

The nuclei are small, uniform, and have hyperchromatic chromatin.

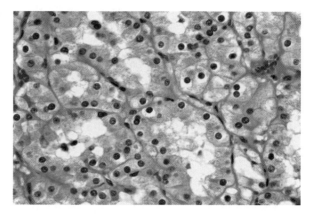

Figure 2-116

CLEAR CELL RENAL CELL CARCINOMA, FUHRMAN NUCLEAR GRADE 2

The nuclei are larger than in nuclear grade 1, with open chromatin and inconspicuous nucleoli that are only visible at high magnification.

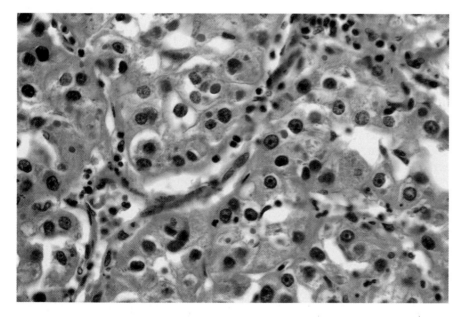

Figure 2-117

CLEAR CELL RENAL CELL CARCINOMA, FUHRMAN NUCLEAR GRADE 3

The nuclei are large and uniform, with open chromatin and prominent nucleoli visible even at low magnification.

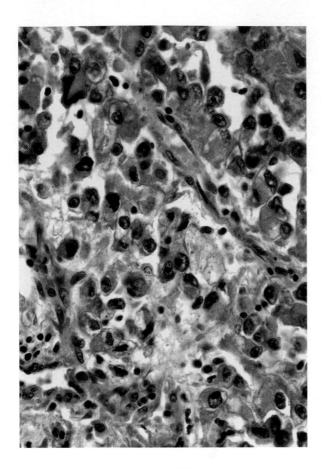

Figure 2-118

CLEAR CELL RENAL CELL CARCINOMA, FUHRMAN NUCLEAR GRADE 4

The tumor nuclei are markedly enlarged, with macronucleoli, irregular nuclear shapes, and pleomorphism.

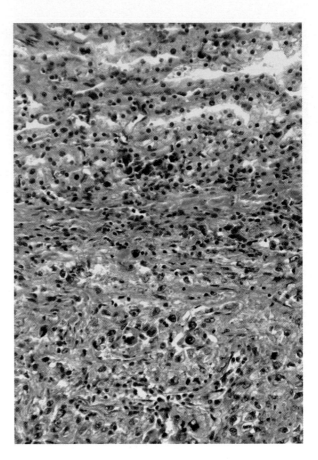

Figure 2-119

CLEAR CELL RENAL CELL CARCINOMA WITH GRADE HETEROGENEITY

There is nuclear grade 2 renal cell carcinoma on the top admixed with nuclear grade 4 renal cell carcinoma on the bottom.

nuclei occupying one high-power field (186). Scattered cells may be discounted, but if several cells within the single focus have the characteristics of the higher grade, then the tumor should be graded accordingly. In contemporary series, the 10-year disease-specific survival rates for patients with nuclear grades 1, 2, 3, and 4 are in the range of 88 to 90 percent, 75 to 82 percent, 40 percent, and 18 percent, respectively (80,197).

Information concerning the biologic behavior of RCCs is weighted toward the clear cell type, since this type comprises 70 percent of renal neoplasms. RCCs grow by direct extension, slowly compressing the adjacent kidney and attenuating the overlying capsule. Historically, most tumors have been large at the time of detection and less than half have been confined to the kidney (26,44). Of those tumors detected before the widespread application of modern imaging techniques, 7 percent were locally invasive, 35 percent metastatic to regional lymph nodes, and 25 percent disseminated. RCCs tend to grow into and propagate along the renal vein (figs. 2-120, 2-121) (44,108,134,202,222). In the past, this phenomenon was common and many cases of vena caval and even right atrial involvement by propagating RCC were observed. Such extensive involvement of the venous system was associated with a significant reduction in patient survival. More recently, intrarenal vein involvement is documented in approximately 16 percent of cases while involvement of the main extrarenal vein and propagation into the vena cava is noted in 8 percent and 7 percent of cases, respectively.

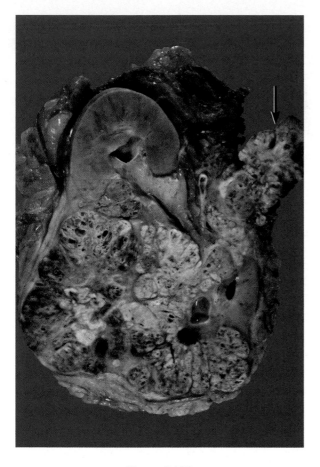

Figure 2-120

RENAL CELL CARCINOMA

This large clear cell renal cell carcinoma has grown into the renal vein (arrow).

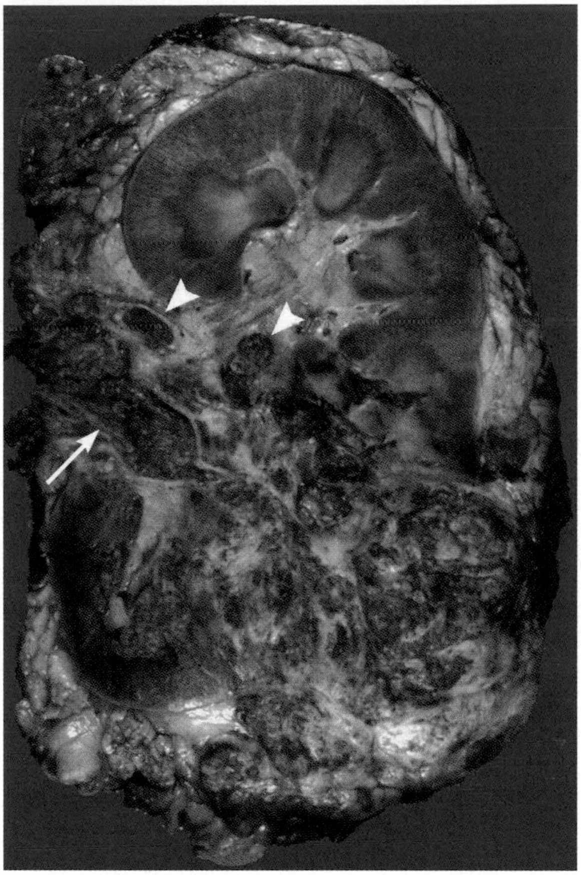

Figure 2-121

RENAL CELL CARCINOMA

A large clear cell renal cell carcinoma with extensive involvement of the main renal vein (arrow) and renal vein tributaries (arrowheads) in the region of the hilum.

When metastases occur, the lung is involved in 55 percent of cases. Other organs are affected in the following descending order of frequency: lymph nodes, liver, bone, adrenal gland, kidney, brain, heart, spleen, intestine, and skin. Compared to other cancers, kidney tumors have a predilection for metastasizing to bone and skin, and metastases to unusual sites are common (26,63,65,113,208,234,302,309).

Prognosis

The prognosis of patients with RCC is influenced by multiple factors, including nuclear grade, tumor size, infiltrative margin, and histologic type, but tumor stage is the most important determinant of outcome (100,283). The clinical features considered to be of proven prognostic significance include clinical stage, symptomatic presentation, weight loss of greater than 10 percent of body weight, Eastern Cooperative Oncology Group performance status of 2 to 3, erythrocyte sedimentation rate greater than 30, hemoglobin of less than 10 g/dL for women and less than 12 g/dL for men, hypercalcemia, and increased alkaline phosphatase level (283). Not all factors are of equal significance and only a few can be considered to have independent significance statistically. Even so, the importance of prognostic factors for renal neoplasms is mitigated by the extremely limited treatment options (essentially surgical excision) as well as the inability to apply the information to the future course for any particular patient.

In general, large carcinomas are more likely to be invasive and metastatic than small lesions. The importance of size is indicated by its inclusion in the American Joint Committee on Cancer (AJCC)/TNM staging system (7,159). An infiltrative margin is an adverse prognostic sign (13,296). A sarcomatoid morphology is associated with an aggressive clinical course, and the greater the proportion of this element, the worse the prognosis (192,262). The presence of necrosis, with or without cystic change, is associated with decreased survival (35,88,180). Lymph node metastases are often microscopic, but have a significant impact upon survival (263,279).

The prognosis can be expressed in terms of histologic subtype, but the effect of subtype is mitigated by its association with grade and stage (8,13,25,30,49,156,206,296,301,305). The histologic type of RCC is included in a postoperative nomogram developed for predicting recurrence (153). The clear cell type is the most common and also the most variable as to stage and grade. The overall survival rate after nephrectomy is 50 percent. The prognosis of patients with the papillary type is significantly better than that for the clear cell type, but the difference is probably because of the lower grade and stage of these tumors at the time of detection (9,49,72,146,229). Still, papillary RCCs have a propensity for late recurrence and metastasis. Although hereditary papillary RCC is associated with low-grade histology, there is a 15 to 26 percent risk of metastases (272). Similar to the papillary type, the chromophobe cell type tends to be localized to the kidney and of nuclear grade 2 at presentation, factors that probably explain its more favorable outlook. In over 300 patients with the chromophobe cell type, only 22 died of disease (2,4,8,32,49,62,255,301). A significant proportion of patients with aggressive chromophobe RCC have tumors with sarcomatoid change (230,255). The classic collecting duct type of RCC is highly aggressive, with more than 50 percent of reported patients dying of disease within 2 years of diagnosis, but it is also a high-grade tumor (43,156). Patients with the lower-grade variants of collecting duct carcinoma have a much better prognosis (190, 236). The medullary type of RCC is both of high grade and stage at diagnosis, and has been almost uniformly fatal, with most patients dead within 1 year of detection (17,81,89,240). The sarcomatoid type, high grade by definition, is highly aggressive regardless of the associated histologic type of RCC; few patients survive long term (192,209,238,262).

Gross invasion of the renal vein by RCC defines category pT3b in the AJCC staging system (7). Patients with gross invasion of the renal vein, and even the vena cava, can survive long term (108,134). The presence of invasion of the renal or vena caval wall is associated with decreased survival in these patients. In many tumors, the presence of microscopic invasion of endothelial-lined spaces is an accepted significant prognostic parameter. Studies on microscopic vascular invasion and its prognostic significance in patients with RCC are limited (115, 276,313), but they suggest that microvascular invasion may be an independent prognostic parameter in localized RCC.

Differential Diagnosis of Renal Cell Carcinoma

Differentiating RCCs from other neoplasms is usually not a diagnostic problem. In those cases where this distinction is problematic, clinical information and certain pathologic characteristics may be useful. The features of the subtypes of RCC are detailed in the previous sections. The RCC marker has been found to be relatively specific for this neoplasm (203). Difficulties arise primarily when tumors are small, papillary, oncocytic, collecting duct type, sarcomatoid type, or metastatic.

Small RCCs can be distinguished from adenomas by their size, pattern, cytoplasmic features, growth, and nuclear anaplasia. All clear cell, chromophobe cell, and collecting duct tumors should be considered carcinomas regardless of their size at diagnosis. Papillary and tubular lesions may represent true adenomas if they lack nuclear anaplasia and are low nuclear grade (1 and 2). According to current criteria, an adenoma should be less than 0.5 cm in greatest dimension; most such lesions have been incidental findings in the past.

When oncocytic cells predominate in a RCC of clear or chromophobe cell type, the tumor must be differentiated from an oncocytoma (Table 2-4). The organoid pattern of an oncocytoma, particularly the presence of nests of cells in a loose fibrous stroma, is characteristic. The

Table 2-4

PATHOLOGIC FEATURES OF ONCOCYTOMA VERSUS CHROMOPHOBE CELL RENAL CELL CARCINOMA

Feature	Oncocytoma	Chromophobe Cell RCC[a] – Eosinophilic Type
Gross appearance	"Mahogany" brown; +/- central scar	Pale tan-brown; +/- zones of necrosis
Architecture	Closely packed nests (periphery) and nests in loose hypocellular stroma; no trabeculae/sheets; +/- tubule formation	Closely packed nests and occasional streaming of cells in myxoid stroma; +/- broad trabeculae/sheets; +/- tubule formation
Nuclear features	Uniform, round; degenerative pleomorphism	Uniform, round, +/- raisinoid; pleomorphism only in high grade
Mitoses	None to rare	Occasional
Cytoplasm	Granular, acidophilic; clearing can be seen	Granular, acidophilic with perinuclear halos; plant-like cells focally in most
Hale's colloidal iron	Negative except at luminal surface in tubular areas	Strongly positive, diffuse
Cytokeratin	Positive; CK7 – strongly positive isolated cells in some	Positive; CK7 – diffusely positive in most
Vimentin	Negative	Negative
Ultrastructure	Numerous mitochondria with lamellar cristae; no microvesicles	Numerous mitochondria with tubulovesicular cristae; interspersed microvesicles

[a]RCC = renal cell carcinoma; CK = cytokeratin.

absence of nuclear anaplasia in these lesions is also important. Oncocytomas may contain areas of nuclear pleomorphism and occasional foci with very large nuclei, but large nucleoli and mitoses are lacking.

Collecting duct carcinomas can be distinguished from the papillary type of RCC by their location, architecture, antigenic expression, and even karyotypic composition. Although infrequent, certain cases have exhibited some urothelial cell–like foci; they differ from urothelial (transitional cell) carcinomas with collecting duct involvement by their architecture. Tumors with mixed urothelial cell and collecting duct features have been described (3).

Most predominantly spindle cell malignant renal neoplasms are sarcomatoid carcinomas rather than purely mesenchymal tumors. Careful microscopic examination of generously sampled lesions almost always reveals foci of epithelial differentiation. Electron microscopy and immunohistochemistry are helpful in selected cases. Spindle cell renal tumors manifesting chondrosarcomatous or osteosarcomatous elements, with or without carcinomatous foci, are designated carcinosarcomas by some, although there is no evidence that these tumors behave

differently from sarcomatoid RCCs without heterologous elements.

Adrenal cortical neoplasms can cause diagnostic difficulty with RCCs. Ipsilateral adrenal metastases are found incidentally in 3 to 4 percent of nephrectomy specimens and incidental adrenal cortical adenomas have also been recorded. This differential diagnosis is particularly problematic when a low-grade clear cell RCC is present in the kidney. Useful features for differentiation are highlighted in Tables 2-5 and 2-6 (38,96,201,274,319).

Rarely, RCCs are confused with metastases to the kidney. The identification of mucopolysaccharides in such cases is diagnostic of a metastasis whereas the simultaneous presence of intracellular glycogen and lipid confirms a RCC. Metastases from RCCs, in contrast, may be extremely difficult to interpret in usual histologic preparations. Radiologic coimaging of the kidney may be necessary to clarify the situation in any particular case. Metastases from sarcomatoid RCC have been confused with primary malignant fibrous histiocytoma of bone; metastatic papillary RCC has been misinterpreted as primary thyroid carcinoma; and metastatic clear cell RCC has been difficult to distinguish

Table 2-5
ADRENAL CORTICAL ADENOMA VERSUS RENAL CELL CARCINOMA: COMPARISON OF PATHOLOGIC FEATURES

Feature	Adrenal Cortical Adenoma	Renal Cell Carcinoma
Number	Usually single; multiple if nodular hyperplasia	Often single; multiple favors metastases
Architecture	Usually nests and alveoli; spindle cell pattern rarely	Nests and alveoli – also tubules, microcysts with proteinaceous fluid or red blood cells
Vasculature	Sinusoidal	Sinusoidal
Nuclei	Usually uniform, round; intranuclear inclusions; bizarre nuclei	Uniform, round; intranuclear inclusions; no bizarre nuclei (except in grade 4 where diagnosis would not be difficult)
Nucleoli	Variable – can be prominent	Depends on grade – low grade, small inconspicuous; high grade, large
Mitoses	None (rare)	Variable – depends on grade
Cytoplasm	Variable clear to acidophilic; cytoplasm is usually fine and microvesicular; acidophilic, may be quite dense	Clear – more water clear than microvesicular although latter can be seen; acidophilic in higher grade, not as dense

Table 2-6
ADRENAL CORTICAL NEOPLASMS VERSUS RENAL CELL CARCINOMA: IMMUNOHISTOCHEMICAL FEATURES

Marker	Adrenal Cortical Neoplasm	Renal Cell Carcinoma (Clear Cell)
Cytokeratin (pan)	Negative (focal weak positivity may be seen)	Positive
CK 7[a]	Negative	Negative
CK 20	Negative	Negative
Inhibin	Positive	Negative
Vimentin	Positive	Positive
Epithelial membrane antigen	Negative	Positive
Melan A (A103)	Positive	Negative
RCC antigen	Negative	Positive

[a]CK = cytokeratin; RCC = renal cell carcinoma.

from certain primary skin and lung tumors. Demonstration of lipid and glycogen without mucopolysaccharides in the cells of such tumors is extremely helpful in confirming a renal origin. Rarely, metastatic RCC may be impossible to distinguish from cerebellar hemangioblastoma. As a rule of thumb, any renal tumor so unusual as to lack features of a known subtype should be considered a metastasis until proven otherwise.

Special Techniques for Diagnosis of Renal Cell Carcinoma

The literature contains an extensive array of special techniques applied to RCC for the purposes of diagnosis and prognosis. To date, those helping in the differential diagnosis have enjoyed more widespread application than those indicating prognosis. As detailed at the beginning of this section, cytogenetics has led the way to the development of the current classification system, and may well have a central role in further refinements. As methodologies such as fluorescent in situ hybridization (FISH) become more widely available, their applicability to differential diagnosis will become more practical. The detection of gross chromosomal anomalies, such as the monosomies characteristic of chromophobe cell carcinoma, is relatively straightforward with FISH and can be used to differentiate this tumor from oncocytoma, for example (213). For the majority of renal tumors, diagnosis is readily apparent using standard histology, and the routine use of karyotyping or molecular genetics is not indicated.

Nuclear grading is a powerful independent prognostic parameter in RCCs. Numerous studies have evaluated the applicability of image-based nuclear morphometry to improve the strength of the nuclear grade and reduce subjectivity (41,87,233,245). In general, these studies have found a variety of nuclear features, such as nuclear roundness factor, mean nuclear area, and mean nuclear perimeter, to be significant predictors of outcome. Their value as independent predictors remains uncertain. Given the limited availability of the technology as well as a variety of technical issues, the ultimate role of nuclear morphometry has yet to be defined.

Total DNA content (ploidy) is also closely related to nuclear grade. Numerous studies over the past 30 years have used image analysis and flow cytometry to determine DNA ploidy in RCCs, but correlations of DNA ploidy with outcome are inconsistent (74,117,265). In only a few studies has an outcome related to DNA ploidy been claimed to be independent of other significant parameters, and for this reason cytometry has not become a routinely applied technique.

Numerous studies of proliferation using flow cytometry and immunohistochemistry for MIB-1, Ki-67, and proliferative cell nuclear antigen (PCNA) demonstrate a fairly consistent correlation between high proliferation rate and decreased survival of patients with RCC (1,70,116, 215,261,298). The value of cellular proliferation determination as an independent parameter has not been proven, however, and its routine use is not yet accepted.

Innumerable other features of RCCs, ranging from growth factor and growth factor receptor expression to suppressor gene mutations and expression, have been studied but all remain experimental and without a defined clinical role in the diagnosis and management of RCC patients (100).

Staging of Renal Cell Carcinoma

Various staging schemes have been applied to RCCs and all have demonstrated a positive

Table 2-7

AMERICAN JOINT COMMITTEE ON CANCER TNM STAGING OF RENAL CELL CARCINOMA (2002)

Primary Tumor (T)

TX	Primary tumor cannot be assessed
T0	No evidence of primary tumor
T1a	Confined to kidney, ≤ 4.0 cm
T1b	Confined to kidney, > 4.0 cm and ≤ 7.0 cm
T2	Confined to kidney, > 7.0 cm
T3a	Tumor invades the perinephric fat or the adrenal gland but not beyond Gerota's fascia
T3b	Tumor grossly extends into the renal vein(s) or vena cava below the diaphragm
T3c	Tumor grossly extends into the renal vein(s) or vena cava above the diaphragm
T4	Tumor invades beyond Gerota's fascia

Regional Lymph Nodes (N)

NX	Regional lymph nodes cannot be assessed
N0	No regional lymph node metastases
N1	Metastasis in a single regional lymph node
N2	Metastasis in more than one regional lymph node

Distant Metastases (M)

MX	Distant metastasis cannot be assessed
M0	No distant metastasis
M1	Distant metastasis

correlation between the extent of tumor at the time of diagnosis and its future behavior (108, 205,206,263). All currently used systems divide RCCs into noninvasive, locally invasive, and metastatic categories. The TNM staging system of the AJCC is recommended (Tables 2-7, 2-8) (7). Multiple studies have confirmed the prognostic significance of this staging system (103,123,144,211,310). In one large series, the 10-year cause-specific survival rates for patients with tumors of T categories T1, T2, T3a, T3b, and T3c were 97, 84, 53, 48, and 29 percent, respectively (103). The maximum size of a RCC that correlates with behavior and should determine stage has been surprisingly controversial over the years. A greatest dimension of 4 cm seems to provide the most acceptable cutoff point (102,103,126,139,329). Application of this new cut-off has demonstrated 10-year cancer-specific survival rates of 98 and 81 percent for the T1a and T1b groups, respectively. Systematic lymphadenectomy may be valuable for staging RCCs, but there is little enthusiasm for this procedure in the surgical community and it is not usually performed.

Table 2-8

AMERICAN JOINT COMMITTEE ON CANCER
TNM STAGING OF RENAL CELL
CARCINOMA (2002): STAGE GROUPINGS

Stage I	T1a/b	N0	M0
Stage II	T2	N0	M0
Stage III	T1a/b	N1	M0
	T2	N1	M0
	T3a	N0	M0
	T3a	N1	M0
	T3b	N0	M0
	T3b	N1	M0
	T3c	N0	M0
	T3c	N1	M0
Stage IV	T4	N0	M0
	T4	N1	M0
	Any T	N2	M0
	Any T	Any N	M1

Selected features of the AJCC staging system are worth clarifying. The T3a category is defined by invasion of the perinephric adipose tissue. Renal tumors commonly bulge into the perinephric fat, but when they are surrounded by a fibrous pseudocapsule this does not represent perinephric fat invasion; demonstration of tumor cells invading the fat itself is necessary (figs. 2-122, 2-123). In marked contrast to the situation in pediatric renal tumors, involvement of renal sinus fat is not specifically addressed in the AJCC system. At least one study indicates that invasion of renal sinus fat is associated with an apparent increase in metastases compared to tumors confined to the kidney, indicating that sinus fat invasion should be included in the T3a category; the issue, however, remains unsettled (31). Adrenal gland involvement in category T3 refers to direct extension of the tumor and not to an adrenal metastasis. When adrenal gland involvement is present, direct invasion must be distinguished from hematogenous spread. For the purpose of staging, renal vein involvement is defined by the presence of a grossly visible tumor thrombus. The thrombus frequently extends beyond the apparent specimen margin of the renal vein grossly, but this should not be interpreted as a positive surgical margin since shrinkage of the vein at transection is a well-known phenomenon. In problematic cases, microscopic evaluation of the "en face" renal vein margin should be used to determine marginal involvement.

RENAL CORTICAL ADENOMA

The notion that a benign epithelial neoplasm of the kidney can be defined and clearly distinguished from a RCC has caused controversy and misunderstanding (24). All neoplasms, whether or not they have the capacity to invade and metastasize, are small at some point during their development and many publications, including Bell's original series, have documented metastases from renal tumors measuring less than 3 cm in greatest dimension (23). With the exception of oncocytoma and metanephric adenoma, it has not been possible to define an unequivocally benign renal cortical neoplasm using histologic, immunohistochemical, and ultrastructural studies (24,82,119). Nevertheless, small renal cortical epithelial neoplasms are frequently found incidentally at autopsy as well as in surgically excised kidneys. These tumors occur more frequently in kidneys scarred from chronic pyelonephritis or renal vascular disease than in normal organs. Their frequency in autopsy studies has been as high as 22 percent. Lesions are reported in children and are a feature of von Hippel-Lindau syndrome. They are usually well demarcated but unencapsulated, pale gray or pale yellow tumors arising in subcapsular portions of the kidney (fig. 2-124). Many have been identified in kidneys with RCC.

The current classification of renal epithelial tumors defines adenoma as a low-grade papillary lesion, 0.5 cm or less in greatest dimension (289). Histologically, renal cortical adenomas consist of densely packed papillae or tubules lined by small, regular, cuboidal cells with rounded, uniform nuclei that lack cytologic anaplasia (e.g., Fuhrman nuclear grades 1 and 2) (figs. 2-125–2-128). Mitoses are rare. In cases with adenomatosis, the epithelial changes may be restricted to single tubules or even partial involvement of tubules. The interface with the normal renal parenchyma ordinarily lacks inflammatory cells and there is no stromal reaction. These neoplasms may contain psammoma bodies or even xanthoma cells.

An unusual reactive process, *adenomatoid metaplasia of the epithelium of Bowman's capsule,* may mimic the changes seen in renal adenomatosis (fig. 2-129). Adenomatoid metaplasia occurs most often in patients with malignancies involving the liver (both primary and secondary) (118,250).

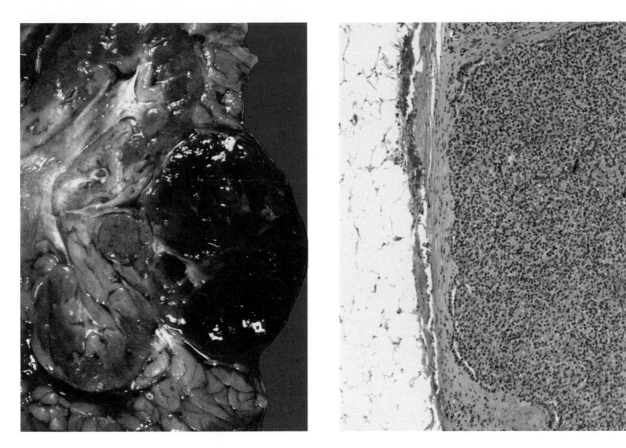

Figure 2-122

RENAL CELL CARCINOMA

Left: This hemorrhagic clear cell renal cell carcinoma is arising near the cortical surface and bulging into the perinephric fat. There is no true invasion of the adipose tissue, however, and this would be staged pT2.

Right: This papillary renal cell carcinoma is bulging into the perinephric adipose tissue but a thin layer of fibrous tissue remains, separating the tumor from the fat. This would be staged as pT2.

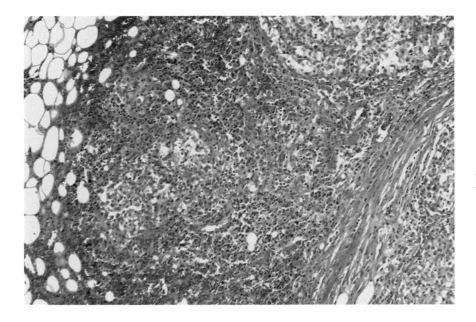

Figure 2-123

RENAL CELL CARCINOMA

Perinephric fat invasion with tumor cells within the adipose tissue (pT3a).

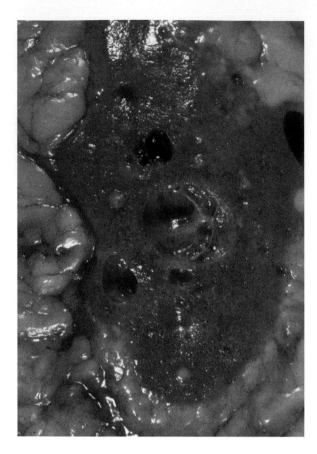

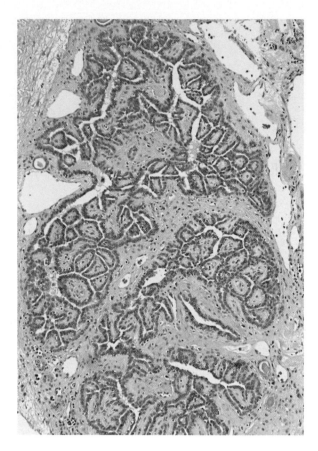

Figure 2-124

PAPILLARY ADENOMA

This kidney involved by acquired cystic kidney disease contains numerous papillary adenomas.

Figure 2-125

PAPILLARY ADENOMA

The tumor is well circumscribed but not encapsulated. Papillary structures are covered by cells having small low-grade nuclei. In this case there is fibrosis of the papillary cores.

Figure 2-126

PAPILLARY ADENOMA

This small papillary adenoma has several psammoma bodies within the central fibrovascular core.

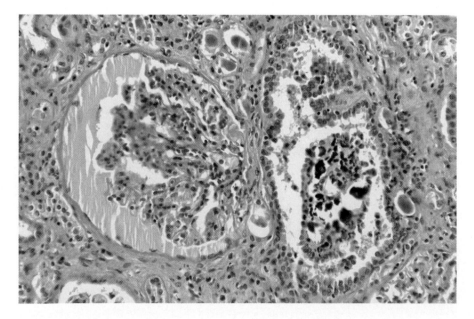

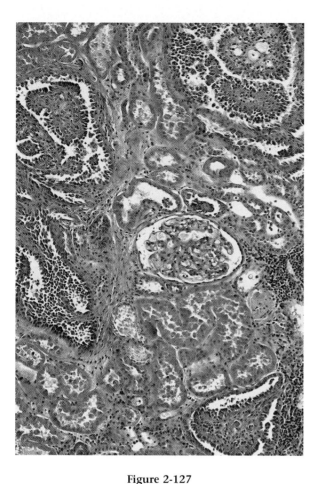

Figure 2-127

PAPILLARY ADENOMA

There are multiple papillary adenomata of varying size.

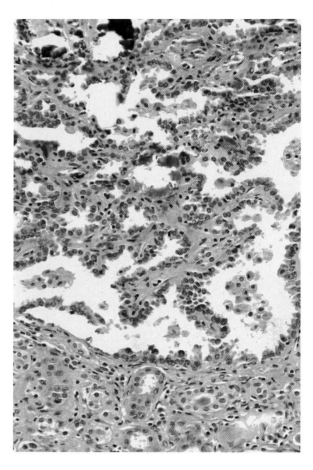

Figure 2-128

PAPILLARY ADENOMA

The interface between the papillary adenoma and the normal kidney shows lack of a capsule.

METANEPHRIC TUMORS

Metanephric renal tumors are more common in children than adults and a complete discussion of these lesions appears in the section on pediatric tumors. These tumors have been categorized according to their histology into three types: adenoma, adenofibroma, and stromal tumor. Metanephric adenofibromas and metanephric stromal tumors almost never occur in adults, so only metanephric adenomas are described in this section (12,14,131).

Metanephric Adenoma

Clinical Features. This rare lesion has been described in detail (66,98,119,149,228) and is more fully discussed in the section on pediatric renal tumors. Some cytogenetic data suggest a relationship with papillary tumors, based on the presence of trisomies 7 and 17, although this is not a consistent finding, which has been disputed recently (36,37a). Metanephric adenomas may be found at any age and occur with a 2 to 1 female predominance. Approximately 50 percent of lesions have been incidental findings, with others detected because of polycythemia, abdominal or flank pain, a mass, or hematuria. Incidental tumors may occur in association with RCC. Two cases with lymph node metastases have been recorded (75,252). In one, the metastasis was related to a papillary carcinoma component (75).

Pathologic Findings. Metanephric adenomas occur in a wide size range, with the largest reported tumor measuring 15 cm. Tumors are well circumscribed, solid or lobulated,

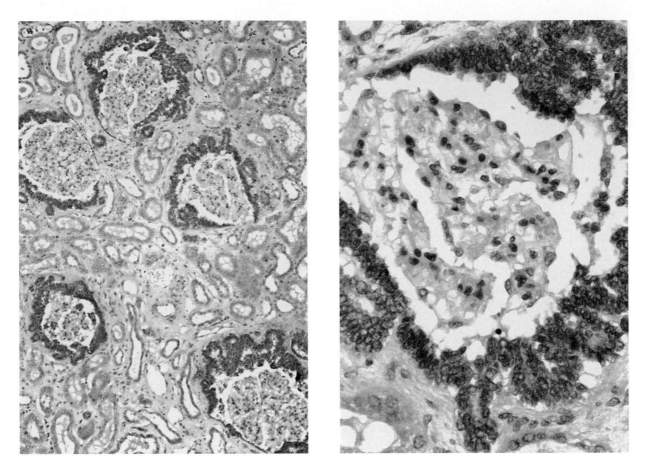

Figure 2-129

ADENOMATOID METAPLASIA OF BOWMAN'S CAPSULE

Low- (left) and high-power (right) photomicrographs illustrate the adenomatous appearance of the lining epithelium of Bowman's capsule. (Courtesy of Dr. D. Ian Turnbull, London, Ontario.)

and gray-white. Small cysts and calcifications may be present. A papillary or microcystic architecture may be present but is uncommon. Hemorrhage and calcification, including psammoma bodies, are frequent. The cells do not contain glycogen and immunohistochemical studies suggest a distal nephron or collecting duct origin (66). Histologically, metanephric adenomas are composed of small, uniform, round tubules embedded in a loose hypocellular stroma (see figs. 1-90–1-92, chapter 1). Individual cells have small, uniform nuclei with absent or inconspicuous nucleoli and scant cytoplasm. Mitoses are rare.

Differential Diagnosis. Metanephric adenoma must be distinguished from papillary RCC and adult nephroblastoma. In contrast to metanephric adenoma, papillary RCC is EMA positive and most tumors are diffusely positive for cytokeratin 7 (Table 2-9). Metanephric adenoma is also positive for WT1 and CD57 (219). Adult nephroblastoma is usually triphasic and includes a blastemal component.

ONCOCYTOMA

Definition. Oncocytomas of the kidney are benign neoplasms that are composed of cells with abundant granular acidophilic cytoplasm, reflecting the presence of numerous mitochondria. The term implies a neoplasm composed entirely of oncocytes with a uniform nested or alveolar pattern.

General and Clinical Features. The term oncocytoma has been applied to tumors arising in a variety of organs, and in many previous reports neither a homogeneous population of oncocytes nor a uniform cytologic grade has

Table 2-9

DIFFERENTIAL DIAGNOSIS OF METANEPHRIC ADENOMA

Feature	Metanephric Adenoma	Papillary Renal Cell Carcinoma	Wilms' Tumor
Age	Children to middle age	Middle to older age	Children, rarely adults
Sex (F:M)	2:1	1:3-4	1:1
Clinical	Incidental; polycythemia	Hematuria; flank pain; mass; incidental	Palpable mass; congenital anomalies
Gross	Single, circumscribed; nodular; gray-tan	Multiple in 50 percent; thick capsule; red-brown	Nodular, bulging; soft, gray-white
Microscopic	Closely packed tubules; small cells, little cytoplasm	Tubulopapillary; basophil/acidophil; foamy histiocytes	Triphasic—epithelial, mesenchymal and blastema
Special studies	Ker + (CK 7 +/–) and Vim +[a] EMA negative; WT1 positive no glycogen	Ker + (CK 7 ++) and Vim +/– EMA+++; WT1 negative glycogen +/–	Epithelium: Ker + (CK7+) and Vim-; EMA +/– WT1 positive

[a]Ker = keratin; CK = cytokeratin; Vim = vimentin; EMA = epithelial membrane antigen.

been required. Thus, when the case series of Klein and Valensi in 1976 (350) resulted in recognition of this neoplasm as a distinctive renal tumor, a certain amount of controversy regarding its histology and biologic potential arose (354,358). Over the years, the controversy has subsided, and there is now general agreement that renal oncocytomas are a homogeneous group of benign neoplasms with gross, microscopic, ultrastructural, and cytogenetic features that tend to distinguish them from other neoplasms of the kidney (365a).

The etiology of oncocytoma is obscure, but immunohistochemical evidence suggests that these neoplasms are differentiating toward the intercalated cells of collecting ducts (355,356). Cytogenetically, a mosaic pattern of normal and aberrant karyotypes is observed (341,352,373). The most common abnormalities include losses of chromosomes 1 and y, deletions from chromosome 14, and rearrangements involving chromosome 11q13 (342,343,356,357). The absence of abnormalities in chromosome 3, aberrations of which occur in the majority of RCCs of the clear cell type, has been a consistent finding in oncocytomas (335,347,356,360).

Oncocytomas account for 3 to 5 percent of kidney tumors in adults (331,336,337,356a). The majority occur in adults over age 50 (median age, 62 years), with a reported age range of 10 to 94 years. Men predominate over women in a ratio of 2-3 to 1. Nearly two thirds of tumors are detected as incidental findings, although pa-

tients may present with hematuria (gross or microscopic), flank pain, or a palpable mass (337). Factors that predispose to the development of an oncocytoma have not been identified. Oncocytoma has been described in patients with the Birt-Hogg-Dube syndrome (358a). In individual cases, oncocytomas may coexist with RCC or angiomyolipoma (337,363).

Oncocytomas are typically detected by radiography performed for an unrelated reason (358,361,371). Considering that these tumors are benign and may be small, there has been considerable interest in identifying characteristic radiographic features (358,361). Although not specific, there may be an identifiable central scar, seen with CT and MRI (figs. 2-130, 2-131) (371). Renal angiography may reveal characteristic features: a "lucent rim"; a homogeneous capillary nephrogram phase; absence of marked disarray in neoplastic vessels; and a spoke-wheel appearance of the feeding arteries (fig. 2-132).

Pathologic Findings. Renal oncocytomas nearly always occur as a homogeneous, well-circumscribed mass. Any part of either kidney may be involved and rarely, the tumor extends into the adjacent fat (332,355,356a,364). Tumors may vary considerably in size: most autopsy lesions are small (median, 2 cm) while the majority of clinical neoplasms are large (median, 6 cm). Solitary lesions are the rule; multiple unilateral or bilateral tumors are recorded in only 5 to 6 percent of cases (337,367,369). When multiplicity occurs, lesions may be microscopic as well as

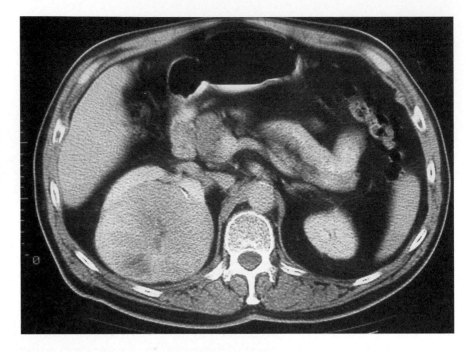

Figure 2-130

ONCOCYTOMA

Computerized tomography demonstrates a renal tumor that is circumscribed and homogeneous except for an irregular central zone which proved to be a central scar. (Fig. 1-205 from Fascicle 11, 3rd Series.)

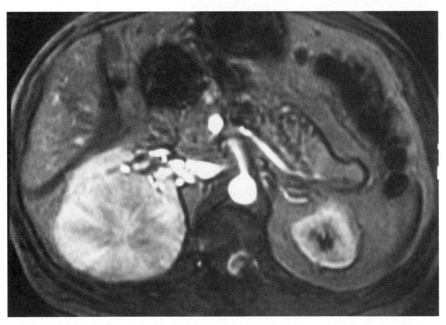

Figure 2-131

ONCOCYTOMA

This is the same tumor as illustrated in figure 2-129, examined by magnetic resonance imaging. In this image the central scar is well visualized. (Fig. 1-206 from Fascicle 11, 3rd Series.)

macroscopic, and oncocytic change may appear in adjacent tubules (349). The term *oncocytosis* is used in such cases (367,369).

Oncocytomas of the kidney are characteristically mahogany brown and have a central stellate scar, but the scar may not be well developed, especially in small lesions (figs. 2-133–2-136). The color is imparted by cytochromes in the mitochondria of the component cells and

may vary depending on the amount of pigment present in any particular tumor. In a few cases, the color of an oncocytoma varied little from that of the adjacent normal kidney. Foci of hemorrhage and cystic degeneration may be seen grossly, but necrosis is not a feature of renal oncocytomas. The gross appearance is so characteristic that many procedures intended to confirm the diagnosis are planned at the time

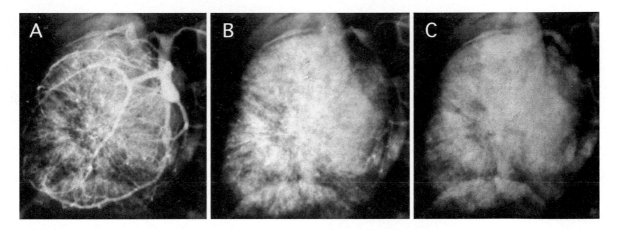

Figure 2-132

ONCOCYTOMA

A: Angiographic examination demonstrates a "spoke wheel" appearance to the tumor's arterial pattern.

B: The tumor is highly vascular without puddling of contrast media or A-V shunting.

C: The later phase demonstrates good encapsulation without venous collateral circulation. (Fig. 1 from Weiner SN, Bernstein RG. Renal oncocytoma: angiographic features of two cases. Radiology 1977;125:633–5).

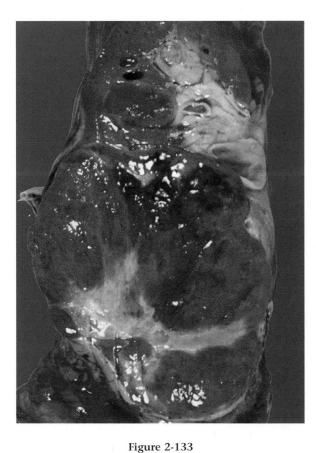

Figure 2-133

ONCOCYTOMA

This large renal oncocytoma has the characteristic dark brown color and a prominent central fibrous scar.

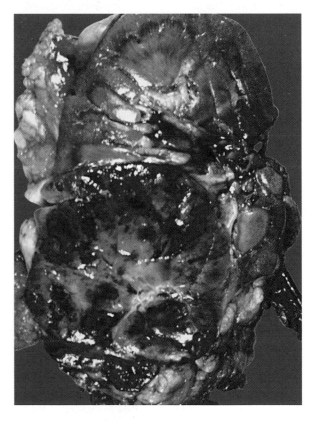

Figure 2-134

ONCOCYTOMA

This renal oncocytoma has the typical brown coloration and central scar. It is unusual in that there is focal hemorrhage present.

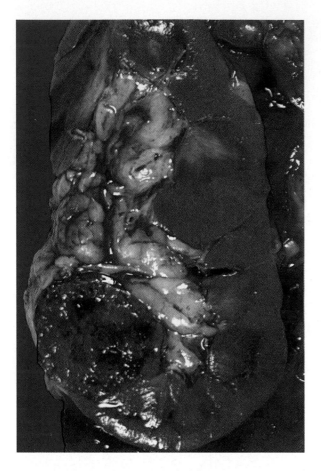

Figure 2-135

ONCOCYTOMA

This small oncocytoma is dark brown but the central scar is not apparent on gross examination.

of gross inspection, and the likelihood that any neoplasm lacking these features is not an oncocytoma is substantial.

In usual histologic preparations, renal oncocytomas have the following features: arrangement of cells in nests (alveoli); composition entirely of oncocytes; and uniform round nuclei (figs. 2-137–2-141). The nests are commonly packed at the periphery and more loosely arranged centrally. Tubular, trabecular, and microcystic patterns are infrequent. Importantly, a sheet-like arrangement of cells is not a feature of renal oncocytoma. Rarely, the cells of oncocytomas extend into the perirenal fat (fig. 2-142) (332,333,356a). The prognostic implications of this finding are unclear, but no patient has died of oncocytoma to date. Extension into perirenal fat occurring in an otherwise typical oncocytoma should probably be reported by the pathologist, preferably in a comment. Labeling such lesions "atypical" without evidence of an adverse biologic potential does not seem warranted. The central scar of an oncocytoma comprises collagenous tissue that may contain cystic areas and even hemorrhage.

The cells of oncocytomas are round to oval, but may appear columnar. Their cytoplasm is homogeneous, acidophilic, and granular in usual histologic preparations. Focal vacuolization, representing intracytoplasmic lumens, occasionally occurs (fig. 2-143) (362). Extracellular hyaline, reminiscent of basement membrane,

Figure 2-136

ONCOCYTOMA

This oncocytoma has prominent cystic change as demonstrated by low-power magnification.

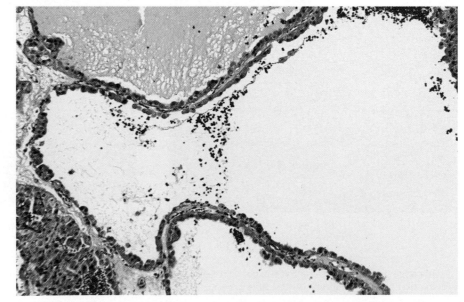

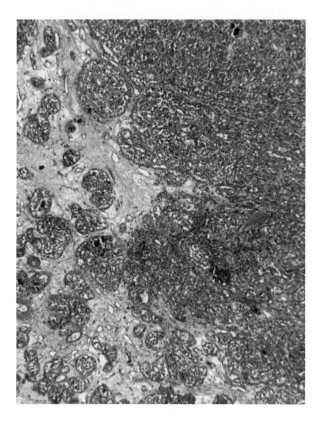

Figure 2-137

ONCOCYTOMA

This low-power view illustrates the more solid areas of the tumor at the upper right, with the cells arranged in well-defined small nests. In the lower left, the nests are becoming separated by a loose hypocellular fibrous stroma. This latter pattern is characteristic of renal oncocytoma.

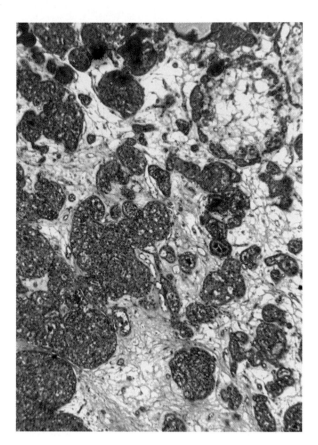

Figure 2-138

ONCOCYTOMA

The oncocytic cells with granular eosinophilic cytoplasm are organized into well-defined solid nests within a loose fibrous stroma.

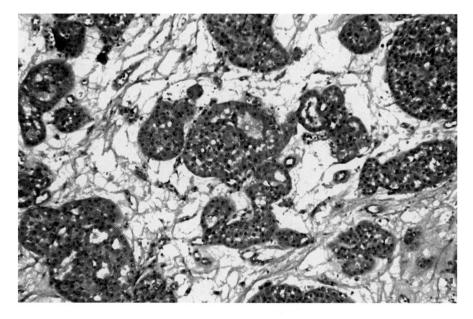

Figure 2-139

ONCOCYTOMA

Within the solid nests of oncocytoma are areas of tubule formation with well-defined lumens.

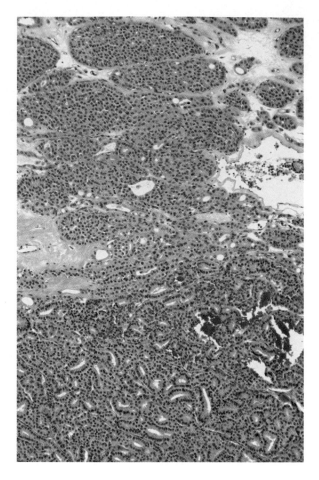

Figure 2-140

ONCOCYTOMA

The tubular differentiation is prominent and involves a large area of the lesion.

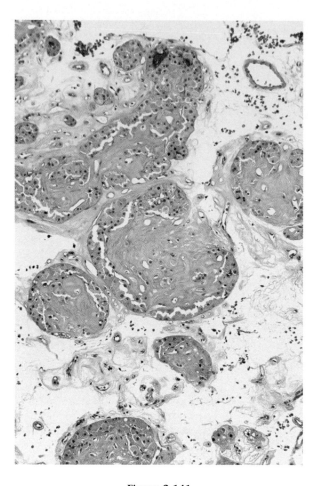

Figure 2-141

ONCOCYTOMA

Hyalinization is associated with the tumor cell nests. The background stroma remains loose.

has been observed and can form globules (345, 349). In contrast, intracellular hyaline is not a feature of renal oncocytomas (344). Cytoplasmic lipochrome can be highlighted by stains for phosphotungstic acid and Sudan black B but the features of oncocytomas are so characteristic in usual preparations that special techniques are not necessary for an accurate interpretation (356a).

The nuclei of renal oncocytoma cells are regular and round to oval, almost always measuring less than 10 μm in greatest dimension (fig. 2-144). They have evenly dispersed, finely granular chromatin. Nucleoli are often present but small. Very rare mitoses may occur but the presence of more than a rare mitosis should suggest another interpretation (332,359,366).

The variations in the cellular features of oncocytomas are limited but well known (356a, 366). In occasional cases, there are scattered foci of cells with immature-appearing nuclei and relatively scant cytoplasm (fig. 2-145) (348). These foci tend to stand out because of the suggestion of increased nuclear density, but their cells gradually blend into the adjacent typical areas. In other cases, cells with pleomorphic and even bizarre nuclei occur singly or in aggregates (fig. 2-146). These nuclei lack both large nucleoli and mitoses, and most authorities consider them to be a degenerative phenomenon similar to cells in endocrine neoplasms. Oncocytomas having these features are biologically benign and the term atypical should not be applied to them. When defined according

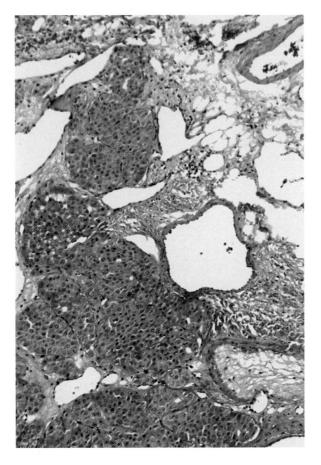

Figure 2-142

ONCOCYTOMA

The tumor extends beyond the confines of the renal capsule into the perirenal fibroadipose tissue.

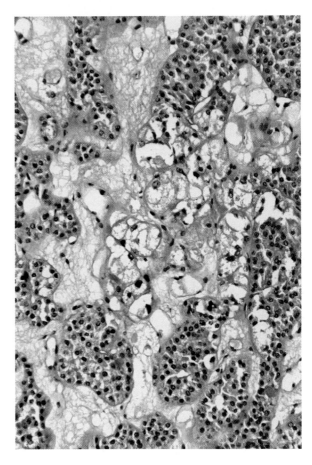

Figure 2-143

ONCOCYTOMA

Vacuolization of the tumor cell cytoplasm produces a focal clear cell appearance.

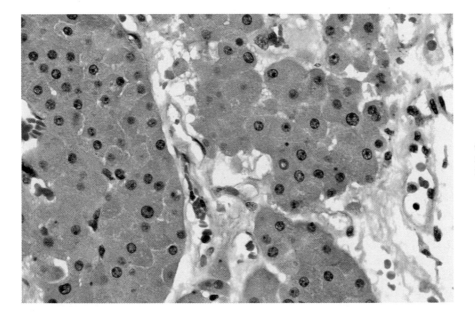

Figure 2-144

ONCOCYTOMA

The typical nuclei in renal oncocytoma are uniform and round, with or without prominent nucleoli.

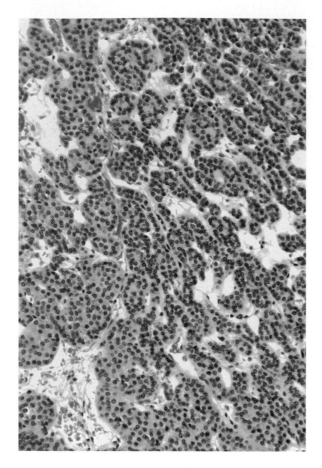

Figure 2-145

ONCOCYTOMA

The cells in this oncocytoma have scanty cytoplasm, resulting in a somewhat immature appearance. The cells are otherwise bland without cytologic atypia.

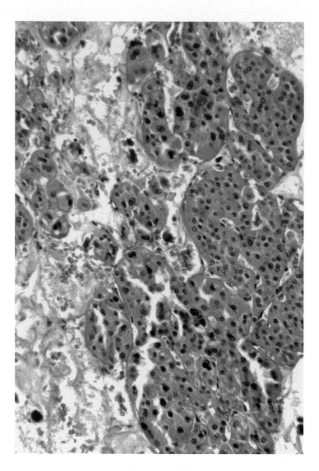

Figure 2-146

ONCOCYTOMA

There are many cells present that contain pleomorphic hyperchromatic nuclei. This is not associated with the presence of mitotic figures.

to the criteria described, oncocytomas do not require further grading or subtyping.

If the designation oncocytoma is to be clinically important, it should confirm the presence of a benign renal neoplasm. Considering that renal tumors commonly have intralesional heterogeneity, confirmation of their nature usually requires evaluation of well-sampled, well-preserved tissue. Sections frozen at the time of a rapid intraoperative consultation do not meet this standard and an unequivocal interpretation of oncocytoma is discouraged.

Oncocytomas have been detected in needle aspirates (fig. 2-147) (360a,370,374). The potential for sampling error due to intralesional heterogeneity generally precludes a definitive diagnosis, but this method of detection has been useful in selected cases where total nephrectomy is contraindicated. The typical cellular features of histologic preparations are observed. Cells are uniform in shape and size, with homogeneous, granular cytoplasm. Nuclei tend to be central and round with even borders; pleomorphism is rare. Large nucleoli are not present.

Immunohistochemical Findings. Immunohistochemically, oncocytomas react with antibodies directed toward constituents of the collecting ducts (e.g., EMA, low molecular weight cytokeratins, and certain lectins) (336,357). They are positive to most pancytokeratin cocktails. A majority of cases react with antibodies to cytokeratin 7, often with scattered, strongly positive single cells, in contrast to the more diffusely strong reactivity in chromophobe cell

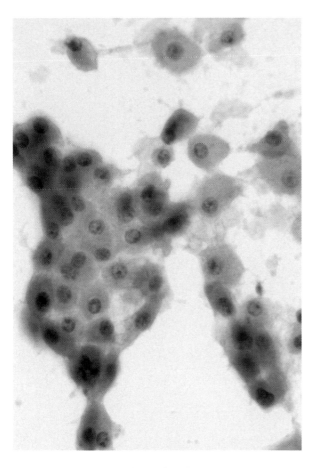

Figure 2-147

ONCOCYTOMA

Fine-needle aspiration biopsy specimen demonstrates small cohesive nests and single cells having abundant granular acidophilic cytoplasm. Nuclei are uniform and round, and some contain small nucleoli.

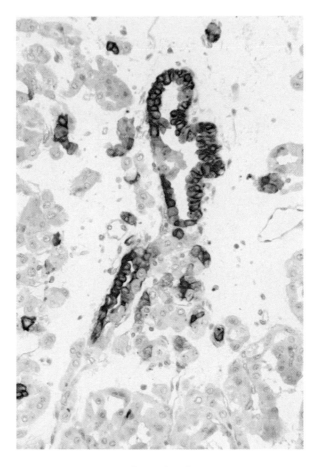

Figure 2-148

ONCOCYTOMA

Immunohistochemical stain for cytokeratin 7 demonstrates intense positivity in scattered, isolated cells and groups of cells. The remaining tumor cells are negative.

RCCs (fig. 2-148) (353,372). There is strong positivity for cytokeratin 14, a finding also present in chromophobe cell RCC but not in clear cell RCC (336a). Expression of cytokeratin 20 varies from none to 80 percent positive (365,366a,372). Reactions for vimentin are positive in a few cases, but the majority of tumors are nonreactive (fig. 2-149). Consistent expression of beta-defensin-1 and parvalbumin is reported (372a). The RCC marker has been negative (355a).

Ultrastructural Findings. Ultrastructurally, oncocytomas are composed exclusively of oncocytes (i.e., cells engorged with mitochondria to the virtual exclusion of other organelles) (fig. 2-150). These mitochondria tend to be uniform and predominantly round, with lamellar cristae, usually in parallel arrays (339,340,366b). Nuclei are uniform and round, and may contain nucleoli. Small globular filamentous bodies composed of cytokeratin are identified in many cases (334). Lipid vacuoles and glycogen are infrequently present and scant when they appear. The cells of oncocytomas have interdigitating cell membranes, with cell junctions and occasional microvilli. In the appropriate setting, ultrastructural analysis is useful for diagnosis but sampling is a potential problem. Occasional oncocytoma cells contain microvesicles characteristic of chromophobe RCC and many clear cell RCCs may be composed of cells with abundant mitochondria (340,351,352a,366b).

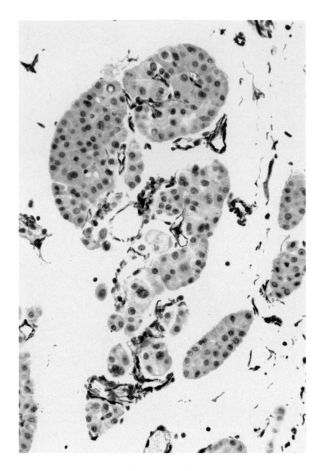

Figure 2-149

ONCOCYTOMA

There is no immunoreactivity for vimentin.

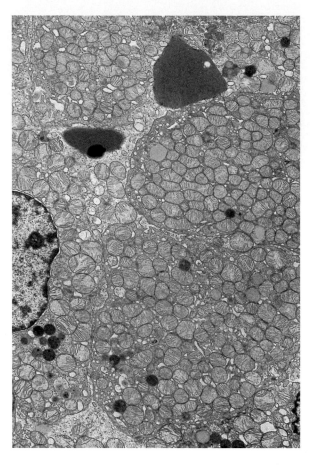

Figure 2-150

ONCOCYTOMA

The cytoplasm of the oncocyte is packed with large mitochondria. (Fig. 1-220 from Fascicle 11, 3rd Series.)

Prognosis. If defined and interpreted according to the guidelines presented here, oncocytomas of the kidney are benign neoplasms. Authorities now agree that cases previously considered aggressive were almost certainly other renal neoplasms, most notably the chromophobe cell variant of RCC (354,356a). It should be noted, however, that survival data are not recorded for every reported case and the implications of certain features (e.g., microscopic involvement of perirenal fat), have not been studied long term. On the other hand, no deaths have been attributed to oncocytomas diagnosed cytologically but not resected.

Differential Diagnosis. Many renal neoplasms contain oncocytic cells, but only oncocytomas are composed entirely of oncocytes. The differential diagnosis begins at the time of gross inspection, where the characteristic brown color combined with a uniform consistency, absence of necrosis, and a central scar, favor oncocytoma (Table 2-10). Histologically, any foci of clear cells, papillae, sheet-like growth, "plant-like" cells, or more than rare mitoses exclude the interpretation of oncocytoma. The presence of foamy macrophages or intracellular hyaline suggests another diagnosis. In the current classification, the clear cell type of RCC can be composed predominantly of acidophilic cells (the granular cell type in previous schemes), but the nuclear grade is usually high and mitoses are readily apparent.

The most perplexing differential diagnostic problem involves the distinction of oncocytoma from the eosinophilic variant of chromophobe cell RCC (see Table 2-4). This almost certainly

Table 2-10

DIFFERENTIAL DIAGNOSIS OF BROWN KIDNEY TUMORS

Tumor	Characteristic Features
Oncocytoma	Circumscribed but no capsule, central scar
Chromophobe RCC[a]	Variegated pale tan, geographic necrosis, small cysts
Papillary RCC	Thick capsule, red-brown, friable
Clear cell RCC	Variegated with yellow areas, necrosis, hemorrhage

[a]RCC = renal cell carcinoma.

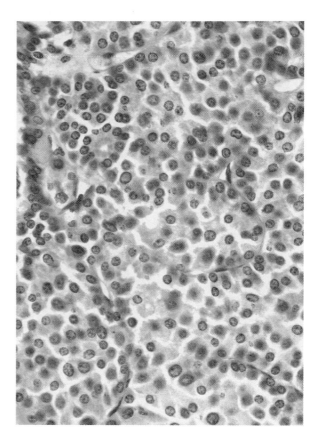

Figure 2-151

ONCOCYTOMA

Hale's colloidal iron faintly stains the cytoplasm. There is more intense staining at the lumenal surface where tubular formation is seen.

accounts for the reported cases of malignant and progressive oncocytomas. In contrast to oncocytomas, even seemingly pure eosinophilic variants of the chromophobe cell type of RCC have a sheet-like growth pattern or a densely packed nested pattern without intervening fibrous stroma, strong cytoplasmic staining with Hale's colloidal iron, perinuclear halos, and raisinoid nuclei. In addition, many have mitotic activity and at least very small foci of typical plant-like cells. There is significant overlap in the immunohistochemical expression profiles of the two. Patients with the Birt-Hogg-Dube syndrome can have so-called hybrid tumors, which have features typical for both oncocytoma and chromophobe cell RCC (358a). In most affected individuals, the tumors are multiple, bilateral, and of different histologic types—important clues to recognizing this syndrome.

Special Techniques. Renal oncocytomas are defined in such a way that most cases do not require special techniques for accurate interpretation. Hale's colloidal iron stain, considered a useful method to exclude chromophobe RCC, is negative in oncocytomas but many laboratories have experienced variable results with this stain (fig. 2-151) (332,336,338,346). Oncocytomas lack mucins and glycogen (338). Cytometry has yielded unexpected results, with tumors having aneuploid populations behaving in a benign fashion (346,368). Renal oncocytomas tend to have consistent, though not necessarily diagnostic, chromosomal abnormalities that tend to distinguish them from other renal neoplasms (341, 352,373). Some of these abnormalities (e.g., loss of chromosomes 1 and y), are readily detected in clinical material but lack diagnostic specificity.

RARE TUMORS WITH EPITHELIAL AND/OR RENAL PARENCHYMAL DIFFERENTIATION

Carcinoid Tumor

Carcinoid tumor was first reported as a primary neoplasm in the kidney in 1966 and a significant number of cases have been recorded since then (392,397,404,418,428,441). Some have developed in renal teratomas (394,444). There is a striking propensity for these tumors to develop in horseshoe kidneys (379,404). The histogenesis is unclear, except for carcinoid tumors arising in teratomas, but the mechanism is considered analogous to that of similar tumors arising in the ovary or testis. Neither argyrophilic cells nor

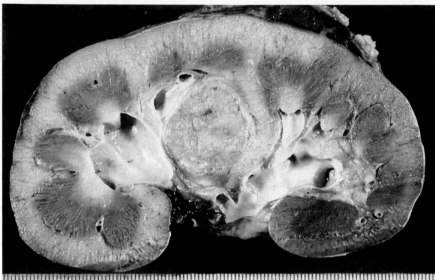

Figure 2-152

CARCINOID TUMOR

The tumor is well circumscribed, homogeneous, and tanyellow. (Courtesy of Dr. Gulcin Altinok, Ankara, Turkey.)

other types of neuroendocrine cells have been documented in the normal kidney (394,400, 407). Prior to accepting a case as primary, the possibility of metastasis should be excluded.

Patients range from 13 to 67 years of age, but most are over 40 years old. There is no significant sex predilection. Most patients have symptoms that could be related to a renal mass; only a few are entirely asymptomatic. At least one reported patient had carcinoid syndrome, but in several cases symptoms were attributed to other hormonal substances (396,401,428). A patient with Cushing's syndrome is the only pediatric case (401).

Carcinoid tumors of the kidney vary in size, but are often large and either well circumscribed or encapsulated (fig. 2-152). Most are solid and yellow-tan, but occasional cysts have been identified. The histologic features are similar to carcinoid tumors at other sites (fig. 2-153). Most tumors are argyrophilic and argentaffin negative. A few are so poorly differentiated that the term carcinoid tumor seems inappropriate and these cases are included among the small cell (neuroendocrine) carcinomas. The immunohistochemical and ultrastructural features of carcinoid tumors of the kidney are characteristic of neuroendocrine neoplasms.

Approximately one third of reported tumors with typical histology have metastasized, predominantly to bone (441). Metastases among the more poorly differentiated tumors or those

with mitotic activity are reported to be more frequent, and the term *atypical carcinoid* is applied (392,394,427).

Small Cell Carcinoma

When defined in current terminology, small cell carcinoma is observed in the renal parenchyma as well as in the renal pelvis (385,392, 393,398,415,418,421,437). Renal pelvic tumors are often associated with more typical urothelial (transitional cell) carcinomas (393). Areas of typical carcinoid tumor rarely occur.

Small cell carcinomas are typically large and locally invasive (figs. 2-154–2-156). Their histologic features do not differ from those of similar tumors at other sites. The differential diagnosis of small blue round cell tumors of the adult kidney is highlighted in Table 2-11. Those cases with an identifiable urothelial carcinoma component, including carcinoma in situ, should be classified as urothelial carcinoma with small cell differentiation arising from the renal pelvis.

Immunohistochemical reactions have yielded variable results. Intermediate-type small cell carcinomas are particularly likely to have antigenic determinants for keratin. Most often, reactions for neurosecretory differentiation are positive and neurosecretory granules can be demonstrated using electron microscopy.

The prognosis is poor: nearly all recorded patients developed metastases and died of their tumors (398,415).

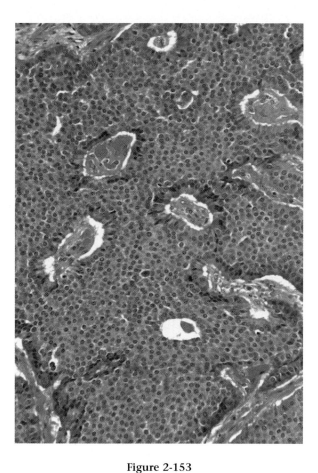

Figure 2-153

CARCINOID TUMOR

This renal carcinoid is growing in solid nests, with individual cells having uniform nuclei and finely granular chromatin.

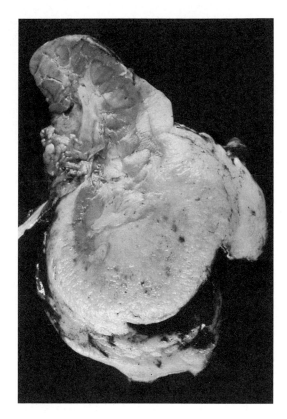

Figure 2-154

SMALL CELL CARCINOMA

This large invasive tumor was pale gray in color. The origin could be the renal pelvis or renal parenchyma. (Fig. 1-227 from from Fascicle 11, 3rd Series.)

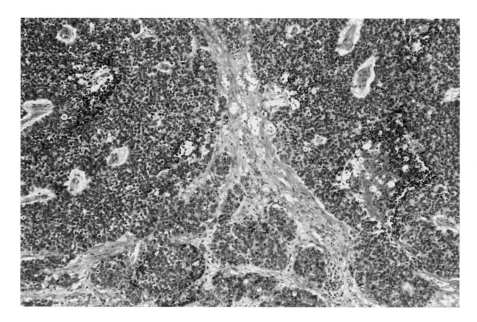

Figure 2-155

SMALL CELL CARCINOMA

A low-power photomicrograph shows sheets of poorly cohesive cells with zonal areas of necrosis.

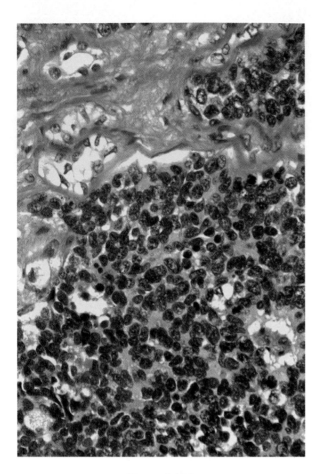

Figure 2-156

SMALL CELL CARCINOMA

Higher-power view of tumor seen in figure 2-155 illustrates typical nuclear features of small cell carcinoma.

Table 2-11
DIFFERENTIAL DIAGNOSIS OF SMALL BLUE ROUND CELL TUMORS IN ADULTS
Small cell carcinoma (urothelial or parenchymal)
Primitive neuroectodermal tumor
Nephroblastoma
Rhabdomyosarcoma
Lymphoma/leukemia
Metastasis

Primitive Neuroectodermal Tumor

Numerous examples of primary primitive neuroectodermal tumor (PNET) of the kidney are documented in the literature (386,388,405). In many cases, the diagnosis is confirmed through demonstration of the *EWS/FLI-1* fusion transcript (426,431,436). These tumors are reported in patients with a wide age range, with most in the second and third decades. They tend to be aggressive and are treated with a multimodal approach similar to that for PNET at other sites (386,405).

Grossly, most PNETs are large and gray to white, with areas of hemorrhage and necrosis. Cystic degeneration is frequent. The microscopic features are similar to those of PNETs at other sites (figs. 2-157, 2-158). Tumor cells have small to intermediate-sized nuclei with scant, clear to acidophilic cytoplasm. The cells are largely arranged in sheets, with perivascular pseudorosettes. There is infiltration of the adjacent renal parenchyma.

Immunohistochemistry has confirmed the expression of the *MIC2* gene product in a membrane pattern in up to 100 percent of cases (405, 415,431). Expression of FLI-1 has been reported in over 50 percent of cases. The tumors also react for vimentin and neuron-specific enolase. In a few cases, cytokeratin positivity has been reported. There is no reactivity for the *WT1* gene product. Ultrastructurally, the cells have cytoplasmic processes and contain scant dense core neurosecretory granules.

Neuroblastoma

Rare examples of intrarenal neuroblastoma are described (430,432). Morphologically, these tumors are identical to adrenal neuroblastoma and it is hypothesized that they arise from adrenal rests or intrarenal sympathetic tissue (see figs. 1-49–1-51, chapter 1) (432).

Paraganglioma/Pheochromocytoma

Rare examples of intrarenal paraganglioma are described (410). The tumors are small and histologically identical to paragangliomas elsewhere.

Juxtaglomerular Cell Tumor

This is a rare neoplasm differentiating toward the modified smooth muscle cells of the juxtaglomerular apparatus (392,429). Recorded patients are 6 to 69 years of age, with a mean age of 27 years (390,416). There is a 1.9 to 1 female to male ratio. Almost all patients are hypertensive, often for many years prior to the detection of

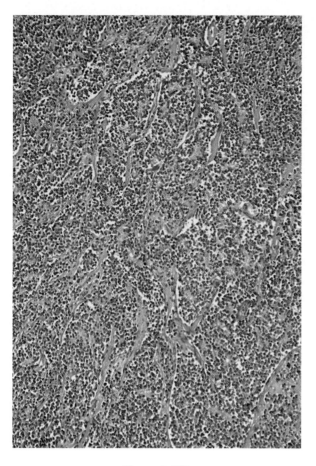

Figure 2-157

PRIMITIVE NEUROECTODERMAL TUMOR

The tumor is composed of poorly cohesive cells having small open nuclei, scant cytoplasm, and in some areas, poorly formed rosettes.

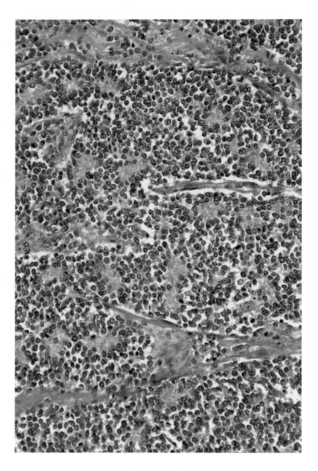

Figure 2-158

PRIMITIVE NEUROECTODERMAL TUMOR

There is focal rosette formation.

the tumor. The hypertension is associated with elevated serum levels of renin and occasionally with increased aldosterone and decreased potassium (hypokalemia). Patients have presented with severe hypertension in pregnancy (402). In over 90 percent of cases, surgical removal of the juxtaglomerular tumor results in a return of the blood pressure to normal levels. Juxtaglomerular tumors are apparently benign, since no local recurrences or metastases have been reported to date, regardless of the type of surgical resection.

In all reported cases, juxtaglomerular cell tumors are unilateral, solitary, and situated in the renal cortex. Most measure less than 4 cm in greatest dimension, but at least one neoplasm measured 9 cm (409). Tumors are usually solid and well circumscribed but scattered small cysts

occur. The cut surface is gray-white to light yellow, with areas of hemorrhage (figs. 2-159–2-162) (392).

Histologically, juxtaglomerular cell tumors are composed of a uniform population of round to polyhedral cells with granular, acidophilic cytoplasm, and are surrounded by a fibrous capsule. Cells may be arranged in irregular trabeculae, organoid patterns, or leaf-like papillae (419). Vascular structures are prominent, with both thin-walled and thick-walled vessels. A hemangiopericytoma-like vascular pattern has been described (416). Cytoplasmic granules are characteristic of both normal and neoplastic juxtaglomerular cells (433). These granules react with PAS and Bowie reagents. The nuclei are generally round to oval and there may be a few mitotic figures.

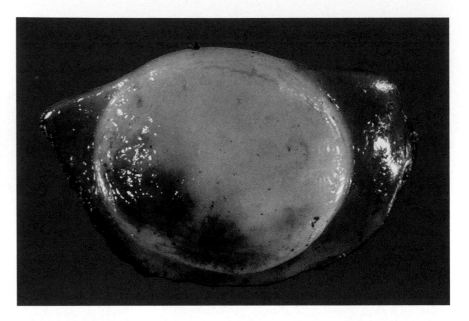

Figure 2-159

JUXTAGLOMERULAR CELL TUMOR

This 1-cm tumor arose in a 17-year-old boy. It is well circumscribed, tan-white, and has focal hemorrhage. (Courtesy of Dr. Janet Poulik, Detroit, MI.)

Immunohistochemically, the tumor cells express smooth muscle and muscle-specific actin as well as CD31. They are nonreactive for cytokeratins, desmin, S-100 protein, HMB-45, chromogranin, and synaptophysin (383,416). Ultrastructurally, the cells often contain rhomboid, renin-specific crystals, similar to those found in the normal juxtaglomerular apparatus (fig. 2-163) (382). Tumor cells are often associated with nonmyelinated nerve fibers (378).

Teratoma

Teratomas rarely occur as primary renal tumors (375,394,407,421,444). Of the few reported cases, three had areas of carcinoid tumor. Two other tumors occurred in dysplastic kidneys. With a single exception, renal teratomas are histologically and clinically benign.

Nephroblastoma

Renal tumors that characteristically arise in children can occur in adults (384,393a,399,403, 406). Most are nephroblastomas (see Nephroblastoma, chapter 1). There are isolated reports of cystic, partially differentiated nephroblastoma; clear cell sarcoma; and rhabdoid tumor occurring in adults (377,381,392a,408,412). Cystic nephroma in adults is best labeled multilocular cyst and considered a distinct entity from that of childhood (392a). The neoplasm that has been reported under the term adult mesoblastic nephroma is also now considered a distinct entity unrelated to that occurring in the pediatric population (see Mixed Epithelial and Stromal Tumor).

Adult nephroblastomas are rare and can be confused with other mixed malignant tumors (figs. 2-164, 2-165). Acceptable cases should contain a blastema. Anaplasia, as defined in pediatric patients, is unusual (403). Identification of nephrogenic rests is rare in adults. In contrast to the situation in most children, adults with nephroblastomas have an adverse prognosis. Metastases have occurred in 13 percent of cases at the time of diagnosis and only half of the patients can be expected to be disease free at 5 years, despite multimodality therapy.

Multilocular Cyst (Cystic Nephroma)

Multilocular cysts are distinctive neoplasms of adults, despite the designation cystic nephroma in previous publications and in the pediatric literature (387,389,392a,413,420a). In adults, multilocular cysts are typically found in middle-aged women (female to male ratio, 7 to 1). They are characteristically situated in the upper pole of the kidney (figs. 2-166, 2-167). Most patients are asymptomatic and the tumors are discovered incidentally. Spontaneous rupture has been reported (395). Coexistence with other renal neoplasms, including angiomyolipoma, has been described (442). By definition, the lesions are solitary and unilateral, and the cysts are multiloculated, with no communication between

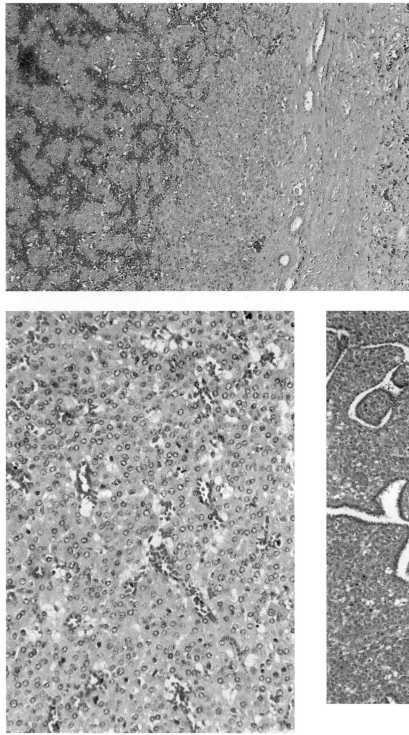

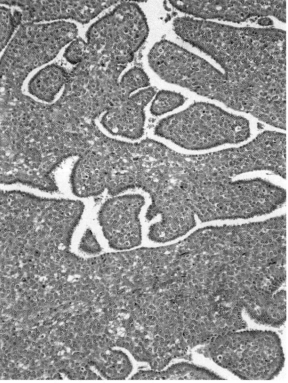

Figure 2-160

JUXTAGLOMERULAR CELL TUMOR

The tumor is encapsulated and consists of small nests of cells that are closely packed. In some areas there is hemorrhage, with red blood cells present between the islands of tumor cells.

Figure 2-161

JUXTAGLOMERULAR CELL TUMOR

The tumor cells have uniform round nuclei and moderate acidophilic cytoplasm. There is a prominent vascular network in the background.

Figure 2-162

JUXTAGLOMERULAR CELL TUMOR

The tumor has a papillary architecture with broad leaf-like papillae. There are flattened epithelial cells on the surface and the cores are filled with uniform cells having acidophilic cytoplasm. (Courtesy of Dr. Bernard Têtú, Quebec City, Quebec.)

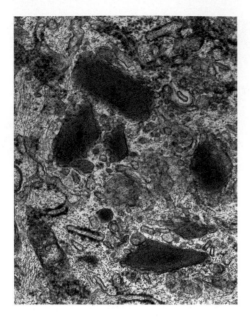

Figure 2-163

JUXTAGLOMERULAR CELL TUMOR

Renin-specific granules are seen in this high-power view. (Fig. 1-232 from Fascicle 11, 3rd Series.)

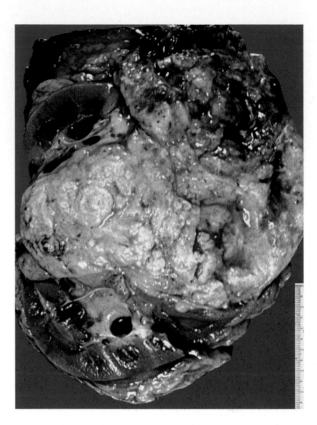

Figure 2-164

ADULT NEPHROBLASTOMA

This adult nephroblastoma has a bulging soft fleshy consistency and is pale gray-white.

locules or with the renal calyces and no renal elements in the cyst walls. The lesions are encapsulated and the adjacent renal parenchyma is normal except for compression-induced changes. If all of these features are not present, entities such as multicystic renal cell carcinoma and cystic dysplastic kidney must be considered.

The cysts are lined by a single layer of epithelial cells, which may be flattened, low cuboidal, or even columnar (figs. 2-168, 2-169). Stratified zones may be present. Occasional lining cells exhibit atypical cytologic features, including nuclear enlargement and hyperchromasia. These cells ordinarily have acidophilic cytoplasm and a hobnail morphology (fig. 2-170). The cells lining the cysts can have clear cytoplasm but this feature alone is insufficient to consider an interpretation of multicystic RCC. The epithelial cells are strongly positive with antibodies to keratins and exhibit a type of lectin binding that suggests that the epithelium lining the cysts is of distal tubule or collecting duct type. The stromal septa between the cysts consist of dense fibrous connective tissue with scattered loose fascicles of smooth muscle but no elements of nephrons. Ovarian-like stroma

may be present (fig. 2-171). Importantly, foci of blastema or nephroblastoma essentially never occur in multilocular cysts of adults. The presence of such elements would define a pediatric-type tumor occurring in an adult and require an interpretation appropriate to such a lesion. If defined according to the criteria presented, multilocular cysts are benign.

Multilocular cysts must be distinguished from multicystic RCC and various types of cystic renal diseases. In multicystic RCC, nests of clear cells are present within the fibrous septa, a feature not seen in multilocular cysts. The presence of thick walls, friable material on the cyst surfaces, and intracystic hemorrhage should heighten the suspicion of a carcinoma with cystic degeneration and prompt more extensive sampling. Non-neoplastic cystic renal diseases are characterized by the presence of remnants of nephrons in the septal walls and abnormal renal architectonics.

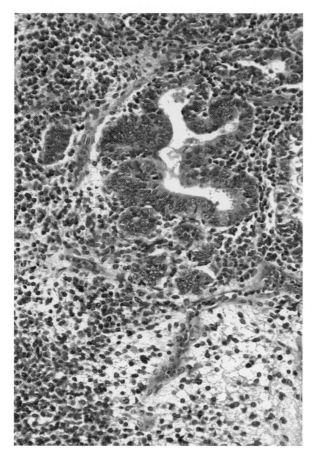

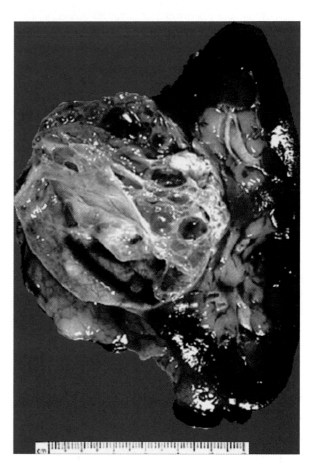

Figure 2-165

ADULT NEPHROBLASTOMA

Adult nephroblastoma with epithelial and blastemal elements.

Figure 2-166

MULTILOCULAR CYST (CYSTIC NEPHROMA)

Nephrectomy specimen shows the typical appearance of a multilocular cyst. The lesion is multiloculated, with thin fibrous septa.

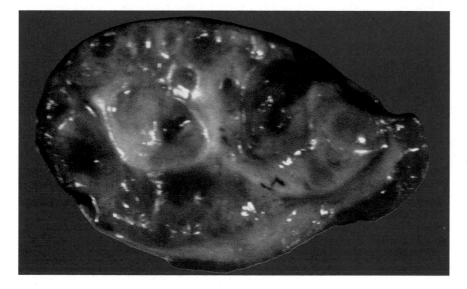

Figure 2-167

MULTILOCULAR CYST (CYSTIC NEPHROMA)

Partial nephrectomy specimen of a multilocular cyst. There are multiple cysts separated by thin fibrous septa.

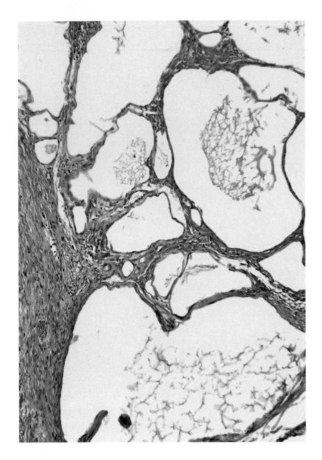

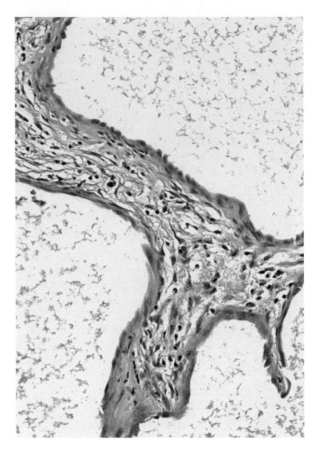

Figure 2-168

MULTILOCULAR CYST (CYSTIC NEPHROMA)

Multiple noncommunicating cysts of varying size with a fibrous capsule (left side of photomicrograph) separate the tumor from the adjacent kidney.

Figure 2-169

MULTILOCULAR CYST (CYSTIC NEPHROMA)

The fibrous septa have a loose myxoid stroma. The lining cells have acidophilic cytoplasm and in this area are compressed against the cyst wall.

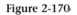

Figure 2-170

MULTILOCULAR CYST (CYSTIC NEPHROMA)

The lining epithelium has a distinctive hobnail morphology. The stroma in the fibrous septa is moderately cellular.

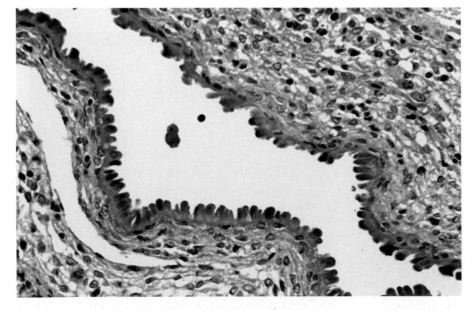

Mixed Epithelial and Stromal Tumor

Renal tumors in adults may be composed of mixtures of epithelial and stromal elements. These rare lesions have received various designations in the literature, perhaps the most popular of which has been adult mesoblastic nephroma (376,391,411,419,420a,423,425,439, 440,443). These tumors occur over a wide age range and are 4 to 5 times more common in women than men. The clinical and epidemiologic features argue against an association with congenital mesoblastic nephroma as do the cytogenetic features (424). Perhaps because of the disparity in incidence between men and women, a hormonal influence on the development of these tumors has been postulated (376). The clinical presentation is similar to that of other renal tumors.

Pathologically, mixed epithelial and stromal tumors are circumscribed or infrequently infiltrative, with a mixed solid and cystic growth pattern (figs. 2-172–2-175). A partial or complete smooth muscle capsule is often present. Tumors can extend into the renal pelvis and even involve the ureter. Spindle cell areas vary from hypocellular and fibrotic to cellular, with a woven pattern reminiscent of ovarian stroma. The epithelial component consists of immature tubules, often with microcystic and macrocystic dilatation. Cells range from low cuboidal to columnar to hobnail, with clear to acidophilic cytoplasm. They may be ciliated or contain mucin (380). Neither the stromal nor the epithelial element has significant cytologic atypia or mitotic activity. A possibly related tumor having a predominantly smooth muscle stroma with a proliferative epithelial component has been described under the term *benign renal angiomyoadenomatous tumor* (418a).

The spindle cells react for vimentin, with variable positivity for actin and desmin, and have positive nuclear reactivity for estrogen and progesterone receptors (in women). In one case, the epithelial cells were also estrogen and progesterone receptor positive, suggesting a possible müllerian origin (380). The epithelial cells are positive for cytokeratins.

Mixed epithelial and stromal tumors must be distinguished primarily from adult nephroblastoma and sarcomatoid RCC. The absence of blastema excludes nephroblastoma

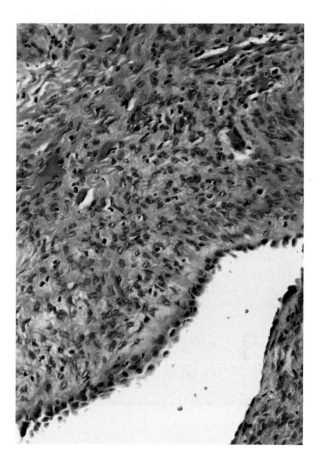

Figure 2-171

MULTILOCULAR CYST (CYSTIC NEPHROMA)

The stroma is cellular but lacks significant cytologic atypia.

and the lack of cellular anaplasia rules out both tumors. To date, all reported cases of mixed epithelial and stromal tumors have been benign. There has been a single report of a tumor having these features, but containing a cytologically malignant focus within the spindle cell component (435); clinically, the tumor did not recur or metastasize.

Spiradenocylindroma

An unusual renal tumor with morphologic features similar to cutaneous cylindroma and apparent somatic mutation of the *CYLD1* gene has been reported (434). The tumor arose in the wall of a renal cyst in a 58-year-old man. Tumor cells were arranged in nodules with solid or trabecular architecture, tubular structures, deposits of PAS-positive material, and focal epidermoid differentiation. The tumor expressed

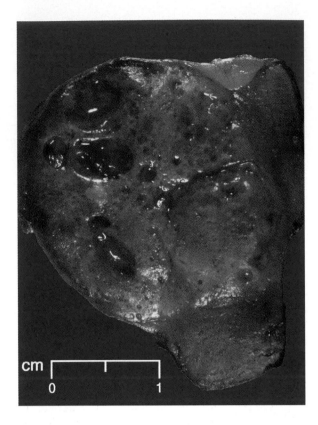

Figure 2-172

MIXED EPITHELIAL AND STROMAL TUMOR

The tumor in this partial nephrectomy specimen is well circumscribed and brown, with variably sized cysts.

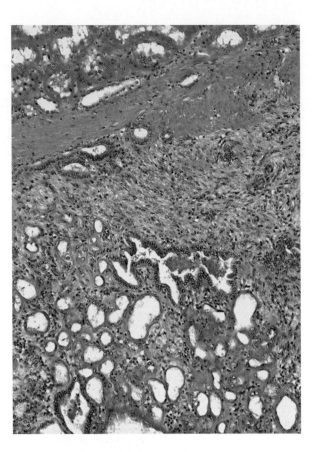
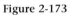

Figure 2-173

MIXED EPITHELIAL AND STROMAL TUMOR

The tumor is surrounded by a well-defined smooth muscle capsule. There is an admixture of spindle cells and epithelial elements. The epithelial elements show a variety of different tubular patterns.

Figure 2-174

MIXED EPITHELIAL AND STROMAL TUMOR

A predominantly mesenchymal area of the lesion with spindle cells arranged in short fascicles. A few tubular elements are located on the lower right.

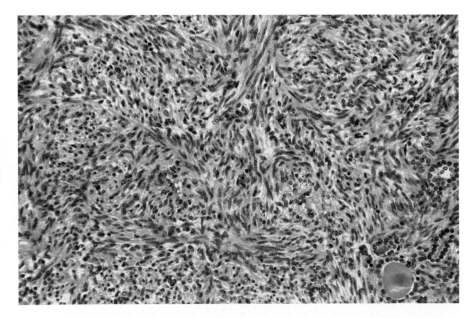

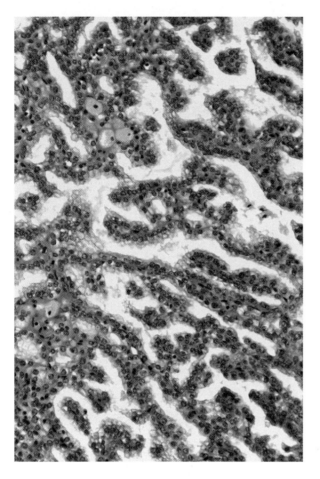

Figure 2-175

MIXED EPITHELIAL AND STROMAL TUMOR

A complex area of the epithelial component in which branching ductal structures are lined by cells with pale acidophilic to clear cytoplasm.

high molecular weight cytokeratin, actin, vimentin, and S-100 protein. The patient was free of disease at 30 months, however, there is insufficient experience with this tumor to determine its biologic behavior.

MESENCHYMAL TUMORS

Angiomyolipoma

Definition. Angiomyolipoma is a neoplasm composed of varying admixtures of blood vessels, smooth muscle cells, and adipose tissue. Most previous classifications have included this tumor among mesenchymal neoplasms.

General and Clinical Features. Angiomyolipoma was considered to represent either a hamartoma or a choristoma in the past, but is now accepted as a neoplasm (451). The evidence for a neoplasm includes monoclonality and the presence of a variety of cytogenetic abnormalities (457, 461,481). The perivascular epithelioid cell is considered to be the cell of origin for this and other related tumors and tumor-like processes (447).

Angiomyolipomas are observed in patients with several hereditary disorders including von Recklinghausen disease, von Hippel-Lindau syndrome, and autosomal dominant (adult) polycystic kidney disease. The latter condition has been reported as the *TSC2/PKD1* contiguous gene syndrome (470). The association of tuberous sclerosis with angiomyolipoma is particularly strong. Whereas angiomyolipomas occur in 80 percent of individuals with tuberous sclerosis, less than half of patients with angiomyolipomas have the tuberous sclerosis complex. Tuberous sclerosis is an autosomal dominant disorder caused by mutation of either the *TSC1* (chromosome 9q34) or *TSC2* (chromosome 16p13) genes (459,470, 481). The products of these two genes, hamartin and tuberin, respectively, interact and are believed to be part of the same molecular pathway (482). In patients with *TSC1* mutations, expression of hamartin is lost and tuberin retained, while in patients with *TSC2* mutations, tuberin expression is lost and hamartin expression retained (474). Mutation of the *TSC2* gene is also seen in lymphangioleiomyomatosis (479).

Angiomyolipomas comprise 0.7 to 2.0 percent of all renal tumors, depending upon whether they are incidental findings or symptomatic tumors, with or without associated tuberous sclerosis (448,453). Unlike with most other types of renal tumors, patients are predominantly women, in a ratio of 2 to 1. The average age at diagnosis is 41 years, although children are also affected (475,480). No racial predilection has been demonstrated. Among symptomatic patients, flank pain related to intratumoral hemorrhage is the most common complaint. Angiomyolipomas are ordinarily detected radiographically, where they can usually be distinguished from other renal tumors (fig. 2-176) (455,465). Fine needle aspiration confirms the diagnosis in many cases, but the cellular changes in aspirates can mimic those of a high-grade neoplasm (455).

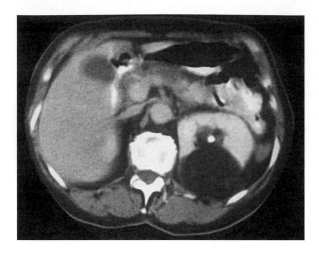

Figure 2-176

ANGIOMYOLIPOMA

By computerized tomography, an angiomyolipoma is visualized with the same radial density as the subcutaneous fat. (Fig. 1-262 from Fascicle 11, 3rd Series.)

Tumors with the histopathologic features of angiomyolipoma have been observed in the renal capsule (capsulomas), attached to the renal capsule but predominantly in the perirenal tissues, localized to the retroperitoneum without renal attachments, and in abdominal organs such as the liver, fallopian tubes, spleen, and regional lymph nodes (449,456,458,462). Most investigators consider the occurrence of these tumors at extrarenal sites to be evidence of multicentricity rather than metastases.

Pathologic Findings. The typical angiomyolipoma is an intrarenal tumor which replaces a portion of the renal parenchyma (figs. 2-177–2-179). Lesions vary considerably in size: capsular lesions rarely measure more than a few millimeters while intrarenal tumors range from 3 to 20 cm (mean, 9.4 cm) in greatest dimension (475). Large masses ordinarily compress the surrounding structures. Rarely, they rupture into the renal calyces or renal vein, and may extend into the renal collecting system, or even the vena cava. Most angiomyolipomas are solitary but multiple tumors are observed in as many as 20 percent of cases (fig. 2-180). In such situations, a large dominant tumor associated with smaller lesions is typical. Massive hemorrhage may occur into an angiomyolipoma (fig. 2-181).

Although circumscribed, angiomyolipomas are not encapsulated and tend to enlarge at the ex-

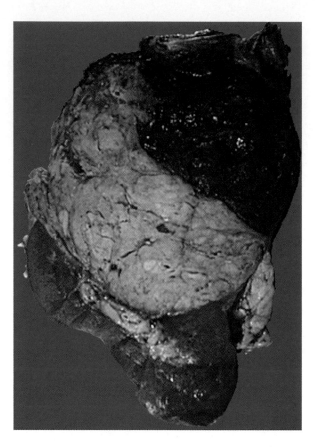

Figure 2-177

ANGIOMYOLIPOMA

Large angiomyolipoma predominantly composed of adipose tissue as indicated by a pale yellow color. There is extensive hemorrhage (upper pole) and this patient presented with an acute retroperitoneal bleed.

pense of the adjacent renal parenchyma, so that elements of normal kidney become surrounded and isolated throughout the tumor. Once entrapped, renal tubular elements may dilate and form cysts. Rarely, this process is so pronounced that tumors appear multicystic (467,473,478). Most such cases occur in patients with tuberous sclerosis. Angiomyolipomas can coexist with other renal neoplasms including clear cell RCC and oncocytoma (459a).

As previously stated, angiomyolipomas are highly associated with the hereditary disease tuberous sclerosis (mental retardation, epilepsy, cutaneous hamartomas, shagreen skin, depigmented spots, and subungual fibromas of the fingers). In most cases, the angiomyolipomas in such patients are multiple and bilateral (fig. 2-182). The association is so close that all patients

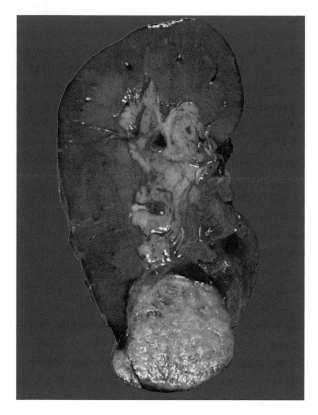

Figure 2-178

ANGIOMYOLIPOMA

This tumor is pale gray-white, corresponding to a predominance of smooth muscle within the neoplasm.

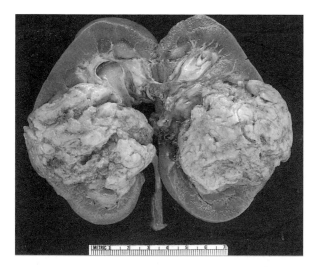

Figure 2-179

ANGIOMYOLIPOMA

The renal pelvis is compressed and distorted by the tumor. (Fig. 1-265 from Fascicle 11, 3rd Series.)

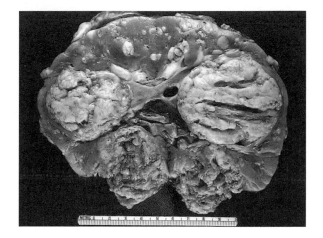

Figure 2-180

ANGIOMYOLIPOMA

This kidney contains numerous tumors of varying sizes. (Fig. 2A from Farrow GM, Harrison EG Jr, Utz DC, Jones DR. Renal angiomyolipoma: a clinicopathologic study of 32 cases. Cancer 1968;22:564–70.)

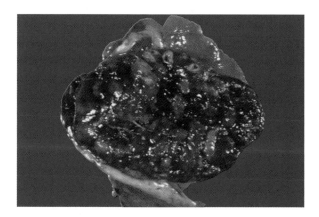

Figure 2-181

ANGIOMYOLIPOMA

Partial nephrectomy specimen shows a hemorrhagic angiomyolipoma having a friable cut surface.

with multiple renal angiomyolipomas should be evaluated for tuberous sclerosis, recognizing that the hereditary syndrome may be only partially expressed (453).

Grossly, angiomyolipomas are ordinarily lobular, yellow, and slightly oily. Tumors consisting primarily of smooth muscle may be pale gray and firm. Hemorrhage is a common finding, especially in symptomatic cases, and may be extensive enough to nearly replace the tumor.

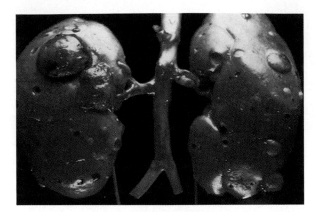

Figure 2-182

ANGIOMYOLIPOMA

The tumors are multiple and bilateral. There are also cortical cysts in this patient with tuberous sclerosis. (Fig. 2C from Farrow GM, Harrison EG Jr, Utz DC, Jones DR. Renal angiomyolipoma: a clinicopathologic study of 32 cases. Cancer 1968;22:564–70.)

Histologically, angiomyolipomas are composed of blood vessels, smooth muscle, and adipose tissue, characteristically admixed in a haphazard fashion (figs. 2-183–2-186). Mature adipose tissue, often associated with fat necrosis, lipophages, and giant cells, ordinarily constitutes the bulk of the tumor but any component may predominate. The smooth muscle cells are often intimately associated with the outer layers of the muscular walls of the blood vessels from which they appear to arise. These muscle cells are arranged in a radial configuration, with the long axis of their elongated nuclei at perpendicular angles to the vessels, imparting a "hair-on-end" appearance. The smooth muscle often courses in interlacing fascicles throughout the neoplasm and is punctuated by islands of adipose tissue and blood vessels. Proliferations may be present within glomerular tufts (463). Lesions at extrarenal sites have a similar histology. In some microscopic fields, wide expanses are composed entirely of smooth muscle. There may be nuclear enlargement, hyperchromasia, and scattered mitoses among the smooth muscle cells (fig. 2-187). Intracytoplasmic granules may be visible microscopically (fig. 2-188). Some tumors have a sizable population of immature smooth muscle cells or leiomyoblasts, with rounded nuclei and cleared cytoplasm, arranged in palisades about a central arteriole (fig. 2-189).

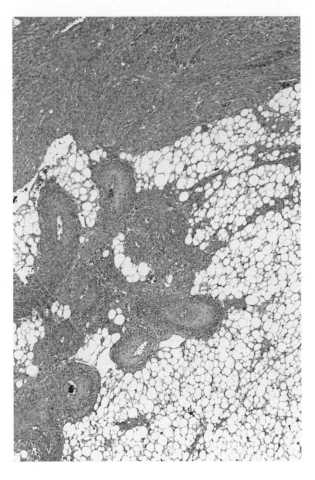

Figure 2-183

ANGIOMYOLIPOMA

The classic triphasic histology of smooth muscle, adipose tissue, and thick-walled blood vessels is shown.

The blood vessels are a striking component of the tumor and typically have very thick, abnormally formed walls. In many areas, the muscular tissue of the blood vessels is replaced by dense fibrous connective tissue of irregular thickness. These vessels resemble arterialized veins like those found in arteriovenous malformations. The internal elastic laminae are generally absent from vascular walls or when present, are fragmented, reduplicated, and frayed. The blood vessels of angiomyolipomas may be extremely tortuous and their walls focally thinned and dilated, creating small cirsoid aneurysms. Specimens obtained by aspiration cytology typically have a mixture of adipose tissue and smooth muscle.

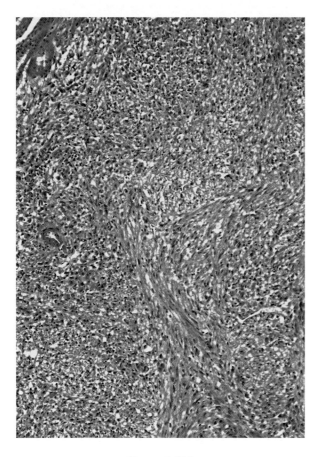

Figure 2-184

ANGIOMYOLIPOMA

A smooth muscle–predominant angiomyolipoma, with cells arranged in broad fascicles.

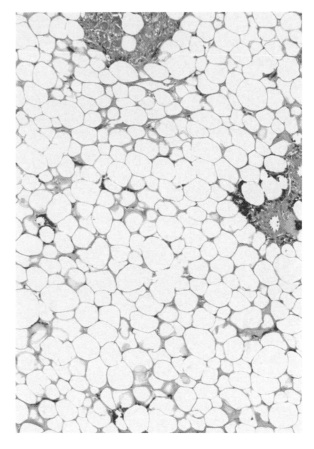

Figure 2-185

ANGIOMYOLIPOMA

This angiomyolipoma consists predominantly of adipose tissue with occasional small blood vessels scattered throughout.

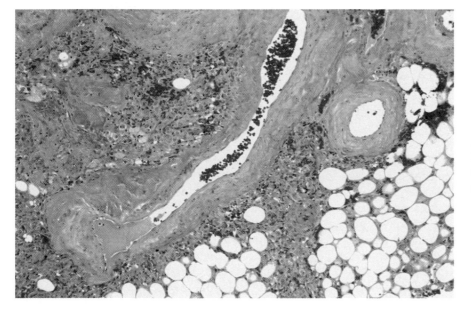

Figure 2-186

ANGIOMYOLIPOMA

Morphologically abnormal blood vessels with variably thickened walls are associated with adipose tissue and smooth muscle.

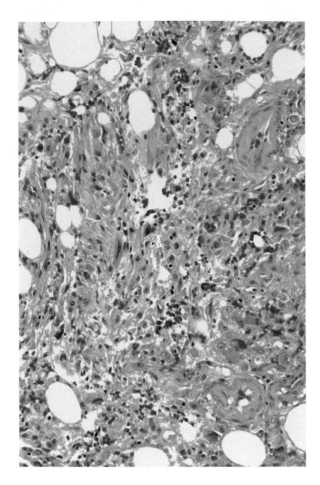

Figure 2-187

ANGIOMYOLIPOMA

Scattered atypical enlarged nuclei within the smooth muscle component of an angiomyolipoma.

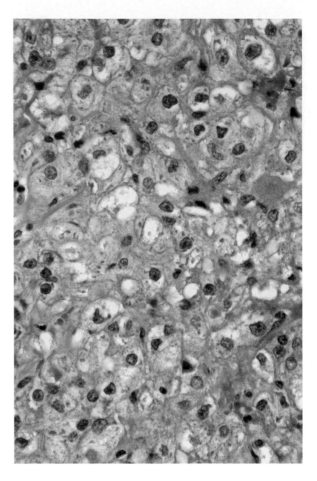

Figure 2-188

ANGIOMYOLIPOMA

Epithelioid smooth muscle cells contain pale basophilic intracytoplasmic granules of variable size and shape.

Ultrastructural studies reveal cells with typical features of smooth muscle and adipocytes. Transitional forms, with features of both cell types, have been identified (473). A spectrum of granules is present, including some with rhomboid and spherical shapes as well as typical premelanosomes (446,460,483).

Prognosis. Despite a heterologous composition and lack of cellular anaplasia, angiomyolipoma is a significant tumor that can predispose to life-threatening complications, the most significant being hemorrhage. The first satisfactorily documented case of malignancy developing in an angiomyolipoma appeared in 1991 (454). In this case, a renal tumor that had extended into the liver and metastasized to the lung exhibited areas of typical angiomyolipoma

along with other foci of transformation into a high-grade spindle cell sarcoma. Patients with tuberous sclerosis have a number of abnormalities that may be life-threatening. Even individuals lacking associated syndromes or malignant transformation may develop progressive renal failure and massive hemorrhage (453,464). New angiomyolipomas have appeared in the remaining kidney after nephrectomy for a contralateral lesion.

Differential Diagnosis. Angiomyolipoma may be confused with leiomyoma, leiomyosarcoma, and sarcomatoid RCC. This is particularly problematic in cases with a predominant smooth muscle component and associated cytologic atypia and necrosis. The presence of characteristic blood vessels and even small amounts of fat

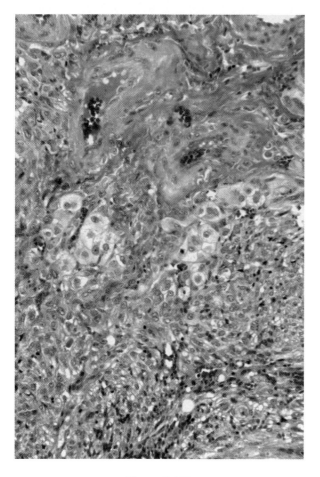

Figure 2-189

ANGIOMYOLIPOMA

Small collections of epithelioid cells within an angiomyolipoma have acidophilic to clear cytoplasm.

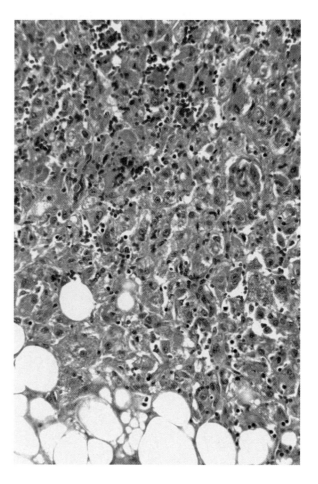

Figure 2-190

EPITHELIOID ANGIOMYOLIPOMA

This otherwise typical angiomyolipoma contains a large area of cells with abundant acidophilic cytoplasm and large nuclei with macronucleoli. (Courtesy of Dr. Peter Engbers, Woodstock, Ontario.)

should separate angiomyolipoma from leiomyoma. Similarly, these features, combined with a paucity of mitotic figures, despite cytologic atypia, distinguish angiomyolipoma from malignant neoplasms. Angiomyolipoma with epithelioid features also must be distinguished from RCC and melanoma. The immunohistochemical profile is useful in difficult cases.

Epithelioid Angiomyolipoma. The documentation of rare angiomyolipomas composed either partially or completely of large epithelioid cells has altered the concept of angiomyolipoma as a completely benign neoplasm (452, 468). The epithelioid cells range from intermediate-sized polygonal cells to giant cells with abundant acidophilic cytoplasm. Clear cell variants similar to "sugar tumor" are also reported (477).

The cells may be mononuclear or multinucleated and have prominent nuclei with macronucleoli, often resembling ganglion cells (figs. 2-190, 2-191). Variable degrees of nuclear pleomorphism are seen and mitotic activity may be brisk. Necrosis is often present. In some cases, the characteristic thick-walled blood vessels and adipose tissue of an angiomyolipoma are absent.

Epithelioid angiomyolipomas are considered to be malignant neoplasms with the capacity to be locally aggressive and metastasize (450, 452,471,472). They occur over a wide age range (6 to 72 years) and in roughly equal numbers of men and women (450). Metastases in some cases have been widespread, involving multiple

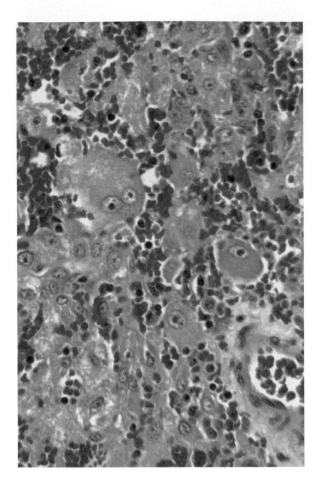

Figure 2-191

EPITHELIOID ANGIOMYOLIPOMA

The epithelioid cells are ganglion-like in morphology, with large nuclei having a single macronucleolus.

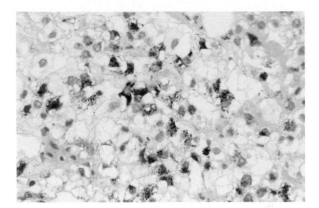

Figure 2-192

EPITHELIOID ANGIOMYOLIPOMA

Positive immunohistochemical staining for HMB-45 within the epithelioid cells of this angiomyolipoma.

organs, with lung and liver the most frequent (450,476). Up to 50 percent of patients with follow-up have died of disease.

Special Techniques. Methods other than immunohistochemistry are not useful in diagnosing angiomyolipoma, but immunohistochemistry is valuable in certain cases. There is consistent expression of muscle markers (muscle-specific actin, smooth muscle actin, desmin) and vimentin (451,466). Almost uniform positivity is seen for melanocytic markers, including HMB-45, MART-1, tyrosinase, and microphthalmia transcription factor (fig. 2-192) (445,466,484). Expression of c-kit (CD117) is seen in all cases (469). Although focal weak reactivity for cytokeratins has been reported, most studies have documented no reactivity (466). Epithelioid angio-

myolipoma has a pattern of immunoreactivity similar to that of the usual angiomyolipoma.

Renomedullary Interstitial Cell Tumor (Medullary Fibroma)

The interstitium of the renal medulla contains a specialized cell type, the interstitial cell, which produces prostaglandins and is believed to serve in the regulation of intrarenal blood pressure (489–491). Ultrastructurally, interstitial cells contain large numbers of electron-dense granules (lipid droplets). It has been suggested that tumors formerly designated medullary fibroma are composed of these renal medullary interstitial cells (489). Interstitial cell tumors are typically small, pale gray, well-circumscribed lesions appearing as incidental findings at autopsy. They are observed in as many as 50 percent of autopsied kidneys and are multiple in approximately 50 percent of cases. Lesions usually occur in adults and are rare in individuals less than 18 years of age. No evidence of systemic function was found in a study comparing heart weight and blood pressure in autopsied patients with interstitial cell tumors compared to a matched control group without these lesions (491).

Grossly, most interstitial cell tumors are less than 0.3 cm in greatest dimension. Lesions measuring more than 0.6 cm are rare, although tumors up to 6.5 cm have been recorded (487, 488). The neoplasms tend to be spade-shaped and occupy the midportion of the medullary pyramids (fig. 2-193).

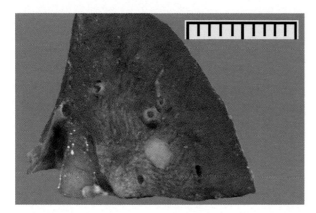

Figure 2-193

RENOMEDULLARY INTERSTITIAL CELL TUMOR

The lesion is a small, relatively circumscribed, gray-white nodule located within the medullary pyramid.

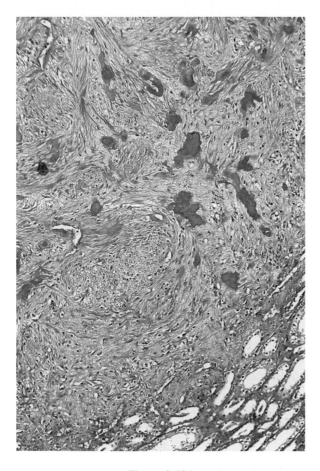

Figure 2-194

RENOMEDULLARY INTERSTITIAL CELL TUMOR

The lesion is well circumscribed but nonencapsulated. Spindle- and stellate-shaped cells are within a hypocellular stroma. Areas of hyalinization are present.

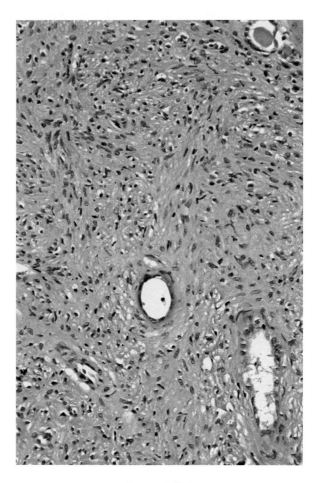

Figure 2-195

RENOMEDULLARY INTERSTITIAL CELL TUMOR

Spindle-shaped cells are in poorly formed fascicles. Note the entrapped renal tubules.

Histologically, interstitial cell tumors consist of a proliferation of small, stellate or polygonal cells in a loose stromal background with entrapped medullary tubules at the periphery (figs. 2-194, 2-195). Some lesions are hyalinized and almost acellular; others contain amyloid. Histochemical studies demonstrate neutral fat, phospholipid, and acid mucopolysaccharides.

Interstitial cell tumors are benign and rarely clinically significant. They should be distinguished from metanephric stromal tumors, rare examples of which have been reported in adults (485,486). Most characteristic of the latter is the formation of concentric rings or collarettes of stromal cells around entrapped renal tubules and blood vessels (see figs. 1-95–1-98, 1-100) (485).

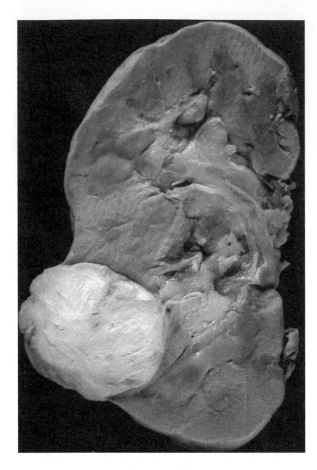

Figure 2-196

LEIOMYOMA

A firm circumscribed tumor with a whorled appearance to the cut surface. (Fig. 1-241 from Fascicle 11, 3rd Series.)

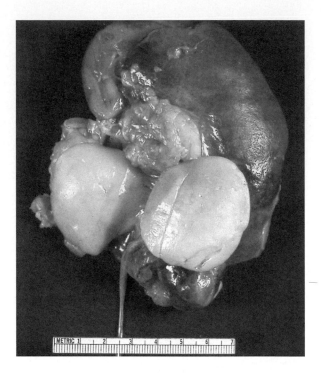

Figure 2-197

LIPOMA

This tumor appears to arise in the hilar adipose tissue rather than the renal parenchyma proper. (Fig. 1-243 from Fascicle 11, 3rd Series.)

Leiomyoma

This is a rare renal neoplasm that occurs in the cortex or capsule (fig. 2-196). Capsular leiomyomas are seen in approximately 5 percent of autopsies, where are usually incidental nodules 0.1 to 0.3 cm in greatest dimension (500). Few patients are symptomatic (497). Some reported tumors may actually represent angiomyolipomas. Renal leiomyomas occur mainly in adults but have been observed in neonates and children (495). The larger, clinically significant tumors are most common in younger women (498,499).

Leiomyomas arising in the kidney do not differ pathologically from similar tumors at other body sites. They may become large and multifocal (493,494,496). Calcification may be seen. No widely accepted criteria for distinction from leiomyosarcoma are available but the presence of mitotic activity, nuclear pleomorphism, or necrosis should raise this possibility (495a). The major entity in the differential diagnosis is smooth muscle–predominant angiomyolipoma.

Leiomyoma of the kidney, and more specifically of apparent capsular origin, has been reported to be HMB-45 positive in addition to expressing the usual smooth muscle markers (492). Tumors occurring in infants must be differentiated from congenital mesoblastic nephroma. Leiomyomas of the kidney are extraordinarily rare, a factor that should be taken into account when considering such an interpretation.

Lipoma

Renal lipomas are very rare tumors, which have been recorded in less than 1 percent of autopsied kidneys (fig. 2-197) (501,502). Very few patients are symptomatic. Most lesions are intrarenal and almost all occur in middle-aged women.

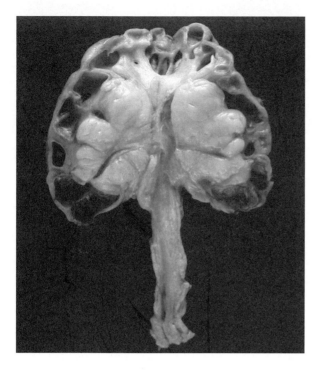

Figure 2-198

PELVIC LIPOMATOSIS

Hydronephrosis and cortical atrophy are associated with an increase in pelvic adipose tissue. (Fig. 1-244 from Fascicle 11, 3rd Series.)

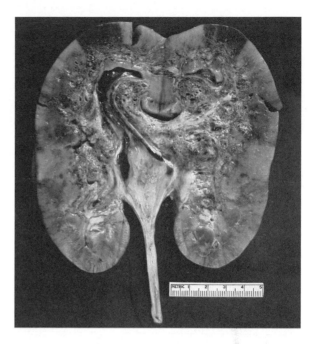

Figure 2-199

HEMANGIOMA

A sponge-like lesion involves much of the kidney and peripelvic tissues. (Fig. 1B from Edward HG, et al. Renal hemangiomas. Mayo Clinic Proc 1962;37:545.)

Most are found incidentally and appear to arise from the renal capsule or the hilar fat.

Intrarenal lipomas must be distinguished from angiomyolipomas. Renal lipomas are true neoplasms and should be differentiated from parapelvic lipomatosis, a condition that occurs following renal cortical atrophy, usually associated with hydronephrosis (fig. 2-198).

Hemangioma

Hemangiomas in the kidney arise in the cortex, medulla, or renal pelvis (fig. 2-199) (504a, 509). Most occur in young and middle-aged adults. Although lesions are usually single, approximately 12 percent are multifocal and a few are bilateral. Some patients with multifocal tumors have symptoms associated with vascular syndromes, such as Klippel-Trenaunay and Sturge-Weber (514). Renal hemangiomas are usually small, asymptomatic, and possibly congenital. Rarely, these tumors present as mass lesions (507,519). The most frequent sign is hematuria. Bleeding may be massive, especially

in large lesions that involve the renal pelvis. Treatment is often surgical, although local cautery of the lesion can be curative (504).

The pathology is similar to that of similar lesions in other organs. Most tumors are small, less than 2 cm in greatest dimension, and red-blue. They are usually found in the medulla but may also involve the cortex and even the capsule (518). Lesions located in perirenal fat can present as a renal mass (505,511). Histologically, the majority of renal hemangiomas are cavernous in type.

Lymphangioma

These tumors are less frequent than hemangiomas and typically occur in young adults complaining of hematuria or a flank mass (fig. 2-200) (506,508,510,512,515–517). Children are affected in approximately one third of cases. Most lymphangiomas are unilateral, with rare bilateral lesions recorded. Most are peripelvic and may actually represent lymphangiectasia due to pelvic inflammation with secondary lymphatic

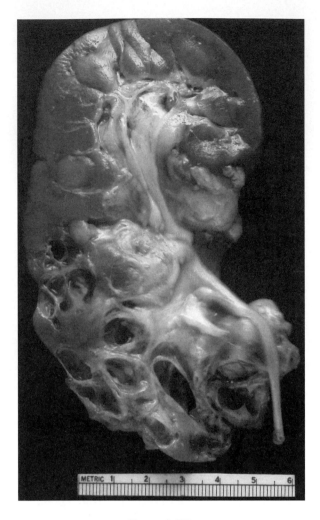

Figure 2-200

LYMPHANGIOMA

This large intrarenal lesion presents a honeycombed appearance. (Fig. 1-248 from Fascicle 11, 3rd Series.)

obstruction. The rare intrarenal lymphangioma has a honeycombed or multicystic gross appearance, with cavernous spaces of varying size. Histologically, the spaces are lined by flattened endothelial cells on a fibrous septum, which may contain elements of smooth muscle. These spaces are filled with lymph.

The major entity in the differential diagnosis is cystic nephroma. The lining cells in lymphangioma have an endothelial cell profile by immunohistochemistry (CD31 and factor VIII–related antigen) (503,513). We are aware of no examples of lymphangiosarcoma of the kidney.

Other Benign Mesenchymal Tumors

Isolated reports of many other benign mesenchymal tumors arising within the kidney have been recorded. These include schwannoma, neurofibroma, perineurioma, benign fibrous histiocytoma, fibroma, and myxoma (520–528a).

Leiomyosarcoma

Sarcomas of the kidney are vanishingly rare. Among primary tumors, leiomyosarcoma is the most frequent, comprising 40 to 60 percent of reported cases (541,544,545a,550,572,576). These tumors are usually situated peripherally and appear to arise from the renal capsule or smooth muscle tissue in the wall of the renal pelvis. Leiomyosarcomas may arise in the smooth muscle of large renal blood vessels but about one third are intrarenal (546). Patients are of a wide age range and a roughly equal sex distribution (544). Overall, the prognosis is poor, with a 3-year survival rate of 20 percent and a median survival period of 18 months in one series (544). Local recurrence and hematogenous spread to bone and lung are frequent.

Leiomyosarcomas of the kidney are pale gray, firm, and fleshy, with a nodular or bosselated surface. Necrosis is common and cystic change may occur (539). Most are large, but size is variable (fig. 2-101) (567). The histologic features are similar to those of leiomyosarcomas at other sites, and various subtypes have been observed (fig. 2-202) (545a). Microscopic vascular invasion is common but extension into large renal veins is unusual. Diagnosis by fine needle aspiration has been reported but should be approached with caution considering that carcinomas with significant spindle cell components are much more common than sarcomas in the kidney (577). Tumors with low-grade histology and a low mitotic rate (less than 5 mitoses per 10 high-power fields) have metastasized (fig. 2-203) (544).

Leiomyosarcoma must be differentiated from sarcomatoid carcinoma and angiomyolipoma. Generous sampling identifies an epithelial component in nearly all cases of sarcomatoid carcinoma. Epithelial markers are usually positive and epithelial features are demonstrable by electron microscopy. Angiomyolipoma can have a nearly pure smooth muscle histology but thick-walled

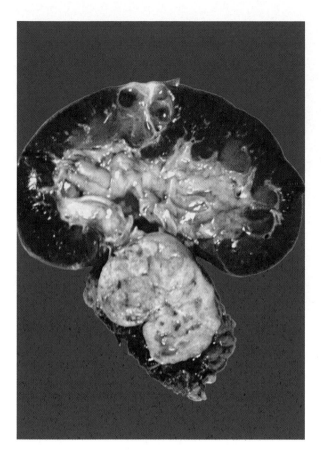

Figure 2-201

LEIOMYOSARCOMA

In this renal leiomyosarcoma the tumor is arising from the renal vein.

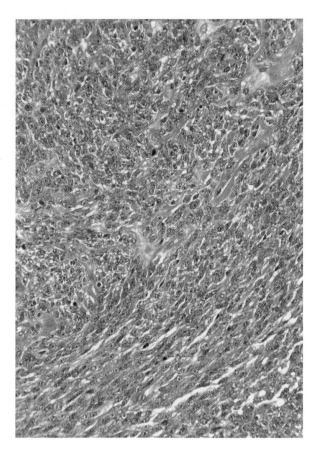

Figure 2-202

LEIOMYOSARCOMA

A leiomyosarcoma with high cellularity, frequent mitotic figures, and moderate cytologic atypia.

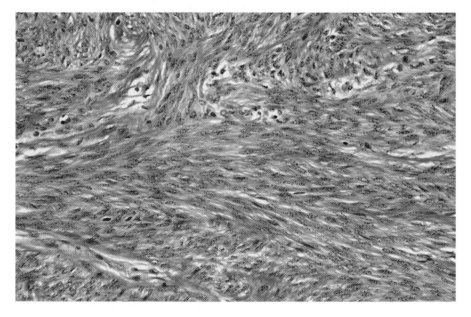

Figure 2-203

LEIOMYOSARCOMA

The tumor is moderately cellular with little nuclear pleomorphism. Only occasional mitotic figures were evident.

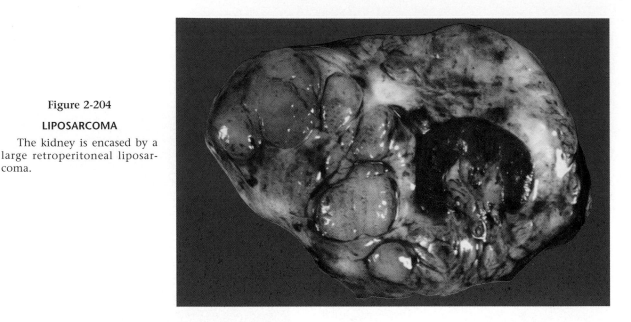

Figure 2-204

LIPOSARCOMA

The kidney is encased by a large retroperitoneal liposarcoma.

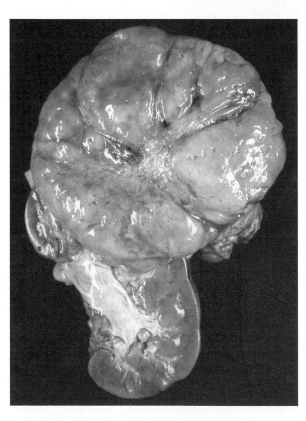

Figure 2-205

LIPOSARCOMA

This large fatty tumor has an intrarenal component but projects from the renal surface. (Fig. 8-82 from Farrow GM. Diseases of the kidney. In: Murphy WM, ed. Urological pathology. Philadelphia: WB Saunders; 1989:409–82.)

vessels and adipose tissue are usually demonstrable, at least focally. HMB-45 positivity supports the diagnosis of angiomyolipoma.

Liposarcoma

Liposarcomas typically occur in the retroperitoneum, with secondary involvement of the kidney, and reviews of the subject have emphasized the difficulty of separating primary renal liposarcoma from secondary involvement by a retroperitoneal tumor (figs. 2-204, 2-205) (533, 545a,547,557,578,580). Liposarcomas also arise in the fat of the renal sinus. Lesions involving only the renal parenchyma are rare. If the contention that liposarcomas may arise within the inner adipose tissue of the renal capsule and be contained by this structure is accepted, then more cases can be included (541,569). Liposarcomas have not always been distinguished from angiomyolipomas in the past.

These cancers do not differ histologically from similar tumors at other body sites. All histologic patterns are observed, the most common being the myxoid type. Complete surgical excision is extremely difficult to achieve, so that local recurrences and eventual tumor-related deaths are the rule. Patients with intrarenal tumors have a better reported prognosis than those with peripheral lesions (557).

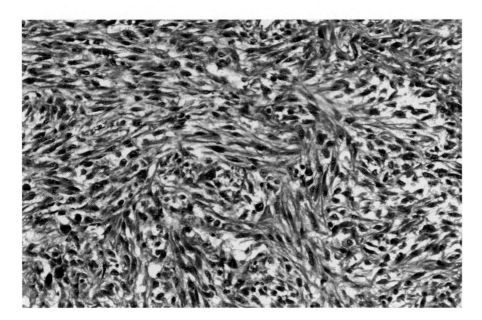

Figure 2-206

MALIGNANT FIBROUS HISTIOCYTOMA

The tumor is composed of pleomorphic spindle cells in a tight storiform architecture.

Solitary Fibrous Tumor

Tumors with the characteristic histologic and immunohistochemical features of solitary fibrous tumor are well described in the kidney (556,579). Patients range in age from 33 to 72 years, with no sex predilection. Presentation is similar to that of other renal masses.

Pathologically, all tumors are solitary, circumscribed, and solid tan-gray, ranging from 3 to 14 cm in greatest dimension. Histologically, the bland spindle cells are arranged haphazardly in short intersecting fascicles or in a hemangiopericytoma-like vascular pattern. Immunohistochemistry reveals positive immunoreactivity for CD34 and vimentin, with variable reactivity for actin, smooth muscle actin, and desmin. These neoplasms are included among mesenchymal malignancies in keeping with their classification in other organs, but all solitary fibrous tumors primary to the kidney have behaved in a benign manner.

Hemangiopericytoma

Hemangiopericytomas have been identified as primary renal neoplasms although about 50 percent of reported cases have arisen in perirenal tissues or in the renal capsule (532,545a, 558,571). A single patient with bilateral renal involvement has been reported (548). Renal lesions are typically large, circumscribed, and fibrous. The histology is essentially the same as for hemangiopericytomas elsewhere. As with hemangiopericytomas in other sites, the criteria for malignancy have not been established. The outlook for long-term survival is better than for those with most other renal sarcomas. Interestingly, in three of the reported cases there was an associated paraneoplastic syndrome of severe hypoglycemia and one patient died in a hypoglycemic coma (531,541).

Fibrosarcoma and Malignant Fibrous Histiocytoma

These tumors may be much less common than the older literature indicates, since many cases of sarcomatoid RCC feature components that closely resemble fibrous histiocytoma and fibrosarcoma (535). The more recent literature includes several well-documented examples, however (552,555,563,564,573). The tendency of these lesions to be large and involve perirenal structures further confounds a determination of primary site. Both fibrosarcoma and malignant fibrous histiocytoma are typically solid, fleshy tumors that exhibit hemorrhage and necrosis. Malignant fibrous histiocytomas are characteristically of the storiform-pleomorphic type, but inflammatory types and giant cell variants have been recorded (fig. 2-206). As with all primary renal sarcomas, sarcomatoid RCC must be excluded. There are too few cases to make any conclusion regarding specific clinical features or prognosis, but reported tumors seem to be aggressive and associated with a very poor prognosis (545a,564).

Rhabdomyosarcoma

Primary rhabdomyosarcoma of the kidney is exceedingly rare in adults (542,545). These tumors are typically large, solid, fleshy, and pale gray (541). Virtually all are of the pleomorphic variety. In most reports, strap cells with cross striations are identified. Sarcomatoid carcinoma should be considered before a diagnosis is rendered.

Angiosarcoma

Primary angiosarcoma is a rare renal neoplasm with very few cases in the literature (fig. 2-207) (529,534,536,537,549,574,575). Almost all occur in older men. Clinical and radiologic findings are nonspecific. These tumors are situated in the renal parenchyma where they form multiple, circumscribed, hemorrhagic masses. A wide range of histologic features has been described, similar to angiosarcomas elsewhere. Areas with identifiable vascular spaces are lined by malignant endothelial cells. Immunohistochemistry may be needed to confirm the nature of the tumor. The outcome has been nearly uniformly fatal, with early metastases to lung, bone, and liver.

Osteosarcoma

Extraosseous osteosarcoma arising in the kidney is a rare but well-documented tumor (fig. 2-208) (540,554,559,562). These cancers tend to occur in elderly patients. The ossification may be identified radiologically. Tumors are typically large and invasive, and consist of osteoid-producing sarcoma cells. Varying degrees of chondrosarcomatous differentiation may also be present. Survival is poor, with the majority of patients dying of their disease within 18 months.

Synovial Sarcoma

The occurrence of synovial sarcoma as a primary neoplasm in the kidney is supported by identification of the *SYT/SSX* fusion product of a t(x:18) translocation in a group of distinctive renal tumors (530,551,553). Most patients are young to middle-aged adults, with a median age of 35 years and a range of 20 to 59 years. There is no sex predilection. Presentation is similar to that of other mass lesions of the kidney.

Pathologically, most tumors are large, necrotic, and grossly cystic. Histologically, they are highly cellular, with short, intersecting fascicles (fig. 2-209). The nuclei are ovoid to fusi-

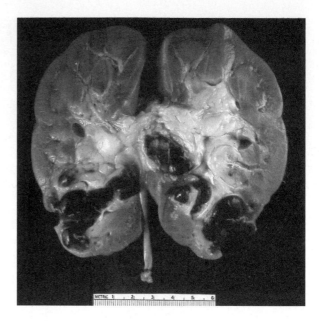

Figure 2-207

ANGIOSARCOMA

There are multiple hemorrhagic tumor masses within the renal parenchyma. (Fig. 1-259 from Fascicle 11, 3rd Series.)

form, with coarse chromatin, variable-sized nucleoli, and frequent mitoses. Cytoplasm is scant and ill-defined. In some cases, the cystic areas are lined by epithelial cells with acidophilic cytoplasm and a hobnail morphology.

The spindle cells are vimentin positive and cytokeratin negative. Focal reactivity for EMA is present in some cases. These tumors are also nonreactive for desmin, muscle-specific actin, CD34, and S-100 protein. Variable reactivity for CD99 has been described. The epithelial component lining the cysts is cytokeratin positive.

The differential diagnosis includes embryonal sarcoma of the kidney, primitive neuroectodermal tumor, and nephroblastoma. The limited clinical data available indicate that these are aggressive neoplasms.

Other Malignant Mesenchymal Tumors

A host of other malignant mesenchymal tumors have been described in the kidney, including chondrosarcoma, low-grade fibromyxoid sarcoma, clear cell sarcoma of soft parts, cystic embryonal sarcoma, malignant mesenchymoma, and malignant schwannoma (538,543, 560,561,565,566,568,570).

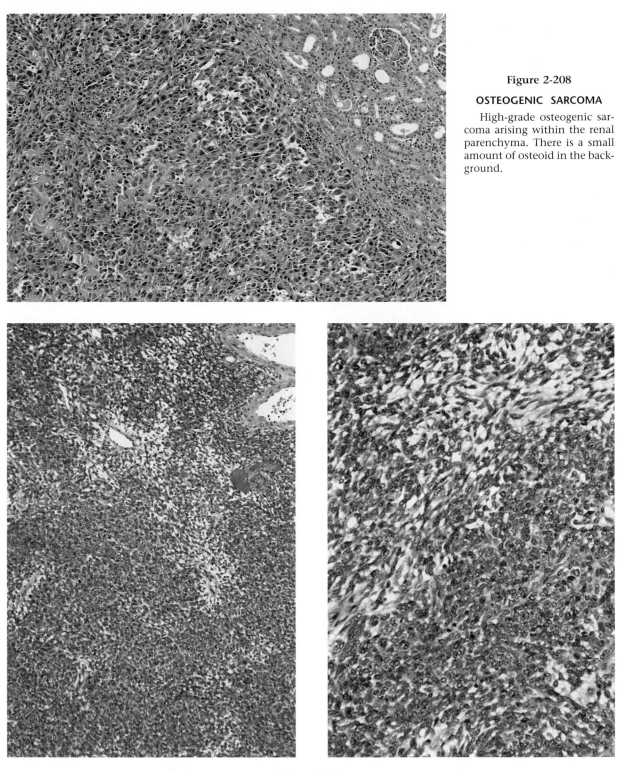

Figure 2-208

OSTEOGENIC SARCOMA

High-grade osteogenic sarcoma arising within the renal parenchyma. There is a small amount of osteoid in the background.

Figure 2-209

SYNOVIAL SARCOMA

Low- (left) and high-power (right) photomicrographs of renal synovial sarcoma. The diagnosis in this case was supported by demonstration of the characteristic t(X:18) translocation. (Courtesy of Dr. Volkan Adsay, Detroit, MI.)

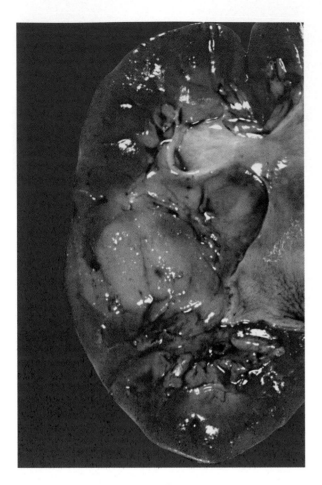

Figure 2-210

MALIGNANT LYMPHOMA

The single, circumscribed, lobulated mass with a fleshy gray-white appearance involves the renal parenchyma.

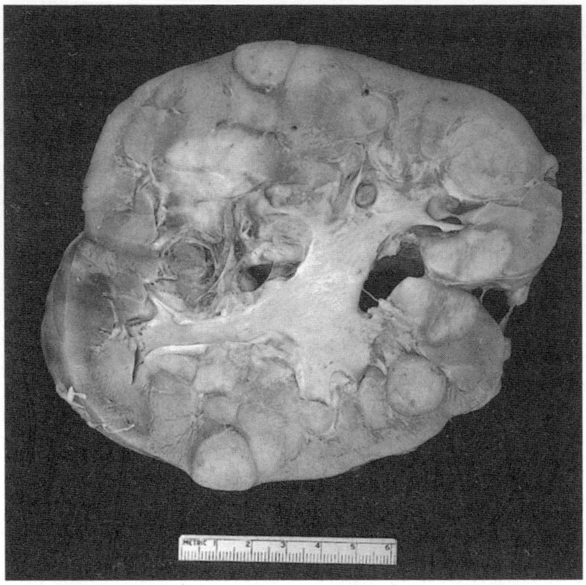

Figure 2-211

MALIGNANT LYMPHOMA

There are multiple tumor nodules in the kidney. (Fig. 2B from Farrow GM, Harrison EG Jr, Utz DC. Sarcomas and sarcomatoid and mixed malignant tumors of the kidney in adults. Part II. Cancer 1968;22:551–5.)

LYMPHOID TUMORS

Lymphoma

Involvement of the kidneys by malignant lymphoma is common in patients with late-stage disease, particularly among those with non-Hodgkin lymphomas having extensive retroperitoneal involvement. Clinical evidence of genitourinary involvement is found in less than 10 percent of cases but this figure increases to nearly 70 percent among autopsy series (584,596, 602). Radiographic studies have also demonstrated a high frequency of renal involvement in late-stage lymphoma (603). Conversely, primary renal lymphoma without evidence of systemic disease is rare, accounting for less than 1 percent of primary extranodal lymphomas (581,584, 586,588,599,604). Clinically, the most frequent presentation is acute renal failure. In such cases, the lymphoma is usually localized to the hilus.

Renal lymphoma may appear as discrete, solitary or multiple nodular parenchymal masses (figs. 2-210, 2-211). Bilateral involvement occurs in over 40 percent of cases and is characterized by diffuse infiltration of the kidneys. Recorded hilar lymphomas are 6 to 11 cm in greatest dimension and encompass the hilar lymph nodes, so that a possible nodal origin cannot be completely excluded. Parenchymal nodules measure up to 15 cm in greatest dimension and are distributed throughout both the cortex and medulla.

Histologically, primary renal lymphomas are usually of the large cell, diffuse type, although almost all subtypes have been described (fig. 2-212) (583,585,589). The tumor cells diffusely permeate the interstitium, tending to spare normal structures, and even cases with grossly circumscribed nodules demonstrate this pattern of growth histologically. Fine needle aspiration biopsy is useful for diagnosing both primary and

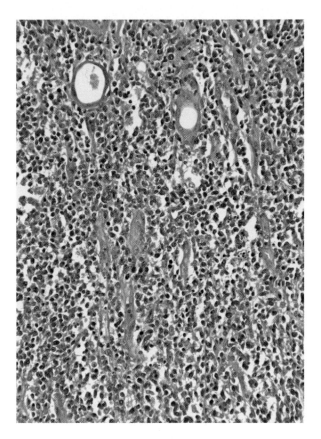

Figure 2-212

MALIGNANT LYMPHOMA

The tumor cells diffusely permeate the renal parenchyma, sparing normal structures. Atrophic residual tubules are seen at the top.

secondary renal lymphomas (605). Extrarenal disease should be excluded at the time of diagnosis of primary renal lymphoma through radiological studies, bone marrow biopsy, and a staging laparotomy (590). The coexistence of renal lymphoma with RCC has been described (606).

Renal involvement also occurs in peripheral T-cell lymphoma and low-grade B-cell lymphoma of mucosa-associated lymphoid tissue (MALT) (593–595,598,600). The microscopic features of these types of lymphoma of the kidney are similar to those in other organs.

Post-Transplant Lymphoproliferative Disorder

Post-transplant lymphoproliferative disorder develops in approximately 1 percent of renal allograft recipients (597). These lesions are characteristically associated with Epstein-Barr virus

(EBV) infection (591), and range from polymorphic plasma cell and B-cell proliferations to monoclonal B-cell lymphomas (most frequent) and myeloma (587,591,597). The histopathologic features vary and depend on the nature of the proliferation (591). Useful findings distinguishing these neoplasms from transplant rejection include the atypical B-cell nature of the cellular infiltrate, an expansile growth pattern, and the presence of serpiginous necrosis in the former (601).

Plasmacytoma

Plasmacytoma is rarely found as a primary tumor in the kidney (592). Most recorded cases are associated with disease in the bones. Amyloidosis has been observed in at least one case. Renal plasmacytomas tend to be solitary mass lesions. A few patients have survived for long periods following resection of the tumor.

Leukemia

Leukemic involvement of the kidney is ordinarily an incidental autopsy finding featuring interstitial infiltration by the neoplastic cells. Rarely, a mass lesion (myeloid sarcoma) occurs in association with acute myeloid leukemia, myeloproliferative disorder, or myelodysplastic syndrome (582).

TUMORS METASTATIC TO THE KIDNEY

In the later stages of evolution of malignant tumors at other locations, metastatic deposits may appear in the kidneys. In autopsy series, the kidneys are involved by metastases in up to 7.2 percent of cases (608,614). Infrequently, the renal metastasis is the primary manifestation (611). The differential diagnosis is ordinarily not a problem since metastatic tumors masquerading as primary renal neoplasms are unusual in well-evaluated patients. The most common primary sites are lung, breast, skin (malignant melanoma), contralateral kidney, gastrointestinal tract, ovary, and testis (612). In most cases, metastases are multiple and bilateral, with well-circumscribed nodules, but they can also be single with infiltrative borders (fig. 2-213). Metastases may be limited to an intraglomerular location, rarely resulting in renal failure (fig. 2-214) (607,609,610). As a rule, the possibility of a metastasis should be considered whenever a

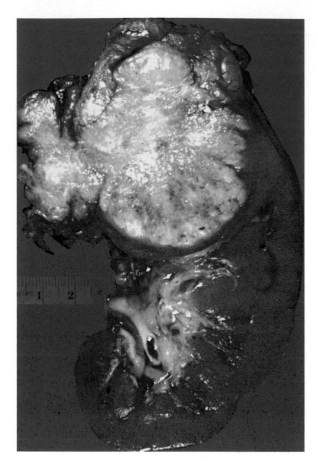

Figure 2-213

METASTATIC CARCINOMA

This is a metastatic poorly differentiated adenocarcinoma of lung origin.

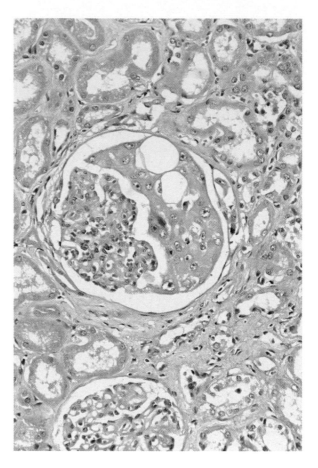

Figure 2-214

METASTATIC CARCINOMA

Metastatic poorly differentiated squamous cell carcinoma of lung origin was confined to the glomeruli throughout the kidney.

renal neoplasm appears unclassifiable as a primary lesion. In some cases, patients with metastases are treated by surgical resection, most often for intractable hematuria.

Metastases also occur to primary renal neoplasms. It is reported that RCC is the most common malignant tumor that acts as the recipient in tumor-to-tumor metastasis (613). The lung is the most common primary site for a tumor metastasizing to a RCC. A case of intravascular lymphomatosis involving RCC has been described (606).

NON-NEOPLASTIC
TUMOROUS CONDITIONS

In its broadest sense, the word "tumor" includes any space-occupying localized enlargement in an anatomic structure. Thus, there are tumors that are not neoplastic but simulate neoplasms clinically and radiologically. A complete discussion of this topic, to include cystic diseases and dysplasias, is beyond the scope of this atlas. It is appropriate, however, to discuss a few conditions that are well recognized for their ability to mimic neoplasms, both clinically and pathologically.

Xanthogranulomatous Pyelonephritis

Xanthogranulomatous pyelonephritis is a distinctive form of subacute and chronic renal inflammation prone to form a mass lesion that may mimic a renal neoplasm. Several collected series of cases have appeared in the literature since the first description in 1916 (619,629,631). Most patients are women in the fourth to sixth decades of life. The most common presenting complaints

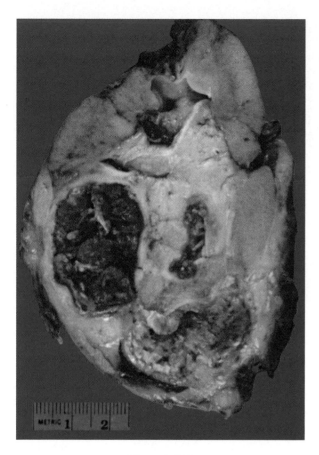

Figure 2-215

XANTHOGRANULOMATOUS PYELONEPHRITIS

The inflammatory process produces a poorly defined mass with a variegated color that includes yellow areas involving the renal parenchyma and perinephric adipose tissue.

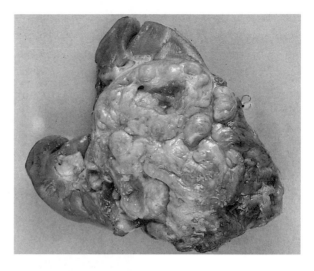

Figure 2-216

XANTHOGRANULOMATOUS PYELONEPHRITIS

A large golden yellow mass replaces much of the kidney and extends into the perirenal tissues. (Fig. 8-23 from Farrow GM. Diseases of the kidney. In: Murphy WM, ed. Uro-logical pathology. Philadelphia: WB Saunders; 1989:409–82.)

are fever, flank pain, and a tender flank mass (621, 624,629,636). Nephrolithiasis is a characteristic associated feature, present in up to 70 percent of patients. As determined by excretory urography, the affected kidney is nonfunctioning in 50 to 70 percent of patients. Common urinary tract bacteria such as *Proteus* and *Escherichia* sp may be isolated from the urine, but the urine culture is negative in as many as 30 percent of cases, even though organisms can be isolated from the lesion itself in 95 percent of cases (623). Because of the mass effect, radiologic findings mimic those of a renal neoplasm (616,622,635,637). The disease is almost always unilateral, but may involve any part or all of the kidney.

In its early stages, xanthogranulomatous pyelonephritis is usually confined to the kidney and appears grossly as golden yellow nodules ranging from a few millimeters to several centimeters in greatest dimension (fig. 2-215). By the time of clinical detection, however, the inflammatory mass is usually very large and may have penetrated Gerota's fascia, mimicking RCC both clinically and pathologically (fig. 2-216).

Histologically, the features of xanthogranulomatous pyelonephritis are variable (figs. 2-217–2-219). Purulent foci with microabscesses and numerous neutrophils may coexist with the more classic histopathology of abundant, lipid-laden macrophages intermixed with lymphocytes and plasma cells. The lipid-laden macrophages (xanthoma cells) may mimic the cells of well-differentiated clear cell RCC. Multinucleated giant cells and spindled fibroblasts may be abundant and such areas can resemble the spindle cell component of a sarcomatoid RCC. These inflammatory elements may have a zonal distribution, with the necrosis and acute inflammation adjacent to the collecting system, surrounded by macrophages with fibrosis and chronic inflammation at the periphery. In a small proportion of cases, Michaelis-Gutmann bodies are found, and when this occurs the designation malakoplakia is appropriate.

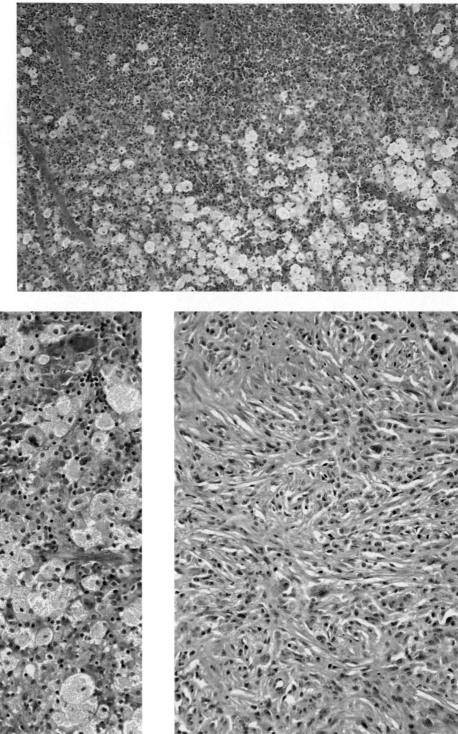

Figure 2-217

XANTHOGRANULOMATOUS PYELONEPHRITIS

A polymorphous inflammation includes numerous foamy macrophages as well as lymphocytes and plasma cells.

Figure 2-218

XANTHOGRANULOMATOUS PYELONEPHRITIS

This polymorphous inflammatory infiltrate includes foamy macrophages, lymphocytes, plasma cells, and a few multinucleated giant cells.

Figure 2-219

XANTHOGRANULOMATOUS PYELONEPHRITIS

There is an area of spindle cell proliferation.

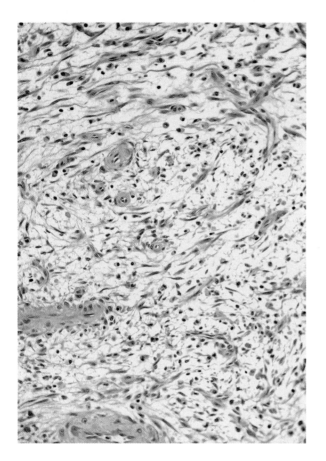

Figure 2-220

INFLAMMATORY PSEUDOTUMOR

This inflammatory myofibroblastic pseudotumor is characterized by a myxoid background with stellate and spindle-shaped cells, and a scattered chronic inflammatory infiltrate. (Courtesy of Dr. John Srigley, Toronto, Ontario.)

Inflammatory Myofibroblastic Pseudotumor

Several examples of inflammatory myofibroblastic pseudotumor have been reported arising in the kidney and perirenal soft tissues (615,620,626,627). Most patients present with a renal mass simulating a neoplasm; one patient had Behçet's syndrome (615). These lesions occur in adults and children, with no sex predilection, and are benign.

Grossly, tumors primarily involving the renal parenchyma are gray-white, unencapsulated, and partially or completely circumscribed. Histologically, three patterns predominate: loosely organized spindle cells in a myxoid background with inflammatory cells and small blood vessels; a spindle cell proliferation with variable amounts

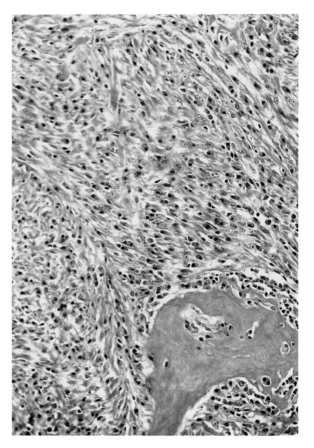

Figure 2-221

INFLAMMATORY PSEUDOTUMOR

There is focal bone formation and moderate cellularity but without significant cytologic atypia. (Courtesy of Dr. John Srigley, Toronto, Ontario.)

of dense collagen, as well as aggregates of lymphocytes and plasma cells; and hypocellular, dense "keloid-like" fibrous tissue with little inflammation (figs. 2-220–2-222) (626).

Immunohistochemistry reveals strong, diffuse positivity for vimentin and variable reactions for smooth muscle actin and muscle-specific actin. Reactions for desmin, CD34, and cytokeratins have been negative in cases studied to date (626).

Perinephric and Sinus Cysts

Cystic masses located in the renal sinus or perinephric adipose tissue may present clinically in such a way that RCC is suspected. These masses usually are organized perirenal hematomas, lymphatic cysts, mesothelial cysts, or peripherally located cortical cysts (617,618,625,630,632).

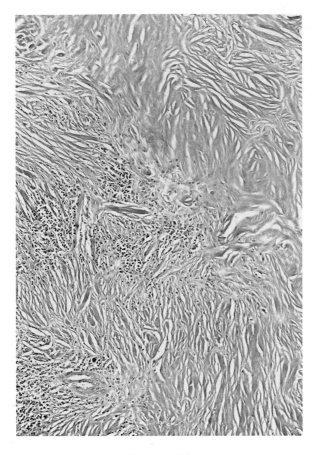

Figure 2-222

INFLAMMATORY PSEUDOTUMOR

There is dense collagenization with a keloid-like appearance and a scattered chronic inflammatory infiltrate. (Courtesy of Dr. John Srigley, Toronto, Ontario.)

The pathologic findings depend on the nature of the cyst. Lymphatic cysts and mesothelial cysts have endothelial and mesothelial linings, respectively. Organizing hematomas and ruptured cortical cysts have a fibrous wall with recent and old hemorrhage and variable degrees of inflammation. In some cases, variably sized ring-shaped structures with double walls and radial striations are found (figs. 2-223, 2-224). These Liesegang-like rings can be confused with cysts or the ova of parasites (633,634). Myospherulosis has also been described in perirenal cysts (628). These cases need to be extensively sampled to exclude the possibility of cystic RCC.

TREATMENT OF PATIENTS WITH RENAL CELL CARCINOMA

Over the past four decades, the survival of patients with RCC has improved significantly, most likely reflecting a stage migration, with an increasing proportion of newly diagnosed tumors being small and of low stage (652). Regardless of the histology, the mainstay of treatment for patients with a renal mass is surgical resection by either partial or radical nephrectomy. Radical nephrectomy includes removal of the kidney with the perinephric fat, encompassed regional lymph nodes, and the ipsilateral adrenal gland (655). In current practice, lymph node dissection is not a routine component of the operation for RCC and is performed at the surgeon's preference. There is no compelling data to indicate

Figure 2-223

PERIRENAL CYST WITH LIESEGANG RINGS

This peripelvic cyst has an inflammatory wall without identifiable epithelium. Within the inflammatory infiltrate are numerous round laminated bodies.

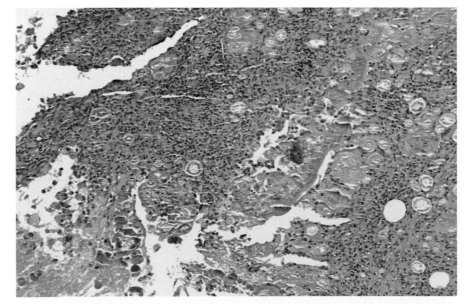

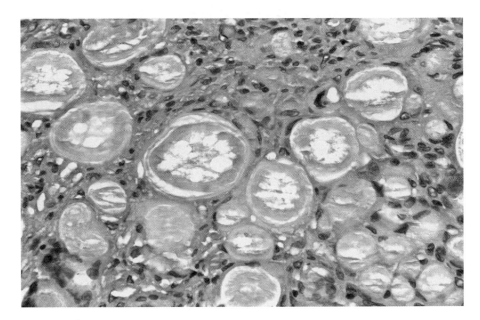

Figure 2-224

PERIRENAL CYST WITH LIESEGANG RINGS

Liesegang rings in the wall of a perirenal cyst give a laminated appearance.

whether inclusion of the lymph nodes impacts on survival of adult patients with renal malignancies (650,654,658). Incidental adrenal metastases have been documented in approximately 5 percent of radical nephrectomy specimens but the clinical value of adrenalectomy as part of nephrectomy is similarly uncertain (656). In patients with smaller tumors, the surgeon may elect not to remove the adrenal gland (653,657).

In the past, partial nephrectomy was restricted to patients with bilateral renal masses, for resection of masses in solitary kidneys, or for patients with diseases associated with an increased risk of renal failure such as diabetes, hypertension, and calculus disease. With improved imaging, increased frequency of detection of small tumors, and improved surgical techniques, partial nephrectomy has gained popularity as an acceptable surgical approach. For technical reasons, partial nephrectomy is optimal with smaller, peripherally located tumors. Numerous studies have demonstrated that this approach is equivalent to radical nephrectomy in suitably selected patients (640,648). The 5-year disease-free survival rates following partial nephrectomy were 98 percent and 96 percent in two contemporary series (640,648).

Laparoscopic nephrectomy or partial nephrectomy is increasingly popular (642,645,651). This procedure may require extensive fragmentation (morcellation) of the tumor-bearing specimen for removal, a process that has the potential to complicate pathologic evaluation. In analyses to date, accurate classification and staging (other than tumor size) has been possible in such specimens (646).

Surgical resection is an accepted approach for patients with renal vein and vena caval involvement. In those cases where the tumor thrombus remains free-floating in the vascular lumen, long-term survival of over 50 percent is expected if there is no associated metastatic disease (643,647,649). If the tumor is adherent to the wall, the prognosis is considered by most to be significantly worse, although this has not been a consistent finding (643,649).

For patients with metastatic RCC, there has been little success in identifying effective adjuvant therapies. In cases of limited metastases, there is some evidence that selected patients benefit from excision of the metastases, particularly if: 1) the metastases developed more than 12 months following nephrectomy; 2) the metastases are isolated; and 3) the metastatic site is the lung (644).

Extensive experience with a broad range of chemotherapeutic agents and a variety of immunologic approaches has not led to a successful cure of metastatic RCC (641). The 3-year disease-free survival rate for patients with untreated metastatic RCC is less than 5 percent. Presently, recombinant human interleukin-2 monotherapy is approved for patients with metastatic RCC. It is believed that this treatment

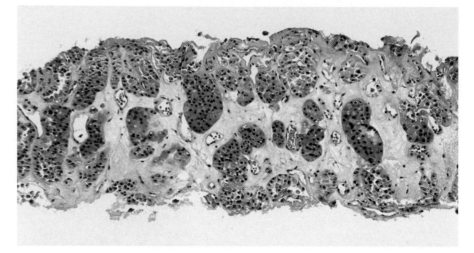

Figure 2-225

ONCOCYTOMA

This needle biopsy specimen from a renal mass shows the characteristic cytologic and architectural features of renal oncocytoma.

might offer improved short-term survival with some long-term durability (652). There is data to support the benefit of nephrectomy prior to immunotherapy in selected patients with metastatic RCC (652). Isolated reports have suggested that some patients with sarcomatoid RCC may respond to aggressive multiagent chemotherapy, however, larger series have failed to demonstrate a significant impact on outcome (638,639).

PROCEDURES FOR PATHOLOGIC EXAMINATION

Renal Biopsy

Historically, percutaneous biopsy of a renal mass has not enjoyed widespread popularity. With the ready availability of thin-needle aspiration as well as small bore core biopsy needles, interest in this technique in selected clinical situations has increased. This interest has grown as the behavior of different tumor types has become better defined.

The two most common scenarios in which percutaneous renal biopsy is advantageous are: 1) for the diagnosis of oncocytoma in patients with one functioning kidney or other reasons for avoiding open surgery; and 2) for evaluation of a complex cystic mass. In up to 70 percent of cases, the benign or malignant nature of complex cystic masses has been resolved through the use of percutaneous needle biopsy (665).

The diagnosis of oncocytoma can be rendered on evaluation of a needle biopsy specimen in selected situations if classic features are present.

These include a pure population of oncocytes and architectural arrangement in nests, in a loose hypocellular stroma (fig. 2-225). Closely packed nests of acidophilic cells are seen in chromophobe cell RCC, but the loose stroma is absent.

Identification of nests of clear cells within the septa of a complex cystic mass on biopsy allows for a definitive diagnosis of multicystic RCC. The presence of hobnail cells, associated with ovarian-like stroma in the septa, is diagnostic of a multilocular cyst. Without unequivocal features, however, a descriptive interpretation is advised.

Partial Nephrectomy

Tumor parameters described below for radical nephrectomy should be used for partial nephrectomy specimens as well. In most cases, a small amount of adipose tissue covers the cortical aspect of the tumor and sections should be submitted to look for fat invasion. Sections must also be submitted to evaluate the parenchymal margin. Often, the amount of renal parenchyma surrounding the tumor is minimal and the yellow color (for clear cell RCC) is visible through the margin (fig. 2-226). The parenchymal margin should be inked and perpendicular sections taken. A margin is considered positive only if tumor directly touches ink. Some authors have advocated a 1-cm margin in partial nephrectomy, but most reports have shown no higher risk of recurrence when less generous margins are obtained (fig. 2-227) (660,670,672,674). In partial nephrectomy specimens of papillary RCC, a small cortical adenoma is occasionally

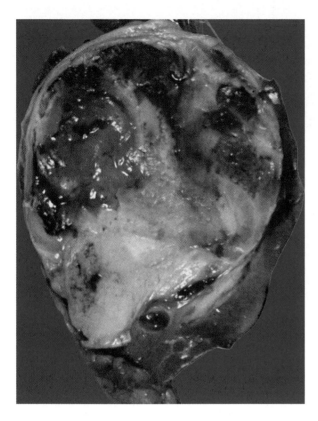

Figure 2-226

RENAL CELL CARCINOMA

This partial nephrectomy specimen contains a clear cell renal cell carcinoma. Note the closeness of the surgical margins to the tumor.

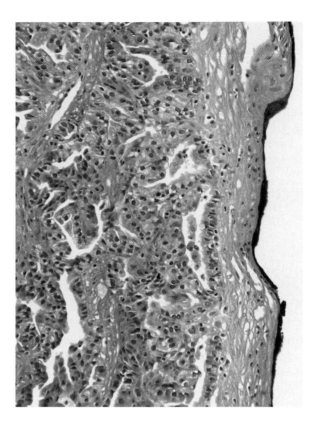

Figure 2-227

RENAL CELL CARCINOMA

The tumor extends close to the inked surgical resection margin in this partial nephrectomy specimen.

present at the inked margin (fig. 2-228). Such a finding is not considered to be a positive margin but it should be noted in a comment.

Radical Nephrectomy

The radical nephrectomy specimen is handled in such a way as to document all the important variables for proper staging and identification of significant prognostic factors. The initial evaluation should assess Gerota's fascia for gross tumor involvement; if areas of adhesions or induration are noted, the foci should be inked. The specimen can be bivalved slightly off center of the hilus to preserve the integrity of the hilar structures. An alternate approach is to remove the perinephric fat, watching for areas of adhesion of the fat to the external surface of the kidney. This may highlight foci of possible perinephric fat invasion (category pT3a) (663). The kidney is then bivalved after removal of the fat.

The hilar area is examined and the renal vein(s) identified and opened. A statement should be made as to whether or not there is gross involvement of the renal vein(s) by tumor. If a tumor thrombus is present, a section should be submitted to confirm that it does represent tumor. If areas of adhesion of the thrombus to the wall are evident, these areas should be sampled as well to further document tumor invasion of the vein wall. The renal vein margin should be assessed; margin involvement is defined by tumor adherent to the wall, not by thrombus extending beyond the margin "floating free" in the lumen (fig. 2-229). The ureter, renal pelvis, and calyces are examined for involvement by tumor. Extension of tumor into the pelvic lumen does not alter tumor stage but should be recorded (fig. 2-230). One report indicates that for localized disease this may represent a significant indicator of poorer prognosis (668a).

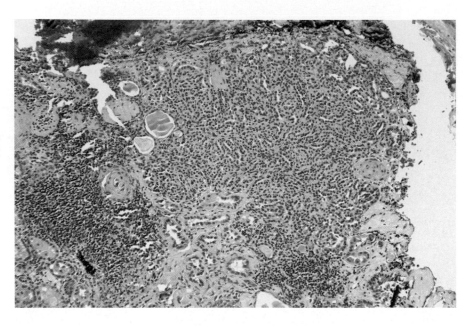

Figure 2-228

RENAL CELL CARCINOMA

A small papillary adenoma is present at the inked margin of this partial nephrectomy specimen that contained a papillary renal cell carcinoma. In this setting, this is not considered a positive surgical margin.

Any areas of nodularity along the pelvis or ureter should be sampled; these may represent metastatic tumor deposits (fig. 2-231).

Evaluation of the tumor as it relates to the perinephric fat and renal sinus is important. Areas of possible fat invasion are usually suspected when the fat does not readily fall away from the cortical interface. If areas suspicious for fat invasion are identified, these should be sampled for microscopic evaluation. If no suspicious areas are noted, one or two sections of the cortical-tumor interface should be randomly submitted.

The dimensions of the kidney and the tumor should be recorded; the latter is important for staging (see Table 2-7). The characteristics of the tumor should be documented. This is important for diagnosis. For example, histologic sections having changes suggestive of an oncocytoma are incongruent with the gross description of a variegated tumor and should prompt further gross examination and sampling. In a variegated tumor, different-appearing areas should be sampled. Gray-white, fleshy areas could indicate a sarcomatoid component, an important prognostic finding. In necrotic cystic masses and complex cystic lesions, extensive sampling may be required to document tumor within the capsular wall. The number of initial sections will depend upon the gross findings.

The hilar adipose tissue should be examined for lymph nodes. In most specimens, no lymph nodes are identified, but if nodules are identified they should be submitted in toto. It has been shown that patients with a histologically documented tumor stage of pN0 have a better prognosis than those with a stage of pNx (673). If grossly involved by tumor, lymph nodes only need to be sampled.

The adrenal gland should be identified and any abnormality sampled. If the adrenal gland is involved, direct extension must be distinguished from metastasis (fig. 2-232).

In many cases, a portion of rib is removed for technical reasons of operative exposure. This should be evaluated histologically, as unsuspected metastases are occasionally found (662).

Frozen Section

In general, frozen section evaluation of kidney biopsy or resection specimens should be limited to cases where the result will impact on the immediate management of the patient. The question most frequently posed at frozen section is whether a renal mass is benign or malignant, with the result determining a partial versus a radical nephrectomy (667,669). Frozen section interpretations of renal masses are often problematic, with false-negative and false-positive rates of 20 percent and 34 percent, respectively (661). For multicystic masses, a false-negative rate of 37 percent has been reported (659). At the present time, partial nephrectomy is considered appropriate "cancer surgery" for properly

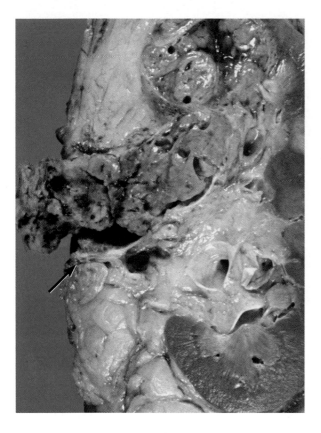

Figure 2-229

RENAL CELL CARCINOMA

Clear cell renal cell carcinoma involving the renal vein. The tumor thrombus extends beyond the cut end of the renal vein. It is the cut end of the renal vein (arrow) that represents the true surgical resection margin, not the thrombus extending beyond.

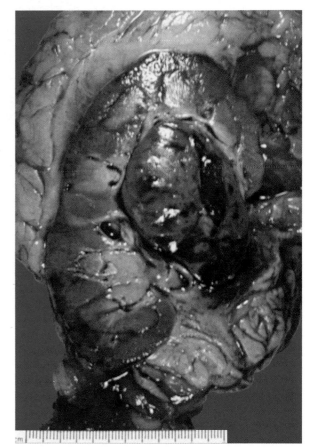

Figure 2-230

RENAL CELL CARCINOMA

This clear cell renal cell carcinoma is growing into and filling the renal calyces and pelvis.

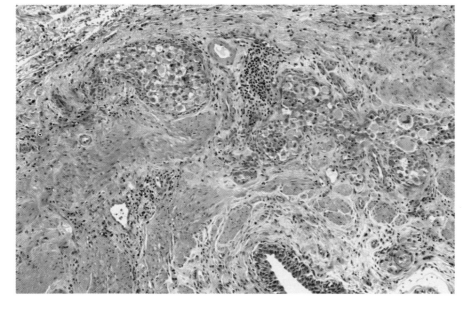

Figure 2-231

RENAL CELL CARCINOMA

Photomicrograph taken from the ureter shows tumor thrombi from a clear cell renal cell carcinoma filling small and intermediate-sized vascular structures.

215

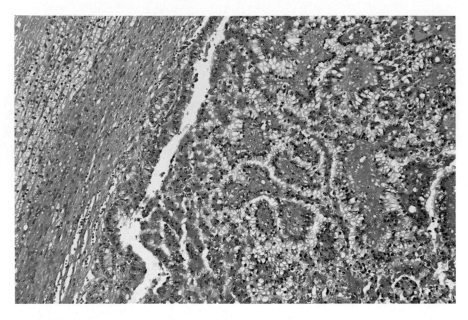

Figure 2-232

METASTATIC RENAL CELL CARCINOMA

Metastatic clear cell renal cell carcinoma involving the adrenal gland. Residual adrenal cortex is present at the left.

Table 2-12

REPORTING OF RENAL CELL CARCINOMA

Histologic type[a]

Nuclear grade (Fuhrman)

Maximum tumor diameter

Presence or absence of perinephric fat invasion

Presence or absence of gross renal vein invasion; if involved, is there invasion of the vein wall by tumor

Microscopic angiolymphatic invasion if identified[b]

Surgical margin status

Status of adrenal gland (if included); if involved—direct invasion or metastasis

Status of regional lymph nodes (if included)

Other significant findings (associated conditions; e.g., acquired cystic kidney disease, adenomata)

---

[a] Although sarcomatoid RCC is not in the classification, if present it should be included in the diagnosis.

[b] This is considered optional but likely has prognostic value.

selected patients and frozen section is not recommended as a determinant of therapeutic approach (661).

Frozen section may have a role in assessing the adequacy of resection margins in partial nephrectomy and some have recommended it as a routine part of such a procedure (672). Problems in the interpretation of frozen section specimens include detached atypical cells and crushed tubules mimicking tumor (668). The use of frozen section has been recommended to evaluate specimens for perinephric fat invasion in order to select ideal candidates for nephron-sparing surgery (666).

Reporting of Resection Specimens

The surgical pathology report must contain appropriate information for accurate staging and prognostication (664,671). A diagnostic interpretation followed by a comment is preferred. This method emphasizes the fact that a pathology report is a consultation rather than a list of observations. Recommended features are detailed in Table 2-12.

REFERENCES

Renal Cell Carcinoma and Adenoma

1. Aaltomaa S, Lipponen P, Ala-Opas M, Eskelinen M, Syrjanen K. Prognostic value of Ki-67 expression in renal cell carcinomas. Eur Urol 1997;31:350–5.
2. Aizawa S, Chigusa M, Ohno Y, Suzuki M. Chromophobe cell renal carcinoma with sarcomatoid component: a report of two cases. J Urol Pathol 1997;6:51–9.
3. Aizawa S, Kikuchi Y, Suzuki M, Furusato M. Renal cell carcinoma of lower nephron origin. Acta Pathol Jpn 1987;37:567–74.
4. Akhtar M, Chantziantoniou N. Flow cytometric and quantitative image cell analysis of DNA ploidy in renal chromophobe cell carcinoma. Hum Pathol 1998;29:1181–8.
5. Akhtar M, Tulbah A, Kardar AH, Ali MA. Sarcomatoid renal cell carcinoma: the chromophobe connection. Am J Surg Pathol 1997;21:1188–95.
6. Al-Saleem T, Wessner LL, Scheithauer BW, et al. Malignant tumors of the kidney, brain and soft tissues in children and young adults with the tuberous sclerosis complex. Cancer 1998;83:2208–16.
7. American Joint Committee on Cancer. AJCC Cancer Staging Manual, 6th ed. Philadelphia: Lippincott-Raven; 2002.
8. Amin MB, Amin MB, Tamboli P, et al. Prognostic impact of histologic subtyping of adult renal epithelial neoplasms: an experience of 405 cases. Am J Surg Pathol 2002;26:281–91.
9. Amin MB, Corless CL, Renshaw AA, Tickoo SK, Kubus J, Schultz DS. Papillary (chromophil) renal cell carcinoma: histomorphologic characteristics and evaluation of conventional pathologic prognostic parameters in 62 cases. Am J Surg Pathol 1997;21:621–35.
10. Argani P, Antonescu CR, Couturier J, et al. PRCC-TFE3 renal carcinomas: morphologic, immunohistochemical, ultrastructural, and molecular analysis of an entity associated with the t(X;1)(p11.2;q21). Am J Surg Pathol 2002;26:1553–66.
11. Argani P, Antonescu CR, Illei PB, et al. Primary renal neoplasms with the ASPL-TFE3 gene fusion of alveolar soft part sarcoma: distinctive tumor entity previously included among renal cell carcinomas of children and adolescents. Am J Pathol 2001;159:179–92.
12. Argani P, Beckwith JB. Metanephric stromal tumor: report of 31 cases of a distinctive pediatric renal neoplasm. Am J Surg Pathol 2000;24:917–26.
13. Arner O, Blanck C, von Schreeb T. Renal adenocarcinoma—grading of malignancy—prognosis. A study of 197 cases. Acta Chir Scand 1965;346(Suppl):1–51.
14. Arroyo MR, Green DM, Perlman EJ, Beckwith JB, Argani P. The spectrum of metanephric adenofibroma and related lesions: clinicopathologic study of 25 cases from the national Wilms Tumor Study Group Pathology Center. Am J Surg Pathol 2001;25:433–44.
15. Auger M, Katz RL, Sella A, Ordonez NG, Lawrence DD, Ro JY. Fine-needle aspiration cytology of sarcomatoid renal cell carcinoma: a morphologic and immunocytochemical study of 15 cases. Diagn Cytopathol 1993;9:46–51.
16. Avery AK, Beckstead J, Renshaw AA, Corless CL. Use of antibodies to RCC and CD10 in the differential diagnosis of renal neoplasms. Am J Surg Pathol 2000;24:203–10.
17. Avery RA, Harris JE, Davis CJ Jr, Borgaonkar DS, Byrd JC, Weiss RB. Renal medullary carcinoma: clinical and therapeutic aspects of a newly described tumor. Cancer 1996;78:128–32.
18. Baer SC, Ro JY, Ordonez NG, et al. Sarcomatoid collecting duct carcinoma: a clinicopathologic and immunohistochemical study of five cases. Hum Pathol 1993;24:1017–22.
19. Balint I, Fischer J, Ljungberg B, Kovacs G. Mapping the papillary renal cell carcinoma gene between loci D17S787 and D17S1799 on chromosome 17q21.32. Lab Invest 1999;79:1713–8.
20. Bannasch P, Krech R, Zerban H. [Morphogenesis and micromorphology of epithelial tumors induced in the rat kidney by nitrosomorpholine. IV. Tubular lesions and basophilic tumors. (author transl)] J Cancer Res Clin Oncol 1980;98:243–65. (German.)
21. Bannasch P, Zerban H. Animal models and renal carcinogenesis. In: Eble JN, ed. Tumors and tumor-like conditions of the kidneys and ureters. New York: Churchill Livingstone; 1990.
22. Bard RH, Lord B, Fromowitz F. Papillary adenocarcinoma of kidney. II. Radiographic and biologic characteristics. Urology 1982;19:16–20.
23. Bell ET. A classification of renal tumors with observations on the frequency of various types. J Urol 1938;39:238–43.
24. Bennington JL. Spectrum of renal adenoma and carcinoma [Abstract]. Am J Surg Pathol 1981;5:194.
25. Bennington JL. Tumors of the kidney. In: Javadpour N, Barsky SH, eds. Surgical pathology of urological diseases. Baltimore: Williams & Wilkins; 1987:106–37.
26. Bennington JL, Beckwith JB. Tumors of the kidney, renal pelvis and ureter. Atlas of Tumor Pathology, 2nd Series, Fascicle 12. Washington, D.C.: Armed Forces Institute of Pathology; 1975.
27. Bertoni F, Ferri C, Benati A, Bacchini P, Corrado F. Sarcomatoid carcinoma of the kidney. J Urol 1987;137:25–8.

28. Bjornsson J, Short MP, Kwiatkowski DJ, Henske EP. Tuberous sclerosis-associated renal cell carcinoma. Clinical, pathological, and genetic features. Am J Pathol 1996;149:1201–8.

29. Blei CL, Hartman DS, Friedman AC, Davis CJ Jr. Papillary renal cell carcinoma: ultrasonic/pathologic correlation. J Clin Ultrasound 1982;10:429–34.

30. Boczko S, Fromowitz FB, Bard RH. Papillary adenocarcinoma of the kidney: a new perspective. Urology 1979;14:491–5.

31. Bonsib SM, Gibson D, Mhoon M, Greene GF. Renal sinus involvement in renal cell carcinoma. Am J Surg Pathol 2000;24:451–8.

32. Bonsib SM, Lager DJ. Chromophobe cell carcinoma: analysis of five cases. Am J Surg Pathol 1990;14:260–7.

33. Boxer RJ, Waisman J, Lieber MM, Mampaso FM, Skinner DG. Non-metastatic hepatic dysfunction associated with renal cell carcinoma. J Urol 1978;119:468–71.

34. Bretan PN Jr, Busch MP, Hricak H, Williams RD. Chronic renal failure: a significant risk factor in the development of acquired renal cysts and renal cell carcinoma. Case reports and review of the literature. Cancer 1986;57:1871–9.

35. Brinker DA, Amin MB, de Peralta-Venturina M, Reuter V, Chan DY, Epstein JI. Extensively necrotic cystic renal cell carcinoma: a clinicopathologic study with comparison to other cystic and necrotic renal cancers. Am J Surg Pathol 2000;24:988–95.

36. Brown JA, Anderl KL, Borell TJ, Qian J, Bostwick DG, Jenkins RB. Simultaneous chromosome 7 and 17 gain and sex chromosome loss provide evidence that renal metanephric adenoma is related to papillary renal cell carcinoma. J Urol 1997;158:370–74.

37. Browne MK, Glashan RW. Multiple pathology in unilateral supernumerary kidney. Br J Surg 1971;58:73–6.

37a. Brunelli M, Eble JN, Zhang S, Martignoni G, Cheng L. Metanephric adenoma lacks the gains of chromosome 7 and 17 and loss of Y that are typical of papillary renal cell carcinoma and papillary adenoma. Mod Pathol 2003;16:1060–3.

38. Busam KJ, Iversen K, Coplan KA, et al. Immunoreactivity for A103, an antibody to melan-A (MART-1), in adrenocortical and other steroid tumors. Am J Surg Pathol 1998;22:57–63.

39. Cao Y, Karsten U, Zerban H, Bannasch P. Expression of MUC1, Thomas-Friedenreich-related antigens, and cytokeratin 19 in human renal cell carcinomas and tubular clear cell lesions. Virchows Arch 2000;436:119–26.

40. Caraway NP, Wojcik EM, Katz RL, Ro JY, Ordonez NG. Cytologic findings of collecting duct carcinoma of the kidney. Diagn Cytopathol 1995;13:304–9.

41. Carducci MA, Piantadosi S, Pound CR, et al. Nuclear morphometry adds significant prognostic information to stage and grade for renal cell carcinoma. Urology 1999;53:44–49.

42. Carney JA. Wilms' tumor and renal cell carcinoma in retroperitoneal teratoma. Cancer 1975;35:1179–83.

43. Chao D, Zisman A, Pantuck AJ, et al. Collecting duct renal cell carcinoma: clinical study of a rare tumor. J Urol 2002;167:71–4.

44. Chatelain C, Jardin A, Bitker MO, Hammoudi Y. Treatment of renal cell carcinoma involving the vena cava and the right atrium. In: deKernion JB, Pavone-Macaluso M, eds. Tumors of the kidney. Baltimore: Williams & Wilkins; 1986:98–110.

45. Chau KY, Pretorius JM, Stewart AW. Myospherulosis in renal cell carcinoma. Arch Pathol Lab Med 2000;124:1476–9.

46. Cherullo EE, Ross JH, Kay R, Novick AC. Renal neoplasms in adult survivors of childhood Wilms tumor. J Urol 2001;165:2013–7.

47. Cheuk W, Lo ES, Chan AK, Chan JK. Atypical epithelial proliferations in acquired renal cystic disease harbor cytogenetic aberrations. Hum Pathol 2002;33:761–5.

48. Cheville JC, Blute ML, Zincke H, Lohse CM, Weaver AL. Stage pT1 conventional (clear cell) renal cell carcinoma: pathological features associated with cancer specific survival. J Urol 2001;166:453–6.

49. Cheville JC, Lohse CM, Zincke H, Weaver AL, Blute ML. Comparisons of outcome and prognostic features among histologic subtypes of renal cell carcinoma. Am J Surg Pathol 2003;27:612–24.

50. Christenson PJ, Craig JP, Bibro MC, O'Connell KJ. Cysts containing renal cell carcinoma in von Hippel-Lindau disease. J Urol 1982;128:798–800.

51. Chow KG, Myles J, Novick AC. The Cleveland Clinic experience with papillary (chromophil) renal cell carcinoma: clinical outcome with histopathological correlation. Can J Urol 2001;8:1223–7.

52. Chow WH, Devesa SS, Warren JL, Fraumeni JF Jr. Rising incidence of renal cell cancer in the United States. JAMA 1999;281:1628–31.

53. Chu PG, Weiss LM. Cytokeratin 14 immunoreactivity distinguishes oncocytic tumour from its renal mimics: an immunohistochemical study of 63 cases. Histopathology 2001;39: 455–62.

54. Chung-Park M, Ricanati E, Lankerani M, Kedia K. Acquired renal cysts and multiple renal cell and urothelial tumors. Am J Clin Pathol 1983;79:238–42.

55. Coffin CM, Swanson PE, Wick MR, Dehner LP. An immunohistochemical comparison of chordoma with renal cell carcinoma, colorectal adenocarcinoma, and myxopapillary ependymoma: a potential diagnostic dilemma in the diminutive biopsy. Mod Pathol 1993;6:531–8.

56. Cohen AJ, Li FP, Berg S, et al. Hereditary renal-cell carcinoma associated with a chromosomal translocation. N Engl J Med 1979;301:592–5.

57. Cohen C, McCue PA, Derose PB. Histogenesis of renal cell carcinoma and renal oncocytoma. An immunohistochemical study. Cancer 1988;62:1946–51.

58. Cohen RJ, McNeal JE, Susman M, et al. Sarcomatoid renal cell carcinoma of papillary origin. A case report and cytogenetic evaluation. Arch Pathol Lab Med 2000;124:1830–2.

59. Cohnheim J. Lectures on general pathology: a handbook for practitioners and students. Translated from 2nd German ed. by McKee AB. London: New Sydenham Society; 1889.

60. Coughlin SS, Neaton JD, Randall B, Sengupta A. Predictors of mortality from kidney cancer in 332,547 men screened for the Multiple Risk Factor Intervention Trial. Cancer 1997;79:2171–7.

61. Cromie WJ, Davis CJ, DeTure FA. Atypical carcinoma of kidney, possibly originating from collecting duct epithelium. Urology 1979;13:315–7.

62. Crotty TB, Farrow GM, Lieber MM. Chromophobe cell renal carcinoma: clinicopathological features of 50 cases. J Urology 1995;154:964–7.

63. Daniels GF, Schaeffer AJ. Renal cell carcinoma involving penis and testis: unusual initial presentations of metastatic disease. Urology 1991;37:369–73.

64. Datta BN. Hyaline intracytoplasmic globules in renal carcinoma. Arch Pathol Lab Med 1977;101:391.

65. Datta MW, Ulbright TM, Young RH. Renal cell carcinoma metastatic to the testis and its adnexa: a report of five cases including three that accounted for the initial clinical presentation. Int J Surg Pathol 2001;9:49–56.

66. Davis CJ Jr, Barton JH, Sesterhenn IA, Mostofi FK. Metanephric adenoma. Clinicopathological study of fifty patients. Am J Surg Pathol 1995;19:1101–14.

67. Davis CJ Jr, Mostofi FK, Sesterhenn IA. Renal medullary carcinoma. The seventh sickle cell nephropathy. Am J Surg Pathol 1995;19:1–11.

68. Deitchman B, Sidhu GS. Ultrastructural study of a sarcomatoid variant of renal cell carcinoma. Cancer 1980;46:1152–7.

69. deKernion JB. Renal tumors. In: Walsh PC, Gittes RF, Perlmutter AD, Stamey TA, eds. Campbell's urology. 5th ed. Philadelphia: WB Saunders; 1986:1294–1342.

70. Delahunt B, Bethwaite PB, Thornton A, Ribas JL. Proliferation of renal cell carcinoma assessed by fixation-resistant polyclonal Ki-67 antibody labelling. Correlation with clinical outcome. Cancer 1995;75:2714–19.

71. Delahunt B, Eble JN. Papillary renal cell carcinoma: a clinicopathologic and immunohisto-chemical study of 105 tumors. Mod Pathol 1997;10:537–44.

72. Delahunt B, Eble JN, McCredie MR, Bethwaite PB, Stewart, JH, Bilous AM. Morphologic typing of papillary renal cell carcinoma: comparison of growth kinetics and patient survival in 66 cases. Hum Pathol 2001;32:590–95.

73. DeLong W, Grignon DJ, Eberwein P, Shum DT, Wyatt JK. Sarcomatoid renal cell carcinoma. An immunohistochemical study of 18 cases. Arch Pathol Lab Med 1993;117:636–40.

74. Di Silverio F, Casale P, Colella D, Andrea L, Seccareccia F, Sciarra A. Independent value of tumor size and DNA ploidy for the prediction of disease progression in patients with organ-confined renal cell carcinoma. Cancer 2000;88:835–43.

75. Drut R, Drut RM, Ortolani C. Metastatic metanephric adenoma with foci of papillary carcinoma in a child: a combined histologic, immunohistochemical, and FISH study. Int J Surg Pathol 2001;9:241–7.

76. Eble JN, Bonsib SM. Extensively cystic renal neoplasms: cystic nephroma, cystic partially differentiated nephroblastoma, multilocular cystic renal cell carcinoma and cystic hamartoma of the renal pelvis. Semin Diagn Pathol 1998;15:2–20.

77. Eble JN, Sauter G, Epstein JI, Sesterhenn IA, eds. World Health Organization classification of tumours: pathology and genetics of tumours of the urinary system and male genital organs. Lyons: IARC Press; 2004.

78. Ekblom P, Miettinen A, Saxen L. Induction of brush border antigens of the proximal tubule in the developing kidney. Dev Biol 1980;74:263–74.

79. Farrow GM, Harrison EG Jr, Utz DC. Sarcomas and the sarcomatoid and mixed malignant tumors of the kidney in adults. III. Cancer 1968;22:556–63.

80. Ficarra V, Righetti R, Martignoni G, et al. Prognostic value of renal cell carcinoma nuclear grading: multivariate analysis of 333 cases. Urol Int 2001;67:130–4.

81. Figenshau RS, Basler JW, Ritter JH, Siegel CL, Simon JA, Dierks SM. Renal medullary carcinoma. J Urol 1998;159:711–3.

82. Fisher ER, Horvat B. Comparative ultrastructural study of so-called renal adenoma and carcinoma. J Urol 1972;108:382–6.

83. Fleming S, Lewi HJ. Collecting duct carcinoma of the kidney. Histopathology 1986;10:1131–41.

84. Fleming S, Lindop GB, Gibson AA. The distribution of epithelial membrane antigen in the kidney and its tumors. Histopathology 1985;9:729–39.

85. Fleming S, Symes CE. The distribution of cytokeratin antigens in the kidney and in renal tumors. Histopathology 1987;11:157–70.

86. Flint A, Cookingham C. Cytologic diagnosis of the papillary variant of renal-cell carcinoma. Acta Cytol 1987;31:325–9.

87. Francois C, Decaestecker C, Petein M, et al. Classification strategies for the grading of renal cell carcinomas, based on nuclear morphometry and densitometry. J Pathol 1997;183:141–50.

88. Frank I, Blute ML, Cheville JC, Lohse CM, Weaver AL, Zincke H. An outcome prediction model for patients with clear cell renal cell carcinoma treated with radical nephrectomy based on tumor stage, size, grade and necrosis: the SSIGN score. J Urol 2002;168:2395–400.

89. Friedrichs P, Lassen P, Canby E, Graham C. Renal medullary carcinoma and sickle cell trait. J Urol 1997;157:1349.

90. Frohmuller HG, Grups JW, Heller V. Comparative value of ultrasonography, computerized tomography, angiography and excretory urography in the staging of renal cell carcinoma. J Urol 1987;138:482–4.

91. Fuhrman SA, Lasky LC, Limas C. Prognostic significance of morphologic parameters in renal cell carcinoma. Am J Surg Pathol 1982;6:655–63.

92. Fukunaga M. Sarcomatoid collecting duct carcinoma. Arch Pathol Lab Med. 1999;123:338–41.

93. Fukuoka T, Honda M, Namiki M, Tada Y, Matsuda M, Sonoda T. Renal cell carcinoma with heterotopic bone formation. Case report and review of the Japanese literature. Urol Int 1987;42:458–60.

94. Fuzesi L, Cober M, Mittermayer C. Collecting duct carcinoma: cytogenetic characterization. Histopathology 1992;21:155–60.

95. Fuzesi L, Gunawan B, Bergmann F, Tack S, Braun S, Jakse G. Papillary renal cell carcinoma with clear cell cytomorphology and chromosomal, loss of 3p. Histopathology 1999;35:157–61.

96. Gaffey MJ, Traweek ST, Mills SE, et al. Cytokeratin expression in adrenocortical neoplasia: an immunohistochemical and biochemical study with implications for the differential diagnosis of adrenocortical, hepatocellular, and renal cell carcinoma. Hum Pathol 1992;23:144–53.

97. Gardner KD Jr. Acquired renal cystic disease and renal adenocarcinoma in patients on long-term hemodialysis. N Engl J Med 1984;310:390.

98. Gatalica Z, Grujic S, Kovatich A, Petersen RO. Metanephric adenoma: histology, immunophenotype, cytogenetics, ultrastructure. Mod Pathol 1996;9:329–33.

99. Gatalica Z, Kovatich A, Miettinen M. Consistent expression of cytokeratin 7 in papillary renal-cell carcinoma: an immunohistochemical study in formalin-fixed, paraffin-embedded tissues. J Urol Pathol 1995;3:205–11.

100. Gelb AB. Renal cell carcinoma: current prognostic factors. Union Internationale Contre le Cancer (UICC) and the American Joint Committee on Cancer (AJCC). Cancer 1997;80: 981–6.

101. Gemmill RM, West JD, Boldog F, et al. The hereditary renal cell carcinoma 3;8 translocation fuses FHIT to a patched-related gene, TRC8. Proc Natl Acad Sci USA 1998;95:9572–7.

102. Gettman MT, Blute ML. Update on pathologic staging of renal cell carcinoma. Urology 2002;60:209–17.

103. Gettman MT, Blute ML, Spotts B, Bryant SC, Zincke H. Pathologic staging of renal cell carcinoma: significance of tumor classification with the 1997 TNM staging system. Cancer 2001;91:354–61.

104. Gibbons RP, Monte JE, Correa RJ Jr, Mason JT. Manifestations of renal cell carcinoma. Urology 1976;8:201–6.

105. Gnarra JR, Tory K, Weng Y, et al. Mutations of the VHL tumour suppressor gene in renal carcinoma. Nat Genet 1994;7:85–90.

106. Gokden N, Nappi O, Swanson PE, et al. Renal cell carcinoma with rhabdoid features. Am J Surg Pathol 2000;24:1329–38.

107. Golde DW, Schambelan M, Weintraub BD, Rosen SW. Gonadotropin-secreting renal carcinoma. Cancer 1974;33:1048–53.

108. Golimbu M, Joshi P, Sperber A, Tessler A, Al-Askari S, Morales P. Renal cell carcinoma: survival and prognostic factors. Urology 1986;27:291–301.

109. Gondos B. Diagnosis of tumors of the kidney: ultrastructural classification. Ann Clin Lab Sci 1981;11:308–15.

110. Granter SR, Perez-Atayde AR, Renshaw AA. Cytologic analysis of papillary renal cell carcinoma. Cancer Cytopathol 1998;84:303–8.

111. Grawitz PA. Die sogennanten lipoma der niere. Virchows Arch Pathol Anat 1883;93:39–63.

112. Green LK, Ayala AG, Ro JY, et al. Role of nuclear grading in stage I renal cell carcinoma. Urology 1989;34:310–5.

113. Green LK, Ro JY, Mackay B, Ayala AG, Luna MA. Renal cell carcinoma metastatic to the thyroid. Cancer 1989;63:1810–15.

114. Gregoire JR, Torres VE, Holley KE, Farrow GM. Renal epithelial hyperplastic and neoplastic proliferation in autosomal dominant polycystic kidney disease. Am J Kidney Dis 1987;9:27–38.

115. Griffiths DF, Verghese A, Golash A, et al. Contribution of grade, vascular invasion and age to outcome in clinically localized renal cell carcinoma. BJU International 2002;90:26–31.

116. Grignon DJ, Abdel-Malak M, Mertens W, et al. Prognostic significance of cellular proliferation in renal cell carcinoma: a comparison of synthesis-phase fraction and proliferating cell nuclear antigen. Mod Pathol 1995;8:18–24.

117. Grignon DJ, Ayala AG, El-Naggar AK, et al. Renal cell carcinoma. A clinicopathologic and DNA flow cytometric analysis of 103 cases. Cancer 1989;64:2133–40.

118. Grignon DJ, Eble JN. Adenomatoid metaplasia of the epithelium of Bowman's capsule. J Urol Pathol 1993;1:293–9.

119. Grignon DJ, Eble JN. Papillary and metanephric adenomas of the kidney. Semin Diagn Pathol 1998;15:41–53.

120. Grignon DJ, Ro JY, Ayala AG. Primary mucin-secreting adenocarcinoma of the kidney. Arch Pathol Lab Med 1988;112:847–49.

121. Grignon DJ, Staerkel G. Surgical diseases of the kidney. In: Silverberg SG, DeLellis RA, Frable WJ eds. Principles and practice of surgical pathology and cytopathology, 3rd ed. New York: Churchill Livingstone; 1997:2135–84.

122. Gritsman AY, Popok SM, Ro JY, Dekmezian RH, Weber RS. Renal-cell carcinoma with intranuclear inclusions metastatic to thyroid: a diagnostic problem in aspiration cytology. Diag Cytopathol 1988;4:125–9.

123. Guinan P, Frank W, Saffrin R, Rubenstein M. Staging and survival of patients with renal cell carcinoma. Semin Surg Oncol 1994;10:47–50.

124. Gunawan B, Bergmann F, Braun S, et al. Polyploidization and losses of chromosomes 1, 2, 6, 10, 13 and 17 in three cases of chromophobe renal cell carcinomas. Cancer Genet Cytogenet 1999;10:57–61.

125. Haddad FS, Shah IA, Manne RK, Costantino JM, Somsin AA. Renal cell carcinoma insulated in the renal capsule with calcification and ossification. Urol Int 1993;51:97–101.

126. Hafez KS, Fergany AF, Novick AC. Nephron sparing surgery for localized renal cell carcinoma: impact of tumor size on patient survival, tumor recurrence and TNM staging. J Urol 1999;162:1930–3.

127. Hai MA, Diaz-Perez R. Atypical carcinoma of kidney originating from collecting duct epithelium. Urology 1982;19:89–92.

128. Haibach H, Burns TW, Carlson HE, Burman KD, Deftos LJ. Multiple hamartoma syndrome (Cowden's disease) associated with renal cell carcinoma and primary neuroendocrine carcinoma of the skin (Merkel cell carcinoma). Am J Clin Pathol 1992;97:705–12.

129. Hand JR, Broders AC. Carcinoma of the kidney: the degree of malignancy in relation to factors bearing on prognosis. J Urol 1932;28:199–216.

130. Hartman DS, Davis CJ Jr, Johns T, Goldman SM. Cystic renal cell carcinoma. Urol 1986;28:145–53.

131. Hennigar RA, Beckwith JB. Nephrogenic adenofibroma. A novel kidney tumor of young people. Am J Surg Pathol 1992;16:325–34.

132. Henson DE, Fielding LP, Grignon DJ, et al. College of American Pathologists Conference XXVI on clinical relevance of prognostic markers in solid tumors. Summary. Members of the Cancer Committee. Arch Pathol Lab Med 1995;119:1109–12.

133. Herts BR, Coll DM, Novick AC, et al. Enhancement characteristics of papillary renal neoplasms revealed on triphasic helical CT of the kidneys. AJR Am J Roentgenol 2002;178:367–72.

133a. Hes O, Hora M, Perez-Montiel DM, et al. Spindle and cuboidal renal cell carcinoma, a tumour having frequent association with nephrolithiasis: report of 11 cases including a case with hybrid conventional renal cell carcinoma/spindle and cuboidal renal cell carcinoma components. Histopathology 2002;41:549–55.

134. Hoehn W, Hermanek P. Invasion of veins in renal cell carcinoma—frequency, correlation and prognosis. Eur Urol 1983;9:276–80.

135. Hosoe S, Brauch H, Latif F, et al. Localization of the von Hippel-Lindau disease gene to a small region of chromosome 3. Genomics 1990;8:634–40.

136. Hughson MD, Buchwald D, Fox M. Renal neoplasia and acquired cystic kidney disease in patients receiving long-term dialysis. Arch Pathol Lab Med 1986;110:592–601.

137. Hughson MD, Johnson LD, Silva FG, Kovacs G. Nonpapillary and papillary renal cell carcinoma: a cytogenetic and phenotypic study. Mod Pathol 1993;6:449–56.

138. Hull MT, Eble JN. Myelinoid lamellated cytoplasmic inclusions in human renal adenocarcinomas: an ultrastructural study. Ultrastruc Pathol 1988;12:41–8.

139. Igarashi T, Tobe T, Nakatsu HO, et al. The impact of a 4 cm. cutoff point for stratification of T1N0M0 renal cell carcinoma after radical nephrectomy. J Urol 2001;165:1103–6.

140. Ishikawa I, Kovacs G. High incidence of papillary renal cell tumors in patients on chronic hemodialysis. Histopathol 1993;22:135–9.

141. Ishikawa I, Saito Y, Shikura N, Kitada H, Shinoda A, Suzuki S. Ten-year prospective study on the development of renal cell carcinoma in dialysis patients. Am J Kid Dis 1990;16:452–8.

142. Jacobs SC, Berg SI, Lawson RK. Synchronous bilateral renal cell carcinoma: total surgical excision. Cancer 1980;46:2341–5.

143. Jagirdar J, Irie T, French SW, Patil J, Schwarz R, Paronetto F. Globular Mallory-like bodies in renal cell carcinoma: report of a case and review of cytoplasmic eosinophilic globules. Hum Pathol 1985;16:949–52.

144. Javidan J, Stricker HJ, Tamboli P, et al. Prognostic significance of the 1997 TNM classification of renal cell carcinoma. J Urol 1999;162:1277–81.

145. Jemal A, Tiwari RC, Murray T, et al. Cancer statistics, 2004. CA Cancer J Clin 2004;54:8–29.

146. Jiang F, Richter J, Schraml P, et al. Chromosomal imbalances in papillary renal cel carcinoma: genetic differences between histological subtypes. Am J Pathol 1998;143:1467–73.

147. Jimenez RE, Eble JN, Reuter VE, et al. Concurrent angiomyolipoma and renal cell neoplasia: a study of 36 cases. Mod Pathol 2001;14:157–63.

148. Johnson WF. Carcinoma in a polycystic kidney. J Urol 1953;69:10–2.

149. Jones EC, Pins M, Dickersin RD, Young RH. Metanephric adenoma of the kidney. A clinicopathological, immunohistochemical, flow cytometric, cytogenetic and electron microscopic study of seven cases. Am J Surg Pathol 1995;19:615–26.

150. Juul N, Torp-Pedersen S, Gronvall S, Holm HH, Koch F, Larsen S. Ultrasonically guided fine needle aspiration biopsy of renal masses. J Urol 1985;133:579–81.

151. Kamishima T, Fukuda T, Emura I, Tanigawa T, Naito M. Pigmented renal cell carcinoma. Am J Surg Pathol 1995;19:350–6.

152. Karstaedt N, McCullough DL, Wolfman NT, Dyer RB. Magnetic resonance imaging of the renal mass. J Urol 1986;136:566–70.

153. Kattan MW, Reuter V, Motzer RJ, Katz J, Russo P. A postopostnostic prognostic nomogram for renal cell carcinoma. J Urol 2001;166:63–7.

154. Kattar MM, Grignon DJ, Sarkar FH, et al. p53 gene expression in sarcomatoid renal cell carcinoma: a clinicopathologic analysis and immunohistochemical study with review of the literature. J Urol Pathol 1996;5:207–21.

155. Kawakami H, Hoshida V, Hanai J, et al. Voided urine cytology of papillary renal cell carcinoma and renal calculus: report of a case with emphasis on the importance of cytologic screening in high-risk individuals. Acta Cytologica 2001;45:771–4.

156. Kennedy S, Merino MJ, Linehan WM, Roberts JR, Robertson CN, Neumann RD. Collecting duct carcinoma of the kidney. Hum Pathol 1990;21:449–56.

157. Kim JK, Frohnert PP, Hui YS, Barnes LD, Farrow GM, Dousa TP. Enzymes of the 3',5'-nucleotide metabolism in human renal cortex and renal adenocarcinoma. Kidney Int 1977;12:172–83.

158. Kim MK, Kim S. Immunohistochemical profile of common epithelial neoplasms arising in the kidney. Appl Immunohistochem Mol Morphol 2002;10:332–8.

159. Kinouchi T, Saiki S, Meguro N, et al. Impact of tumor size on the clinical outcomes of patients with Robson Stage I renal cell carcinomas. Cancer 1999;85:689.

160. Kiuru M, Launonen V, Hietala M, et al. Familial cutaneous leiomyomatosis is a two-hit condition associated with renal cell cancer of characteristic histopathology. Am J Pathol 2001;159:825–9.

161. Kmetec A, Kaplan-Pavlovcic S, Ferluga D. Renal cell carcinoma in nonfunctioning transplanted kidney. Am J Nephrol 2001;21:256–8.

162. Koga S, Yamasaki A, Nishikido M, et al. Multiloculated renal cell carcinoma. Int Urol Nephrol 1993;23:423–8.

163. Kolonel LN. Association of cadmium with renal cancer. Cancer 1976;37:1782–7.

164. Kovacs G. Papillary renal cell carcinoma. A morphologic and cytogenetic study of 11 cases. Am J Pathol 1989;134:27–34.

165. Kovacs G, Akhtar M, Beckwith BJ, et al. The Heidelberg classification of renal cell tumours. J Pathol 1997;183:131–3.

166. Kovacs G, Szucs S, De Riese W, Baumgartel H. Specific chromosome aberration in human renal cell carcinoma. Int J Cancer 1987;40:171–8.

167. Krishnan B, Truong LD. Renal epithelial neoplasms: the diagnostic implications of electron microscopic study in 55 cases. Hum Pathol 2002;33:68–79.

168. Kumar S, Cederbaum AI, Pletka PG. Renal cell carcinoma in polycystic kidneys: case report and review of the literature. J Urol 1980;124:708–9.

169. Kuroda N, Inoue K, Guo L, et al. Expression of CD9/motility-related protein 1 (MPR-1) in renal parenchymal neoplasms: consistent expression in papillary and chromophobe renal cell carcinomas. Hum Pathol 2001;32:1071–7.

170. Lack EE, Cassady JR, Sallan SE. Renal cell carcinoma in childhood and adolescence: a clinical and pathological study of 17 cases. J Urol 1985;133:822–8.

171. Lager DJ, Huston BJ, Timmerman TG, Bonsib SM. Papillary renal tumors. Morphologic, cytochemical, and genotypic features. Cancer 1995;76:669–73.

172. Landier JF. Desligneres S, Debre B, Boccon-Gibod L, Steg A. Papillary renal cell carcinoma. Ann Urol (Paris) 1980;14:205–8.

173. Lang EK. Angio-computed tomography and dynamic computed tomography in staging of renal cell carcinoma. Radiology 1984;151:149–55.

174. Latham B, Dickersin GR, Oliva E. Subtypes of chromophobe cell renal carcinoma. An ultrastructural and histochemical study of 13 cases. Am J Surg Pathol 1999;23:530–5.

175. Latif F, Tory K, Gnarra J, et al. Identification of the von Hippel-Lindau disease tumor suppressor gene. Science 1993;260:1317–20.

176. Launonen V, Vierimaa O, Kiuru M, et al. Inherited susceptibility to uterine leiomyomas and renal cell cancer. Proc Natl Acad Sci U S A 2001;98:3387–92.

177. La Vecchia C, Negri E, D'Avanzo B, Franceschi S. Smoking and renal cell carcinoma. Cancer Res 1990;50:5231–3.

178. Leary T. Crystalline ester cholesterol and adult renal tumors. Arch Pathol 1950;50:151–78.

179. Lei JY, Middleton LP, Guo XD, et al. Pigmented renal cell carcinoma with melanocytic differentiation. Hum Pathol 2001;32:233–6.

180. Leibovitch I, Lev R, Mor Y, Golomb J, Dotan ZA, Ramon J. Extensive necrosis in renal cell carcinoma specimens: potential clinical and prognostic implications. Isr Med Assoc J 2001;3:563–5.

181. Lendvay TS, Broecker B, Smith EA. Renal cell carcinoma in a 2-year-old child with tuberous sclerosis. J Urol 2002;168:1131–2.

182. Leroy X, Zini L, Leteurtre E, et al. Morphologic subtyping of papillary renal cell carcinoma: correlation with prognosis and differential expression of MUC1 between the two subtypes. Mod Pathol 2002;15:1126–30.

183. Linehan WM, Lerman MI, Zbar B. Identification of the von Hippel-Lindau (VHL) gene. Its role in renal cancer. JAMA 1995;273:564–70.

184. Liu J, Fanning CV. Can renal oncocytomas be distinguished from renal cell carcinoma on fine-needle aspiration specimens? A study of conventional smears in conjunction with ancillary studies. Cancer Cytopathol 2001;93:390–7.

185. Ljungberg B, Holmberg G, Sjodin JG, Hietala SO, Stenling R. Renal cell carcinoma in a renal cyst: a case report and review of the literature. J Urol 1990;143:797–9.

186. Lohse CM, Blute ML, Zincke H, Weaver AL, Cheville JC. Comparison of standardized and nonstandardized nuclear grade of renal cell carcinoma to predict outcome among 2,042 patients. Am J Clin Pathol 2002;118:877–86.

187. Lu TC, Lim PS, Hsu WM, Wang TH, Liu ST. Renal oncocytoma in acquired renal cystic disease. J Formos Med Assoc 2001;100:488–91.

188. Lubensky IA, Schmidt L, Zhuang Z. Hereditary and sporadic papillary renal carcinomas with c-met mutations share a distinct morphological phenotype. Am J Pathol 1999;155:517–26.

189. Macke RA, Hussain MB, Imray TJ, Wilson RB, Cohen SM. Osteogenic and sarcomatoid differentiation of a renal cell carcinoma. Cancer 1985;56:2452–7.

190. MacLennan GT, Farrow GM, Bostwick DG. Low-grade collecting duct carcinoma of the kidney: report of 13 cases of low-grade mucinous tubulocystic renal carcinoma of possible collecting duct origin. Urology 1997;50:679–84.

191. Maclure M, Willett W. A case-control study of diet and risk of renal adenocarcinoma. Epidemiology 1990;1:430–40.

192. Mai KT, Blew B, Collins JP. Renal cell carcinoma with extensive and minimal sarcomatoid change: prognostic significance and relationship with subtypes of renal cell carcinoma. J Urologic Pathol 1999;11:35–46.

193. Mai KT, Burns BF. Chromophobe cell carcinoma and renal cell neoplasms with mucin-like changes. Acta Histochem 2000;102:103–13.

194. Malchoff CD, Sarfarazi M, Tendler B, et al. Papillary thyroid carcinoma associated with papillary renal neoplasia: genetic linkage analysis of a distinct heritable tumor syndrome. J Clin Endocrinol Metab 2000;85:1758–64.

195. Mancilla-Jimenez R, Stanley RJ, Blath RA. Papillary renal cell carcinoma: a clinical, radiologic, and pathologic study of 34 cases. Cancer 1976;38:2469–80.

196. Marcus PB, Kemp CB. Ectopic renal cell carcinoma: pathologist's problem. Urology 1978;12:453–7.

197. Matas AJ, Simmons RL, Kjellstrand CM, Buselmeier TJ, Najarian JS. Increased incidence of malignancy during chronic renal failure. Lancet 1975;1:883–5.

198. Matson MA, Cohen EP. Acquired cystic kidney disease: occurrence, prevalence, and renal cancers. Medicine 1990;69:217–26.

199. Mauri MF, Bonzanini M, Luciani L, Dalla Palma P. Renal collecting duct carcinoma. Report of a case with urinary cytologic findings. Acta Cytol 1994;38:755–8.

200. Mauro MA, Wadsworth DE, Stanley RJ, McClennan BL. Renal cell carcinoma: angiography in the CT era. AJR Am J Roentgenol 1982;139:1135–8.

201. McCluggage WG, Burton J, Maxwell P, Sloan JM. Immunohistochemical staining of normal, hyperplastic and neoplastic adrenal cortex with a monoclonal antibody against alpha inhibin. J Clin Pathol 1998;51:114–6.

202. McDonald JR, Priestly JT. Malignant tumors of the kidney—surgical and prognostic significance of tumor thrombosis of the renal vein. Surg Gynecol Obstet 1943;77:295–306.

203. McGregor DK, Khurana KK, Cao C, et al. Diagnosing primary and metastatic renal cell carcinoma. The use of the monoclonal antibody "renal cell carcinoma marker." Am J Surg Pathol 2001;25:1485–92.

204. McLaughlin JK, Mandel JS, Blot WJ, Schuman LM, Mehl ES, Fraumeni JF Jr. A population—based case—control study of renal cell carcinoma. J Natl Cancer Inst 1984;72:275–84.

205. McNichols DW, Segura JW, DeWeerd JH. Renal cell carcinoma: long-term survival and late recurrence. J Urol 1981;126:17–23.

206. Medeiros LJ, Gelb AB, Weiss LM. Renal cell carcinoma. Prognostic significance of morphologic parameters in 121 cases. Cancer 1988;61:1639–51.

207. Medeiros LJ, Michie SA, Johnson DE, Warnke RA, Weiss LM. An immunoperoxidase study of renal cell carcinoma: correlation with nuclear grade, cell type, and histologic pattern. Hum Pathol 1988;19:980–7.

208. Melnick SJ, Amazon K, Dembrow V. Metastatic renal cell carcinoma presenting as a parotid tumor: a case report with immunohistochemical findings and a review of the literature. Hum Pathol 1989;20:195–7.

209. Mian BM, Bhadkamkar N, Slaton JW, et al. Prognostic factors and survival of patients with sarcomatoid renal cell carcinoma. J Urol 2002;167:65–70.

209a. Michal M, Hes O, Havlicek F. Benign renal angiomyoadenomatous tumor: a previously unreported renal tumor. Ann Diagn Pathol 2000;4:311–5.

210. Mittal BV, Cotton RE. Severely atypical changes in renal epithelium in biopsy and graft nephrectomy specimens in two cases of cadaver renal transplantation. Histopathology 1987;11:833–41.

211. Moch H, Gasser T, Amin MB, Torhorst J, Sauter G, Mihatsch MJ. Prognostic utility of the recently recommended histologic classification and revised TNM staging system of renal cell carcinoma: a Swiss experience with 588 tumors. Cancer 2000;89:604–14.

212. Moder KG, Litin SC, Gaffey TA. Renal cell carcinoma associated with sarcoidlike tissue reaction. Mayo Clin Proc 1990;65:1498–501.

213. Mohamed AN, Koppitch FC, El-Nagaar M, Bakdounes KM, Grignon DJ. Chromosome analysis of six chromophobe renal cell carcinomas. J Urol Pathol 1998;9:223–31.

214. Moon TD, Dexter DF, Morales A. Synchronous independent primary osteosarcoma and adenocarcinoma of kidney. Urology 1983;21:608–10.

215. Morell-Quadreny L, Clar-Blanch F, Fenollosa-Enterna, Perez-Bacete M, Martinez-Lorente A, Lombart-Bosch A. Proliferating cell nuclear antigen (PCNA) as a prognostic factor in renal cell carcinoma. Anticancer Res 1998;18:677–82.

216. Mourad WA, Nestok BR, Saleh GY, Solez K, Power RF, Jewell LD. Dysplastic tubular epithelium in "normal" kidney associated with renal cell carcinoma. Am J Surg Pathol 1994;18:1117–24.

217. Moyad MA. Obesity interrelated mechanisms, and exposures and kidney cancer. Semin Urologic Oncol 2001;19:270–9.

218. Moyad MA. Review of potential risk factors for kidney (renal cell) cancer. Semin Urol Oncol 2001;19:280–93.

219. Muir TE, Cheville JC, Lager DJ. Metanephric adenoma, nephrogenic rests, and Wilms' tumor: a histologic and immunophenotypic comparison. Am J Surg Pathol 2001;25:1290–6.

220. Murad T, Komaiko W, Oyasu R, Bauer K. Multilocular cystic renal cell carcinoma. Am J Clin Pathol 1991;95:633–7.

221. Murphy WM, Beckwith JB, Farrow GM. Tumors of the Kidney, bladder and related urinary structures. Atlas of Tumor Pathology, 3rd series, Fascicle 11. Washington, DC: Armed Forces Institute of Pathology; 1994.

222. Myers GH Jr, Fehrenbaker LG, Kelalis P. Prognostic significance of renal vein invasion by hypernephroma. J Urol 1968;100:420–3.

223. Nassir A, Jollimore J, Gupta R, Bell D, Norman R. Multilocular cystic renal cell carcinoma: a series of 12 cases and review of the literature. Urology 2002;60:421–7.

224. Ng RC, Suki WN. Renal cell carcinoma occurring in a polycystic kidney of a transplant recipient. J Urol 1980;124:710–2.

225. Ngan KW, Ng KF, Chuang CK. Solid variant of papillary renal cell carcinoma. Chang Gung Med J 2001;24:582–6.

226. Nguyen GK, Schumann GB. Cytopathology of renal collecting duct carcinoma in urine sediment. Diag Cytopathol. 1997;15:446–9.

227. Nielsen B, Braide I, Hasselbalch H. Evidence for an association between hairy cell leukemia and renal cell and colorectal carcinoma. Cancer 1992;70:2087–90.

228. Nonomura A, Mizukami Y, Hasegawa T, Ohkawa M. Metanephric adenoma of the kidney: an electron microscopic and immunohistochemical study with quantitative DNA measurement by image analysis. Ultrastruct Pathol 1995;19:481–8.

229. Onishi T, Ohishi Y, Goto H, Suzuki M, Miyazawa Y. Papillary renal cell carcinoma: clinicopathological characteristics and evaluation of prognosis in 42 patients. BJU Int 1999;83:937–43.

230. Onishi T, Oishi Y, Yanada S, Abe K, Hasegawa T, Maeda S. Prognostic implications of histological features in patients with chromophobe cell renal carcinoma. BJU Int 2002;90:529–32.

231. Ono K, Nishino E, Nakamine H. Renal collecting duct carcinoma. Report of a case with cytologic findings on fine needle aspiration. Acta Cytol 2000;44:380–4.

232. Ornstein DK, Lubensky IA, Venzon D, Zbar B, Linehan WM, Walther MM. Prevalence of microscopic tumors in normal appearing renal parenchyma of patients with hereditary papillary renal cancer. J Urol 2000;163:431–3.

233. Ozer E, Yorukoglu K, Sagol O, et al. Prognostic significance of nuclear morphometry in renal cell carcinoma. BJU International 2002;90:20–5.

234. Pagano S, Ruggeri P, Franzoso F, Brusamolino R. Unusual renal cell carcinoma metastasis to the gallbladder. Urology 1995;45:867–9.

235. Parker L, Kollin J, Vicario D, Nguyen T. Hemihypertrophy as possible sign of renal cell carcinoma. Urology 1992;40:286–8.

236. Parwani AV, Husain AN, Epstein JI, Beckwith JB, Argani P. Low-grade myxoid renal epithelial neoplasms with distal nephron differentiation. Hum Pathol 2001;32:506–12.

237. Pavlovich CP, Walther MM, Eyler RA, et al. Renal tumors in the Birt-Hogg-Dube syndrome. Am J Surg Pathol 2002;26:1542–52.

238. de Peralta-Venturina M, Moch H, Amin M, et al. Sarcomatoid differentiation in renal cell carcinoma: a study of 101 cases. Am J Surg Pathol 2001;25:275–84.

239. Pinto JA, Menolascino F, Daboin I, Romero K, Hernandez S. Ductal carcinoma of the kidney with extensive signet ring cell mucosecreting areas. A case report with immunohistochemical analysis. Pathol Res Pract 2001;197:827–32.

240. Pirich LM, Chou P, Walterhouse DO. Prolonged survival of a patient with sickle cell trait and metastatic medullary carcinoma. J Pediatr Hematol Oncol 1999;21:67–9.

241. Pitz S, Moll R, Storkel S, Thoenes W. Expression of intermediate filament proteins in subtypes of renal cell carcinomas and in renal oncocytomas. Distinction of two classes of renal cell tumors. Lab Invest 1987;56:642–53.

242. Polascik TJ, Cairns P, Epstein JI, et al. Distal nephron renal tumors: microsatellite allelotype. Cancer Res 1996;56:1892–5.

243. Porena M, Vespasiani G, Rosi P, et al. Incidentally detected renal cell carcinoma: role of ultrasonography. J Clin Ultrasound 1992;20:395–400.

244. Poulakis V, Witzsch U, de Vries R, Becht E, Altmannsberger HM, Storkel S. Alpha-fetoprotein producing renal cell carcinoma. Urol Int 2001;67:181–3.

245. Pound CR, Partin AW, Epstein JI, Simons JW, Marshall FF. Nuclear morphometry predicts recurrence in clinically localized renal cell carcinoma. Urology 1993;42:243–8.

246. Press GA, McClennan BL, Melson GL, Weyman PJ, Mauro MA, Lee JK. Papillary renal cell carcinoma: CT and sonographic evaluation. AJR Am J Roentgenol 1984;143:1005–9.

247. Presti JC Jr, Rao PH, Chen Q, et al. Histopathological, cytogenetic, and molecular characterization of renal cortical tumors. Cancer Res 1991;51:1544–52.

248. Rakozy C, Schmahl GE, Bogner S, Storkel S. Low-grade tubular-mucinous renal neoplasms: morphologic, immunohistochemical, and genetic features. Mod Pathol 2002;15:1162–71.

249. Reddy ER. Bilateral renal cell carcinoma—unusual occurrence in three members of one family. Br J Radiol 1981;54:8–11.

250. Reidbord HE. Metaplasia of the parietal layer of Bowman's capsule. Am J Clin Pathol 1968;50:240–2.

251. Renshaw AA, Corless CL. Papillary renal cell carcinoma. Histology and immunohistochemistry. Am J Surg Pathol 1995;19:842–9.

252. Renshaw AA, Freyer DR, Hammers YA. Metastatic metanephric adenoma in a child. Am J Surg Pathol 2000;24:570–4.

253. Renshaw AA, Granter SR, Fletcher JA, Kozakewich HP, Corless CL, Perez-Atayde AR. Renal cell carcinomas in children and young adults: increased incidence of papillary architecture and unique subtypes. Am J Surg Pathol 1999;23:795–802.

254. Renshaw AA, Granter SR. Fine needle aspiration of chromophobic renal cell carcinoma. Acta Cytol 1996;40:867–72.

255. Renshaw AA, Henske EP, Loughlin KR, Shapiro C, Weinberg DS. Aggressive variants of chromophobe renal cell carcinoma. Cancer 1996;78:1756–61.

256. Renshaw AA, Lee KR, Madge R, Granter SR. Accuracy of fine needle aspiration in distinguishing subtypes of renal cell carcinoma. Acta Cytol 1997;41:987–94.

257. Reuter VE, Presti JC Jr. Contemporary approach to the classification of renal epithelial tumors. Semin Oncol 2000;27:124–37.

258. Reutzel D, Mende M, Naumann S, et al. Genomic imbalances in 61 renal cancers from the proximal tubulus detected by comparative genomic hybridization. Cytogenet Cell Genet 2001;93:221–7.

259. Richards FM, Payne SJ, Zbar B, Affara NA, Ferguson-Smith MA, Maher ER. Molecular analysis of de novo germline mutations in the von Hippel-Lindau disease gene. Hum Mol Genet 1995;4:2139–43.

260. Rioux-Leclercq NC, Epstein JI. Renal cell carcinoma with intratumoral calcium oxalate crystal deposition in patients with acquired cystic disease of the kidney. Arch Pathol Lab Med 2003;127:E89–92.

261. Rioux-Leclercq N, Turlin B, Bansard JY, et al. Value of immunohistochemical Ki-67 and p53 determinations as predictive factors of outcome in renal cell carcinoma. Urology 2000;55:501–5.

262. Ro JY, Ayala AG, Sella A, Samuels ML, Swanson DA. Sarcomatoid renal cell carcinoma: clinicopathologic. A study of 42 cases. Cancer 1987;59:516–26.

263. Robson CJ, Churchill BM, Anderson W. The results of radical nephrectomy for renal cell carcinoma. J Urol 1969;101:297–301.

264. Rodriguez-Jurado R, Gonzalez-Crussi F. Renal medullary carcinoma: immunohistochemical and ultrastructural observations. J Urol Pathol 1996;4:191–203.

265. Ruiz-Cerda JL, Hernandez M, Gomis F, et al. Value of deoxyribonucleic acid ploidy and nuclear morphometry for prediction of disease progression in renal cell carcinoma. J Urol 1996;155:459–65.

266. Rumpelt HJ, Storkel S, Moll R, Scharfe T, Thoenes W. Bellini duct carcinoma: further evidence for this rare variant of renal cell carcinoma. Histopathology 1991;18:115–22.

267. Saito S, Hatano T, Hayakawa M, Koyama Y, Ohsawa A, Iwamasa T. Studies on alpha-feto-protein produced by renal cell carcinoma. Cancer 1989;63:544–9.

268. Sakai N, Kanda F, Kondo K, Fukuoka H, Tanaka T. Sonographically detected malignant transformation of a simple renal cyst. Int J Urol 2001;8:23–5.

269. Sanders ME, Mick R, Tomaszewski JE, Barr FG. Unique pattern of allelic imbalance distinguish type 1 from type 2 sporadic papillary renal cell carcinoma. Am J Pathol 2002;161:997–1005.

270. Schmidt L, Duh F, Chen F, et al. Germline and somatic mutations in the tyrosine kinase domain of the MET proto-oncogene in papillary renal carcinomas. Nat Genet 1997;16:68–73.

271. Schmidt L, Junker K, Nakaigawa N, et al. Novel mutations of the MET proto-oncogene in papillary renal carcinomas. Oncogene 1999;18:2343–50.

272. Schmidt L, Lubensky I, Linehan WM, et al. Hereditary papillary renal carcinoma: pathology and pathogenesis. 1999;128:11–27.

273. Schraml P, Muller D, Bednar R, et al. Allelic loss at the D9S171 locus on chromosome 9p13 is associated with progression of papillary renal cell carcinoma. J Pathol 2000;190:457–61.

274. Schroder S, Padberg BC, Achilles E, Holl K, Dralle H, Kloppel G. Immunocytochemistry in adrenocortical tumors: a clinicopathologic study of 72 neoplasms. Virchows Arch A Pathol Anat Histopathol 1992;420:65–70.

275. Selli C, Amorosi A, Vona G, et al. Retrospective evaluation of c-erbB-2 oncogene amplification using competitive pcr in collecting duct carcinoma of the kidney. J Urol 1997;158:245–7.

276. Sevinc M, Kirkali Z, Yorukoglu K, Mungan U, Sade M. Prognostic significance of microvascular invasion in localized renal cell carcinoma. Eur Urol 2000;38:728–33.

277. Shah IA, Mellstrom M, Wheeler L, Haddad FS. CD 68 immunoreactivity in renal cell carcinoma: an aid to diagnosis and histogenesis. J Urol Pathol 1996;5:193–206.

277a. Shannon BA, Cohen RJ. Rhabdoid differentiation of chromophobe renal cell carcinoma. Pathology 2003;35:228–30.

278. Sidhar SK, Clark J, Gill S, et al. The t(X;1)(p11.2;q21.2) translocation in papillary renal cell carcinoma fuses a novel gene PRCC to the TFE3 transcription factor gene. Hum Mol Genet 1996;5:1333–8.

279. Siminovitch JP, Montie JE, Straffon RA. Lymphadenectomy in renal adenocarcinoma. J Urol 1982;127:1090–1.

280. Skinner DG, Colvin RB, Vermillion CD, Pfister RC, Leadbetter WF. Diagnosis and management of renal cell carcinoma. A clinical and pathological study of 309 cases. Cancer 1971;28:1165–77.

281. Solomon D, Schwartz A. Renal pathology in von Hippel-Lindau disease. Hum Pathol 1988;19:1072–9.

282. Srigley JR, Eble JN. Collecting duct carcinoma of the kidney. Semin Diagn Pathol 1998;15:54–67.

283. Srigley JR, Hutter RV, Gelb AB, et al. Current prognostic factors—renal cell carcinoma: Workgroup No. 4 Union Internationale Contre le Cancer (UICC) and the American Joint Committee on Cancer (AJCC). Cancer 1997; 80:994–6.

284. Srigley JR, Kapusta L, Reuter V, et al. Phenotypic, molecular and ultrastructural studies of a novel low-grade epithelial neoplasm possibly related to the loop of Henle [Abstract]. Mod Pathol 2002;15:182A.

285. Stahlschmidt J, Cullinane C, Roberts P, Picton SV. Renal medullary carcinoma: prolonged remission with chemotherapy, immunohistochemical characterization and evidence of ber/abl rearrangement. Med Pediatr Oncol 1999;33:551–7.

286. Stanisic TH, Donovan J. Prolactin secreting renal cell carcinoma. J Urol 1986;136:85–6.

287. Steffens J, Bock R, Braedel HU, Isenberg E, Buhrle CP, Ziegler M. Renin-producing renal cell carcinoma. Eur Urol 1990;18:56–60.

288. Steiner G, Cairns P, Polascik TJ, et al. High-density mapping of chromosomal arm 1q in renal collecting duct carcinoma: region of minimal deletion at 1q32.1-32.2. Cancer Res 1996;56:5044–6.

289. Storkel S, Eble JN, Adlakha K, Amin M, Blute ML, Bostwick DG. Classification of renal cell carcinoma: Workgroup No. 1. Union Internationale Contre le Cancer (UICC) and the American Joint Committee on Cancer (AJCC). Cancer 1997;80:987–9.

290. Storkel S, Steart PV, Drenckhahn D, Thoenes W. The human chromophobe cell renal carcinoma: its probable relation to intercalated cells of the collecting duct. Virchows Arch B Cell Pathol Incl Mol Pathol 1989;56:237–45.

291. Sufrin G, Chasan S, Golio A, Murphy GP. Paraneoplastic and serologic syndromes of renal adenocarcinoma. Semin Urol 1989;7:158–71.

292. Sufrin G, Mirand EA, Moore RH, Chu TM, Murphy GP. Hormones in renal cancer. J Urol 1977;117:433–8.

293. Sukosd F, Digon B, Fischer J, Pietsch T, Kovacs G. Allelic loss at 10q23.3 but lack of mutation of PTEN/MMAC1 in chromophobe renal cell carcinoma. Cancer Gen Cytogen 2001;128:161–3.

294. Sukosd F, Kuroda N, Beothe T, Kaur AP, Kovacs G. Deletion of chromosome 3p14.2-p25 involving the VHL and FHIT genes in conventional renal cell carcinoma. Cancer Res 2003;63:455–7.

295. Swartz MA, Karth J, Schneider DT, Rodriguez R, Beckwith JB, Perlman EJ. Renal medullary carcinoma: clinical, pathologic, immunohistochemical, and genetic analysis with pathogenetic implications. Urology 2002;60:1083–9.

296. Syrjanen K, Hjelt L. Grading of human renal adenocarcinoma. Scand J Urol Nephrol 1978;12:49–55.

297. Takahashi M, Kahnoski R, Gross D, Nicol D, Teh BT. Familial adult renal neoplasia. J Med Genet 2002;39:1–5.

298. Tannapfcl A, Hahn HΛ, Katalinic Λ, Fietkau RJ, Kuhn R, Wittekind CW. Prognostic value of ploidy and proliferation markers in renal cell carcinoma. Cancer 1996;77:164–71.

299. Teh BT, Giraud S, Sari NF, et al. Familial non-VHL non-papillary clear-cell renal cancer. Lancet 1997;349:848–9.

300. Thoenes W, Storkel S, Rumpelt HJ. Human chromophobe cell renal carcinoma. Virchows Arch B Cell Pathol Incl Mol Pathol 1985;48:207–17.

301. Thoenes W, Storkel S, Rumpelt HJ, Moll R, Baum HP, Werner S. Chromophobe cell renal carcinoma and its variants—a report on 32 cases. J Pathol 1988;155:277–87.

302. Thompson LD, Heffess CS. Renal cell carcinoma to the pancreas in surgical pathology material. Cancer 2000;89:1076–88.

303. Tickoo SK, Amin MB, Zarbo RJ. Colloidal iron staining in renal epithelial neoplasms, including chromophobe renal cell carcinoma: emphasis on technique and patterns of staining. Am J Surg Pathol 1998;22:419–24.

304. Tickoo SK, Lee MW, Eble JN, et al. Ultrastructural observations on mitochondria and microvesicles in renal oncocytoma, chromophobe renal cell carcinoma, and eosinophilic variant of conventional (clear cell) renal cell carcinoma. Am J Surg Pathol 2000;24:1247–56.

305. Tomera KM, Farrow GM, Lieber MM. Sarcomatoid renal carcinoma. J Urol 1983;130:657–9.

306. Toro JR, Glenn G, Duray P, et al. Birt-Hogg-Dube syndrome: a novel marker of kidney neoplasia. Arch Dermatol 1999;135:1195–202.

307. Tosaka A, Yoshida K, Kobayashi N, Takeuchi S, Uchijima Y, Saitoh H. [A report of two cases of multilocular cystic renal cell carcinoma: review of 51 cases reported and the results of a prognostic survey.] Hinyokika Kiyo 1992;38:1045–50. (Japanese.)

308. Treiger BF, Khazan R, Goldman SM, Marshall FF. Renal cell carcinoma with situs inversus totalis. Urology 1993;41:455–7.

309. Troncoso A, Ro JY, Grignon DJ, et al. Renal cell carcinoma with acrometastasis: report of two cases and review of the literature. Mod Pathol 1991;4:66–9.

310. Tsui K, Shvarts O, Smith RB, Figlin RA, deKernion JB, Belldegrun A. Prognostic indicators for renal cell carcinoma: a multivariate analysis of 643 patients using the revised 1997 TNM staging criteria. J Urol 2000;163:1090–5.

311. Ulrich W, Horvat R, Krisch K. Lectin histochemistry of kidney tumours and its pathomorphological relevance. Histopathology 1985;9:1037–50.

312. Val-Bernal JF, Gomez-Roman JJ, Vallina T, Villoria F, Mayorga M, Garcia-Arranz P. Papillary (chromophil) renal cell carcinoma with mucinous secretion. Pathol Res Prac 1999;195:11–17.

313. Van Poppel H, Vandendriessche H, Boel K, et al. Microscopic vascular invasion is the most relevant prognosticator after radical nephrectomy for clinically nonmetastatic renal cell carcinoma. J Urol 1997;158:45–9.

314. Velickovic M, Delahunt B, Storkel S, Grebem SK. VHL and FHIT locus loss of heterozygosity is common in all renal cancer morphotypes but differs in pattern and prognostic significance. Cancer Res 2001;61:4815–9.

315. Wang S, Filipowicz EA, Schnadig VJ. Abundant intracytoplasmic hemosiderin in both histiocytes and neoplastic cells: a diagnostic pitfall in fine-needle aspiration of cystic papillary renal-cell carcinoma. Diagn Cypathol 2000;24:82–5.

316. Weeks DA, Beckwith JB, Mierau GW, Zuppan CW. Renal neoplasms mimicking rhabdoid tumor of kidney. A report from the National Wilms' Tumor Study Pathology Center. Am J Surg Pathol 1991;15:1042–54.

317. Wenz W. Tumors of the kidney following retrograde pyelography with colloidal thorium dioxide. Ann N Y Acad Sci 1967;145:806–10.

318. Wick MR, Cherwitz DL, Manivel JC, Sibley R. Immunohistochemical findings in tumors of the kidney. In: Eble JN, ed. Tumors and tumor-like conditions of the kidneys and ureters. New York: Churchill Livingstone; 1990:207–47.

319. Wick MR, Cherwitz DL, McGlennan RC, Dehner LP. Adrenocortical carcinoma. An immunohistochemical comparison with renal cell carcinoma. Am J Pathol 1986;122:343–52.

320. Wu SL, Fishman IJ, Shannon RL. Chromophobe renal cell carcinoma with extensive calcification and ossification. Ann Diagn Pathol 2002;6:244–7.

321. Wynder EL, Mabuchi K, Whitmore WF Jr. Epidemiology of adenocarcinoma of the kidney. J Natl Cancer Inst 1974;53:1619–34.

322. Yoshida M, Yao M, Ishikawa I, et al. Somatic von Hippel-Lindau disease gene mutation in clear-cell renal carcinomas associated with end-stage renal disease/acquired cystic disease of the kidney. Genes Chromosomes Cancer 2002;35:359–64.

323. Yoshida MA, Ohyashiki K, Ochi H, et al. Cytogenetic studies of tumor tissue from patients with nonfamilial renal cell carcinoma. Cancer Res 1986;46(4 Pt 2):2139–47.

324. Yoshida SO, Imam A, Olson CA, Taylor CR. Proximal renal tubular surface membrane antigens identified in primary and metastatic renal cell carcinomas. Arch Pathol Lab Med 1986;110:825–32.

325. Young AN, de Oliveira Salles PG, Lim SD, et al. Beta defensin-1, parvalbumin, and vimentin: a panel of diagnostic immunohistochemical markers for renal tumors derived from gene expression profiling studies using cDNA microarrays. Am J Surg Pathol 2003;27:199–205.

326. Zbar B, Brauch H, Talmadge C, Linehan M. Loss of alleles of loci on the short arm of chromosome 3 in renal cell carcinoma. Nature 1987;327:721–4.

327. Zincke H, Swanson SK. Bilateral renal cell carcinoma: influence of synchronous and asynchronous occurrence on patient survival. J Urol 1982;128:913–5.

328. Zisman A, Chao DH, Pantuck AJ, et al. Unclassified renal cell carcinoma: clinical features and prognostic impact of a new histological subtype. J Urol 2002;168:950–5.

329. Zisman A, Pantuck AJ, Chao DH, et al. Reevaluation of the 1997 TNM classification for renal cell carcinoma: T1 and T2 cutoff point at 4.5 rather than 7 cm. better correlates with clinical outcome. J Urol 2001;166:54–8.

330. Zisman A, Pantuck AJ, Dorey F, et al. Improved prognostication of renal cell carcinoma using an integrated staging system. J Clin Oncol 2001;19:1649–57.

Oncocytoma

331. Alanen KA, Ekfors TO, Lipasti JA, Nurmi MJ. Renal oncocytoma: the incidence of 18 surgical and 12 autopsy cases. Histopathology 1984;8:731–7.

332. Amin MB, Crotty TB, Tickoo SK, Farrow GM. Renal oncocytoma: a reappraisal of morphologic features with clinicopathologic findings in 80 cases. Am J Surg Pathol 1997;21:1–12.

333. Barnes CA, Beckman EN. Renal oncocytoma and its congeners. Am J Clin Pathol 1983;79:312–8.

334. Bonsib SM, Bray C. Cytokeratin-containing globular filamentous bodies in renal oncocytoma. Ultrastruct Pathol 1991;15:521–9.

335. Brauch H, Tory K, Linehan WM, Weaver DJ, Lovell MA, Zbar B. Molecular analysis of the short arm of chromosome 3 in five renal oncocytomas. J Urol 1990;143:622–4.

336. Cochand-Priollet B, Molinie V, Bougaran J, et al. Renal chromophobe cell carcinoma and oncocytoma. A comparative morphologic, histochemical, and immunohistochemical study of 124 cases. Arch Pathol Lab Med 1997;121:1081–6.

336a. Chu PG, Weiss LM. Cytokeratin 14 immunoreactivity distinguishes oncocytic tumour from its renal mimics: an immunohistochemical study of 63 cases. Histopathology 2001;39:455–62.

337. Dechet CB, Bostwick DG, Blute ML, Bryant SC, Zincke H. Renal oncocytoma: multifocality, bilateralism, metachronous tumor development and coexistent renal cell carcinoma. J Urol 1999;162:40–2.

338. DeLong WH, Sakr WA, Grignon DJ. Chromophobe renal cell carcinoma: A comparative histochemical and immunohistochemical study. J Urol Pathol 1996;4:1–8.

339. Eble JN, Hull MT. Morphologic features of renal oncocytoma: a light and electron microscopic study. Hum Pathol 1984;15:1054–61.

340. Erlandson RA, Shek TW, Reuter VE. Diagnostic significance of mitochondria in four types of renal epithelial neoplasms: an ultrastructural study of 60 tumors. Ultrastruct Pathol 1997;21:409–17.

341. Fleming S. The impact of genetics on the classification of renal carcinoma. Histopathology 1993;22:89–92.

342. Fuzesi L, Gunawan B, Braun S, Boeckmann W. Renal oncocytoma with a translocation t(9;11)(p23;q13). J Urol 1994;152:471–2.

343. Fuzesi L, Gunawan B, Braun S, et al. Cytogenetic analysis of 11 renal oncocytomas: further evidence of structural rearrangements of 11q13 as a characteristic chromosomal anomaly. Cancer Genet Cytogenet 1998;107:1–6.

344. Gatalica Z, Miettinen M, Kovatich A, McCue PA. Hyaline globules in renal cell carcinomas and oncocytomas. Hum Pathol 1997;28:400–3.

345. Guarino M, Zuccoli E, Garda E, et al. Extracellular matrix globules in renal oncocytoma. Pathol Res Pract 2001;197:245–52.

346. Hartwick RW, el-Naggar AK, Ro JY, et al. Renal oncocytoma and granular renal cell carcinoma. A comparative clinicopathologic and DNA flow cytometric study. Am J Clin Pathol 1992;98:587–93.

347. Herbers J, Schullerus D, Chudek J, et al. Lack of genetic changes at specific genomic sites separates renal oncocytomas from renal cell carcinomas. J Pathol 1998;184:58–62.

348. Hes O, Michal M, Boudova L, Mukensnabl P, Kinkor Z, Miculka P. Small cell variant of renal oncocytoma—a rare and misleading type of benign renal tumor. Int J Surg Pathol 2001;9:215–22.

349. Hes O, Michal M, Sulc M, Kocova L, Hora M, Rousarova M. Glassy hyaline globules in granular renal cell carcinoma, chromophobe cell carcinoma, and oncocytoma of the kidney. Ann Diagn Pathol 1998;2:12–8.

350. Klein MJ, Valensi QJ. Proximal tubular adenomas of the kidney with so-called oncocytic features. A clinicopathologic study of 13 cases of a rarely reported neoplasm. Cancer 1976;38:906–14.

351. Koller A, Kain R, Haitel A, Mazal PR, Asboth F, Susani M. Renal oncocytoma with prominent intracytoplasmic vacuoles of mitochondrial origin. Histopathology 2000;37:264–8.

352. Kovacs G. Molecular differential pathology of renal cell tumors. Histopathology 1993;22:1–8.

352a. Latham B, Dickersin GR, Oliva E. Subtypes of chromophobe cell renal carcinoma. An ultrastructural and histochemical study of 13 cases. Am J Surg Pathol 1999;23:530–5.

353. Leroy X, Moukassa D, Copin MC, Saint F, Mazeman E, Gosselin B. Utility of cytokeratin 7 for distinguishing chromophobe renal cell carcinoma from renal oncocytoma. Eur Urol 2000;37:484–7.

354. Lieber MM, Tomera KM, Farrow GM. Renal oncocytoma. J Urol 1981;125:481–5.

355. Lyzak JS, Farhood A, Verani R. Intracytoplasmic lumens in renal oncocytoma and possible origin from intercalated cells of the collecting duct. J Urol Pathol 1994;2:135–51.

355a. McGregor DK, Khurana KK, Cao C, et al. Diagnosing primary and metastatic renal cell carcinoma. The use of the monoclonal antibody "renal cell carcinoma marker." Am J Surg Pathol 2001;25:1485–92.

356. Morra MN, Das S. Renal oncocytoma: a review of histogenesis, histopathology, diagnosis and treatment. J Urol 1993;150:295–302.

356a. Murphy WM, Beckwith JB, Farrow GM. Tumors of the Kidney, bladder and related urinary structures. Atlas of Tumor Pathology, 3rd series, Fascicle 11. Washington, D.C.: Armed Forces Institute of Pathology; 1994.

357. Neuhaus C, Dijkhuizen T, van den Berg E, et al. Involvement of the chromosomal region 11q13 in renal oncocytoma: case report and literature review. Cancer Genet Cytogenet 1997;94:95–8.

358. Newhouse JH, Wagner BJ. Renal oncocytomas. Abdom Imaging 1998;23:249–55.

358a. Pavlovich CP, Walther MM, Eyler RA, et al. Renal tumors in the Birt-Hogg-Dube syndrome. Am J Surg Pathol 2002;26:1542–52.

359. Perez-Ordonez B, Hamed G, Campbell S, et al. Renal oncocytoma: a clinicopathologic study of 70 cases. Am J Surg Pathol 1997;21:871–83.

360. Presti JC Jr, Rao PH, Chen Q, et al. Histopathological, cytogenetic, and molecular characterization of renal cortical tumors. Cancer Res 1991;51:1544–52.

360a. Renshaw AA, Lee KR, Madge R, Granter SR. Accuracy of fine needle aspiration in distinguishing subtypes of renal cell carcinoma. Acta Cytol 1997;41:987–94.

361. Rofsky NM, Bosniak MA. MR imaging in the evaluation of small (< or =3.0 cm) renal masses. Magn Reson Imaging Clin N Am 1997;5:67–81.

362. Shimasaki H, Tanaka H, Aida S, et al. Renal oncocytoma with intracytoplasmic lumina: a case report with ultrastructural findings of "oncoblasts." Ultrastruct Pathol 2001;25:153–8.

363. Siracusano S, Zanon M, D'Aloia G, Plaino F, Trombetta C, Bussani R. Rare association of renal angiomyolipoma and oncocytoma. Urology 1998;51:837–9.

364. Slagel D, Bonsib SM. Renal oncocytoma with unusual features: case report and review of morphologic variants of oncocytoma. J Urol Pathol 1995;3:223–33.

365. Stopyra GA, Warhol MJ, Multhaupt HA. Cytokeratin 20 immunoreactivity in renal oncocytoma. J Histochem Cytochem 2001;49:919–20.

365a. Storkel S, Eble JN, Adlakha K, Amin M, Blute ML, Bostwick DG. Classification of renal cell carcinoma: Workgroup No. 1. Union Internationale Contre le Cancer (UICC) and the American Joint Committee on Cancer (AJCC). Cancer 1997;80:987–9.

366. Tickoo SK, Amin MB. Discriminant nuclear features of renal oncocytoma and chromophobe renal cell carcinoma. Analysis of their potential ability in the differential diagnosis. Am J Clin Pathol 1998;110:782–7.

366a. Tickoo SK, Amin MB, Zarbo RJ. Colloidal iron staining in renal epithelial neoplasms, including chromophobe renal cell carcinoma: emphasis on technique and patterns of staining. Am J Surg Pathol 1998;22:419–24.

366b. Tickoo SK, Lee MW, Eble JN, et al. Ultrastructural observations on mitochondria and microvesicals in renal oncocytoma, chromophobe renal cell carcinoma, and eosinophilic variant of conventional (clear cell) renal cell carcinoma. Am J Surg Pathol 2000;24:1247–56.

367. Tickoo SK, Reuter VE, Amin MB, et al. Renal oncocytosis: a morphologic study of fourteen cases. Am J Surg Pathol 1999;23:1094–101.

368. Veloso JD, Solis OG, Barada JH, Fisher HA, Ross JS. DNA ploidy of oncocytic-granular renal cell carcinomas and renal oncocytomas by image analysis. Arch Pathol Lab Med 1992;116:154–8.

369. Warfel KA, Eble JN. Renal oncocytomatosis. J Urol 1982;127:1179–80.

370. Wiatrowska BA, Zakowski MF. Fine-needle aspiration biopsy of chromophobe renal cell carcinoma and oncocytoma: comparison of cytomorphologic features. Cancer 1999;87:161–7.

371. Wildberger JE, Adam G, Boeckmann W, et al. Computed tomography characterization of renal cell tumors in correlation with histopathology. Invest Radiol 1997;32:596–601.

372. Wu SL, Kothari P, Wheeler TM, Reese T, Connelly JH. Cytokeratins 7 and 20 immunoreactivity in chromophobe renal cell carcinomas and renal oncocytomas. Mod Pathol 2002;15:712–7.

372a. Young AN, de Oliveira Salles PG, Lim SD, et al. Beta defensin-1, parvalbumin, and vimentin: a panel of diagnostic immunohistochemical markers for renal tumors derived from gene expression profiling studies using cDNA microarrays. Am J Surg Pathol 2003;27:199–205.

373. Zambrano NR, Lubensky IA, Merino MJ, Linehan WM, Walther MM. Histopathology and molecular genetics of renal tumors toward unification of a classification system. J Urol 1999;162:1246–58.

374. Zardawi IM. Renal fine needle aspiration cytology. Acta Cytol 1999;43:184–90.

Rare Tumors with Epithelial and/or Renal Parenchymal Differentiation

375. Aaronson IA, Sinclair-Smith C. Multiple cystic teratomas of the kidney. Arch Pathol Lab Med 1980;104:614.

376. Adsay NV, Eble JN, Srigley JR, Jones EC, Grignon D. Mixed epithelial and stromal tumor of the kidney. Am J Surg Pathol 2000;24:958–70.

377. Amin MB, de Peralta-Venturina MN, Ro JY, et al. Clear cell sarcoma of the kidney in an adolescent and in young adults: a report of four cases with ultrastructural, immunohistochemical, and DNA flow cytometric analysis. Am J Surg Pathol 1999;23:1455–63.

378. Barajas L. The development and ultrastructure of the juxtaglomerular cell granule. J Ultrastruct Res 1966;15:400–13.

379. Begin LR, Guy L, Jacobson SA, Aprikian AG. Renal carcinoid and horseshoe kidney: a frequent association of two rare entities—a case report and review of the literature. J Surg Oncol 1998;68:113–9.

380. Beiko DT, Nickel JC, Boag AH, Srigley JR. Benign mixed epithelial stromal tumor of the kidney of possible mullerian origin. J Urol 2001;166:1381–2.

381. Benchekroun A, Ghadouane M, Zannoud M, Alami M, Iken A, Faik M. Clear cell sarcoma of the kidney in an adult. A case report. Ann Urol 2002;36:33–5.

382. Biava CG, West M. Fine structure of normal human juxtaglomerular cells. II. Specific and nonspecific cytoplasmic granules. Am J Pathol 1966;49:955–79.

383. Bonsib SM, Hansen KK. Juxtaglomerular cell tumors: a report of two cases with negative HMB-45 immunostaining. J Urol Pathol 1998;9:61–72.

384. Byrd RL, Evans AE, D'Angio GJ. Adult Wilms' tumor: effect of combined therapy on survival. J Urol 1982;127:648–51.

385. Capella C, Eusebi V, Rosai J. Primary oat cell carcinoma of the kidney. Am J Surg Pathol 1984;8:855–61.

386. Casella R, Moch H, Rochlitz C, et al. Metastatic primitive neuroectodermal tumor of the kidney in adults. Eur Urol 2001;39:613–7.

387. Castillo OA, Boyle ET Jr, Kramer SA. Multilocular cysts of the kidney. A study of 29 patients and a review of the literature. Urology 1991;37:156–62.

388. Chan YF, Llewellyn H. Intrarenal primitive neuroectodermal tumour. Br J Urol 1994;73;326–7.

389. Davila RM, Kissane JM, Crouch EC. Multilocular renal cyst. Immunohistochemical and lectin-binding study. Am J Surg Pathol 1992;16:508–14.

390. Dunnick NR, Hartman DS, Ford KK, Davis CJ Jr, Amis ES Jr. The radiology of juxtaglomerular cell tumors. Radiology 1983;147:321–6.

391. Durham JR, Bostwick DG, Farrow GM, Ohorodnik JM. Mesoblastic nephroma of adulthood. Report of three cases. Am J Surg Pathol 1993;17:1029–38.

392. Eble JN. Unusual renal tumors and tumor-like conditions. In: Eble JN, ed. Tumors and tumor-like conditions of the kidneys and ureters. New York: Churchill Livingstone; 1990:145–76.

392a. Eble JN, Bonsib SM. Extensively cystic renal neoplasms: cystic nephroma, cystic partially differentiated nephroblastoma, multilocular cystic renal cell carcinoma and cystic hamartoma of the renal pelvis. Semin Diagn Pathol 1998;15:2–20.

393. Essenfeld H, Manivel JC, Benedetto P, Albores-Saavedra J. Small cell carcinoma of the renal pelvis: a clinicopathologic, morphologic and histochemical study of 2 cases. J Urol 1990;144:344–7.

393a. Farrow GM, Harrison EG Jr, Utz DC. Sarcomas and the sarcomatoid and mixed malignant tumors of the kidney in adults. III. Cancer 1968;22:556–63.

394. Fetissof F, Benatre A, Dubois MP, Lanson Y, Arbeille-Brassart B, Jobard P. Carcinoid tumor occurring in a teratoid malformation of the kidney. An immunohistochemical study. Cancer 1984;54:2305–8.

395. Fujimoto K, Samma S, Fukui Y, Yamaguchi A, Hirayama A, Kikkawa A. Spontaneously ruptured multilocular cystic nephroma. Int J Urol 2002;9:183–6.

396. Gleeson MH, Bloom SR, Polak JM, Henry K, Dowling RH. Endocrine tumor in kidney affecting small bowel structure, motility, and absorptive function. Gut 1971;12:773–82.

397. Goldblum JR, Lloyd RV. Primary renal carcinoid. Case report and literature review. Arch Pathol Lab Med 1993;117:855–8.

398. Gonzalez-Lois C, Madero S, Redondo P, Alonso I, Salas A, Angeles Montalban M. Small cell carcinoma of the kidney: a case report and review of the literature. Arch Pathol Lab Med 2001;125:796–8.

399. Grignon DJ, Ro JY, Ayala AG. Mesenchymal tumors of the kidney. In: Eble JN, ed. Tumors and tumor-like conditions of the kidneys and ureters. New York: Churchill Livingstone; 1990:123–44.

400. Guy L, Begin LR, Oligny LL, Brock GB, Chevalier S, Aprikian AG. Searching for an intrinsic neuroendocrine cell in the kidney. An immunohistochemical study of the fetal, infantile and adult kidney. Pathol Res Pract 1999;195:25–30.

401. Hannah J, Lippe B, Lai-Goldman M, Bhuta S. Oncocytic carcinoid tumor of the kidney associated with periodic Cushing's syndrome. Cancer 1988;61:2136–40.

402. Henderson NL, Mason RC. Juxtaglomerular cell tumor in pregnancy. Obstet Gynecol 2001;98:943–5.

403. Huser J, Grignon DJ, Ro JY, Ayala AG, Shannon RL, Papadopoulos NJ. Adult Wilms' tumor: a clinicopathologic study of 11 cases. Mod Pathol 1990;3:321–6.

404. Isobe H, Takashima H, Higashi N, et al. Primary carcinoid tumor in a horseshoe kidney. Int J Urol 2000;7:184–8.

405. Jimenez RE, Folpe AL, Lapham RL, et al. Primary Ewing's sarcoma/primitive neuroectodermal tumor of the kidney: a clinicopathologic and immunohistochemical analysis of 11 cases. Am J Surg Pathol 2002;26:320–7.

406. Kilton L, Matthews MJ, Cohen MH. Adult Wilms tumor: a report of prolonged survival and review of literature. J Urol 1980;124:1–5

407. Kojiro M, Ohishi H, Isobe H. Carcinoid tumor occurring in a cystic teratoma of the kidney: a case report. Cancer 1976;38:1636–40.

408. Kumar R, Seth A, Dinda AK. Incidental cystic, partially differentiated nephroblastoma in an adult. J Urol 2001;165:1622.

409. Kuroda N, Moriki T, Komatsu F, et al. Adult-onset giant juxtaglomerular cell tumor of the kidney. Pathol Int 2000;50:249–54.

410. Lagace R, Tremblay M. Non-chromaffin paraganglioma of the kidney with distant metastases. Can Med Assoc J 1968;99:1095–98.

411. Levin NP, Damjanov I, Depillis VJ. Mesoblastic nephroma in an adult patient: recurrence 21 years after removal of the primary lesion. Cancer 1982;49:573–7.

412. Lowe W, Weiss RM, Todd MB, True LD. Malignant rhabdoid tumor of the kidney in an adult. J Urol 1990;143:110–12.

413. Madewell JE, Goldman SM, Davis CJ Jr, Hartman DS, Feigin DS, Lichtenstein JE. Multilocular cystic nephroma: a radiographic-pathologic correlation of 58 patients. Radiology 1983;146:309–21.

414. Majhail NS, Elson P, Bukowski RM. Therapy and outcome of small cell carcinoma of the kidney: report of two cases and a systematic review of the literature. Cancer 2003;97:1436–41.

415. Marley EF, Liapis H, Humphrey PA, et al. Primitive neuroectodermal tumor of the kidney—another enigma: a pathologic, immunohistochemical, and molecular diagnostic study. Am J Surg Pathol 1997;21:354–9.

416. Martin SA, Mynderse LA, Lager DJ, Cheville JC. Juxtaglomerular cell tumor: a clinico-pathologic study of four cases and review of the literature. Am J Clin Pathol 2001;116:854–63.

417. Masuda T, Oikawa H, Yashima A, Sugimura J, Okamoto T, Fujioka T. Renal small cell carcinoma (neuroendocrine carcinoma) without features of transitional cell carcinoma. Pathol Int 1998;48;412–5.

418. McCaffrey JA, Reuter VV, Herr HW, Macapinlac HA, Russo P, Motzer RJ. Carcinoid tumor of the kidney. The use of somatostatin receptor scintography in diagnosis and management. Urol Oncol 2000;5;108–11.

418a. Michal M, Hes O, Havlicek F. Benign renal angiomyoadenomatous tumor: a previously unreported renal tumor. Ann Diagn Pathol 2000;4:311–5.

419. Michal M, Syrucek M. Benign mixed epithelial and stromal tumor of the kidney. Pathol Res Pract 1998;194:445–8.

420. Mills SE, Wolfe JT 3rd, Weiss MA, et al. Small cell undifferentiated carcinoma of the urinary bladder. A light microscopic, immunocytochemical, and ultrastructural study of 12 cases. Am J Surg Pathol 1987;11:606–17.

420a. Murphy WM, Beckwith JB, Farrow GM. Tumors of the Kidney, bladder and related urinary structures. Atlas of Tumor Pathology, 3rd series, Fascicle 11. Washington, D.C.: Armed Forces Institute of Pathology; 1994.

421. Otani M, Tsujimoto S, Miura M, Nagashima Y. Intrarenal mature cystic teratoma associated with renal dysplasia: case report and literature review. Pathol Int 2001;51;560–4.

422. Parham DM, Roloson GJ, Feely M, Green DM, Bridge JA, Beckwith JB. Primary malignant neuroepithelial tumors of the kidney: a clinicopathologic analysis of 146 adult and pediatric cases from the National Wilms' Tumor Study Group Pathology Center. Am J Surg Pathol 2001;25:133–46.

423. Pawade J, Soosay GN, Delprado W, Parkinson MC, Rode J. Cystic hamartoma of the renal pelvis. Am J Surg Pathol 1993;17:1169–75.

424. Pierson CR, Schober MS, Wallis T, et al. Mixed epithelial and stromal tumor of the kidney lacks the genetic alterations of cellular congenital mesoblastic nephroma. Hum Pathol 2001;32:513–29.

425. Prats Lopez J, Palou Redorta J, Morote Robles J, Martinez Perez E, Ruiz Marcellan C. Leiomyomatous renal hamartoma in an adult. Eur Urol 1988;14:80–2.

426. Quezado M, Benjamin DR, Tsokos M. EWS/FLI-1 fusion transcripts in three peripheral primitive neuroectodermal tumors of the kidney. Hum Pathol 1997;28:767–71.

427. Raslan WF, Ro JY, Ordonez NG, et al. Primary carcinoid of the kidney. Immunohistochemical and ultrastructural studies of five patients. Cancer 1993;72:2660–6.

428. Resnick ME, Unterberger H, McLoughlin PT. Renal carcinoid producing the carcinoid syndrome. Med Times 1966;94:895–6.

429. Robertson PW, Klidjian A, Harding LK, Walters G, Lee MR, Robb-Smith AH. Hypertension due to a renin-secreting renal tumor. Am J Med 1967;43:963–76.

430. Rolonson GJ, Beckwith JB. Primary neuroepithelial tumors of the kidney in children and adults: a report from the NWTS Pathology Center. Mod Pathol 1993;6:67A.

431. Sheaff M, McManus A, Scheimberg I, Paris A, Shipley J, Baithun S. Primitive neuroectodermal tumor of the kidney confirmed by fluorescence in situ hybridization. Am J Surg Pathol 1997;21:461–8.

432. Shende A, Wind ES, Lanzkowsky P. Intrarenal neuroblastoma mimicking Wilms' tumor. N Y State J Med 1979;79:93.

433. Squires JP, Ulbright TM, DeSchryver-Kecskemeti K, Engleman W. Juxtaglomerular cell tumor of the kidney. Cancer 1984;53:516–23.

434. Strobel P, Zettl A, Ren Z, et al. Spiradenocylindroma of the kidney: clinical and genetic findings suggesting a role of somatic mutation of the CYLD1 gene in the oncogenesis of an unusual renal neoplasm. Am J Surg Pathol 2002;26:119–24.

435. Svec A, Hes O, Michal M, Zachoval R. Malignant mixed epithelial and stromal tumor of the kidney. Virchows Arch 2001;439:700–2.

436. Takeuchi T, Iwasaki H, Ohjimi Y, et al. Renal primitive neuroectodermal tumor: an immunohistochemical and cytogenetic analysis. Pathol Int 1996;46:292–7.

437. Tetu B, Ro JY, Ayala AG, Ordonez NG, Johnson DE. Small cell carcinoma of the kidney. A clinicopathologic, immunohistochemical and ultrastructural study. Cancer 1987;60:1809–14.

438. Tetu B, Vaillancourt L, Camilleri, Bruneval P, Bernier L, Tourigny R. Juxtaglomerular cell tumor of the kidney: report of two cases with papillary pattern. Hum Pathol 1993;24:1168–74.

439. Trillo AA. Adult variant of congenital mesoblastic nephroma. Arch Pathol Lab Med 1990;114:533–5.

440. Truong LD, Williams R, Ngo T, et al. Adult mesoblastic nephroma: expansion of the morphologic spectrum and review of the literature. Am J Surg Pathol 1998;22:827–39.

441. Unger PD, Russell A, Thung SN, Gordon RE. Primary renal carcinoid. Arch Pathol Lab Med 1990;114:68–71.

442. Val-Bernal JF, Hernandez-Nieto E, Garijo MF. Association of cystic nephroma with angiomyolipoma in the same kidney. Pathol Res Pract 2000;196:583–8.

443. Van Velden DJ, Schneider JW, Allen FJ. A case of adult mesoblastic nephroma: ultrastructure and discussion of histogenesis. J Urol 1990;143:1216–9.

444. Yoo J, Park S, Jung Lee H, Jin Kang S, Kee Kim B. Primary carcinoid tumor arising in a mature teratoma of the kidney: a case report and review of the literature. Arch Pathol Lab Med 2002;126:979–81.

Angiomyolipoma

445. Ashfaq R, Weinberg AG, Albores-Saavedra J. Renal angiomyolipomas and HMB-45 reactivity. Cancer 1993;71:3091–7.

446. Barnard M, Lajoie G. Angiomyolipoma: immunohistochemical and ultrastructural study of 14 cases. Ultrastruct Pathol 2001;25:21–9.

447. Bonetti F, Pea M, Martignoni G, et al. Clear cell ("sugar") tumor of the lung is a lesion strictly related to angiomyolipoma—the concept of a family of lesions characterized by the presence of the perivascular epithelioid cells (PEC). Pathology 1994;26:230–6.

448. Blute ML, Malek RS, Segura JW. Angiomyolipoma: clinical metamorphosis and concepts for management. J Urol 1988;139:20–4.

449. Chen KT, Bauer V. Extrarenal angiomyolipoma. J Surg Oncol 1984;25:89–91.

450. Cibas ES, Goss GA, Kulke MH, Demetri GD, Fletcher CD. Malignant epithelioid angiomyolipoma ("Sarcoma ex angiomyolipoma") of the kidney: a case report and review of the literature. Am J Surg Pathol 2001;25:121–6.

451. Eble JN. Angiomyolipoma of kidney. Semin Diagn Pathol 1998;15:21–40.

452. Eble JN, Amin MB, Young RH. Epithelioid angiomyolipoma of the kidney: a report of five cases with a prominent and diagnostically confusing epithelioid smooth muscle component. Am J Surg Pathol 1997;21:1123–30.

453. Farrow GM, Harrison EG Jr, Utz DC, Jones DR. Renal angiomyolipoma. A clinicopathologic study of 32 cases. Cancer 1968;22:564–70.

454. Ferry JA, Malt RA, Young RH. Renal angiomyolipoma with sarcomatous transformation and pulmonary metastases. Am J Surg Pathol 1991;15:1083–8.

455. Glenthoj A, Partoft S. Ultrasound-guided percutaneous aspiration of renal angiomyolipoma. Report of two cases diagnosed by cytology. Acta Cytol 1984;28:265–8.

456. Goodman ZD, Ishak KG. Angiomyolipomas of the liver. Am J Surg Pathol 1984;8:745–50.

457. Green AJ, Sepp T, Yates JR. Clonality of tuberous sclerosis hamartomas shown by non-random X-chromosome inactivation. Hum Genet 1996;97:240–3.

458. Hulbert JC, Graf R. Involvement of the spleen by renal angiomyollpoma: metastasis or multicentricity? J Urol 1983;130:328–9.

459. Identification and characterization of the tuberous sclerosis gene on chromosome 16. The European Chromosome 16 Tuberous Sclerosis Consortium. Cell 1993;75:1305–15.

459a. Jimenez RE, Eble JN, Reuter VE, et al. Concurrent angiomyolipoma and renal cell neoplasia: a study of 36 cases. Mod Pathol 2001;14:157–63.

460. Kaiserling E, Krober S, Xiao JC, Schaumburg-Lever G. Angiomyolipoma of the kidney. Immunoreactivity with HMB-45. Light- and electron-microscopic findings. Histopathology 1994;25:41–8.

461. Kattar MM, Grignon DJ, Eble JN, et al. Chromosomal analysis of renal angiomyolipoma by comparative genomic hybridization: evidence for clonal origin. Hum Pathol 1999;30:295–9.

462. Katz DA, Thom D, Bogard P, Dermer MS. Angiomyolipoma of the fallopian tube. Am J Obstet Gynecol 1984;148:341–3.

463. Kilicaslan I, Gulluoglu MG, Dogan O, Uysal V. Intraglomerular microlesions in renal angiomyolipomas. Hum Pathol 2000;31:1325–8.

464. Klapproth HJ, Poutasse EF, Hazard JB. Renal angiomyolipomas—report of 4 cases. Arch Pathol 1959;67:400–41.

465. Kutcher R, Rosenblatt R, Mitsudo SM, Goldman M, Kogan S. Renal angiomyolipoma with sonographic demonstration of extension into the inferior vena cava. Radiology 1982;143:755–6.

466. L'Hostis H, Deminiere C, Ferriere JM, Coindre JM. Renal angiomyolipoma: a clinicopathologic, immunohistochemical, and follow-up study of 46 cases. Am J Surg Pathol 1999;23:1011–20.

467. Lynne CM, Carrion HM, Bakshandeh K, Nadji M, Russel E, Politano VA. Renal angiomyolipoma, polycystic kidney, and renal carcinoma in a patient with tuberous sclerosis. Urology 1979;14:174–6.

468. Mai KT, Perkins DG, Collins JP. Epithelioid cell variant of renal angiomyolipoma. Histopathology 1996;28:277–80.

469. Makhlouf HR, Remotti HE, Ishak KG. Expression of KIT (CD117) in angiomyolipoma. Am J Surg Pathol 2002;26:493–7.

470. Martignoni G, Bonetti F, Pea M, Tardanico R, Brunelli M, Eble JN. Renal disease in adults with TSC2/PKD1 contiguous gene syndrome. Am J Surg Pathol 2002;26:198–205.

471. Martignoni G, Pea M, Bonetti F, et al. Carcinomalike monotypic epithelioid angiomyolipoma in patient without evidence of tuberous sclerosis: a clinicopathologic and genetic study. Am J Surg Pathol 1998;22:663–72.

472. Martignoni G, Pea M, Rigaud G, et al. Renal angiomyolipoma with epithelioid sarcomatous transformation and metastases: demonstration of the same genetic defects in the primary and metastatic lesions. Am J Surg Pathol 2000;24:889–94.

473. Perez-Atayde AR, Iwaya S, Lack EE. Angiomyolipomas and polycystic renal disease in tuberous sclerosis. Ultrastructural observations. Urology 1981;17:607–10.

474. Plank TL, Logginidou H, Klein-Szanto A, Henske EP. The expression of hamartin, the product of the TSC1 gene, in normal human tissues and in TSC1- and TSC2-linked angiomyolipomas. Mod Pathol 1999;12:539–45.

475. Price EB, Mostofi FK. Symptomatic angiomyolipoma of the kidney. Cancer 1965;18:761-74.

476. Radin R, Ma Y. Malignant epithelioid renal angiomyolipoma in a patient with tuberous sclerosis. J Computer Assist Tomogr 2001;25:873–5.

477. Saito K, Fujii Y, Kasahara I, Kobayashi N, Kasuga T, Kihara K. Malignant clear cell "sugar" tumor of the kidney: clear cell variant of epithelioid angiomyolipoma. J Urol 2002;168:2533–4.

478. Silpananta P, Michel RP, Oliver JA. Simultaneous occurrence of angiomyolipoma and renal cell carcinoma. Clinical and pathologic (including ultrastructural) features. Urology 1984;23:200–4.

479. Smolarek TA, Wessner LL, McCormack FX, Mylet JC, Menon AG, Henske EP. Evidence that lymphangiomyomatosis is caused by TSC2 mutations: chromosome 16p13 loss of heterozygosity in angiomyolipomas and lymph nodes from women with lymphangiomyomatosis. Am J Hum Genet 1998;62:810–5.

480. Stapleton FB, Johnson D, Kaplan GW, Griswold W. The cystic renal lesion in tuberous sclerosis. J Pediatr 1980;97:574–9.

481. van Slegtenhorst M, de Hoogt R, Hermans C, et al. Identification of the tuberous sclerosis gene TSC1 on chromosome 9q34. Science 1997;277:805–8.

482. van Slegtenhorst M, Nellist M, Nagelkerken B, et al. Interaction between hamartin and tuberin, the TSC1 and TSC2 gene products. Hum Mol Genet 1998;7:1053–7.

483. Yum M, Ganguly A, Donohue JP. Juxtaglomerular cells in renal angiomyolipoma. Ultrastructural observation. Urology 1984;24:283–6.

484. Zavala-Pompa A, Folpe AL, Jimenez RE, et al. Immunohistochemical study of microphthalmia transcription factor and tyrosinase in angiomyolipoma of the kidney, renal cell carcinoma, and renal and retroperitoneal sarcomas: comparative evaluation with traditional diagnostic markers. Am J Surg Pathol 2001;25:65–70.

Renomedullary Interstitial Cell Tumor (Medullary Fibroma)

485. Argani P, Beckwith JB. Metanephric stromal tumor: report of 31 cases of a distinctive pediatric neoplasm. Am J Surg Pathol 2000;24:917–26.
486. Bluebond-Langner R, Pinto PA, Argani P, Chan TY, Halushka M, Jarrett TW. Adult presentation of metanephric stromal tumor. J Urol 2002;168:1482–3.
487. Dall'Era M, Das S. Benign medullary fibroma of the kidney. J Urol 2000;164:2018.
488. Glover SD, Buck AC. Renal medullary fibroma: a case report. J Urol 1982;127:758–60.
489. Lerman RJ, Pitcock JA, Stephenson P, Muirhead EE. Renomedullary interstitial cell tumor (formerly fibroma of the renal medulla). Hum Pathol 1972;3:559–68.
490. Mandal AK. The renal papilla and hypertension: an up-to-date review. Pathol Annu 1981;16(Pt 2):295–313.
491. Stuart R, Salyer WR, Salyer DC, Heptinstall RH. Renomedullary interstitial cell lesions and hypertension. Hum Pathol 1976;7:327–32.

Leiomyoma

492. Bonsib SM. HMB-45 reactivity in renal leiomyomas and leiomyosarcomas. Mod Pathol 1996;9:664–9.
493. Clinton-Thomas CL. A giant leiomyoma of the kidney. Br J Surg 1956;43:497–501.
494. Dasgupta P, Sandison A, Parks C, Worth P. Case report: renal leiomyoma with unusual calcification. Clin Radiol 1998;53:857–8.
495. Fisher KS, van Blerk PJ. Childhood leiomyoma of kidney. Urology 1983;21:74–5.
495a. Grignon DJ, Ro JY, Ayala AG. Mesenchymal tumors of the kidney. In: Eble JN, ed. Tumors and tumor-like conditions of the kidneys and ureters. New York: Churchill Livingstone; 1990:123–44.
496. Mohammed AY, Matthew L, Harmse JL, Lang S, Townell NH. Multiple leiomyoma of the renal capsule. Scand J Urol Nephrol 1999;33:138–9.
497. Petersen RO. Urologic pathology. Philadelphia: JB Lippincott; 1986:121.
498. Steiner M, Quinlan D, Goldman SM, et al. Leiomyoma of the kidney: presentation of 4 new cases and the role of computerized tomography. J Urol 1990;143:994–8.

499. Tessler FN, Tublin ME, Rifkin MD. US case of the day. Renal leiomyoma. Radiographics 1998;18:791–3.
500. Xipell JM. The incidence of benign renal nodules (a clinicopathologic study). J Urol 1971;106:503–6.

Lipoma

501. Dineen MK, Venable DD, Misra RP. Pure intrarenal lipoma—report of a case and review of the literature. J Urol 1984;132:104–7.
502. Hamilton I, Reis L, Bilimoria S, Long RG. A renal lipoma. Br Med J 1980;281:1323–4.

Hemangioma/Lymphangioma

503. Anderson C, Knibbs DR, Ludwig ME, Ely MG 3rd. Lymphangioma of the kidney: a pathologic entity distinct from solitary multilocular cyst. Hum Pathol 1992;23:465–8.
504. Daneshmand S, Huffman JL. Endoscopic management of renal hemangioma. J Urol 2002;167:488–9.
504a. Grignon DJ, Ro JY, Ayala AG. Mesenchymal tumors of the kidney. In: Eble JN, ed. Tumors and tumor-like conditions of the kidneys and ureters. New York: Churchill Livingstone; 1990:123–44.
505. Haas CA, Resnick MI, Abdul-Karim FW. Cavernous hemangioma presenting as a renal hilar mass. J Urol 1998;160:2139–40.
506. Honma I, Takagi Y, Shigyo M, et al. Lymphangioma of the kidney. Int J Urol 2002;9:178–82.
507. Hull GW 3rd, Genega EM, Sogani PC. Intravascular capillary hemangioma presenting as a solid renal mass. J Urol 1999;162:784–5.
508. Joost J, Schafer R, Altwein JE. Renal lymphangioma. J Urol 1977;118(Pt 1):22–4.
509. Moros Garcia M, Martinez Tello D, Ramon Y Cajal Junquera S, Valdivia Uria G, Romero Aguirre F, Ortego Fernandez de Retana J. Multiple cavernous hemangiomas of the kidney. Eur Urol 1988;14:90–2.
510. Nakai Y, Namba Y, Sugao H. Renal lymphangioma. J Urol 1999;162:484–5.
511. Okuno T, Ando M, Arisawa C, Okano T. A case of perirenal hemangioma mimicking renal cell carcinoma. Int J Urol 1999;6;104–6.
512. Pickering SP, Fletcher BD, Bryan PJ, Abramowsky CR. Renal lymphangioma: a cause of neonatal nephromegaly. Pediatr Radiol 1984;14:445–8.
513. Ramani P, Shah A. Lymphangiomatosis. Histologic and immunohistochemical analysis of four cases. Am J Surg Pathol 1993;17:329–35.
514. Schofield D, Zaatari GS, Gay BB. Klippel-Trenaunay and Sturge-Weber syndromes with renal hemangioma and double inferior vena cava. J Urol 1986;136:442–5.

515. Schwarz A, Lenz T, Klaen R, Offermann G, Fiedler U, Nussberger J. Hygroma renale: pararenal lymphatic cysts associated with renin-dependent hypertension (Page kidney). Case report on bilateral cysts and successful therapy by marsupialization. J Urol 1993;150:953–7.
516. Singer DR, Miller JD, Smith G. Lymphangioma of kidney. Scott Med J 1983;28:293–4.
517. Varela JR, Bargiela A, Requejo I, Fernandez R, Darriba M, Pombo F. Bilateral renal lymphangiomatosis: US and CT findings. Eur Radiol 1998;8:230–1.
518. Wang T, Palazzo JP, Mitchell D, Petersen RO. Renal capsular hemangioma. J Urol 1993;149:1122–3.
519. Zaidi SZ, Mor Y, Scheimberg I, Quimby GF, Mouriquand PD. Renal haemangioma presenting as an abdominal mass in a neonate. Br J Urol 1998;82:763–4.

Other Benign Mesenchymal Tumors

520. Alvarado-Cabrero I, Folpe AL, Srigley JR, et al. Intrarenal schwannoma: a report of four cases including three cellular variants. Mod Pathol 2000;13:851–6.
521. Freund ME, Crocker DW, Harrison JH. Neurofibroma arising in a solitary kidney. J Urol 1967;98:318–21.
522. Kahn DG, Duckett T, Bhuta SM. Perineurioma of the kidney. Report of a case with histologic, immunohistochemical, and ultrastructural studies. Arch Pathol Lab Med 1993;117:654–7.
523. Kobayashi S, Yamadori I, Ohmori M, Akaeda T. Benign fibrous histiocytoma of the renal capsule. Acta Pathol Jpn 1992;42:217–20.
524. Lopes M, Raciti G, Maira A, Magro G. Cortical benign fibromatous tumor (fibroma) of the kidney. Urol Int 1999;62:34–6.
525. Magro G, Lopes M, Giannone G. Benign fibromatous tumor (fibroma) of the kidney: a case report. Pathol Res Pract 1998;194:123–7.
526. Melamed J, Reuter VE, Erlandson RA, Rosai J. Renal myxoma. A report of two cases and review of the literature. Am J Surg Pathol 1994;18:187–94.
527. Sakakibara N, Seki T, Maru A, Koyanagi T. Benign fibrous histiocytoma of the kidney. J Urol 1989;142:1558–9.
528. Val-Bernal JF, Hernando M, Garijo MF, Villa P. Renal perineurioma in childhood. Gen Diagn Pathol 1997;143;75–81.
528. Wang T, Palazzo JP, Mitchell D, Petersen RO. aRenal capsular hemangioma. J Urol 1993;149: 1122–3.

Sarcomas

529. Aksoy Y, Gursan N, Ozbey I, Bicgi O, Keles M. Spontaneous rupture of a renal angiosarcoma. Urol Int 2002;68:60–2.
530. Argani P, Faria P, Epstein JI, et al. Primary renal synovial sarcoma: molecular and morphologic delineation of an entity previously included among embryonal sarcomas of the kidney. Am J Surg Pathol 2000;24:1087–96.
531. Asa SL, Bedard YC, Buckspan MB, Klotz PG, Bain J, Steinhardt MI. Spontaneous hypoglycemia associated with hemangiopericytoma of the kidney. J Urol 1981;125:864–7.
532. Bowers DL, Te A, Hibshoosh H, Sawczuk IS. Renal hemangiopericytoma. Case report and review of the literature. Urol Int 1995;55;162–6.
533. Cano JY, D'Altorio RA. Renal liposarcoma: case report. J Urol 1976;115:747–9.
534. Cason JD, Waisman J, Plaine L. Angiosarcoma of kidney. Urology 1987;30:281–3.
535. Cavaliere A, Fratini D, Legittimo C, Tosi F, Lolli E. Renal fibrosarcoma. Single case in a ten-year survey. Pathologica 1984;76:615–21.
536. Cerilli LA, Huffman HT, Anand A. Primary renal angiosarcoma: a case report with immunohistochemical, ultrastructural, and cytogenetic features and review of the literature. Arch Pathol Lab Med 1998;122:929–35.
537. Chatterjee D, Powell A. Renal hemangioendothelioma. Int Surg 1982;67:373–5.
538. Delahunt B, Beckwith JB, Eble JN, Fraundorfer MR, Sutton TD, Trotter GE. Cystic embryonal sarcoma of kidney: a case report. Cancer 1998;82:2427–33.
539. Dominici A, Mondaini N, Nesi G, Travaglini F, Di Cello V, Rizzo M. Cystic leiomyosarcoma of the kidney: an unusual clinical presentation. Urol Int 2000;65:229–31.
540. Dudhat S, Desai S, Borges A, Shinde S. Retroperitoneal extraosseous osteosarcoma. A case report and review of literature. Indian J Cancer 1999;36:186–9.
541. Farrow GM, Harrison EG Jr, Utz DC, ReMine WH. Sarcomas and sarcomatoid and mixed malignant tumors of the kidney in adults. Part I. Cancer 1968;22:545–50.
542. Gaboardi F, Carbone M, Bozzola A, Galli L. Rhabdomyosarcoma of the kidney. Arch Esp Urol 1990;43:205–6.
543. Gomez-Brouchet A, Soulie M, Delisle MB, Escourrou G. Mesenchymal chondrosarcoma of the kidney. J Urol 2001;166:2305.
544. Grignon DJ, Ayala AG, Ro JY, el-Naggar A, Papadopoulos N. Primary sarcomas of the kidney. A clinicopathologic and DNA flow cytometric study of 17 cases. Cancer 1990;65:1611–8.
545. Grignon DJ, McIsaac GP, Armstrong RF, Wyatt JK. Primary rhabdomyosarcoma of the kidney. A light microscopic, immunohistochemical and electron microscopic study. Cancer 1988;62:2027–32.
545a. Grignon DJ, Ro JY, Ayala AG. Mesenchymal tumors of the kidney. In: Eble JN, ed. Tumors and tumor-like conditions of the kidneys and ureters. New York: Churchill Livingstone; 1990:123–44.

546. Grignon DJ, Ro JY, Papadopoulos NE, Ayala AG. Leiomyosarcoma of renal vein. Urology 1991;38:255–8.

547. Helenon O, Merran S, Paraf F, et al. Unusual fat-containing tumors of the kidney: a diagnostic dilemma. Radiographics 1997;17:129–44.

548. Heppe RK, Donohue RE, Clark JE. Bilateral renal hemangiopericytoma. Urology 1991;38:249–53.

549. Johnson VV, Gaertner EM, Crothers BA. Fine-needle aspiration of renal angiosarcoma. Arch Pathol Lab Med 2002;126:478–80.

550. Kavantzas N, Pavlopoulos PM, Karaitianos I, Agapitos E. Renal leiomyosarcoma: report of three cases and review of the literature. Arch Ital Urol Androl 1999;71:307–11.

551. Kim DH, Sohn JH, Lee MC, et al. Primary synovial sarcoma of the kidney. Am J Surg Pathol 2000;24:1097–104.

552. Kim SJ, Ahn BC, Kim SR, et al. Primary malignant fibrous histiocytoma of the kidney. Yonsei Med J 2002;43:399–402.

553. Koyama S, Morimitsu Y, Morokuma F, Hashimoto H. Primary synovial sarcoma of the kidney: report of a case confirmed by molecular detection of the SYT-SSX2 fusion transcripts. Pathol Int 2001;51:385–91.

554. Leventis AK, Stathopoulos GP, Boussiotou AC, Papadimitriou KP, Kehayas PC. Primary osteogenic sarcoma of the kidney—a case report and review of the literature. Acta Oncol 1997;36:775–7.

555. Lopez JI, Angulo JC, Flores N, Toledo JD. Malignant fibrous histiocytoma of the renal capsule and synchronous transitional cell carcinoma of the bladder. Path Res Pract 1996;192:468–71.

556. Magro G, Cavallaro V, Torrisi A, Dell'Albani M, Lanzafame S. Intrarenal solitary fibrous tumor of the kidney: report of a case with emphasis on the differential diagnosis in the wide spectrum of monomorphous spindle cell tumors of the kidney. Pathol Res Pract 2002;198:37–43.

557. Mayes DC, Fechner RE, Gillenwater JY. Renal liposarcoma. Am J Surg Pathol 1990;14:268–73.

558. Merchant SH, Mittal BV, Desai MS. Haemangiopericytoma of kidney: a report of 2 cases. J Postgrad Med 1998;44:78–80.

559. Mortensen PH. Primary osteogenic sarcoma of the kidney. Br J Urol 1989;63:101–2.

560. Naslund MJ, Dement S, Marshall FF. Malignant renal schwannoma. Urology 1991;38:447–9.

561. Nativ O, Horowitz A, Lindner A, Many M. Primary chondrosarcoma of the kidney. J Urol 1985;134:120–1.

562. O'Malley FP, Grignon DJ, Shepherd RR, Harker LA. Primary osteosarcoma of the kidney. Report of a case studied by immunohistochemistry, electron microscopy, and DNA flow cytometry. Arch Pathol Lab Med 1991;115:1262–5.

563. Papadopoulos I, Rudolph P. Primary renal malignant fibrous histiocytoma: a case report. Urol Int 1999;63:136–8.

564. Ptochos A, Karydas G, Iosifidis N, Tyrothoulakis E, Papazafiriou G, Kehagia-Koutoufari T. Primary renal malignant fibrous histiocytoma. A case report and review of the literature. Urol Int 1999;63:261–4.

565. Quinn CM, Day DW, Waxman J, Krausz T. Malignant mesenchymoma of the kidney. Histopathology 1993;23:86–8.

566. Romics I, Bach D, Beutler W. Malignant schwannoma of kidney capsule. Urology 1992:40:453–5.

567. Roy C, Pfleger D, Tuchmann C, et al. Small leiomyosarcoma of the renal capsule. CT findings. Eur Radiol 1998;8:224–7.

568. Rubin BP, Fletcher JA, Renshaw AA. Clear cell sarcoma of soft parts: report of a case primary in the kidney with cytogenetic confirmation. Am J Surg Pathol 1999;23:589–94.

569. Sasagawa I, Suzuki K, Ishizaki M, et al. Liposarcoma of the renal capsule. Urol Int 1992;48:223–5.

570. Silverman JF, Nathan G, Olson PR, Prichard J, Cohen JK. Fine-needle aspiration cytology of low-grade fibromyxoid sarcoma of the renal capsule (capsuloma). Diagn Cytopathol 2000;23:279–83.

571. Siniluoto TM, Paivansalo MJ, Hellstrom PA, Leinonen AS, Kyllonen AP. Hemangiopericytoma of the kidney: a case with preoperative ethanol embolization. J Urol 1988;140:137–8.

572. Srinivas V, Sogani PC, Hajdu SI, Whitmore WF Jr. Sarcomas of the kidney. J Urol 1984;132:13–6.

573. Tarjan M, Cserni G, Szabo Z. Malignant fibrous histiocytoma of the kidney. Scand J Urol Nephrol 2001;35:518–20.

574. Terris D, Plaine L, Steinfeld A. Renal angiosarcoma. Am J Kidney Dis 1986;8:131–3.

575. Tsuda N, Chowdhury PR, Hayashi T, et al. Primary renal angiosarcoma: a case report and review of the literature. Pathol Int 1997;47:778–83.

576. Tsukamoto T, Lieber MM. Sarcomas of the kidney, urinary bladder, prostate, spermatic cord, paratestis and testis in adults. In: Raaf JH, ed. Soft tissue sarcomas: diagnosis and treatment. St. Louis: Mosby Year Book; 1992:201–26.

577. Villanueva RR, Nguyen-Ho P, Nguyen GK. Leiomyosarcoma of the kidney. Report of a case diagnosed by fine needle aspiration cytology and electron microscopy. Acta Cytol 1994;38:568–72.

578. Wang LJ, Wong YC, Chen CJ, See LC. Computerized tomography characteristics that differentiate angiomyolipomas from liposarcomas in the perinephric space. J Urol 2002;167:490–3.

579. Wang J, Arber DA, Frankel K, Weiss LM. Large solitary fibrous tumor of the kidney: report of two cases and review of the literature. Am J Surg Pathol 2001;25:1194–9.

580. Yaman O, Soygur T, Ozer G, Arikan N, Yaman LS. Renal liposarcoma of the sinus renalis. Int Urol Nephrol 1996;28:477–80.

Lymphoid Tumors

581. Arranz Arija JA, Carrion JR, Garcia FR, et al. Primary renal lymphoma: report of 3 cases and review of the literature. Am J Nephrol 1994;14: 148–53.

582. Bagg MD, Wettlaufer JN, Willadsen DS, Ho V, Lane D, Thrasher JB. Granulocytic sarcoma presenting as a diffuse renal mass before hematological manifestations of acute myelogenous leukemia. J Urol 1994;152:2092–3.

583. Chin KC, Perry GJ, Dowling JP, Thomson NM. Primary T-cell-rich B-cell lymphoma in the kidney presenting with acute renal failure and a second malignancy. Pathology 1999;31:325–7.

584. Da'as N, Polliack A, Cohen Y, et al. Kidney involvement and renal manifestations in non-Hodgkin's lymphoma and lymphocytic leukemia: a retrospective study in 700 patients. Eur J Haematol 2001;67:158–64.

585. D'Agati V, Sablay LB, Knowles DM, Walter L. Angiotropic large cell lymphoma (intravascular malignant lymphomatosis) of the kidney: presentation as minimal change disease. Hum Pathol 1989;20:263–8.

586. Dimopoulos MA, Moulopoulos LA, Costantinides C, Deliveliotis C, Pantazopoulos D, Dimopoulos C. Primary renal lymphoma: a clinical and radiological study. J Urol 1996;155:1865–7.

587. Dunphy CH, Gardner LJ, Grosso LE, Evans HL. Flow cytometric immunophenotyping in posttransplant lymphoproliferative disorders. Am J Clin Pathol 2002;117:24–8.

588. Ferry JA, Harris NL, Papanicolaou N, Young RH. Lymphoma of the kidney. A report of 11 cases. Am J Surg Pathol 1995;19:134–44.

589. Ferry JA, Harris NL, Picker LJ, et al. Intravascular lymphomatosis (malignant angioendotheliomatosis). A B-cell neoplasm expressing surface homing receptors. Mod Pathol 1988;1:444–52.

590. Harris GJ, Lager DJ. Primary renal lymphoma. J Surg Oncol 1991;46:273–7.

591. Harris NL, Ferry JA, Swerdlow SH. Posttransplant lymphoproliferative disorders: summary of Society for Hematopathology Workshop. Semin Diagn Pathol 1997;14:8–14.

592. Igel TC, Engen DE, Banks PM, Keeney GL. Renal plasmacytoma: Mayo Clinic experience and review of the literature. Urology 1991;37:385–9.

593. Jindal B, Sharma SC, Das A, Banerjee AK. Indolent behaviour of low-grade B cell lymphoma of mucosa-associated lymphoid tissue arising in the kidney. Urol Int 2001;67:91–3.

594. Lee SC, Roth LM, Brashear RE. Lymphomatoid granulomatosis. A clinicopathologic study of four cases. Cancer 1976;38:846–53.

595. Lipford EH, Margolick JB, Longo DL, Fauci AS, Jaffe ES. Angiocentric immunoproliferative lesions: a clinicopathologic spectrum of post-thymic T-cell proliferations. Blood 1988;72: 1674–81.

596. Martinez-Maldonado M, Ramirez de Arellano GA. Renal involvement in malignant lymphomas: a survey of 49 cases. J Urol 1966;95:485–8.

597. Muti G, De Gasperi A, Cantoni S, et al. Incidence and clinical characteristics of posttransplant lymphoproliferation disorders: report from a single center. Transpl Int 2000;13(Suppl 1):S382–7.

598. Nichols PW, Koss M, Levine AM, Lukes RJ. Lymphomatoid granulomatosis: a T-cell disorder? Am J Med 1982;72:467–71.

599. Osborne BM, Brenner M, Weitzner S, Butler JJ. Malignant lymphoma presenting as a renal mass: four cases. Am J Surg Pathol 1987;11: 375–82.

600. Parveen T, Navarro-Roman L, Medeiros LJ, Raffeld M, Jaffe ES. Low-grade B-cell lymphoma of mucosa-associated lymphoid tissue arising in the kidney. Arch Pathol Lab Med 1993;117:780–3.

601. Randhawa P, Demetris AJ, Pietrzak B, Nalesnik M. Histopathology of renal posttransplant lymphoproliferation: comparison with rejection using the Banff schema. Am J Kidney Dis 1996;28:578–84.

602. Richmond J, Sherman RS, Diamond HD, Craver LF. Renal lesions associated with malignant lymphomas. Am J Med 1962;32:184–207.

603. Sheeran SR, Sussman SK. Renal lymphoma: spectrum of CT findings and potential mimics. AJR Am J Roentgenol 1998;171:1067–72.

604. Stallone G, Infante B, Manno C, Campobasso N, Pannarale G, Schena FP. Primary renal lymphoma does exist: case report and review of the literature. J Nephrol 2000;13:367–72.

605. Truong LD, Caraway N, Ngo T, Laucirica R, Katz R, Ramzy I. Renal lymphoma. The diagnostic and therapeutic roles of fine-needle aspiration. Am J Clin Pathol 2001;115:18–31.

606. Wang BY, Strauchen JA, Rabinowitz D, Tillem SM, Unger PD. Renal cell carcinoma with intravascular lymphomatosis: case report of unusual collision tumors with review of the literature. Arch Pathol Lab Med 2001;125:1239–41.

Metastatic Tumors to the Kidneys

607. Belghiti D, Hirbec G, Bernaudin JF, Pariente EA, Martin N. Intraglomerular metastases. Report of two cases. Cancer 1984;54:2309–12.

608. Bracken RB, Chica G, Johnson DE, Luna M. Secondary renal neoplasms: an autopsy study. South Med J 1979;72:806–7.

609. Melato M, Laurino L, Bianchi P, Faccini L. Intraglomerular metastases. A possibly maldiagnosed entity. Zentralbl Pathol 1991;137:90–2.

610. Naryshkin S, Tomaszewski JE. Acute renal failure secondary to carcinomatous lymphatic metastases to kidneys. J Urol 1991;146:1610–12.

611. Payne RA. Metastatic renal tumors. Br J Surg 1960;48:310–15.

612. Petersen RO. Kidney: metastatic neoplasms. In: Urologic pathology. Philadelphia: JB Lippincott; 1986:134–6.

613. Sella A, Ro JY. Renal cell cancer: best recipient of tumor-to-tumor metastasis. Urology 1987;30:35–8.

614. Wagle DG, Moore RH, Murphy GP. Secondary carcinomas of the kidney. J Urol 1975;114:30–3.

Non-neoplastic Tumorous Conditions

615. Aessopos A, Alatzoglou K, Koroveis K, Tassiopoulos S, Lefakis G, Ismailou-Parassi A. Renal pseudotumor simulating malignancy in a patient with Adamantiades-Behcet's disease: case report and review of the literature. Am J Nephrol 2000;20:217–21.

616. Becker JA. Xanthogranulomatous pyelonephritis. A case report with angiographic findings. Acta Radiol Diagn (Stockh) 1966;4:139–44.

617. Blue PW, Ratajczak KJ, Ghaed N. Intraparenchymal perirenal pseudocyst following trauma. Clin Nuc Med 1982;7:472–3.

618. Brkovic D, Moehring K, Doersam J, et al. Aetiology, diagnosis and management of spontaneous perirenal hematomas. Eur Urol 1996;29:302–7.

619. Ceccarelli FE Jr, Wurster JC, Chandor SB. Xanthogranulomatous pyelonephritis in an infant. J Urol 1970;104:755–7.

620. Fisch AE, Brodey PA. Plasma cell granuloma of kidney. Urology 1976;8:89–91.

621. Flynn JT, Molland EA, Paris AM, Blandy JP. The underestimated hazards of xanthogranulomatous pyelonephritis. Br J Urol 1979;51:443–4.

622. Gerber WL, Catalona WJ, Fair WR, Michigan S, Melson L. Xanthogranulomatous pyelonephritis masquerading as occult malignancy. Urology 1978;11:466–71.

623. Goodman M, Curry T, Russell T. Xanthogranulomatous pyelonephritis (XGP): a local disease with systemic manifestations. Report of 23 patients and review of the literature. Medicine (Baltimore) 1979;58:171–81.

624. Grainger RG, Longstaff AJ, Parsons MA. Xanthogranulomatous pyelonephritis: a reappraisal. Lancet 1982;1:1398–401.

625. Hayami S, Adachi Y, Ishigooka M, et al. Retroperitoneal cystic lymphangioma diagnosed by computerized tomography, magnetic resonance imaging and thin needle aspiration. Int Urol Nephrol 1996;28:21–6.

626. Kapusta LR, Weiss MA, Ramsay J, Lopez-Beltran A, Srigley JR. Inflammatory myofibroblastic tumors of the kidney: a clinicopathologic and immunohistochemical study of 12 cases. Am J Surg Pathol 2003;27:658–66.

627. Kobayashi TK, Ueda M, Nishino T, Kushima R, Nakajima S, Kaneko C. Inflammatory pseudo-tumor of the kidney: report of a case with fine needle aspiration cytology. Acta Cytol 2000;44:478–80.

628. Le Gall F, Huerre M, Cipolla B, Shalev M, Ramee MP. A case of myospherulosis occurring in the perirenal adipose tissue. Path Res Pract 1996;192:172–8.

629. Malek RS, Elder JS. Xanthogranulomatous pyelonephritis: a critical analysis of 26 cases and of the literature. J Urol 1978;119:589–93.

630. Nahm AM, Ritz E. The renal sinus cyst—the great imitator. Nephrol Dial Transplant 2000;15:913–4.

631. Noyes WE, Palubinskas AJ. Xanthogranulomatous pyelonephritis. J Urol 1969;101:132–6.

632. Smith VC, Edwards RA, Jorgensen RA, et al. Unilocular retroperitoneal cyst of mesothelial origin presenting as a renal mass. Arch Pathol Lab Med 2000;124:766–9.

633. Sneige N, Dekmezian RH, Silva EG, Cartwright J Jr, Ayala AG. Pseudoparasitic Liesegang structures in perirenal hemorrhagic cysts. Am J Clin Pathol 1988;89:148–53.

634. Sneige N, Dekmezian R, Zaatari GS. Liesegang-like rings in fine needle aspirates of renal/perirenal hemorrhagic cysts. Acta Cytol 1988;32:547–51.

635. Tiguert R, Gheiler EL, Yousif R, et al. Focal xanthogranulomatous pyelonephritis presenting as a renal tumor with vena caval thrombus. J Urol 1998;160:117–8.

636. Tolia BM, Iloreta A, Freed SZ, Fruchtman B, Bennett B, Newman HR. Xanthogranulomatous pyelonephritis: detailed analysis of 29 cases and a brief discussion of atypical presentations. J Urol 1981;126:437–42.

637. Vinik M, Freed TA, Smellie WA, Weidner W. Xanthogranulomatous pyelonephritis: angiographic considerations. Radiology 1969;92:537–40.

Treatment

638. Bangalore N, Bhargava P, Hawkins MJ, Bhargava P. Sustained response of sarcomatoid renal-cell carcinoma to MAID chemotherapy: case report and review of the literature. Ann Oncol 2001;12:271–4.

639. Escudier B, Droz JP, Rolland F, et al. Doxorubicin and ifosfamide in patients with metastatic sarcomatoid renal cell carcinoma: a phase II study of the Genitourinary Group of the French Federation of Cancer Centers. J Urol 2002;168:959–61.

640. Fergany A, Hafez KS, Novick AC. Long-term results of nephron sparing surgery for localized renal cell carcinoma: 10-year followup. J Urol 2000;163:442–5.

641. Figlin RA. Renal cell carcinoma: management of advanced disease. J Urol 1999;161:381–7.

642. Gill I, Meraney A, Schweizer D, et al. Laparoscopic radical nephrectomy in 100 patients: a single center experience from the United States. Cancer 2001;92:1843–55.

643. Hatcher PA, Anderson EE, Paulson DF, Carson CC, Robertson JE. Surgical management and prognosis of renal cell carcinoma invading the vena cava. J Urol 1991;145:20–3.

644. Kavolius JP, Mastorakos DP, Pavlovich C, Russo P, Burt ME, Brady MS. Resection of metastatic renal cell carcinoma. J Clin Oncol 1998;16:2261–6.

645. Kavoussi LR, Kerbl K, Capelouto CC, McDougall EM, Clayman RV. Laparoscopic nephrectomy for renal neoplasms. Urology 1993;42:603–8.

646. Landman J, Lento P, Hassen W, Unger P, Waterhouse R. Feasibility of pathological evaluation of morcellated kidneys after radical nephrectomy. J Urol 2000;164:2086–9.

647. Langenburg SE, Blackbourne LH, Sperling JW, et al. Management of renal tumors involving the inferior vena cava. J Vasc Surg 1994;20:385–8.

648. Lee C, Katz J, Shi W, Thaler HT, Reuter VE, Russo P. Surgical management of renal tumors 4 cm. or less in a contemporary cohort. J Urol 2000;163:730–6.

649. Ljungberg B, Stenling R, Osterdahl B, Farrelly E, Aberg T, Roos G. Vein invasion in renal cell carcinoma: impact on metastatic behavior and survival. J Urol 1995;154:1681–4.

650. Minervini A, Lilas L, Morelli G, et al. Regional lymph node dissection in the treatment of renal cell carcinoma: is it useful in patients with no suspected adenopathy before or during surgery? BJU Int 2001;88:169–72.

651. Ono Y, Kinukawa T, Hattori R, Gotoh M, Kamihira O, Ohshima S. The long-term outcome of laparoscopic radical nephrectomy for small renal cell carcinoma. J Urol 2001;165:1867–70.

652. Pantuck AJ, Zisman A, Belldegrun AS. The changing natural history of renal cell carcinoma. J Urol 2001;166:1611–23.

653. Paul R, Mordhorst J, Leyh H, Hartung R. Incidence and outcome of patients with adrenal metastases of renal cell cancer. Urology 2001;57:878–82.

654. Phillips E, Messing EM. Role of lymphadenectomy in the treatment of renal cell carcinoma. Urology 1993;41:9–15.

655. Robson CJ. Radical nephrectomy for renal cell carcinoma. J Urol 1963;89:37–42.

656. Sagalowsky AI, Kadesky KT, Ewalt DM, Kennedy TJ. Factors influencing adrenal metastases in renal cell carcinoma. J Urol 1994;151:1181–4.

657. Shalev M, Cipolla B, Guille F, Staerman F, Lobel B. Is ipsilateral adrenalectomy a necessary component of radical nephrectomy? Pathol Res Pract 1996;192:172–8.

658. Wood DP. Role of lymphadenectomy in renal cell carcinoma. Urol Clin N Am 1991;18:421–6.

Procedures for Pathologic Evaluation and Reporting

659. Bielsa O, Lloreta J, Gelabert-Mas A. Cystic renal cell carcinoma: pathological features, survival and implications for treatment. Br J Urol 1998;82:16–20.

660. Castilla EA, Liou LS, Abrahams NA, et al. Prognostic importance of resection margin width after nephron-sparing surgery for renal cell carcinoma. Urology 2002;60:993–7.

661. Dechet CB, Sebo T, Farrow G, Blute ML, Engen DE, Zincke H. Prospective analysis of intraoperative frozen needle biopsy of solid renal masses in adults. J Urol 1999;162:1282–4; discussion 1284–5.

662. Delong WH, Grignon DJ. Pathologic findings in ribs removed at the time of radical nephrectomy for renal cell carcinoma. Int J Surg Pathol 1994;1:177–80.

663. Eble JN. Recommendations for examining and reporting tumor-bearing kidney specimens from adults. Semin Diagn Pathol 1998;15:77–82.

664. Farrow G, Amin MB. Protocol for the examination of specimens from patients with carcinomas of renal tubular origin, exclusive of Wilms tumor and tumors of urothelial origin: a basis for checklists. Cancer Committee College of American Pathologists. Arch Pathol Lab Med 1999;123:23–7.

665. Lang EK, Macchia RJ, Gayle B, et al. CT-guided biopsy of indeterminate renal cystic masses (Bosniak 3 and 2F): accuracy and impact on clinical management. Eur Radiol 2002;12:2518–24.

666. Lerner SE, Tsai H, Flanigan RC, Trump DL, Fleischmann J. Renal cell carcinoma: consideration for nephron-sparing surgery. Urology 1995;45:574–7.

667. Maatman TJ, Novick AC, Tancinco BF, et al. Renal oncocytoma: a diagnostic and therapeutic dilemma. J Urol 1984;132:878–81.

668. McHale T, Malkowicz SB, Tomaszewski JE, Genega EM. Potential pitfalls in the frozen section evaluation of parenchymal margins in nephron-sparing surgery. Am J Clin Pathol 2002;118:903–10.

668a. Palapattu GS, Pantuck AJ, Dorey F, Said JW, Figlin RA, Belldegrun AS. Collecting system invasion in renal cell carcinoma: impact on prognosis and future staging strategies. J Urol 2003;170:768–72.

669. Pfannkuch F, Leistenschneider W, Nagel R. Problems of assessment in the surgery of renal adenomas. J Urol 1981;125:95–8.

670. Piper NY, Bishoff JT, Magee C, et al. Is a 1-CM margin necessary during nephron-sparing surgery for renal carcinoma? Urology 2001;58:849–52.

671. Recommendations for reporting resected neoplasms of the kidney. Association of Directors of Anatomic and Surgical Pathology. Mod Pathol 1996;9:865–8.

672. Thrasher JB, Robertson JE, Paulson DF. Expanding indications for conservative renal surgery in renal cell carcinoma. Urology 1994;43:160–8.

673. Ward JF, Blute ML, Cheville JC, Lohse CM, Weaver AL, Zincke H. The influence of pNx/pN0 grouping in a multivariate setting for outcome modeling in patients with clear cell renal cell carcinoma. J Urol 2002;168:56–60.

674. Zucchi A, Mearini L, Mearini E, Costantini E, Vivacqua C, Porena M. Renal cell carcinoma: histological findings on surgical margins after nephron sparing surgery. J Urol 2003;196:905–8.

3 TUMORS OF THE URINARY BLADDER

NORMAL ANATOMY

The urinary bladder forms during the first 12 weeks of gestation as the result of three events (7). The trigone (base) develops by dilatation, fusion, and eventual incorporation of portions of the mesonephric ducts into the urogenital sinus, forming a triangular area that receives the terminal portions of the future ureters. The müllerian ducts are close to this area but their influence, if any, on the formation of the trigone is not known. In the second event, the posterior walls, dome, and portions of the lateral walls arise from mesenchyme surrounding the urogenital sinus when that space is transected by the urorectal septum. Thirdly, the anterior wall and portions of the lateral walls develop in conjunction with closure of the infraumbilical portion of the abdominal wall. The bulk of the resulting organ is derived from tissue at the rostral portion of the urogenital sinus.

Despite the embryologic continuity of the urogenital sinus with the allantois and urachus, neither of these structures is involved in the formation of the urinary bladder. The allantois is an embryonic structure lined by endoderm that is connected to the urachus. It is rudimentary in humans. The urachus is formed during the descent of the anterior abdominal wall, when the rostral portion of the urogenital sinus is attenuated into a tubular structure. This tube is torn apart as the embryo elongates, but remnants persist in the anterior abdominal wall and, occasionally, in the bladder wall of the fully developed human. These remnants may be lined by various types of epithelium, most often urothelium (transitional cell). They rarely connect directly to the adult bladder lumen. The most embryologically complicated portion of the bladder is its base, a fact that may help explain the propensity for all types of tumors to arise in this area.

The fully developed urinary bladder is designed to store and expel urine. Anchored deep in the pelvis, the organ consists of a meshwork of thick muscle bundles that surround a highly vascular lamina propria lined by stratified epithelium (fig. 3-1) (13). In usual histologic preparations, the muscles of the wall (detrusor muscles) exist in rounded bundles separated by an interstitium that contains scant collagen. At

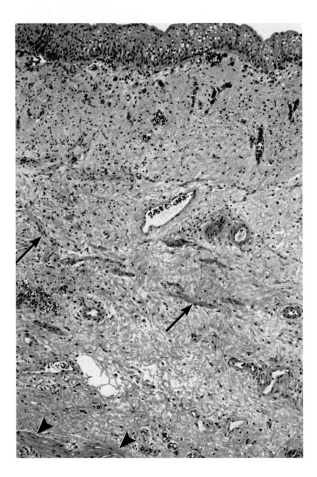

Figure 3-1

NORMAL URINARY BLADDER

Wisps of smooth muscle (arrows) occur in the lamina propria. Their configuration is different from the muscle bundles of the detrusor (arrowheads). A well-developed muscularis mucosae is not present as a continuous layer in human urinary bladders.

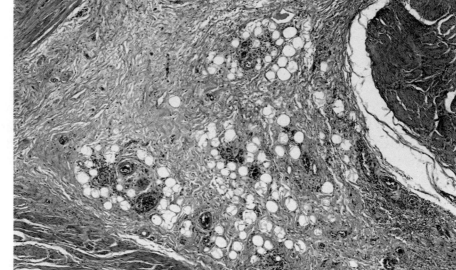

Figure 3-2

INTERSTITIAL FAT IN URINARY BLADDER

Fat commonly occurs in the urinary bladder, both between muscle fascicles and in the lamina propria.

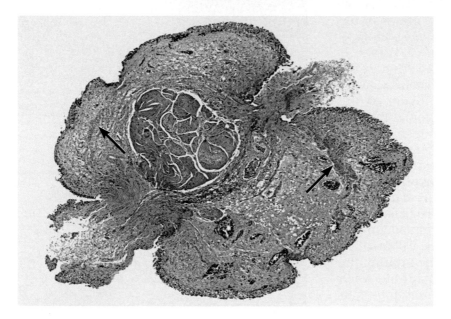

Figure 3-3

TYPICAL CONFIGURATION OF BLADDER BIOPSY SPECIMEN

Bladder tissue tends to round up in fixatives. This has essentially no effect on the architecture at the surfaces but may cause tangential planes in the deeper tissues. Vestigial remnants of muscularis mucosae (arrows) do not form a plane sufficiently distinctive for substaging the lamina propria.

the bladder periphery, bundles of muscularis propria may slightly interdigitate with the surrounding paravesical fat. In the bladder neck, these muscle bundles tend to become small and uniform, a feature that facilitates their recognition in tissue samples. Foci of adipose tissue frequently occur in the interstitium (fig. 3-2).

The lamina propria is a layer of loose connective tissue which normally contains a few lymphocytes and a network of thin-walled blood vessels. Some of these vessels are so closely applied to the epithelial lining that any process that

denudes or ulcerates the mucosa results in abnormal numbers of red blood cells in the urine. In well-oriented specimens, the lamina propria can sometimes be divided into inner and outer zones by a discontinuous layer of thick-walled blood vessels and wispy muscle fibers, reminiscent of the muscularis mucosae of the gastrointestinal tract (fig. 3-3) (6,12). In focal areas, these structures may seem to define compartments within the lamina propria, but an anatomic layer identical to the muscularis mucosae of the gut does not exist in the human

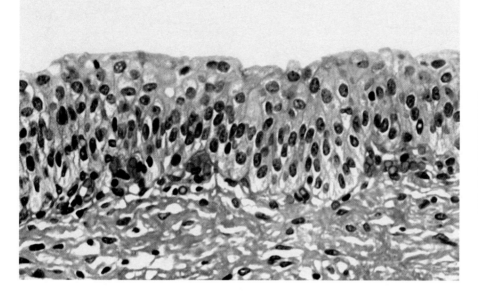

Figure 3-4

NORMAL UROTHELIUM

A single layer of large, occasionally binucleated superficial cells covers multiple layers of intermediate and basal cells. Note the even distribution and polarization of the nuclei. Fixation in picric acid–based solutions tends to accentuate nucleoli, which would not be apparent in formalin-fixed preparations.

urinary bladder. In contrast to the well-defined, rounded fascicles of the detrusor muscle, muscle fibers in the lamina propria are small and irregular. When viewed en face, they often appear plaited, with serrated ends. Distinction of the vestigial remnants resembling muscularis mucosae from portions of muscularis propria is important for the accurate pathologic staging of bladder neoplasms. Like the muscularis propria, the lamina propria commonly contains foci of adipose tissue, another feature with potential implications for pathologic staging (11).

The bladder is lined by multiple layers of relatively flat cells, like squamous mucosa, in which the superficial elements are large and secrete small amounts of mucin, like glandular mucosa. Perhaps for this reason, the term "transitional cell" epithelium has become deeply entrenched in the medical lexicon. A more preferred term for this mucosa is "urothelium." In fact, a family of membrane proteins called uroplakins has been shown to be specific for the urothelia of a variety of mammalian species (15).

Several features of the urothelium are important to an understanding of bladder neoplasms (8). At the structural level, invaginated nests of urothelial cells (Brunn nests) may occur throughout the urothelium but are most common at the bladder base. Their greater frequency in adults than in newborns and late-stage fetuses suggests an acquired phenomenon, per-haps as a reaction to trauma or infection. The exact number of layers in the normal human bladder urothelium is unknown but varies between three and seven, depending on the degree of bladder distension. An increase in the number of cell layers is not in itself neoplastic but is considered abnormal, especially when the mucosal thickening occurs on a fibrovascular stalk. Urothelial cell proliferation is almost always accompanied by morphologic changes in the nuclei, so that recognition of a neoplasm based solely on increased layering is rarely a problem.

At the cellular level, normal urothelial cells are of two distinctive types (fig. 3-4): cells of the superficial layer and cells comprising the underlying intermediate and basal layers. The cells comprising all but the superficial layer are small and uniform, with well-defined borders and amphophilic cytoplasm rich in glycogen. The glycogen often dissolves in usual preparations, leaving cleared areas which have sometimes been erroneously described as vacuoles. These cells have sparse desmosomes, facilitating their ability to flatten and slide over one another during bladder distension (8). They also manifest blood group isoantigens and cytokeratins (especially 7, 8, 18, and 19) of molecular weights ranging from 40 to 70 kD (3,4,9). Epidermal growth factor receptors are on the surfaces of the deepest cells and urothelial cells normally produce certain interleukins and growth factors (1,5,10).

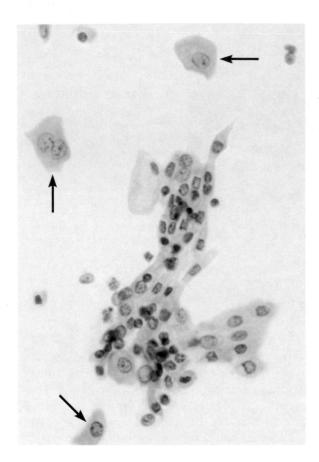

Figure 3-5

NORMAL UROTHELIAL CELLS

Superficial cells (arrows) retain their shape in urinary specimens. They are much larger and have larger nucleoli than the intermediate and basal cells.

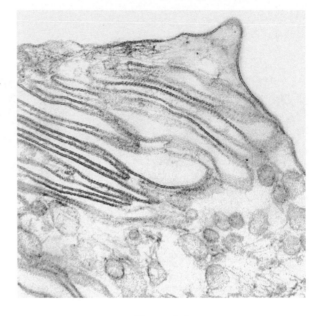

Figure 3-6

NORMAL UROTHELIAL ULTRASTRUCTURE

Transmission electron microscopy reveals the microridges created by uroplakin-rich plaques as well as the intracytoplasmic infolding of the surface membrane of a superficial urothelial cell.

In tissue sections, the architecture of urothelium is largely determined by the orientation and shape of the nuclei of subsuperficial intermediate and basal cells. These nuclei are ovoid, with the long axis oriented at right angles to the surface. Nuclei are regularly arranged in the epithelium. They have evenly dispersed, finely granular chromatin which accentuates the regularly contoured nuclear borders. Nucleoli are small and inapparent in tissue fixed in formalin but are often revealed by fixatives that better preserve cellular detail. The normal urothelium has an estimated turnover time of approximately 1 year and it is unusual to see mitoses.

The superficial layer of urothelium is composed of a specialized group of cells that could be considered terminally differentiated. These cells are much larger than the underlying elements; this, plus their location and shape, have suggested the term "umbrella" cells. Superficial cells tend to have acidophilic cytoplasm and store small amounts of neutral mucin, but are primarily modified to maintain the integrity of the mucosa during expansion and contraction as well as to prevent urine transport into the stroma. These cells have a rigid surface membrane which maintains its shape after exfoliation (figs. 3-5, 3-6). In young and early middle-aged individuals, the surface membrane is reinforced with plaques of asymmetric unit membrane alternating with sections of symmetric surface (8,15). This structure tends to break down with age and is lost early in carcinogenesis, but may reform after successful therapy.

Superficial cells may manifest blood group antigens, uroplakins, and cytokeratins but lack epidermal growth factor receptors. A few are binucleate. The nuclei are large even though the nuclear-cytoplasmic ratios are low. They have evenly dispersed chromatin and regularly contoured borders; they often have nucleoli, appreciated even in formalin-fixed specimens. As the first layer of epithelial defense, superficial cells are exposed to various noxious substances and often appear reactive. In such cases, their nuclei are enlarged and their chromatin more coarsely clumped. Nucleoli may be prominent. Mitoses are rare in superficial cells, even in situations of great stimulation. In general, the presence of superficial cells is a sign of relatively normal maturation and differentiation. Neoplasms that manifest superficial cells are usually not aggressive.

The molecular composition of normal bladder tissue is mind-boggling in its complexity (2,4,5,10,14,15). Growth factors, adhesion molecules, kinases, cytokeratins, cytokines, and a variety of yet to be discovered substances all interact in a constant dynamic. Most of these substances have been found in altered forms in bladder neoplasms, suggesting that some at least may be important for understanding tumorigenesis and possible responses to treatment. The likelihood that each human bladder is composed of a slightly different mix of these substances only adds to the problem of deciphering the "normal" condition at the molecular level. The currently available data strongly indicate that carcinogenesis in human bladders involves cellular machinery already in place.

CLASSIFICATION

Classification schemes for bladder tumors, especially for the urothelial (transitional cell) neoplasms that constitute the majority of cases, have evolved over the past several decades and there is no reason to assume that they will not continue to change as information regarding genomics and proteomics accumulates (16–23). The classification preferred in this Fascicle is presented in Table 3-1. The portion referring to urothelial neoplasms is adopted from the 1998 World Health Organization (WHO)/International Society of Urological Pathology (ISUP) scheme (18). This formulation recognizes two very important features of urothelial neoplasms: 1) a significant percentage are of such low cytologic grade and such nonaggressive behavior that they cannot be considered malignant, i.e., carcinomas and 2) the majority of true urothelial carcinomas are of high cytologic grade. This scheme also requires diagnosticians to distinguish low-grade from high-grade neoplasms, rather than allowing the utilization of hybrid designations such as grade 1-2 or 2-3. Further, it includes urinary cytopathology as an important aspect of the evaluation of urothelial neoplasms. In slight contrast to the 1998 WHO/ISUP scheme, the urothelial neoplasms in Table 3-1 are not separated according to the presence or absence of invasion nor are they categorized according to configuration (papillary and infiltrating). Depending on cytologic grade, papillary noninvasive neoplasms can share both phenotypic and genetic features with infiltrating invasive lesions, and many urothelial neoplasms have papillary, infiltrating, and even flat components.

The process of classification is governed by certain general principles, the understanding of which should help practitioners to assess the practical value of future alterations.

- Classification schemes are devices, often determined by consensus rather than fact, by which we attempt to better understand the biologic nature of disease.

- The ultimate goal of classification is to separate patients into homogeneous groups whose neoplasms will have similar, if not identical, natural courses and respond similarly to available therapeutic regimens.

- The principal assumption underlying pathologic classification is that biologic processes are reflected in morphologic changes as viewed through a light microscope, and that the relationship is not only causal but timely. As knowledge of genomic and proteomic processes accumulates, both this assumption and classification by histology are being challenged.

- All classification schemes have limitations, both in concept and in application. In general, interpretive reproducibility among pathologists is inversely proportional to the number of discriminations required and the complexity of the definitions. Systems that have few decision points or that rely upon instruments programmed to make few actual measurements, e.g., diploid versus aneuploid, are more reproducible than schemes having multiple categories, each having a complex definition.

- The factors that determine how a pathologist classifies any particular case have

Table 3-1

CLASSIFICATION OF URINARY BLADDER TUMORS

Epithelial Neoplasms	Nonepithelial Neoplasms
Urothelial (transitional cell) neoplasms	Mesenchymal tumors
Papilloma	Benign
Inverted	Malignant
Exophytic	Pheochromocytoma (paraganglioma)
Papillary urothelial neoplasm of low malignant potential	Lymphoma
Carcinoma	Plasmacytoma
Low grade	Germ cell neoplasms
High grade	
Carcinoma in situ	**Non-Neoplastic Tumorous Conditions**
Dysplasia/atypia	Condyloma acuminatum-squamous papilloma
Variants of urothelial carcinoma	Metaplasia
Urothelial carcinoma with gland-like (microcystic)	Squamous
lumens	Intestinal
Urothelial carcinoma, nested type	Nephrogenic
Urothelial carcinoma, sarcomatoid type	Inflammation
Homologous	Inflammatory pseudotumor (pseudosar-
Heterologous (carcinosarcoma)	comatous fibromyxoid tumor)
Urothelial carcinoma, micropapillary type	Malakoplakia
Squamous cell carcinoma	Xanthogranulomatous cystitis
Verrucous carcinoma	Granulomas
Adenocarcinoma	"Cystitis"
Villous tumor	Glandularis et cystica
Poorly differentiated small cell carcinoma	Follicular
Rare neoplasms	Bullous
Carcinoid tumor	Polypoid/papillary
Melanoma	Emphysematous
Lymphoepithelial carcinoma	Interstitial
Large cell neuroendocrine carcinoma	Eosinophilic
Giant and spindle cell carcinoma	Amyloid
Plasmacytoid/lymphomatoid carcinoma	Rests, choristomas, hamartomas, vascular lesions
Rhabdoid tumor	Cysts
Basaloid carcinoma	Endometriosis and endocervicosis
	Ectopic prostate
	Paraganglionic tissue
	Extramedullary hematopoiesis
	Hamartoma
	Vascular lesions

never been adequately understood and the result represents an individual interpretation, not a fact. Variations in categorization among pathologists using the same classification scheme are currently inevitable.

BLADDER NEOPLASMS

Neoplasia in the human urinary bladder is nearly always addressed in terms of carcinogenesis and carcinoma, since more than 99 percent of bladder tumors are epithelial neoplasms. The subject is extraordinarily complex and not necessarily illuminated by the volumes of literature currently available. Factors reportedly in-volved in urothelial carcinogenesis alone include at least four cell cycle regulators, multiple proliferation (onco)genes, five types of growth factors, four families of adhesion molecules, four classes of proteases, multiple kinases, abnormalities of at least 13 chromosomes, overexpression of telomerase, aberrant cytokeratins, and a number of yet to be elucidated abnormalities in protein expression probably related to structurally normal but functionally misregulated genes (30, 41,45,48,49). Roles for specific chromosomes and genes in the pathogenesis of urothelial neoplasms have been claimed but the evidence is not compelling. Aberrations in the structure of chromosomes, especially chromosome 9, and overexpression of p53 protein have been extensively studied without conclusive results. The involvement of host factors is very poorly understood (57). A generally accepted common pathway describing the molecular biology of urothelial carcinogenesis does not yet exist.

The pathways governing the development of a neoplasm in any particular individual may be unique to that individual, even though the evolving lesions themselves often share sufficient morphologic characteristics with others to allow for a group classification by light microscopy (25,31,40,52). Current theories suggest that human carcinomas arise in an environment of growth restraint, a situation that promotes abnormal regulation among certain clones of cells (34). If normal regulation cannot be re-established, then further selection occurs among the abnormal clones, followed eventually by heterogeneous differentiation to form a neoplasm that may not be easily destroyed using unimodal approaches. This misregulation may involve a limited number of genetic pathways but evidence suggests that a threshold number, rather than a specific type, of genetic or perhaps proteomic aberrations must occur before a patient comes to harm. Many studies suggest that human carcinomas arise from reactive/regenerative epithelium and that normal cells are not an appropriate baseline for the study of neoplasia. Information in this area is so rapidly accumulating that all summaries must be considered incomplete.

As a practical matter for patient care, the literature suggests that perceptions of urothelial carcinogenesis fall into two broad categories. Those who subscribe to the traditional approach envision a system wherein a neoplasm is established early in the process and will progress over time unless treated. Progression is manifested morphologically by increasing architectural distortion and cellular anaplasia. Neoplasms detected subsequent to treatment of the initial tumor represent progressive events related to that tumor. In this view, the range of morphologic changes between normal and invasive carcinoma is described as "intraurothelial neoplasia." Small or low-grade lesions are considered "early" and the development of an adverse outcome in a patient presenting with a low-grade noninvasive lesion is considered evidence of "progression" of the initial, previously resected tumor. Death from disease is considered evidence that the initial neoplasm was malignant, regardless of its grade and stage at the time of resection and pathologic examination.

A somewhat contrary notion contends that a neoplasm is established relatively late in the process and that the biologic potential for the aggressive behavior of any particular neoplasm is reflected in its morphology. Those who hold this view see little compelling evidence that the lower-grade intraepithelial abnormalities represent committed neoplasms and reject the term intraurothelial neoplasia. They note that even anaplastic intraepithelial lesions seem to lack the capacity to invade the immediately underlying stroma. Likewise, very low-grade papillary urothelial neoplasms seem to lack the capacity to invade and metastasize. The majority of patients presenting with such tumors do not develop bladder neoplasms in the future. When subsequent tumors do occur, they almost always have the same morphologic appearance as the initial lesion, as if the host were adequately managing the misregulated clones. According to this view, most of the processes that might predispose a patient to an adverse outcome have already occurred by the time a urothelial neoplasm is clinically detected. Patients rarely suffer from disseminated low-grade lesions, and adverse events are almost always related to high-grade cancers that are established at the time of initial diagnosis. In fact, the grade and stage of any particular neoplasm must represent the establishment of a stable (not static) relationship between carcinogenic factors and host resistance; otherwise, these two factors would not be consistently reliable prognostic indicators.

In the following discussion, bladder neoplasms differentiating toward normal urothelium are labeled urothelial (transitional cell), although terms such as epithelioma and epidermoid carcinoma have been used in the past. A significant percentage of urothelial neoplasms are benign in the sense that their cells have many features of normal urothelium and, once these tumors are removed, approximately 90 to 95 percent of affected patients do not develop higher-grade neoplasms, invasion of the muscular wall, or metastases. Urothelial neoplasms with the capacity to invade and metastasize, i.e., true carcinomas, are divided into a small group with features of low cytologic grade and a larger group with features of high cytologic grade. Correlations among classification schemes identifying 3, 4, or 5 grades of urothelial neoplasms are not exact and direct extrapolations among categories cannot be made. In general, almost all papillary urothelial neoplasms of low malignant potential (PUNLMP) in this atlas would be included among the grade 1 carcinomas in the 1973 WHO system (42). In contrast, approximately half of the high-grade tumors described here would be included among grade 2 lesions using the 1973 WHO system.

In organs lined by urothelium, only urothelial neoplasms can be considered well differentiated. Bladder carcinomas recapitulating the epithelium of colon (adenocarcinoma) or skin (squamous cell carcinoma) are considered poorly differentiated regardless of how much they resemble the normal epithelium of these organs. The aggressive behavior of the majority of glandular and squamous carcinomas supports this view, although exceptions like verrucous carcinoma exist. Therefore, grading of glandular and squamous cell neoplasms has not been widely accepted.

The category of "mixed carcinoma" has been deleted from this text, since there is little evidence that this category encompasses tumors of distinctive behavior. Urothelial tumors with foci of malignant squamous or glandular differentiation are essentially always high-grade lesions whose clinical course, stage for stage, is not different from that of a high-grade urothelial carcinoma without such heterogeneity. These types of tumors are discussed and illustrated in the text but are not included in Table 3-1.

The issue of what constitutes a variant of urothelial carcinoma is somewhat controversial. Many authors list all of the heterogeneities separately, suggesting that variations in differentiation (squamous, glandular, trophoblastic, giant cell, etc) or stromal response (spindle cell, desmoplastic) represent entities that should be included in the pathologic diagnosis. While pathologists should most certainly be aware of these histologic variations, nearly all such lesions occur as part of a high-grade, high-stage carcinoma and most represent histologic nu-

ances that have no clinical significance. In this Fascicle, the listed variants of urothelial carcinoma are limited to those whose misinterpretation could have adverse consequences for patient care. Other variations are described and illustrated in the text but not included in the classification table.

Some influential classification schemes seem to restrict the grading of urothelial neoplasms to papillary and noninvasive lesions. This may have some merit, considering that the depth of invasion and the presence or absence of extravesical dissemination are more indicative of the patient's future course than grade, once invasion has been documented. Nevertheless, confining grade to noninvasive urothelial neoplasms seems unnecessarily restrictive and could deprive patients of important information in certain situations. Therefore, all urothelial neoplasms should be graded.

Intraepithelial lesions are not tumors in the classic sense of space-occupying masses, but many are neoplastic based on clinical and cytologic criteria. The terms used for intraepithelial lesions are influenced by the previously described controversy over carcinogenesis. Carcinoma in situ is defined as a flat, noninvasive urothelial lesion composed of cells with significant anaplasia. Such lesions include those with cellular maturation toward the surface, often termed severe dysplasia in other systems.

Intraepithelial lesions comprising cellular atypia of mild and moderate degrees, so-called dysplasia or atypical hyperplasia, have been difficult to define in morphologic terms. Slight and moderate degrees of urothelial dysplasia may occur in bladders that will never develop carcinoma and the biologic nature of these lesions is highly controversial. They may or may not be neoplasms according to the definition of the 1998 WHO/ISUP system but no discussion of intraepithelial neoplasms would be complete without their inclusion. Intraepithelial carcinomas of squamous and glandular types have not been well defined in the urothelium and are only briefly discussed.

A few names merely reflect common English usage. The term metaplasia ordinarily connotes the transition from one morphologically normal tissue to another and is not used in reference to malignant tumors. Undifferentiated is a somewhat misleading term when coupled with carcinoma, since the lesion in question must be differentiated to some degree or it could not be identified as a carcinoma. Malignancies classified into this category in other formulations are termed poorly differentiated in this atlas.

Superficial carcinoma is a term firmly entrenched in the lexicon of urologists to describe a urothelial neoplasm that has not invaded into the detrusor muscle. Used in this way, the category of superficial carcinoma includes a variety of pathologic lesions ranging from cytologically benign papillomas to high-grade cancers of any histologic type, some of which have invaded the lamina propria. This designation has some clinical merit but does not describe a single pathologic entity and should be employed with appropriate modifiers; it is not further discussed.

General Features of Bladder Neoplasms

Bladder tumors comprise a heterogeneous group of lesions; however, since all arise in an organ of relatively simple structure and function, general statements concerning their characteristics are justified (43). Approximately 95 percent of all bladder neoplasms are epithelial tumors and 80 to 90 percent of these differentiate as urothelial (transitional cell) lesions. Among the remainder, squamous cell carcinomas comprise 2 to 15 percent; adenocarcinomas less than 2 percent; and poorly differentiated carcinomas less than 0.5 percent. Given these statistics, it is not surprising that the best studied bladder tumors are urothelial neoplasms and most of our knowledge in this area applies to them.

The etiology of human bladder neoplasms is essentially unknown (Table 3-2) (28,29). In its function as a reservoir for urine, the bladder is exposed to a complex array of chemicals, often in concentrated forms. Although unproven, many experts believe that the majority of tumors result primarily from environmental factors. This theory is supported by the increased frequency of bladder tumors in patients living in industrial areas, especially in areas associated with petrochemicals, and by the proven relationship between bladder carcinoma and exposure to both tobacco smoke and arylamines. Nitrosamines, metabolites of the nitrates commonly added to processed meats, are well-established carcinogens in laboratory rodents but

Table 3-2
CARCINOGENIC FACTORS IN HUMAN BLADDER CANCER

Established
Beta-naphthylamine (2-naphthylamine, 2-amino-naphthalene, 2-naphthalene)
4-Aminobiphenyl
Chlornaphazine
Tobacco smoke

Suspected
Schistosomiasis
Cyclophosphamide
Phenacetin
Bladder stones
Chronic irritation
Bladder outlet obstruction
Benzidine
Auramine
Aluminum products
Chlorinated drinking water

Theorized/Unproved
Arsenic compounds
Coffee/caffeine
Radiation
Dietary fats and oils
Nitrate/nitrite/nitrosamine
Urinary tract infection
Paints
Azathioprine
Motor exhaust fumes
Hair dyes

their role in human carcinogenesis is unclear. Other environmental factors associated with an increased relative risk of bladder tumors in humans include exposure to benzidine, auramine, high-dose phenacetin, cyclophosphamide, and radiation. The calcified eggs of *Schistosoma hematobium* in individuals having persistent cystitis, for example, probably represent such a combination, since the highest frequency of bladder carcinoma worldwide occurs in areas where the population is exposed to this parasite and affected bladders are chronically inflamed (33). In fact, nearly any factor that results in long-term bladder outlet obstruction or chronic inflammation can increase the risk of urothelial neoplasms, albeit slightly.

The list of putative risk factors for human bladder cancer is long and changing. For example, epidemiologic studies have not supported an increased risk for individuals ingesting saccharin or cyclamate (29). Nor have transmissible agents such as polyomavirus been strongly supported by the data (27). Dietary factors remain controversial. Epidemiologic evidence depends on what is recognized as a bladder cancer. In the past, epidemiologic evidence has been based on classifications that included almost all urothelial neoplasms among the carcinomas. The 1998 WHO/ISUP classification now recognizes that approximately 20 percent of urothelial neoplasms are either benign or of very low malignant potential, an adjustment that should result in more accurate epidemiologic assessments.

Except for the arylamine class of chemicals and perhaps the calcified eggs of *S. hematobium*, a substantial role in bladder cancer has not been proven for any environmental factor. Even in experimental situations, animals must be exposed to high doses over prolonged periods and the majority of the resulting neoplasms do not metastasize. Current concepts of human carcinogenesis and the empirical observation that few individuals exposed to any suspected environmental factor actually develop bladder neoplasms strongly suggest that the human host has important mechanisms to defend against all phases of the process. It is likely that neoplasms in humans are not solely a function of environmental overdose but result from a combination of exposure to cancerous stimuli and defects in host resistance.

The histogenesis of epithelial neoplasms has been studied in both experimental animals and humans (47). Animal studies demonstrate that neoplasms arise through a time-sequenced series of cellular changes of increasing degrees of anaplasia. The histologic type of tumor and its growth pattern depend upon both the species of animal and the type of chemical carcinogen used, another indication of the importance of the host in the process. In contrast to humans, animals can be exposed to such large, continuous doses of chemicals that almost all develop carcinomas, a situation in which any host resistance has been artificially overcome. In experimental systems of chemical carcinogenesis, the initial epithelial changes consist of generalized hyperplasia with slight nuclear atypia (atypical hyperplasia). The epithelial cells develop in a disordered fashion, which includes abnormalities of cellular arrangement and atypical nuclear changes (dysplasia). The earliest point in this process at which cellular changes reflect the establishment of a neoplasm remains unknown.

Studies of bladder tumor histogenesis in humans have been largely limited to monitoring small populations exposed to chemicals in the workplace and histologic examination of the grossly normal urothelium of patients who already have neoplasms elsewhere in the bladder (39,46,53). Workers exposed to suspected carcinogens may develop overt bladder malignancies but have often remained free of neoplasms throughout the study period. Even those shedding malignant-looking cells into their urine may not develop clinical cancer. The cystoscopically "normal" mucosa in bladders containing papillary or nodular tumors is often abnormal when examined histologically (46). This might mean that bladder neoplasms arise through a field change phenomenon wherein the entire epithelium is reactive to carcinogenic stimuli but in which lesions develop at different rates. Such a thesis is supported by studies of microsatellite aberrations in selected chromosomes (25,31). These studies indicate that the urothelium of each individual may develop neoplasms by pathways unique to that person. It is likely that most areas of abnormal epithelium not overtly malignant at diagnosis either temporarily or permanently lack the capacity to develop into true carcinomas. Whatever thinking is correct, the evolution of bladder neoplasms from low grade and noninvasive to high grade and disseminated is apparently unusual, having been observed in only a small percentage of clinical cases (36).

Bladder tumors may arise via intravesical seeding of the normal mucosa by cells from an existing neoplasm. This theory is supported by laboratory studies documenting colonization of urothelium by highly anaplastic cultured tumor cells and observations in humans of an increased frequency of new tumors at the bladder dome after surgical resection (24,54). It is further supported by the finding of similar chromosomal aberrations in multiple coexistent bladder tumors from the same patients (41). The concept of intravesical seeding has been challenged by studies documenting polyclonality among multiple tumors in the same bladder and even among cells from the same tumor (26,49).

Intravesical seeding does not account for the development of the initial neoplasm nor does it adequately explain the mechanism by which tumor cells might survive in urine with sufficient energy to invade normal epithelium and replicate. Further, there is no convincing clinical evidence that procedures that might facilitate intravesical seeding, for example, multiple surgical interventions, increase the frequency of new tumors in bladders harboring urothelial neoplasms.

The subject remains controversial but a growing body of evidence suggests that most urothelial neoplasms can be separated into two fairly well-defined categories based primarily upon cytologic grade (36–38). The thesis that configuration (i.e., papillary versus flat) is an essential component of urothelial carcinogenesis has not yet withstood critical examination (56). The lower-grade lesions (papilloma, PUNLMP) must be papillary to be recognized histologically as neoplastic. Flat lesions of this cytologic grade have been difficult to define and nodular tumors composed entirely of lower-grade neoplastic cells are essentially nonexistent. Almost all lower-grade urothelial neoplasms manifest many features of normal differentiation. They are associated with an excellent long-term prognosis. Patients presenting with these lesions, who do not develop a high-grade carcinoma, can expect a normal lifespan (36). In contrast, high-grade tumors are usually nodular, but may be papillary or flat. Nearly all manifest many features of abnormal differentiation, and 85 to 90 percent of deaths related to urothelial neoplasms occur among patients with high-grade tumors. Even when patients having high-grade urothelial carcinomas do not die of their cancers, they do not have a normal life expectancy.

Clinical Features of Bladder Neoplasms

The clinical features of bladder tumors vary in different parts of the world (43). In countries where *S. hematobium* is endemic and the most prevalent histologic type is squamous cell carcinoma, patients present with hematuria and symptoms of chronic irritation. Bladder carcinoma is a leading cause of cancer-related deaths in these areas (33). In other locations, different frequencies and environmental relationships exist. Many of the clinical characteristics discussed here can be generally applied, but one should

be aware that they are drawn primarily from studies in the United States.

In the United States, the demographics associated with bladder tumors have not changed appreciably in more than three decades (29, 35,51,55). Bladder neoplasms comprise 2 to 6 percent of all tumors. Men are affected more often than women (2.7 to 1) and Caucasians more often than people of other racial backgrounds. A familial predisposition may exist (50). According to statistics from the Surveillance, Epidemiology, and End Results (SEER) databank, the incidence has been rising steadily over the last three decades and more than 60,000 new cases/year are expected. In contrast, the estimated death rate has remained relatively constant at 9,000 to 12,000/year during this period. Variations in survival among subgroups of the population are documented but the reasons are not entirely clear. Urinary tract tumors account for 3 to 5 percent of cancer-related deaths in the United States.

Bladder neoplasms are primarily encountered in men aged 50 to 70 years (median and mean, 64 to 68 years). With the exception of certain myosarcomas, bladder tumors are rare in children and adults less than 40 years of age. The traditional wisdom that urothelial neoplasms occurring in the young are predominantly low-grade and noninvasive has been challenged by more recent data suggesting that there are no differences in clinical stage and only slight variations in biologic potential based solely on age at presentation (58). Adjusted for age, the incidence of bladder tumors in the population over 40 years is approximately 35/100,000, making them the fourth most common tumor among men and the tenth most frequent among women (32,35).

Patients with bladder neoplasms have non-specific signs and symptoms (32). Those with epithelial tumors usually experience gross or microscopic hematuria. Those with intraepithelial lesions often complain of dysuria, frequency, and suprapubic pain. Mass lesions, with or without a feeling of pelvic fullness, are associated primarily with sarcomas.

The majority of bladder tumors, whether neoplastic or non-neoplastic, benign or malignant, occur at the base (trigone), a region that includes the ureteral orifices and extends into the bladder neck. At least 60 percent of primary bladder neoplasms occur as single lesions and nearly

80 percent of all tumors are localized to the bladder base at clinical diagnosis. Based on cystoscopic estimates, over half of the primary lesions are less than 2.5 cm in greatest dimension. Fewer than 10 percent of patients present with metastases. In contrast to the location of primary tumors, "recurrent" bladder neoplasms commonly occur at sites other than that of the initial lesion, such as the dome (24). Most lesions arising subsequent to resection of a primary bladder neoplasm do not occupy the exact same site and are therefore not recurrences but new tumors.

Since almost all bladder tumors are treated soon after diagnosis, the natural history of these lesions cannot be studied. Observations of treated patients document a relationship between prognosis and histologic type. In general, nonurothelial carcinomas tend to be progressive and are often associated with an adverse outcome. This is also true for urothelial cancers of high cytologic grade and tumors containing mixtures of high-grade urothelial and other components, such as squamous, glandular, or small cell carcinomas. In contrast, adverse patient outcome is unusual if the initial lesion is a urothelial tumor of low cytologic grade, despite the tendency of patients presenting with these lesions to develop new tumors.

Detection and Monitoring

Procedures for the detection and monitoring of bladder neoplasms can be considered in three categories: 1) established procedures with an extensive database grounded in long tradition or compelling data; 2) methods with limited databases but future promise; and 3) techniques whose clinical value has yet to be confirmed (43). Items 2 and 3 are discussed in the section on Special Techniques. Among the established methods are bimanual palpation, cystoscopy with or without random or selected-site biopsies, and urinary cytology (32,38,44). All have limitations and none can detect the presence of a neoplasm in every instance; they are best used in combination.

Bimanual examination and cystoscopy are clinical techniques that allow the examiner to detect mass lesions and assess their extent in the tissue. Cystoscopic examination facilitates not only the identification of a tumor but its multiplicity, location, size, and configuration.

This method is of limited value for detecting flat, noninvasive mucosal abnormalities; very small tumors; and lesions at certain bladder sites. The sensitivity of cystoscopy is high but its specificity rather low.

Bladder neoplasms are defined according to their histologic characteristics and histologic examination is the most specific method for assessing these lesions. Using this approach, neoplasms can be typed, graded, and staged. The major limitation of histologic examination is inadequate sampling and suboptimal methods of tissue preparation and processing.

Urinary cytopathology is especially useful for the detection and monitoring of patients with epithelial neoplasms (38,44). This approach is best applied to high-grade neoplasms, where nearly all of the features usually ascribed to cancerous cells can be appreciated in adequate samples. Urinary cytopathology is less useful for the detection and monitoring of very low-grade neoplasms, primarily because most of these tumors are composed of cells that lack features of malignancy, but also because not all of the cells have all of the features usually ascribed to low-grade neoplasms, even when these cells are present in the sample. Using urinary cytopathology, nearly all aggressive urothelial neoplasms can be detected in adequately sampled bladders, whether these neoplasms occur as primary or recurrent tumors. It is not rare for malignant cells to appear in a urinary sample months to years before the neoplasm is detected cystoscopically or histologically. The cytologic method is used to monitor patients with suspected urothelial carcinoma in situ at various sites, including the bladder, distal ureters, urethra, and prostatic ducts. It is valuable for patients having urinary diversions. The inability to detect low-grade neoplasms is not a major limitation to the use of urinary cytopathology, since low-grade lesions are rarely aggressive and can be readily detected cystoscopically. More important limitations to urinary cytopathology include the inability to localize lesions, determine the presence of invasion, and identify tumors of the kidney and prostate gland. Further, the method is insensitive for screening the normal population. Even in positive specimens, the tumor cells in the urinary sample do not always correlate exactly with the grade or type of neoplasm in the corresponding tissue biopsy. Considering the limitations of the methodology, urinary specimens are best classified in four basic categories: 1) negative, to include reactive cellular changes; 2) dysplastic cells, rule out low-grade neoplasm; 3) cells suspicious for a high-grade neoplasm; 4) malignant tumor cells consistent with a high-grade neoplasm. Its limitations notwithstanding, urinary cytopathology is an important technique and should be integrated into every detection and monitoring program for neoplasms of the urinary bladder.

UROTHELIAL (TRANSITIONAL CELL) NEOPLASMS

The subject of urothelial neoplasms cannot be adequately addressed without reference to interobserver variability in interpretation. Whether a particular grade of tumor is considered rare or common, aggressive or benign, is not only dependent upon its definition but also upon how the tissues and cells in a specimen are interpreted by individual pathologists (179,186,187,191, 197,201,221). The pathologic assessment of such specimens is not a laboratory test, in the sense of a result produced by a high precision machine. A pathologic diagnosis is an interpretation (i.e., the result of a complex integration of factors) influenced as much by the comfort level and diagnostic aggressiveness of the observer as by his or her knowledge of the subject. Considering that pathologists are required to furnish interpretations relating to the type and likely behavior of neoplasms occurring in populations of genetically diverse patients with varying lifestyles, and that the interpretation must ordinarily be made on very small amounts of tissue furnished at only a single point in the patient's disease, it is extraordinary that the level of interobserver variation is as low as it is.

Interobserver variability in interpretation is inevitable and probably cannot be reduced to less than 10 percent, regardless of how lesions are defined or how thoroughly pathologists are educated (100,179). Depending on which tumors are to be separated, the degree of variation can be reduced by recognizing and combining categories that cannot be reliably distinguished. In the 1998 WHO/ISUP formulation (102), for example, both evidence and per-

sonal experience suggest that pathologists virtually never confuse very low-grade tumors like papillary urothelial neoplasm of low malignant potential (PUNLMP) with tumors like high-grade carcinoma. Conversely, pathologists tend to have problems distinguishing lesions of similar histology, like PUNLMP and low-grade carcinoma. Considering that the clinical approach to urothelial neoplasms tends to be influenced primarily by stage and that lower grade neoplasms are almost always noninvasive whereas invasive neoplasms are nearly always high-grade, the case for combining the categories of papilloma, PUNLMP, and low-grade carcinoma into a single group of "low-grade neoplasm" contrasted to a category of "high-grade carcinoma" seems to have merit. The proposition has not been adopted because many experts are reluctant to combine categories of tumors associated with slightly different long-term risks to patients even though these tumors cannot be reliably distinguished by currently available methods. Regardless of which classification of urothelial neoplasm one prefers, the problem of distinguishing among the grades, especially the lower grades, remains. The following discussion of urothelial neoplasms should be read with this in mind.

Urothelial (Transitional Cell) Papilloma

Urothelial (transitional cell) papillomas are pathologically and clinically benign neoplasms arising in urothelial-lined organs. Urothelial (transitional cell) papillomas may be inverted or exophytic, and all current classification schemes that recognize these tumors use the same pathologic definitions.

Inverted Papilloma. Inverted papilloma is a benign tumor comprising less than 1 percent of urothelial neoplasms (167,168). It is distinctive both grossly and microscopically (fig. 3-7). Cystoscopically, inverted papilloma is a solitary, raised, pedunculated or polypoid lesion with a smooth surface. Most are under 3 cm in greatest dimension but rare lesions are as large as 8 cm. Histologically, cords of urothelial cells appear as if a papillary lesion had invaginated into the lamina propria. The central portions of the cords contain maturing urothelial cells and the surrounding tissue is stroma, exactly the opposite of an exophytic papilloma, where the central stroma is surrounded by the epithelial cells.

Figure 3-7

INVERTED UROTHELIAL PAPILLOMA

A: The tumor appears grossly as a small submucosal nodule (arrow). (Courtesy of Dr. George M. Farrow, Rochester, MN.)

B: In contrast to exophytic papilloma, the epithelial cells are oriented toward the central portions of the trabeculae as if the fingers of a glove had been invaginated into its hand.

C: Nuclear atypia is common in inverted papillomas but has no known effect upon the behavior of the neoplasm.

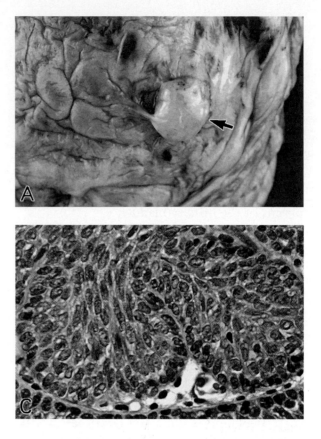

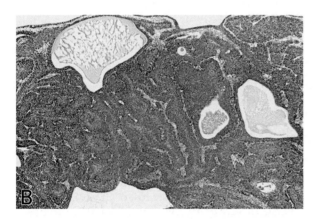

Inverted papillomas grow as expansile masses and do not infiltrate the muscular wall. They rarely coexist with carcinomas. Conversely, carcinomas occasionally have intertwining invasive papillae which resemble an inverted papilloma. Cystic areas and foci of squamous metaplasia are common in inverted papillomas. Neuroendocrine differentiation has been recorded (214). Tumors with DNA aneuploid cells and tumors with cells overexpressing p53 protein have been reported (88). Occasionally, inverted papillomas exist in association with florid proliferations of Brunn nests (147). Both histologic patterns may represent host reactions to similar stimuli but their exact histogenetic relationship is unclear.

Cellular atypia and a measurable population of cells synthesizing DNA are common in inverted papillomas, but true anaplasia is rare (88). Atypical nuclear changes may result from compression of cells within tightly packed trabeculae. This theory is supported by cytologic studies in which features of malignancy have not been recognized among disaggregated urothelial cells from bladders harboring inverted papillomas (76). The ultrastructure, antigenic composition, molecular biology, and DNA content of inverted papilloma cells have been noncontributory to the diagnosis and prognosis in the few evaluated cases (59).

If the diagnosis of inverted papilloma is confined to the prototype lesion discussed and illustrated here, these tumors are benign. Recurrent lesions are unusual, and progression from pure inverted papilloma to carcinoma has not been documented. The temptation to expand the definition of inverted papilloma to include all polypoid lesions with predominantly subsurface growth patterns, such as florid proliferations of Brunn nests, should be resisted.

Inverted papillomas are histologically distinctive tumors that must be differentiated primarily from exophytic papilloma and PUNLMP. Nuclear atypia may not be important in this differentiation as long as the atypia is primarily manifested by increased nuclear size and coarsely granular chromatin not associated with pleomorphism, and the configuration of the lesion is characteristic. Any exophytic component in a papillary urothelial neoplasm essentially excludes inverted papilloma.

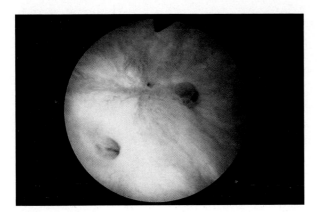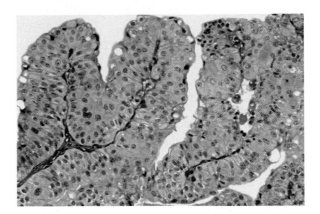

Figure 3-8

EXOPHYTIC UROTHELIAL PAPILLOMA

Left: Cystoscopic photograph. (Courtesy of Dr. Mark S. Soloway, Miami, FL.)
Right: Urothelial papilloma. By definition, these neoplasms have architecturally and cytologically unremarkable urothelium arranged on delicate fibrovascular stalks. In specimens such as this, fixed in picric acid–based solutions, nucleoli seem prominent.

Exophytic Papilloma. As defined in the 1998 WHO/ISUP scheme (102), exophytic papilloma is a very uncommon urothelial neoplasm that many pathologists never encounter (fig. 3-8) (85,102). Exophytic urothelial papillomas are composed of architecturally and cytologically normal urothelium arranged on delicate fibrovascular stalks. Despite a general feeling that these tumors occur in young individuals and are associated with little or no risk to the patient, the literature on the subject is fragmentary. Few individuals have been followed for prolonged periods, even in large studies. Whether or not the histologic normality extends to the molecular biology of these lesions remains to be seen.

Distinguishing exophytic papilloma from other urothelial tumors would seem to be straightforward. Still, the appreciation of the normal range of architecture and cytology may well differ among observers, and one person's papilloma may be another's PUNLMP. Interobserver variability in this area of the morphologic spectrum is unlikely to have clinical significance, since both tumors are associated with a very favorable prognosis.

Papillary Urothelial Neoplasm of Low Malignant Potential

Definition and General Features. This rather cumbersome term was chosen by the consensus conferees after the term "papilloma" had been assigned to the lesions previously discussed (102). It describes a papillary, low-grade urothelial neoplasm that apparently lacks the capacity to invade or metastasize (86,101,102,198). As illustrated in this atlas, PUNLMPs conform to nearly all of the tumors designated as papilloma in the third series Fascicle of the Armed Forces Institute of Pathology (AFIP) (173), most of the lesions termed transitional cell carcinoma grade 1 in the 1973 WHO system (168), and some of the tumors classed as grade 1 carcinoma in the 1999 WHO scheme (167). Exact extrapolations of terminology among classification systems cannot be achieved and not all grade 1 carcinomas in other formulations qualify as PUNLMPs.

Depending upon how the tumors in any particular formulation are categorized, PUNLMPs have many features in common with normal urothelium. The histologic architecture of the cells on the stalks is preserved and the nuclear features are only slightly abnormal (116,170). Almost all cells have structurally normal chromosomes and diploid DNA. Expression of normal blood group ABH antigens occurs in over 80 percent of tumors. Proliferative activity is either within or only slightly outside the normal range, as is the expression of genes and gene products (90,138,184,194). Lacking significant nuclear anaplasia, PUNLMP cells are difficult to recognize in urinary samples. These tumors are considered neoplastic primarily because of the propensity of patients having them to develop

Table 3-3

GUIDELINES FOR EVALUATING UROTHELIAL NEOPLASMS[a]

| | Configuration | | Cell Distribution | | Pleomor- phism | Nuclear Features Chromatin | | Large Nucleoli |
	Papillary	Nodular	Even	Clustered		Fine	Coarse	
PUNLMP[b]	+++[c]	0	+++	0	+	+++	0	±
Carcinoma								
low grade	++	+	+++	0	+	++	±	+
high grade	+	+++	0	+++	+++	+	+++	++

[a]Modified from Murphy WM. Urothelial neoplasia. In: Weinstein RS, Gardner WA Jr, eds. Pathology and pathobiology of the urinary bladder and prostate. Baltimore: William & Wilkins; 1992:77–111.
[b]PUNLMP = papillary urothelial neoplasm of low malignant potential.
[c]Key to features: 0 = absent; + = may occur sporadically; ± = occurs in some tumors but not consistent; ++ = occurs in most tumors; +++ = characteristic feature that occurs in all or almost all cases.

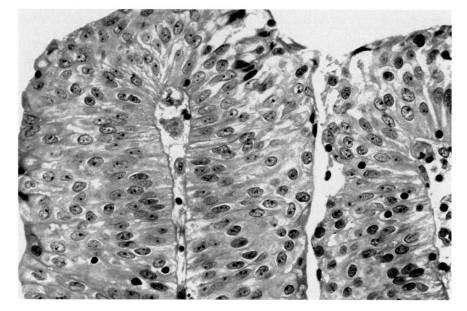

Figure 3-9

PAPILLARY UROTHELIAL NEOPLASM OF LOW MALIGNANT POTENTIAL

In contrast to a urothelial papilloma, the nuclei of these tumors are slightly atypical, even though the architectural pattern is largely preserved. The cells in specimens such as this, fixed in a picric acid–based solution, seem to have prominent nucleoli.

new, histologically similar lesions (recurrences) and because of the slightly increased risk for an adverse patient outcome (123).

Pathologic Findings. In histologic preparations, PUNLMPs are composed of multiple layers of cells which retain their superficial cell layer and cover delicate fibrovascular stalks (Table 3-3; figs. 3-9–3-13). Neoplastic cells often extend onto flat areas of urothelium adjacent to the bases of the stalks (fig. 3-13). The number of cell layers is not an important diagnostic feature, except in the rare instance where the cells appear normal by light microscopy and the only abnormality is an increased number of cell layers (70). The stalks of PUNLMPs may have di-

lated blood vessels, edema, or even foamy macrophages, but structures with broad stalks rich in connective tissue are not neoplasms.

The cells of PUNLMPs tend to be evenly distributed on the stalks. They have moderately distinct borders and homogeneous, amphophilic to acidophilic cytoplasm. Cytoplasmic clearing is almost always reduced when compared to normal cells from the same patient. Nuclei may be round or elongated, and they tend to maintain their normal perpendicular orientation to the surface and basal lamina (fig. 3-12). Irregularities of nuclear borders are common and best appreciated in cytologic samples. Chromatin is evenly dispersed and finely granular. Nucleoli are

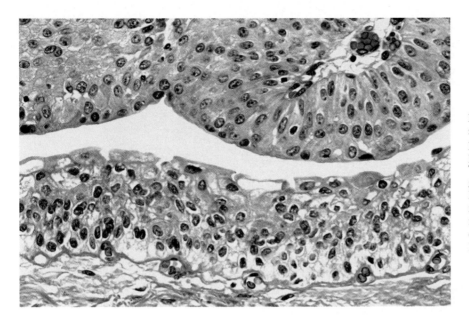

Figure 3-10

PAPILLARY UROTHELIAL NEOPLASM OF LOW MALIGNANT POTENTIAL

The cells of a low-grade papillary urothelial neoplasm are similar to normal. They differ primarily in their lack of cytoplasmic clearing and larger size. The nuclei of even very low-grade urothelial neoplasms are larger and slightly more irregular than normal. (Fig. 3-22C from Murphy WM. Urinary cytopathology. Chicago: ASCP Press; 2000:39.)

Figure 3-11

PAPILLARY UROTHELIAL NEOPLASM OF LOW MALIGNANT POTENTIAL

In histologic preparations, the architectural pattern of cells arranged on a delicate fibrovascular stalk defines a low-grade neoplasm. When these cells are disaggregated from the stalk into cytologic samples, they often appear unremarkable. (Fig. 3-24 from Murphy WM. Urinary cytopathology. Chicago: ASCP Press; 2000:41.)

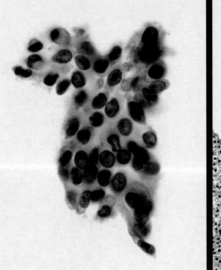

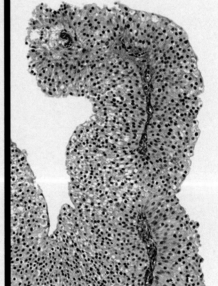

small or absent. Mitoses may occur, especially in tissue fixed in picric acid–based solutions, but are not numerous.

When separated from the stalk and either exfoliated or washed into cytologic samples, the cells of PUNLMPs cannot always be distinguished from normal elements. In most cases, the unequivocal diagnosis of a neoplasm cannot be made and the cells have been recognized as abnormal in only 24 to 60 percent of cases (fig. 3-14) (68,143,158,172). Occasionally, urinary samples contain cells characteristic of a PUNLMP

(fig. 3-15). In many specimens, abundant cells are the principal clue to the presence of a PUNLMP. Detection of these elements is best achieved with Papanicolaou preparations (Table 3-4).

Recognizable neoplastic cells are larger than the normal basal and intermediate cells essentially always present in the same specimen. They may be isolated or aggregated. Tight papillary clusters may occur but are not an important diagnostic feature. Cytoplasmic vacuolization is not ordinarily a feature of low-grade neoplastic cells although cytoplasmic degeneration may occur.

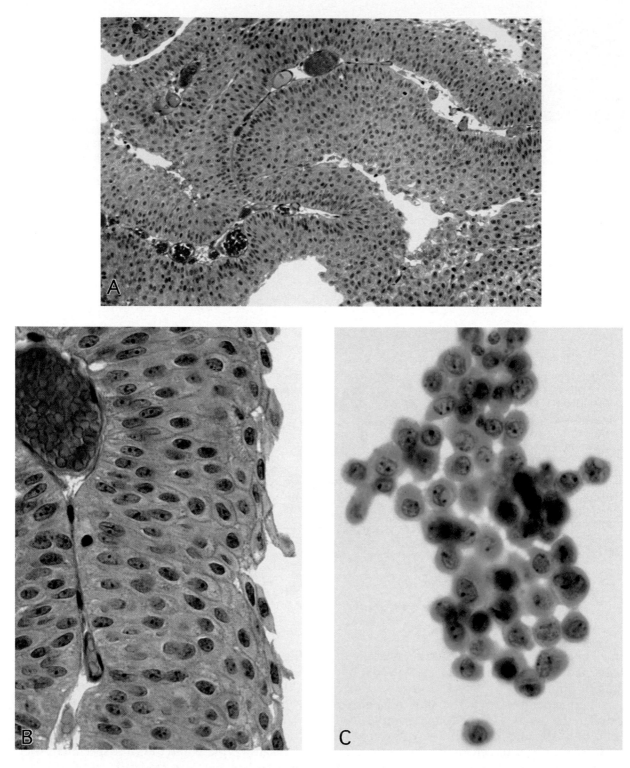

Figure 3-12

PAPILLARY UROTHELIAL NEOPLASM OF LOW MALIGNANT POTENTIAL

A: Nuclei are evenly spaced and not densely arranged at low magnification.

B: The preservation of architecture is apparent at higher magnification.

C: The disaggregated cells in a urinary specimen appear nearly normal.

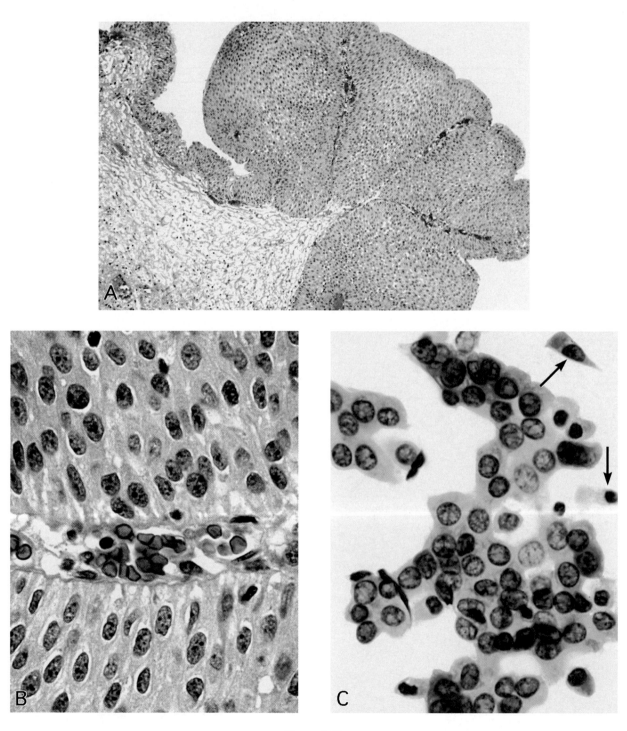

Figure 3-13

PAPILLARY UROTHELIAL NEOPLASM OF LOW MALIGNANT POTENTIAL

A: The papillae are broad and the neoplastic cells extend down the stalk onto the adjacent flat urothelium.

B: At high magnification, the architecture is preserved but the nuclei are large and irregular with more granular than normal chromatin. Interobserver variation for the distinction between PUNLMP and low-grade carcinoma is substantial and some may interpret this lesion as a low-grade carcinoma. The cytologic changes in C tend to support the lower-grade interpretation.

C: The abnormalities of nuclear size, shape, and chromatin among disaggregated cells in a urinary specimen can be compared to the features of normal elements (arrows). (Fig. 3-22 from Murphy WM. Urinary cytopathology. Chicago: ASCP Press: 2000:39.)

Table 3-4

CELLULAR FEATURES OF UROTHELIAL NEOPLASMS[a]

		Low Grade/Dysplastic	High Grade
Cells	Arrangement	Papillary and loose clusters	Isolated and loose clusters
	Size	Increased, uniform	Increased, pleomorphic
	Number	Often numerous	Variable
Cytoplasm		Homogeneous	Variable
N-C ratio[b]		Increased	Increased
Nuclei	Position	Eccentric	Eccentric
	Size	Enlarged	Variable
	Morphology	Variable within aggregates	Variable
	Borders	Irregular notches (creases)	Irregular
	Chromatin	Fine, even	Coarse, uneven
Nucleoli		Small, absent	Variable

[a]Table 2 from Murphy WM, Soloway MS, Jukkola AF, Crabtree WN, Ford KS. Urinary cytology and bladder cancer. Cancer 1984;53:1555-65.
[b]N-C ratio = nuclear-cytoplasmic ratio.

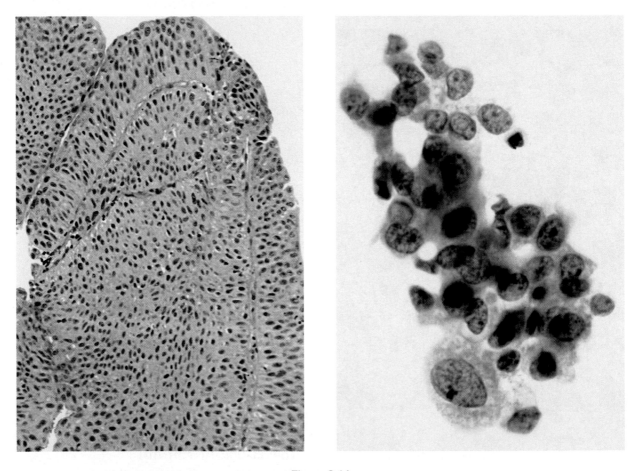

Figure 3-14

PAPILLARY UROTHELIAL NEOPLASM OF LOW MALIGNANT POTENTIAL

Left: Compressed papillae.
Right: The corresponding cells in a urinary specimen. These cells have features best interpreted as "dysplastic cells, a low-grade neoplasm cannot be excluded." (Fig. 3-20A,C from Murphy WM. Urinary cytopathology. Chicago: ASCP Press; 2000:37.)

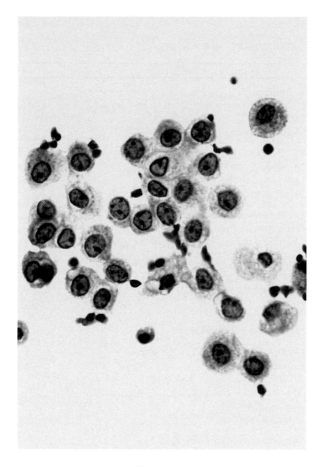

Figure 3-15

**PAPILLARY UROTHELIAL NEOPLASM
OF LOW MALIGNANT POTENTIAL**

Cells such as these in a urinary specimen are characteristic of a papillary urothelial neoplasm of low malignant potential.

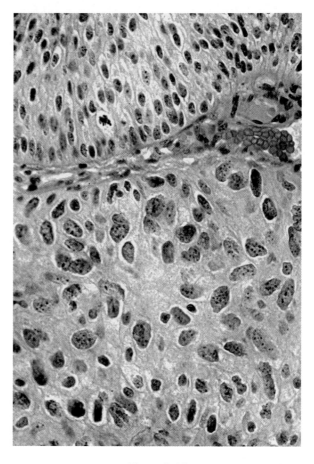

Figure 3-16

UROTHELIAL CARCINOMA, HIGH GRADE

Foci of high-grade cells occasionally appear in otherwise low-grade papillary neoplasms. Such tumors have the aggressive potential of a high-grade carcinoma.

Nuclear-cytoplasmic ratios are greater than 1 to 2 and the nuclei often occupy an extremely eccentric position in the cells. Many nuclei have irregular borders. These most commonly appear as shallow depressions, notches, or creases, and correlate with morphometrically calculated abnormalities expressed as the nuclear shape index. Nucleoli are inconspicuous or absent. Although most often indicative of a PUNLMP, cells with these characteristics may occasionally be exfoliated or washed from the surfaces of low-grade carcinomas or dysplastic lesions (Table 3-5).

Immunohistochemistry and electron microscopy do not contribute significantly to the diagnosis or prognosis of patients with urothelial neoplasms, including PUNLMP. Molecular and other factors that may identify urothelial neoplasms are not in general use and are discussed in the section, Special Techniques.

Prognosis. Most authorities believe that if untreated, PUNLMPS have the capacity to grow and dedifferentiate into aggressive cancers, but the evidence for this opinion is anecdotal. Well-documented cases of aggressive PUNLMPs are rare if they exist at all. This is not to say that tumors with small foci of high-grade carcinoma or truly carcinomatous lesions could not be (mis)-interpreted as PUNLMPs (fig. 3-16). Interobserver variability for the distinction of PUNLMPs from low-grade carcinomas in at least one study was 39 to 50 percent (179). The possibility of interobserver discrepancy notwithstanding, histologically confirmed PUNLMPs are ordinarily single,

Table 3-5

CYTOLOGIC CLASSIFICATION OF GENITOURINARY NEOPLASMS[a]

Cells	Histologic Correlates[b]
Normal or reactive	**Normal** **Inflammation** PUNLMP[c] Urothelial papilloma
Dysplastic cells, rule out low-grade neoplasm	**PUNLMP** **Urothelial carcinoma, low grade** Dysplasia (atypia) Inflammation
Suspicious for high-grade neoplasm	**Urothelial carcinoma, high grade** **Carcinoma in situ** Urothelial carcinoma, low grade
Positive – consistent with low-grade neoplasm	**Urothelial carcinoma, low grade** Urothelial carcinoma, high grade Carcinoma in situ Dysplasia PUNLMP Squamous cell carcinoma
Positive – consistent with high-grade neoplasm	**Urothelial carcinoma, high grade** **Carcinoma in situ** Urothelial carcinoma, low grade Squamous cell carcinoma Adenocarcinoma Other carcinoma
Positive – consistent with squamous cell carcinoma	**Squamous cell carcinoma**
Positive – consistent with adenocarcinoma	**Adenocarcinoma**

[a]Modified from Table 2-1 from reference 172.
[b]Correlates in order of expected frequency; bold indicates most common. 1998 WHO/ISUP histologic classification of urothelial neoplasms.
[c]PUNLMP = papillary urothelial neoplasm of low malignant potential.

small tumors that are completely resected as the only initial treatment. In most current series, new tumors (recurrences) occur in less than 50 percent of patients and 80 percent of these new tumors are also PUNLMPs (86,132). The first new tumors usually develop within 3 years after the index lesion, but "late recurrences" are well documented. Overall, less than 8 percent of patients whose initial bladder neoplasm is a PUNLMP have an adverse outcome and, unless patients develop a high-grade lesion, they can expect a normal lifespan (81,123,132,134,151). Both progression and death from disease for patients presenting with a PUNLMP are essentially always due to a high-grade carcinoma.

Differential Diagnosis. The principal problems in the differential diagnosis involve the distinction of PUNLMPs from exophytic papillomas and low-grade carcinomas. The slight architectural and cytologic abnormalities of PUNLMPs distinguish them from exophytic papillomas, papillomas being completely normal. Distinction from low-grade carcinoma relies on more subtle features (173,198). At low and intermediate magnification in histologic sections, the cells of low-grade carcinoma are smaller and more densely arranged on the fibrovascular stalks than the cells of PUNLMP. Their nuclei tend to round up, thus creating a slight distortion of the cellular architecture. At high magnification, a slight degree of nuclear pleomorphism may be appreciated. Similar to PUNLMP, the nuclear chromatin of low-grade carcinoma is finely granular and evenly distributed. As previously

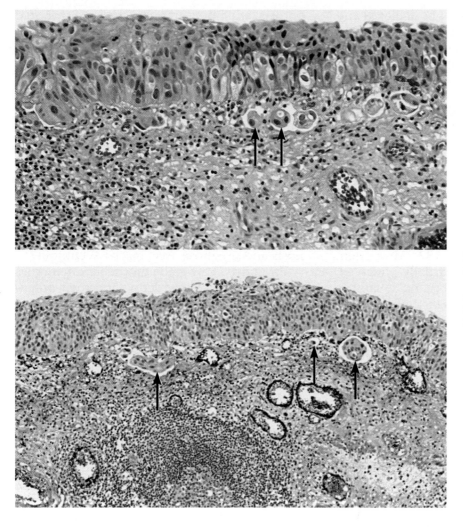

Figure 3-17

PSEUDOVASCULAR INVASION OF A UROTHELIAL NEOPLASM

Top: The spaces surrounding the urothelial nests (arrows) are artifacts.

Bottom: The artifactual nature of the spaces is confirmed by a negative immunohistochemical reaction for factor VIII (arrows).

discussed, interobserver variation in the distinction of PUNLMP from low-grade carcinoma is high enough to support combining these lesions into a single category of "low-grade neoplasm." Immunohistochemical analyses are unlikely to be helpful in the differential diagnosis (60).

In a very few cases, papillary tumors with features of a PUNLMP contain foci of high-grade carcinoma and these neoplasms act like high-grade carcinomas (fig. 3-16) (132). In such cases, the high-grade cells are most likely to occur at the stromal/epithelial interface. Pseudovascular spaces containing nests of cells lacking high-grade features may also occur at the stromal/epithelial interface (fig. 3-17) (150). Such foci should not be interpreted as vascular invasion or high-grade carcinoma. The basal surface of papillary urothelial neoplasms should be thor-

oughly examined before an interpretation of PUNLMP or low-grade carcinoma is rendered.

Urothelial (Transitional Cell) Carcinoma, Low Grade

Definition and General Features. Urothelial (transitional cell) carcinoma, low grade, is a predominantly papillary urothelial neoplasm resembling PUNLMP architecturally and cytologically (see Table 3-3). It is included among the malignancies because of its capacity to invade and (rarely) metastasize. As defined and illustrated here, low-grade urothelial carcinomas could be included among the grade 1 transitional cell carcinomas but most authorities group them with the grade 2, grade 2a, or grade A tumors of other formulations (75,159,167,168). It should be emphasized that exact extrapolations among classification schemes cannot be achieved and that interobserver variability in interpretation affects the categorization of any particular lesion. Figures will undoubtedly vary in published series, but 12 to 25 percent of urothelial neoplasms are low-grade lesions (122,132). Like other tumors, low-grade carcinomas ordinarily present at the bladder base and are usually solitary. Their molecular biology is incompletely characterized; available data indicate low frequencies of DNA synthesis, DNA aneuploidy, and genetic aberrations (75,122,175).

Pathologic Findings. Histologically, nearly all low-grade urothelial carcinomas are papillary. Invasive components are documented in less than 20 percent of cases (132). Most often, the superficial cell layer is partially preserved. Rarely, small foci of glandular and squamous differentiation occur, although these patterns are more common in high-grade urothelial tumors. Low-grade urothelial carcinomas have a characteristic light microscopic appearance at low-power magnification (figs. 3-18–3-20). The cells are uniform in size and evenly distributed but densely packed in tissue sections. They have indistinct borders and little or no cytoplasmic clearing. Nuclei often retain a semblance of normal orientation but are rounded and slightly pleomorphic. Nuclear borders are irregular, a feature most easily appreciated in cytologic preparations. Chromatin is evenly dispersed and finely granular. Large nucleoli may occupy some nuclei but are not a prominent feature of low-grade carcinomas. Mitoses may be numerous, especially in preparations fixed in picric acid–based solutions, but are not an important diagnostic feature. They are often scattered throughout the tumor rather than concentrated in basal areas.

In cytologic samples, neoplastic cells from low-grade urothelial carcinomas may or may not be readily appreciated, depending upon whether the tumor is differentiating toward the lower (PUNLMP) or the upper (high-grade carcinoma) part of the histologic spectrum for this category (see Table 3-4) (143,172,197). In untreated cases, numerous cells may appear in cytologic samples and this in itself is abnormal. Most tumor cells occur in loose clusters and have the high nuclear-cytoplasmic ratios, markedly eccentric nuclei, irregular nuclear

borders, and finely granular, evenly distributed chromatin characteristic of low-grade neoplasms. These features are accentuated in cells from low-grade carcinomas as compared to cells from PUNLMPs, but they often differ more in degree than in kind. Therefore, PUNLMPs, low-grade carcinomas, and even dysplastic lesions cannot always be differentiated in cytologic samples (Table 3-5). It is not uncommon for a few cells disaggregated from a low-grade carcinoma to have the coarse chromatin and large nucleoli of a high-grade neoplasm.

Ultrastructural and immunohistochemical studies of low-grade urothelial carcinomas have not yet contributed significantly to their diagnosis and prognosis (see Special Techniques).

Prognosis. Low-grade urothelial carcinomas are difficult to closely define and their potential for aggressive behavior is correspondingly uncertain. The available evidence tends to confirm a very favorable outcome for patients whose initial tumor is a low-grade carcinoma or its equivalent in other formulations (87,123, 132). Both progression and death from disease occur in less than 15 percent of patients. Adverse events may occur late in the course but are not currently predictable. In fact, the difference in outcome of patients presenting with a low-grade carcinoma and those presenting with a PUNLMP is only 8 to 15 percent, suggesting that pathologic similarities reflect biologic similarities. As with nearly all carcinomas, the prognosis for groups of patients tends to be influenced by tumor stage at detection. Whether or not prognosis is influenced by molecular factors remains to be established (see Special Techniques).

Differential Diagnosis. The problem of distinguishing low-grade carcinoma from PUNLMP has been discussed in the section on PUNLMP. The distinction between low-grade carcinoma and high-grade carcinoma is more straightforward and associated with a very low level of interobserver variation (179). Nearly all invasive urothelial carcinomas are high grade, at least in the foci of invasion, whether the invasion is confined to the lamina propria or includes the muscularis propria. In addition, the nuclei of high-grade carcinoma cells tend to cluster in tissue sections. They exhibit marked variation in shape, not necessarily in size, and have coarsely clumped, unevenly distributed

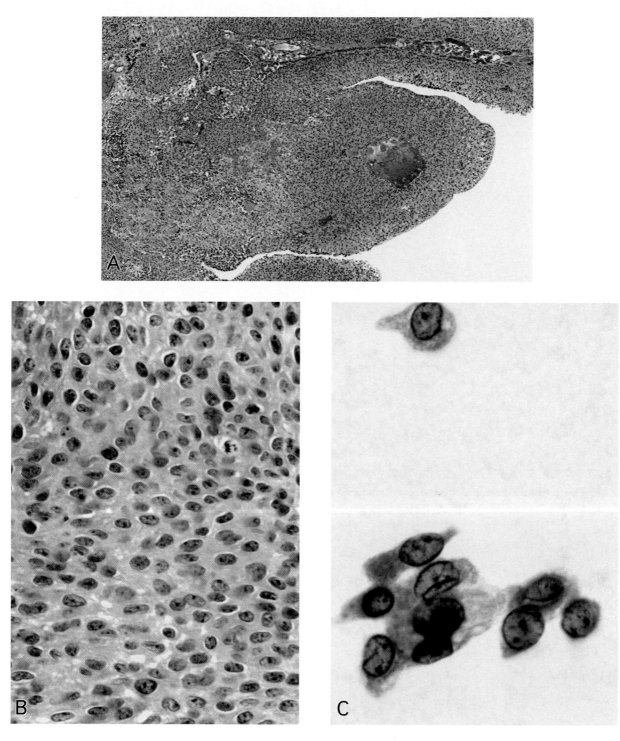

Figure 3-18

UROTHELIAL CARCINOMA, LOW GRADE

A: At low magnification, the nuclei are evenly distributed but more dense than those of a papillary urothelial neoplasm of low malignant potential.

B: The nuclei tend to be evenly distributed but irregular, thus disturbing the architectural pattern.

C: In cytologic preparations, the nuclei are markedly eccentric and large; the nuclear-cytoplasmic ratios are high. (Fig. 3-2 from Murphy WM. Urinary cytopathology. Chicago: ASCP Press; 2000:19.)

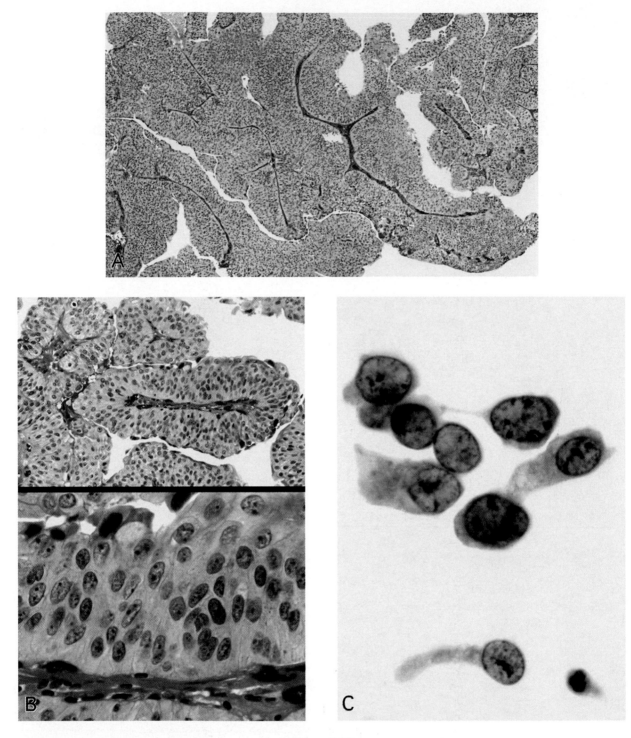

Figure 3-19

UROTHELIAL CARCINOMA, LOW GRADE

A: Dense nuclei at low magnification.

B: Intermediate and high magnifications confirm the preservation of the architectural pattern but appreciable nuclear abnormalities are seen.

C: Nuclear abnormalities are readily identified in cytologic preparations. The appearance of cytoplasm surrounding only a portion of the nucleus is characteristic.

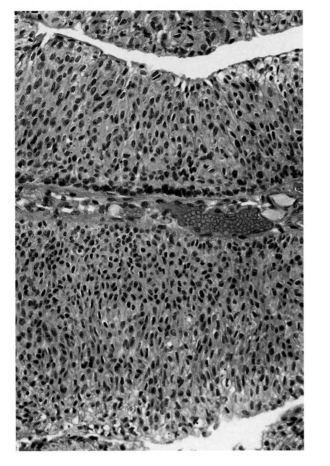 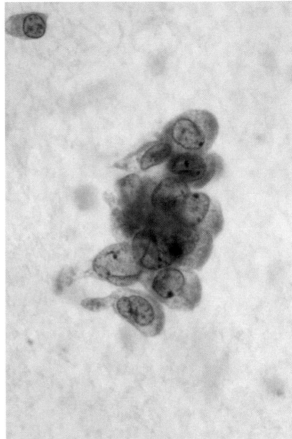

Figure 3-20

UROTHELIAL CARCINOMA, LOW GRADE

Left: Densely packed but uniformly distributed cells with small nuclei and high nuclear-cytoplasmic ratios are characteristic.
Right: Tumor cells in urinary specimens are often admixed with normal elements. Note the normal nuclei both within the aggregate and at the upper left.

chromatin. Nucleoli may be helpful if they are large and numerous but this is unusual in urothelial carcinomas. Mitoses are not an important differential diagnostic feature. As in the differential diagnosis of PUNLMPs, foci of high-grade cells in a predominantly low-grade carcinoma should alter the interpretation to high-grade carcinoma.

Urothelial (Transitional Cell) Carcinoma, High Grade

Definition and General Features. Urothelial (transitional cell) carcinoma, high grade, is a malignant neoplasm that is often invasive; it is either papillary, nodular, or both (see Table 3-3; fig. 3-21). As defined here, at least 50 percent of all urothelial neoplasms and 60 to 80 percent of all true carcinomas are high-grade urothelial carcinomas (101,102,122,132). These tumors include all grade 3 and approximately half of grade 2 carcinomas in other classification systems (167,168). Almost all high-grade urothelial carcinomas have elevated proliferation indices and DNA synthesis as well as abnormal antigenic and genetic expression (90,138,170,184).

Pathologic Findings. In histologic preparations, high-grade urothelial carcinomas are usually infiltrating neoplasms whose cells are arranged in sheets, nests, and broad cords (figs. 3-22–3-25). Papillary and flat components are common but do not usually predominate. Rarely, small portions of a low-grade papillary

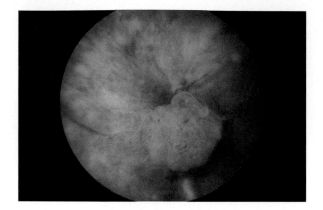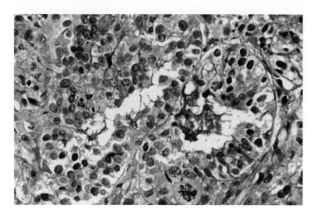

Figure 3-21

UROTHELIAL CARCINOMA, HIGH GRADE

Left: Cystoscopic appearance of this high-grade urothelial carcinoma. (Courtesy of Dr. Mark S. Soloway, Miami, FL.)
Right: Pleomorphic and clustered nuclei are characteristic.

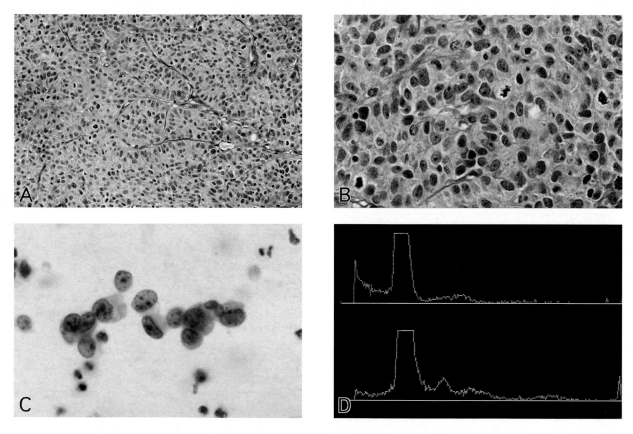

Figure 3-22

UROTHELIAL CARCINOMA, HIGH GRADE

A: Urothelial carcinoma, high grade, at low magnification.
B: Characteristic nuclear changes at high magnification.
C: Urinary cytology obtained during follow-up; high-grade neoplastic cells.
D: Flow cytometric histograms obtained at different times during follow-up. In the top histogram, 24 percent of the cells examined fell outside the normal G1G0 range (hyperdiploidy). The bottom histogram was created from the same specimen as in C. In contrast to the previous histogram (top), this specimen illustrates aneuploidy.

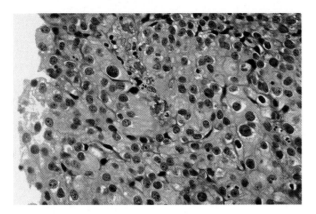

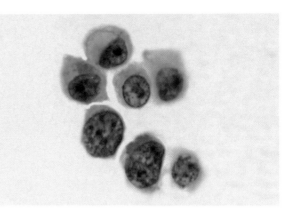

Figure 3-23

UROTHELIAL CARCINOMA, HIGH GRADE

Left: Intermediate magnification.
Right: Cytologic specimen; high-grade neoplastic cells.

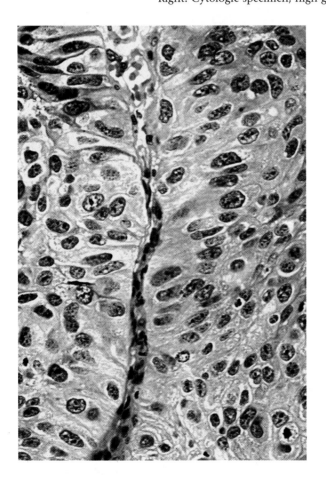

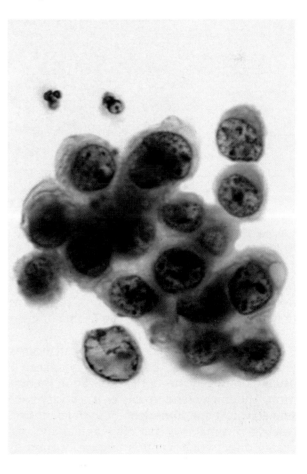

Figure 3-24

UROTHELIAL CARCINOMA, HIGH GRADE

Left: Intermediate magnification.
Right: High-grade neoplastic cells. (Fig. 3-1 from Murphy WM. Urinary cytopathology. Chicago: ASCP Press; 2000:17.)

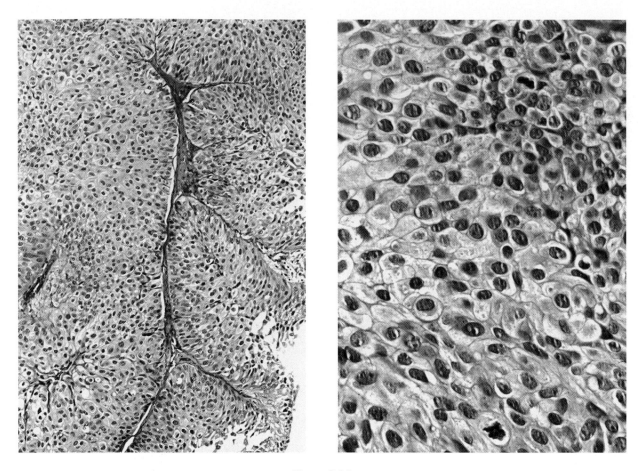

Figure 3-25

UROTHELIAL CARCINOMA, HIGH GRADE

Left: Low magnification.
Right: The tendency for uniformity in nuclear size and shape might be interpreted as evidence of a low-grade carcinoma but the nuclear clustering and coarse chromatin granularity militate in favor of a high-grade tumor.

neoplasm are composed of high-grade carcinoma; at low-power magnification the lesion may seem to be a low-grade carcinoma or even a PUNLMP (see fig. 3-16.)

The cells of high-grade urothelial carcinomas tend to have indistinct borders. The cytoplasm is usually homogeneous but vacuolization is common. The nuclei tend to cluster. They vary considerably in shape, although not so much in size. Nuclear chromatin is coarsely granular and unevenly dispersed, a feature more easily appreciated in formalin-fixed than in picric acid–fixed tissues. Large nucleoli appear in some nuclei. Mitoses are common and may be abnormal.

Urothelial carcinomas of high cytologic grade may manifest heterogeneous elements of both epithelial and stromal origin (148,156,

232,238). Intracellular and extracellular mucins are most often encountered, followed by foci of malignant glandular and squamous differentiation (figs. 3-26–3-28). When foci of nonurothelial differentiation are prominent, the cancers have been designated "mixed" or "metaplastic" in some formulations. Not all heterogeneous elements are malignant.

Rarely, high-grade urothelial and even other types of bladder carcinomas manifest giant cells of stromal origin or pseudosarcomatous stromal spindle cells (232,238). When these elements are prominent, many pathologists choose to highlight the lesions with designations such as "carcinoma with osteoclast-type giant cells" or "carcinoma with spindle cell stroma" (fig. 3-29). Such variations should be recognized by

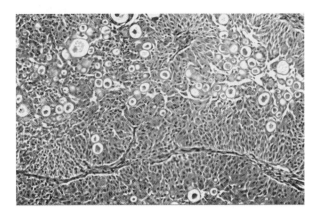
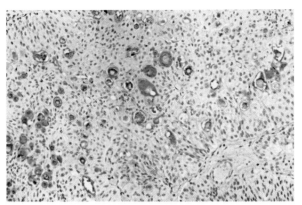

Figure 3-26

UROTHELIAL CARCINOMA, LOW GRADE WITH INTRACELLULAR MUCIN

Left: Hematoxylin and eosin (H&E)–stained specimen.
Right: Alcian blue stain for mucins.

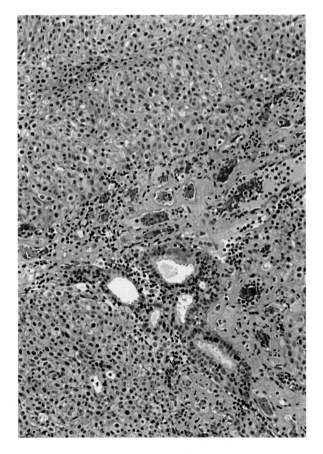

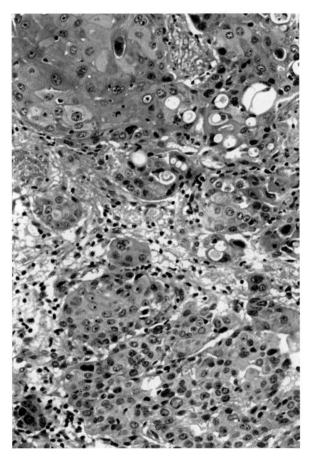

Figure 3-27

**UROTHELIAL CARCINOMA
WITH GLANDULAR DIFFERENTIATION**

Tumors with histologic patterns such as this can be considered "mixed," but the biologic behavior tends to be based upon the grade of the urothelial element.

Figure 3-28

**UROTHELIAL CARCINOMA WITH
SQUAMOUS DIFFERENTIATION**

(Fig. 84 from Murphy WM. Atlas of bladder carcinoma. Chicago: ASCP Press; 1986:67.)

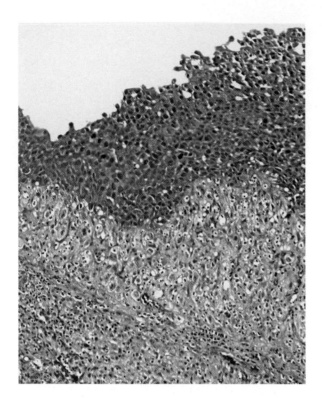

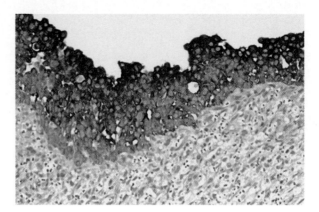

Figure 3-29

**UROTHELIAL CARCINOMA
WITH SPINDLE CELL STROMA**

Left: A dense spindle cell proliferation underlies the urothelial carcinoma.

Above: An immunohistochemical reaction for pancy-tokeratins highlights the epithelium and confirms that the stromal cells are not epithelial.

the pathologist to avoid interpretive errors but they have no other known implications for patient care and there is no compelling reason to include subtype designations such as these in the diagnosis, where their presence might confuse the unsophisticated.

High-grade urothelial carcinomas may produce hormones, the most common of which is beta-human chorionic gonadotropin (ß-HCG) (fig. 3-30) (74,96,127,234). This hormone has been detected in the serum of 10 to 30 percent of bladder cancer patients and in more than 50 percent of individuals with disseminated disease. Tissue localization is much less frequent, probably because the hormone is not stored in secretory granules but released soon after production. Since the free beta subunit has no endocrine function, signs and symptoms related to hormonal abnormalities are rare. The almost exclusive association of increased serum ß-HCG levels with bladder tumors that are predominantly of urothelial differentiation (not choriocarcinomas), and the production of this hormone by normal urothelial cells in culture, suggest a relationship at the genetic transcriptional level. It is tempting to consider urothelial carcinomas that produce ß-HCG as a distinctive variant. The

distinction is lost at the histologic level, however, where tumors associated with increased serum ß-HCG cannot be reliably distinguished from those lacking the hormone. The value of ß-HCG in identifying a subgroup of patients with a poor prognosis has been disputed, undoubtedly because most patients with elevated hormone levels already have advanced disease (74,127).

Adequate cytologic samples from bladders harboring high-grade urothelial carcinomas almost always contain readily recognizable anaplastic cells (see figs. 3-22–3-24; Table 3-4) (143, 172). Diagnostic elements may be scarce and more poorly preserved in voided urine samples than in bladder washings. Inadequate sampling is probably the major source of the often cited "false-negative" interpretations found in the literature, but the subject of endoscopic sampling of bladder lesions has rarely been addressed (158). Neoplastic elements are isolated or loosely clustered. They may be associated with a background of degenerating blood, cellular debris, and inflammation, but this so-called tumor diathesis is not a reliable diagnostic feature. In fact, invasion cannot be accurately predicted by cytologic analysis. Cytoplasmic degeneration and vacuolization are common in

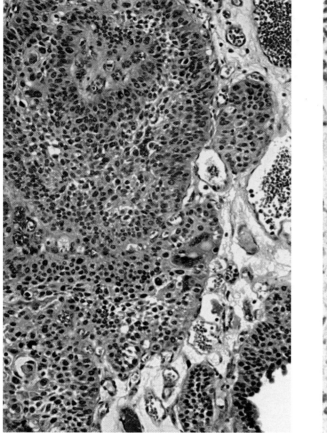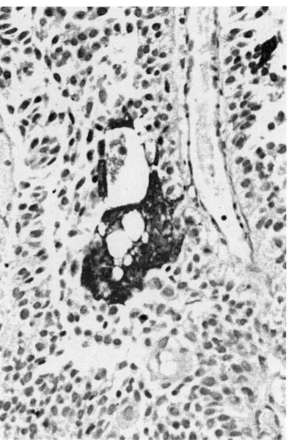

Figure 3-30

UROTHELIAL CARCINOMA WITH SYNCYTIOTROPHOBLASTIC GIANT CELLS

Left: Cells with bizarre nuclei are relatively common in high-grade urothelial carcinomas.
Right: Only a few cells react with antibodies to human chorionic gonadotropin. The positive reaction may be seen in giant cells as well as smaller, mononucleated cells. (Courtesy Dr. J. I. Epstein, Baltimore, MD.)

high-grade neoplastic cells. High-grade neoplastic cells characteristically have moderate to high nuclear-cytoplasmic ratios. Cells with very anaplastic-appearing nuclei but very low nuclear-cytoplasmic ratios may be difficult to distinguish from superficial cells that are affected by topical chemotherapy, and should not form the sole basis for a diagnostic interpretation. As in histologic preparations, nuclear pleomorphism is the most reliable diagnostic feature. Chromatin is coarsely granular and nearly always irregularly dispersed. Large nucleoli occur in some high-grade neoplastic cells. In usual cytologic preparations, high-grade urothelial tumor cells cannot always be distinguished from the cells of other high-grade lesions, such as adenocarcinomas.

In contrast to PUNLMPs and low-grade urothelial carcinomas, high-grade urothelial carcinomas have more cellular heterogeneity. Electron microscopy has not been particularly useful for the recognition of high-grade urothelial carcinomas. The immunohistochemical profile is broad, with no marker yet having sufficient sensitivity and specificity for reliable identification (110).

High-grade urothelial carcinomas grow via local invasion into the bladder wall as well as intramucosal spread into Brunn nests and the prostatic urethra. Concomitant carcinoma in situ at adjacent or distant sites is common in bladders harboring high-grade carcinomas and residual disease after "complete" surgical resection has been documented in many cases (139,177).

Figure 3-31

TRUNCATED PAPILLARY TUMOR AFTER TOPICAL THERAPY

The denuded papillary cores can be recognized by their residual lumens (arrows). (Fig. 2-57 from Murphy WM. Diseases of the urinary bladder, urethra, ureters, and renal pelves. In: Murphy WM, ed. Urological pathology. Philadelphia: WB Saunders; 1997:94.)

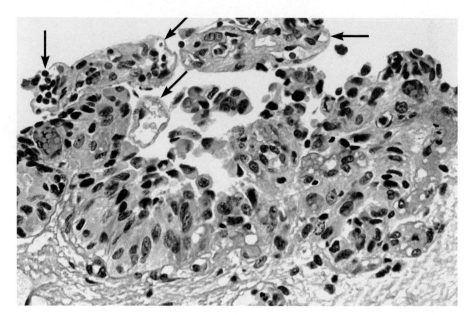

Involvement of prostatic ducts has been documented in up to 40 percent of cystectomy specimens (230). Metastases to regional lymph nodes have been recorded in 20 percent of cases from at least one cancer referral center but are probably less frequent in the bladder cancer population as a whole (118). Of course, the frequency of documented metastases could be a reflection of the thoroughness of the lymph node dissection. Distant metastases are relatively infrequent and can appear in unlikely places. The recorded frequency of distant metastatic sites in decreasing order is: lung, liver, bone, other organs (109).

Prognosis. The prognosis for patients with high-grade urothelial carcinoma is in sharp contrast to the favorable long-term outlook for patients with papillomas, PUNLMPs, and low-grade carcinomas. Almost all disease-related deaths from bladder neoplasms are due to high-grade tumors and in at least 85 percent of cases, the high-grade lesion was the initial neoplasm (132,136). Patient outcome is apparently dependent on multiple factors, most of which have been established by the time of initial clinical detection. Multifocal disease, concomitant carcinoma in situ, depth of invasion into the bladder wall, invasion of the prostatic stroma, metastases, and failure to respond to topical therapy are well established as high-risk factors (104,170). Death from disease in such cases can be as high as 65 percent. The value of subcellular markers,

such as *p53* and its protein product, remains to be established (see Special Techniques).

The outcome can be influenced by treatment, primarily surgery, but 20 percent of patients with noninvasive tumors at initial diagnosis develop progressive lesions and at least 12 percent die of disease (120,152). High-grade tumors that have invaded into the lamina propria are associated with even higher percentages of progression and death (91,235). Patient outcome does not seem to be affected by the substage of the lamina propria invasion, although the data indicate that invasive urothelial neoplasms abutting the muscularis propria are associated with a more adverse outlook than those hugging the mucosa (140).

Most deaths from high-grade urothelial carcinomas occur during the first 5 years of follow-up but adverse outcomes are recorded after many years of patient monitoring. In general, the prognosis for patients with high-grade urothelial carcinomas is poor. Disease-free intervals can be prolonged with early medical intervention but even when rendered disease free, patients cannot expect normal longevity (120,132).

Differential Diagnosis. High-grade urothelial carcinomas are distinguished from low-grade carcinomas by their nuclear clustering, pleomorphism, and chromatin pattern (Table 3-3). Since an intermediate grade of urothelial tumor cell has not been defined, the category of

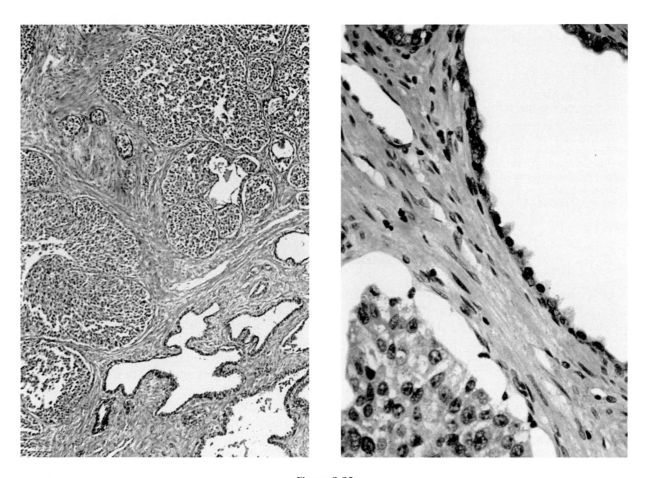

Figure 3-32

UROTHELIAL CARCINOMA INVOLVING PROSTATIC DUCTS

Left: H&E–stained specimen.
Right: Negative prostate-specific antigen immunohistochemical reaction in the tumor cells.

high-grade encompasses a spectrum of morphologic changes, and at least half of the tumors ordinarily graded 2 (of 3) in the 1973 WHO system (168) are classed as high grade in the 1998 WHO/ISUP scheme (102). The papillae of a high-grade carcinoma in patients treated with topical agents are often denuded and collapsed, creating a picture that resembles carcinoma in situ (fig. 3-31). Recognition of capillaries attached to the surface of an undulating high-grade lesion is essential to the correct interpretation.

Differential diagnostic problems may arise when high-grade urothelial carcinomas involve prostatic ducts or when prostatic carcinomas have invaded the bladder base, especially when the primary site is unknown or is unrecorded (fig. 3-32). The nuclei of malignant urothelial

cells are large and pleomorphic, with coarsely granular chromatin and only a few nucleoli. In contrast, the nuclei of prostatic carcinomas are round and relatively uniform, with finely granular chromatin and prominent nucleoli. If necessary, immunohistochemical reactions for prostate-specific antigen can be helpful (185). Reactions for cytokeratins 7 and 20, carcinoembryonic antigens, or cocktails including thrombomodulin, 34ßE12, and cytokeratin 20 are not as specific (89,110,192). Reactions for uroplakin III are potentially specific but not particularly sensitive (135,192).

The appearance of squamous, glandular, or histologically benign stromal elements in a high-grade urothelial carcinoma does not alter the basic interpretation, although their presence

Figure 3-33

UROTHELIAL CARCINOMA IN SITU

Cystoscopically, CIS may appear as normal urothelium (left) or as erythematous urothelium (right) in different patients at different times in the course of their disease. (Courtesy of Dr. Mark S. Soloway, Miami, FL.)

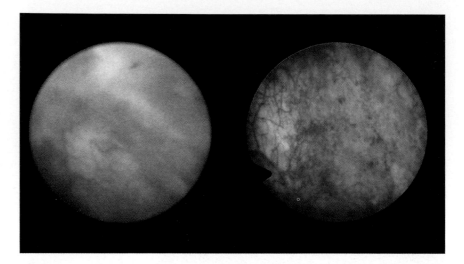

could be mentioned in a comment. Foci of small cell carcinoma, with or without polypeptide production, may be important and should be included in the diagnostic interpretation.

Carcinoma in Situ

Definition and General Features. Urothelial carcinoma in situ (CIS) is a flat, noninvasive neoplasm composed of cells of high cytologic grade (164). Glandular variants have been described but are rare and difficult to define (79). Squamous CIS is equally difficult to characterize. Anaplastic cells appear in all layers but do not always replace the full thickness of the urothelium. Similar lesions have been called moderate and severe dysplasia in other formulations. CIS may vary in its degree of cytologic anaplasia and a range of morphologic changes can be appreciated; nevertheless, grading is not recommended.

Clinical Features. The clinical features of urothelial CIS differ from those of other urothelial neoplasms. Primary lesions are rare, occurring in less than 1 percent of individuals with urinary symptoms (107). In contrast, foci of CIS have been identified in nearly every bladder removed for invasive carcinoma (144). CIS is unusual in association with low-grade papillary lesions but quite common in bladders harboring high-grade carcinomas. The tendency for patients to have symptoms for years prior to diagnosis and for lesions to persist without invasion for years after detection has been observed frequently (107,163). CIS is usually multifocal, often involving the urothelium in areas other than the bladder base (84).

The signs and symptoms of patients with primary CIS are more suggestive of an infection than a neoplasm; they are essentially the same as those of interstitial cystitis. The severity of symptoms tends to parallel the extent of the lesion. Hematuria is common but patients are more discomfited by dysuria, frequency, and suprapubic pain. At cystoscopy, CIS may appear as either erythematous or normal mucosa (fig. 3-33).

Pathologic Findings. Histologically, CIS exists in several patterns (144,190). Most often, cells with high nuclear-cytoplasmic ratios, amphophilic cytoplasm, and indistinct borders are irregularly arranged over discrete areas of urothelium (figs. 3-34–3-36). The demarcation between CIS and the adjacent mucosa is nearly always sharp, even when coexistent epithelial atypicalities are present. Hyperplasia (more than seven cell layers) is unusual, and multilayered neoplastic urothelium should be suspected of representing the base of a papillary lesion. Slight maturation may occur as cells progress toward the epithelial surface and remnants of the superficial cell layer may be preserved. Nuclear pleomorphism is prominent. Nuclei are large and irregular, with coarsely granular, irregularly dispersed chromatin. Many have large nucleoli. Mitoses are variable and occasionally abnormal. Very rarely, cells with nuclei characteristic of CIS are small and densely aggregated, a pattern that has sometimes been called the small cell variant. The term "small cell" used in this regard is purely descriptive and does not connote neuroendocrine differentiation.

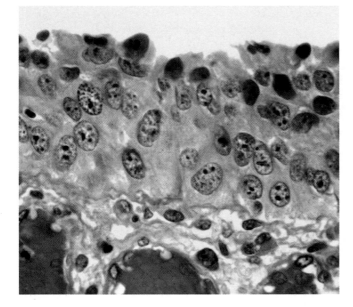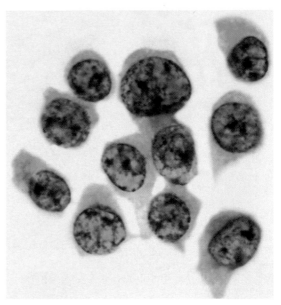

Figure 3-34

UROTHELIAL CARCINOMA IN SITU

Left: Histology of a lesion with little dyscohesion.
Right: In cytologic preparations, these cells are indistinguishable from those of any other high-grade urothelial neoplasm.

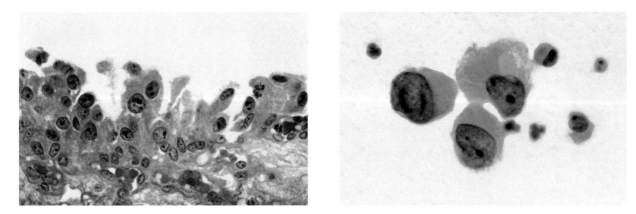

Figure 3-35

UROTHELIAL CARCINOMA IN SITU

Left: Characteristic appearance of CIS in a bladder biopsy. There is considerable cellular dyscohesion. Normal nuclei are scattered among the neoplastic elements.
Right: High-grade neoplastic cells. (Fig. 2-1 from Murphy WM. Urinary cytopathology. Chicago: ASCP Press; 2000:7.)

In approximately 10 percent of cases, CIS is composed of large cells with relatively low nuclear-cytoplasmic ratios, fairly well-defined borders, and slightly acidophilic cytoplasm (fig. 3-37) (190). When seen en face, this lesion resembles extramammary Paget's disease and has been called the pagetoid variant. So-called pagetoid CIS is rarely, if ever, the primary lesion and usually comprises only small foci in a CIS of the usual pattern.

All histologic variants of CIS may be associated with marked inflammation of the lamina propria and vascular ectasia. The relationship of the inflammation to the neoplasm is not completely clear but is almost certainly nonspecific.

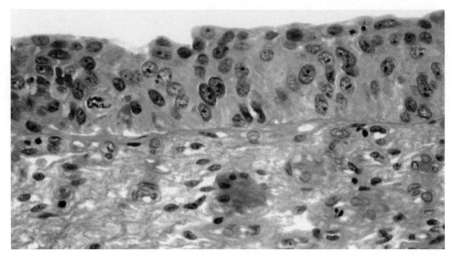

Figure 3-36

**UROTHELIAL
CARCINOMA IN SITU**

Top: This specimen might be construed as representing the lower end of the histologic spectrum.

Bottom: High-grade neoplastic cells.

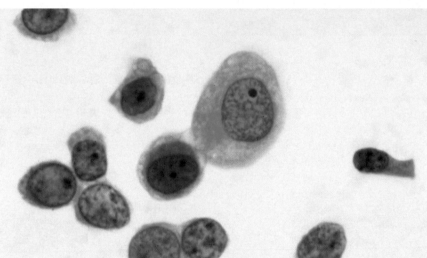

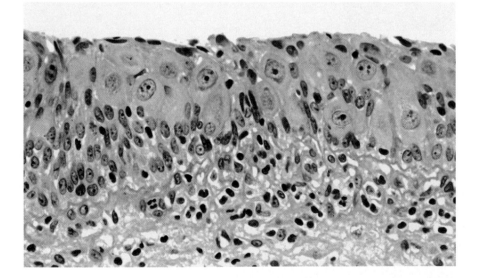

Figure 3-37

**UROTHELIAL CARCINOMA
IN SITU, PAGETOID TYPE**

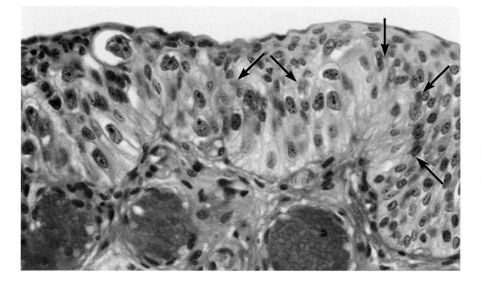

Figure 3-38

UROTHELIAL CARCINOMA IN SITU, UNDERMINING ADJACENT UROTHELIUM

The neoplastic cells have grown along the basement membrane, creating a sharp demarcation with the overlying normal urothelium (arrows).

A common feature of urothelial CIS is the lack of intercellular cohesion, resulting in extensive denudation of the epithelium in tissue sections. In such cases, the pathologist should resist the temptation to interpret the material as "negative" as if no abnormality were present; the term "denudation" is more appropriate. When the urothelium is markedly denuded in a patient being followed for bladder cancer or denuding cystitis, not only should the remaining epithelial cells be examined for cytologic anaplasia, but urinary specimens should be reviewed for malignant cells.

Cytologic samples from untreated patients with urothelial CIS often contain numerous high-grade neoplastic cells. With few exceptions, these cells have features of any high-grade bladder neoplasm. In our experience, in situ lesions cannot be reliably distinguished from invasive tumors using urinary cytology alone. Malignant tumor cells are readily identified in urinary samples and despite an inability to determine location or depth of invasion, cytology remains the most reliable method for detection of both primary and recurrent/persistent cancer in this group of patients.

Abnormalities in the molecular biology of CIS are myriad but none has been widely accepted as crucial to either diagnosis or prognosis (see Special Techniques) (92,113). If anything, the cells of this noninvasive lesion seem more disturbed than those of deeply invasive, high-grade urothelial carcinomas. These changes further document the extreme cellular derangement of CIS and suggest that invasion and metastasis require more than aberrations of tumor cells alone.

CIS grows by intramucosal extension and can spread throughout the ductular system of the prostate and even into the seminal vesicles (fig. 3-38). As previously noted, prostatic involvement by urothelial carcinoma has been documented in up to 40 percent of cystectomy specimens (230). There is little evidence to suggest that CIS spontaneously regresses, but the lesions may never invade. The conditions that favor invasion are unknown but must not include mechanical disruption of the basement membrane, since mucosal biopsies do not result in an increased frequency of invasive tumors at the biopsy sites.

Prognosis. The literature on CIS is confounded by the tendency of most authors to group patients with previous and coincident urothelial neoplasms plus CIS with cases in which CIS is the primary lesion. The fact that the previous neoplasms may have been papillary and noninvasive is not necessarily mitigating, since nearly all of these papillary lesions would have been of high cytologic grade and the prognosis of patients presenting with high-grade, noninvasive urothelial carcinoma is not good. When urothelial CIS is the initial bladder neoplasm, patients seem to have a favorable prognosis (106,189). In arguably the best

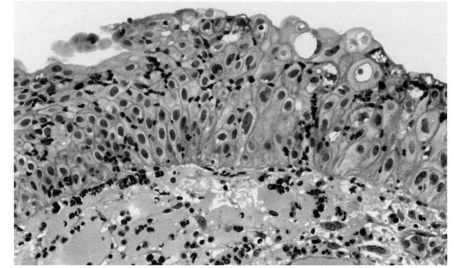

Figure 3-39

REACTIVE UROTHELIUM SECONDARY TO X-RAY THERAPY

X-ray therapy delivered to adjacent organs such as the prostate gland can create urothelial changes resembling the pagetoid variant of CIS.

documented study, invasion at the time of cystectomy was almost always limited to the lamina propria and usually occurred at only one site; the frequency was 34 percent (106). Only 6 percent of patients in this study died of bladder cancer. Even when case studies include patients having previous noninvasive neoplasms, the cancer-specific 15-year survival rate is 74 percent (84). In contrast, it has been the general experience that patients with multifocal CIS, CIS in conjunction with high-grade invasive urothelial carcinomas, CIS unresponsive to topical therapy, and CIS involving the prostatic ducts do poorly (107,170,196).

Differential Diagnosis. When adequately sampled and of typical histology, urothelial CIS is a distinctive neoplasm that is easily recognized by knowledgeable pathologists. Often, however, the lesion is markedly denuded or represented by only a small group of cells in an otherwise normal or reactive epithelium. In such cases, the most reliable approach to diagnosis is to examine the bladder washings that should have been obtained prior to any bladder manipulation and biopsy. Even a few high-grade tumor cells in a urinary specimen from a patient treated and followed for bladder cancer are diagnostic. Immunohistochemical reactions for various markers may be helpful in certain cases but none of these markers is as sensitive and specific as the discriminating capacity of the confident diagnostician (162).

CIS must be distinguished from intraepithelial abnormalities of lesser degrees of cellular anaplasia, so-called dysplasia or atypia (102). The point at which cells lack the morphology of carcinoma has not been adequately determined and a certain level of interobserver variability at the low end of the CIS spectrum must be expected (202). Antibodies that identify abnormal intracellular structures or DNA seem to offer promise but their utility remains to be established (113).

The histologic changes caused by irradiation can be difficult to distinguish from those of CIS, especially when the patient's history is either lacking or erroneously recorded on the pathology transmittal slip (fig. 3-39). Radiation changes in the urothelium may manifest as cells with enlarged, pleomorphic nuclei with nucleoli but, since this is a reactive/regenerative process, the cells tend to be cohesive and may have distinctive cellular borders. Urinary cytology is negative. When radiation reactions occur in the urothelium, the component cells often resemble those of the pagetoid variant of CIS and it is important to remember that this variant essentially never occurs as the primary lesion. The nuclei of pagetoid CIS tend to be more pleomorphic than those of reactive urothelium but the nuclear-cytoplasmic ratios of both lesions may be low.

Dysplastic Intraepithelial Lesions

Definition and General Features. Dysplasia and atypia are the most commonly used terms to describe a group of urothelial changes that resemble lesions of similar names in other organs. This terminology is highly controversial but essential to any discussion of urothelial neoplasms, since these lesions tend to define the limits of the qualitative light microscopic approach to the subject. The concept that all carcinomas arise from preexisting epithelium is widely accepted, but the processes by which intraepithelial neoplasms develop in humans are largely unknown. Until the carcinogenic process is better understood, controversy concerning epithelial changes of lesser degrees of morphologic anaplasia than CIS is inevitable (102). No single term seems to encompass all facets of the problem and various designations have been proposed: dysplasia, CIS grade 1, atypical hyperplasia, atypia, simple hyperplasia, and urothelial intraepithelial neoplasia all refer to the same lesions. As defined here, urothelial dysplasia describes a spectrum of histologic changes occurring in flat, noninvasive urothelium. These changes may arise from a variety of stimuli, including neoplastic and non-neoplastic, but can be distinguished morphologically from other lesions recognized as either reactive, regenerative, or CIS (Table 3-6) (82,83,102,174).

Clinical Features. The clinical features associated with dysplastic urothelial abnormalities are poorly characterized. Almost all cases are uncovered in bladders that have already developed carcinomas (107,144,177). The incidence of dysplastic lesions in the general population is unknown but the frequency among bladder cancer patients varies from 20 to 86 percent. Lesions are more easily documented and probably much more common in association with advanced disease. Experiences in clinic and hospital populations, where patients were only partially selected because of known bladder neoplasms, suggest that the frequency of dysplastic changes among noncancer patients is probably less than 5 percent (83,170). The lack of visible cystoscopic abnormalities, obvious cytologic changes, and serum markers make early detection of this lesion a sporadic, serendipitous event.

Concern about the importance of dysplastic urothelial lesions centers upon the following observations: dysplastic lesions are often observed in bladders harboring carcinomas; the cells in dysplastic lesions morphologically resemble those in low-grade papillary tumors; experimental animals exposed to large doses of chemical carcinogens develop carcinomas through a series of intraepithelial changes of increasing cytologic severity; the ultrastructural and antigenic composition of dysplastic lesions more closely resemble CIS than normal urothelium; and the appearance of urothelial dysplasia in patients with a history of bladder cancer may increase the risk of an adverse outcome (83,177). This information is somewhat tempered by the following: urinary dysplasia has not been well defined and a great deal of interobserver variation in interpretation can be expected; dysplastic lesions are uncommon, if not rare, in noncancer patients; the frequency and severity of dysplasia seems to parallel rather than precede advanced neoplastic disease; few studies have documented an increased risk of an adverse outcome among patients with mildly dysplastic lesions; and only 3 to 10 percent of patients with dysplasia in the best-documented studies died from bladder cancer over a 10- to 25-year period (83,170,177,205).

Current information indicates that urothelial abnormalities described as dysplasia may be risk factors for an adverse outcome among patients with previous or coincident neoplasms, but the degree of risk is apparently small. Until methods to identify these lesions in patients without bladder neoplasms are developed, their clinical significance will likely remain obscure.

Pathologic Findings. Dysplastic cells are recognized in histologic preparations by the disorientation and clustering of their nuclei (fig. 3-40). When compared to normal cells in other areas of the specimen, dysplastic cells have a more homogeneous cytoplasm and larger nuclei. Nuclei may seem to overlap. The notches, creases, and shallow depressions of nuclear borders seen in PUNLMPs are present but less pronounced. Chromatin is finely granular and evenly dispersed. Nucleoli are absent or small. Mitoses are rare.

Dysplastic cells are seen in urinary samples (172). Not surprisingly, they resemble the changes previously described for PUNLMPs. In fact, the nuclear changes in cells from flat dysplastic lesions are so similar to those in cells from low-grade papillary lesions that distinction probably cannot be made in most cases.

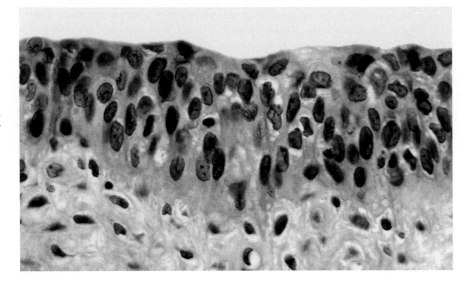

Figure 3-40

UROTHELIAL DYSPLASIA

Large, clustered nuclei with irregular borders create disordered urothelium.

Prognosis. The pathways of growth and progression of dysplastic lesions are not known. It is tempting to believe that dysplastic lesions represent a phase in the development of CIS and many experts have expressed this theory with the term "intraurothelial neoplasia." The evidence that dysplastic lesions are precursors of either flat or papillary urothelial neoplasms in humans is scant (80,93,211,226). Putative markers of abnormal development have not been generally present in lesions interpreted as dysplasia by light microscopy, whereas some of these markers have been identified in histologically normal urothelium (115,128,226,229). Even in selected examples, the rate of progression associated with primary urothelial dysplasia is low and death from bladder cancer is lower still (83,206,237). When urothelial carcinomas do develop, they do not seem to arise preferentially from the sites of the previously diagnosed dysplasia (83). In fact, a significant majority of individuals having biopsies interpreted as primary urothelial dysplasia never develop a more serious histologically documented urothelial abnormality. Given the evidence, urothelial dysplasia cannot be confirmed as either a neoplasm or a precursor.

Differential Diagnosis. If urothelial dysplasia is not considered to represent the low end of the morphologic spectrum of CIS, then it is important to distinguish the two lesions (Table 3-6). The distinction rests primarily on the recognition of nuclear anaplasia as manifested by enlarged nuclei with irregular borders and coarsely granular chromatin, often with one or more large nucleoli. Accurate interpretation becomes more difficult when anaplastic cells are scattered or exist in only a single small focus in the epithelium. It is important to remember that abnormal nuclei must be in the subsuperficial cell layers of the urothelium for an interpretation of CIS. Superficial cells can have nuclei with all the features commonly ascribed to carcinoma and yet still be reactive. The distinction between dysplasia and CIS can be facilitated by urinary cytology, where the high-grade tumor cells of CIS tend to be easily distinguished from the cells of dysplasia. As with CIS, dysplastic lesions are essentially never hyperplastic and the presence of an apparently hyperplastic dysplasia should raise the suspicion that one is viewing the flat component of a papillary tumor.

At the opposite end of the morphologic spectrum, dysplastic lesions tend to resemble reactive processes resulting from a variety of stimuli, including preparation artifacts. In many cases, urothelial dysplasia can be differentiated from reactive atypias by nuclear clustering, nuclear border irregularities, granular chromatin, and the absence of prominent nucleoli. The variations in the histologic definition of urothelial dysplasia reported in the literature have tended to cause more confusion than clarity, and recognition of dysplastic urothelial lesions in pathologic specimens is likely to remain problematic.

Table 3-6

COMPARISON OF DYSPLASIA TO CARCINOMA IN SITU AND REACTIVE UROTHELIUM[a]

	CIS[b]	Dysplasia	Reactive
Cell layers	Variable	Variable	Variable
Mucosal infiltrate	Absent	Absent	Variable
Polarization	Abnormal	Slightly abnormal	Slightly abnormal
Cytoplasm	Homogeneous	Homogeneous	Vacuolated
N-C ratio[c]	Increased	Slightly increased	Normal, slightly increased
Nuclei			
Position	Variable	Clustered	Normal
Borders	Pleomorphic	Notches, creases	Regular, smooth
Chromatin	Coarse	Fine	Fine, dusty
Distribution	Uneven	Even	Even
Nucleoli	Large	Small, absent	Prominent
Mitoses	Variable	Variable	Variable

[a]Modified from Table 2-10 from Murphy WM. Diseases of the urinary bladder, urethra, ureters, and renal pelves. In: Murphy WM, ed. Urological pathology. Philadelphia: WB Saunders; 1989:96.
[b]CIS = Carcinoma in situ.
[c]N-C ratio = nuclear-cytoplasmic ratio.

Two categories of atypia are recognized in the 1998 WHO/ISUP classification (82,102,198). These designations were probably accepted for the sake of completeness and as a counterpoint to dysplasia and CIS. In any case, they do not describe neoplasms or preneoplastic states.

A category of papillary urothelial hyperplasia is also recognized in the 1998 WHO/ISUP classification. This is a controversial and as yet poorly accepted lesion. Illustrations tend to depict a growth pattern with rather stubby, broad stalks that is difficult to distinguish from an undulating but basically flat mucosa. Very likely, most of these lesions would be included among other categories of urothelial disease or given little credence by the majority of pathologists.

Variants of Urothelial (Transitional Cell) Carcinoma

Variants of urothelial carcinoma are neoplasms differentiating toward urothelium but having unexpected histologic patterns (see Table 3-1) (170,232). The unexpected element, whether a gland-like lumen (microcyst), cell nest, or focus of "papillary" cells, may occur as a minor component in many urothelial neoplasms. The variation becomes noteworthy only when it is florid or when awareness of it will avoid diagnostic error.

Urothelial tumors with heterologous elements, mixed epithelial differentiation, and hormone production have been discussed in the section on high-grade urothelial carcinomas. Spindle cells in the stroma of a urothelial neoplasm can be benign or carcinomatous, an especially important factor when the tissue sample lacks epithelial elements. Anecdotal reports of variations, such as urothelial carcinoma with optically clear cell features, appear sporadically in the literature (146). In the following sections, well-characterized variants of urothelial carcinoma are discussed.

Urothelial Carcinoma with Gland-Like Lumens (Microcystic Variant). This is an uncommon tumor characterized by the presence of prominent intercellular or intracellular lumens that are surrounded by neoplastic urothelial or squamous cells (figs. 3-41, 3-42) (95,97,232, 233). It is important primarily for accurate differentiation from adenocarcinoma. Lumens may occur in all grades of urothelial carcinoma but are more frequent in high-grade tumors. They are usually small but may reach cystic proportions. Most appear empty in usual histologic

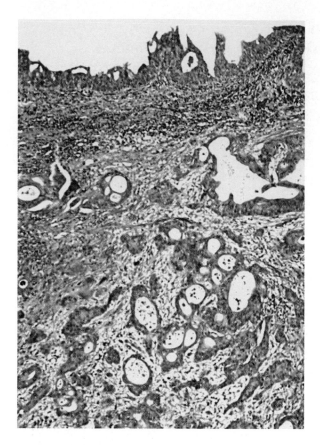

Figure 3-41

UROTHELIAL CARCINOMA, HIGH GRADE, WITH GLAND-LIKE LUMENS

preparations but some contain granular acidophilic material or necrotic tumor cells. Appropriate histochemical reactions reveal small amounts of predominantly acid mucins in almost all cases. Ultrastructural studies have confirmed the light microscopic findings. In most instances, these gland-like structures probably reflect a genetically programmed ability of urothelial cells to form and line spaces (like bladders). The glandular debris and necrotic cells found in a few lumens suggest a degenerative etiology in some cases. The presence of gland-like spaces has no known prognostic significance.

The distinction of urothelial carcinomas with gland-like lumens from urothelial tumors with glandular differentiation and adenocarcinomas is somewhat arbitrary, since it might be argued that the arrangement of epithelial cells around a lumen constitutes a gland, regardless of whether or not substances are produced by the cells. Nevertheless, the distinctions described here are important when the urothelial neoplasm is of low cytologic grade. They are also important because an adenocarcinoma appearing in bladder tissue may represent direct extension from a primary cancer of the gastrointestinal tract. Adenocarcinomas of the bladder do not seem to differ pathologically from those of the gastrointestinal tract; all variations occur. In contrast, the histologic architecture of the gland-like variant of urothelial carcinoma is distinctly urothelial. Extracellular lumens are lined by flattened cells rather than goblet cells and the pattern is reminiscent of cystitis glandularis et cystica.

Urothelial Carcinoma, Nested Type. This is a rare bladder tumor in which neoplastic urothelial cells are arranged in structures resembling proliferations of Brunn nests (figs. 3-43, 3-44) (99,216). It is only important because its seemingly benign architecture and cytology belie its potentially aggressive behavior. Therefore, high-grade neoplasms with focal nests and tumors with an overlying surface of CIS should not be included among cases of this variant.

Almost all reported cases of the nested variant have occurred in men, aged 53 to 97 years, who presented with hematuria, urgency, or signs of ureteral obstruction. Lesions tend to be small and multifocal; they are often localized to ureteral orifices. The overlying urothelium is ordinarily histologically normal. The distinctive feature of this variant is the arrangement of tumor cells in nests and abortive tubules, suggestive of cystitis glandularis et cystica. The nests can be compact or separated. Degenerative changes may result in a microcystic appearance. Most of the neoplastic cells are only slightly atypical but scattered anaplastic elements are found in every case. Often, the degree of nuclear anaplasia increases with the depth of invasion. In half the cases, a urothelial neoplasm of more usual type is present (99).

Urothelial carcinoma, nested type, grows by invasion of the bladder wall. Persistent disease is the rule and death from disease has been documented in about 25 percent of patients. Cystectomy may be beneficial but the history of the treated patients with this rare tumor remains to be elucidated.

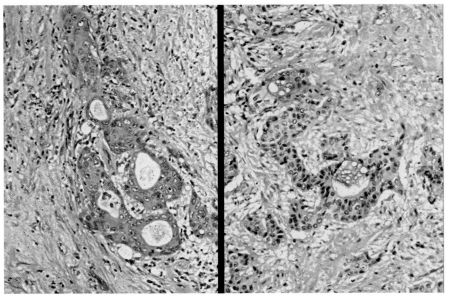

Figure 3-42

UROTHELIAL CARCINOMA, HIGH GRADE, WITH GLAND-LIKE LUMENS

Left: The cells surrounding the lumens have an architectural pattern reminiscent of urothelium rather than colon.

Right: Mucins are present in the lumens; goblet cells are not identified.

Figure 3-43

UROTHELIAL CARCINOMA, NESTED TYPE

(Courtesy of Dr. Daniel M. Lundblad, Parkersburg, WV.)

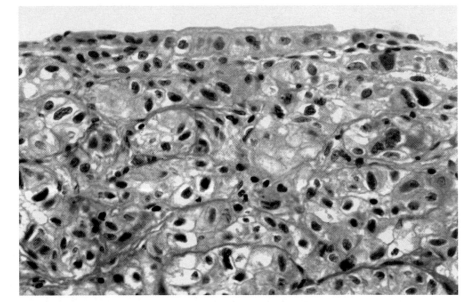

Urothelial carcinoma, nested type, can be differentiated from prostatic carcinoma by its location, histology, and negative reactions for prostate-specific antigen and prostatic acid phosphatase. A lack of colonic differentiation distinguishes it from adenocarcinoma. These tumors differ from proliferations of Brunn nests by their invasive growth pattern and focal nuclear anaplasia. They are distinguished from nephrogenic metaplasia by their multilayering, even in tubular foci; the tubules of nephrogenic metaplasia are always lined by a single layer of cells.

Urothelial Carcinoma, Sarcomatoid Type. This unusual tumor is composed predominantly of spindle cells that surround isolated islands of pure or mixed urothelial carcinoma (fig. 3-45) (126,131,200,228,232). It is important primarily because of its distinction from sarcoma, a distinction initially claimed using immunohistochemistry to identify cytokeratins among the spindle cells. The range of phenotypic changes that are included in the category "sarcomatoid" has varied over time. In many previous publications, for example, bladder tumors with a combination

285

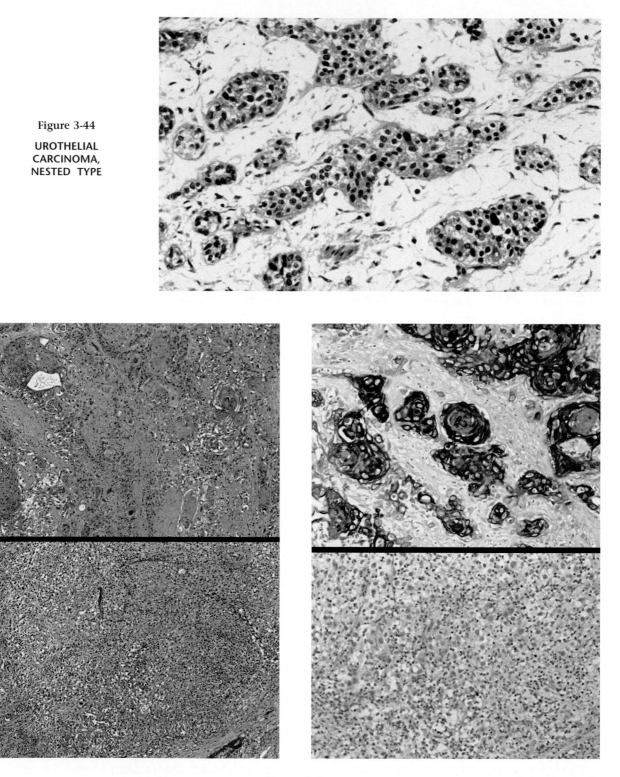

Figure 3-44

UROTHELIAL CARCINOMA, NESTED TYPE

Figure 3-45

UROTHELIAL CARCINOMA, HOMOLOGOUS SARCOMATOID TYPE

Left: Islands of malignant epithelial differentiation (top) should be sought among the predominantly spindle cell neoplasm.
Right: The islands of epithelial differentiation react for pancytokeratins (top) whereas the spindle cell elements may not.

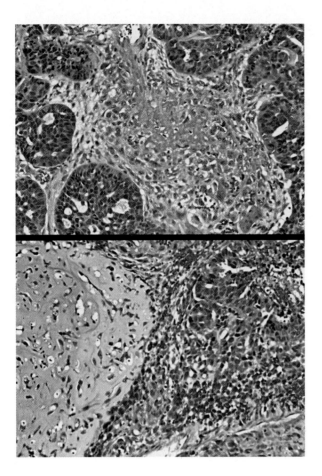

Figure 3-46

UROTHELIAL CARCINOMA, HETEROLOGOUS SARCOMATOID TYPE (CARCINOSARCOMA)

The heterologous element is usually chondrosarcomatous but may be an osteosarcoma. Other types are less common.

of urothelial and mesenchymal differentiation have been separately classified as carcinosarcoma or malignant mixed mesodermal tumor (fig. 3-46) (67,133,155,231). The more recent preference is to include these lesions among the sarcomatoid carcinomas, adding the descriptor "with heterologous differentiation" (101).

The clinical features of patients with sarcomatoid carcinoma, with or without heterologous differentiation, do not differ significantly from those of high-grade urothelial carcinomas, except perhaps for a slightly lower male to female ratio. Cystoscopically, lesions tend to be infiltrative with a polypoid surface. Microscopically, the tumors often resemble malignant fibrous histiocytomas, but some are reminiscent of pseudosar-

comatous fibromyxoid tumors (inflammatory pseudotumors) while others contain separate foci of high-grade urothelial carcinoma and malignant mesenchymal elements such as cartilage or bone. Myxoid and sclerosing areas have been described (131). Multiple tissue sections may be necessary to uncover the islands of epithelial differentiation or foci of CIS that are diagnostic. A previous history of urothelial carcinoma may be helpful, as is a diffusely positive reaction for cytokeratins, but focal positivity for cytokeratins can occur in true sarcomas.

These cancers grow by invasion of the bladder wall. Most urothelial carcinomas of the sarcomatoid type are high stage at diagnosis and the 5-year survival rate is less than 30 percent. Individuals with low-stage disease have a more favorable outlook. Treatment is variable, consisting of surgical resection with or without radiation and chemotherapy.

The homologous type of the sarcomatoid variant is best recognized by the identification of malignant epithelial islands within the spindle cells or CIS in the overlying mucosa. Immunohistochemistry can be helpful but may be confusing as well. Differentiation from pseudosarcomatous lesions is achieved by appreciating the presence of both malignant epithelial islands and malignant spindle cells.

Urothelial Carcinoma, Micropapillary Type. This is an unusual variant that may be more common in practice than the reported cases suggest (fig. 3-47) (62,130,161). It is important because of its aggressive behavior, even when present in only a few foci. The tumors are histologically reminiscent of a papillary serous cystadenocarcinoma of the ovary. The papillary component appears as clusters of cells with peripherally arranged nuclei, creating a rosette-like pattern. Many of the spaces surrounding the clusters are artifacts but vascular invasion is common. Mucins tend to be absent. Nuclei may vary in degree of anaplasia but most are high grade. The molecular characteristics of these tumors are poorly understood, probably due to their rarity.

The micropapillary variant grows by invasion and dissemination. Importantly, the micropapillary pattern is retained in metastases. Involvement of the muscular wall should be assumed whether or not a portion of muscularis propria appears in the tissue sample. Prognosis is

287

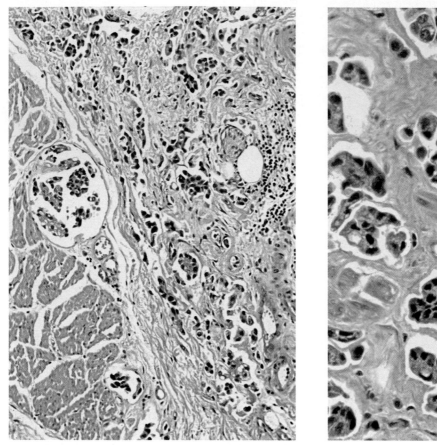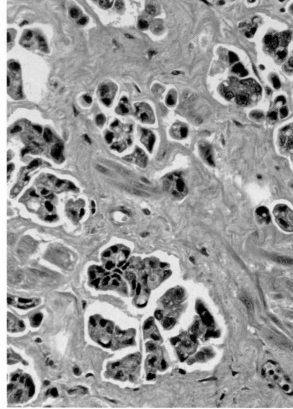

Figure 3-47

UROTHELIAL CARCINOMA, MICROPAPILLARY TYPE

Left: Invasion of the muscular wall is usual in tumors manifesting this variation.
Right: Mucins are either not present or present in very small amounts.

particularly poor and has not been affected by treatment. Distinction from other entities has not been a problem for those aware of this variant.

Special Techniques

Urothelial tissues and cells can be examined for their total DNA (ploidy), quantitative morphometric features, structural antigenic composition, genetic and chromosomal constitution, gene protein products, and presence and rate of DNA synthesis. Information is often obtained using immunohistochemistry and the light microscope. Other methods include enzyme-linked immunoabsorbent assay, fluorescence in situ hybridization and in situ hybridization, silver impregnation, instrumentation using computerized programs for capturing and reconstructing light scatter from dyes exposed to laser beams,

laser capture microdissection, DNA (RNA) microarray analysis, and polymerase chain reactions. Many of these techniques are not new; they become "special" primarily in contrast to "routine" methodologies. The role of so-called special techniques in the assessment of human bladder tumors is evolving but clarity in this area remains elusive. Quite simply, there is too much information to handle and more data appear in the literature daily. At times, it seems that both medical and lay communities have convinced themselves that technology has brought us to the brink of a new era in clinical medicine and we intend to make it so as a matter of faith, if not fact. This attitude tends to be reinforced by a system that demands and rewards newness, seemingly for its own sake. The environment invites misuse if not abuse and great caution should be employed by anyone trying to use this information for patient care (124,154,171,202).

The value of special techniques tends to be confounded by a traditional laxity in the use of medical terminology. The term "bladder cancer" in a medical report, for example, with all of its frightening connotations, includes lesions that are probably not malignant or are associated with a very low likelihood of an adverse outcome. The term "superficial bladder cancer" encompasses neoplasms of a wide range of potential behavior. We say that a tumor has "progressed" when in fact that tumor has usually been completely excised and any future events for the patient are due to a new tumor that developed. These new tumors are traditionally termed "recurrences," as if the original lesion had developed a life of its own when in fact the mere presence of a new tumor does not necessarily mean bad things for patients. Applying special techniques to the detection of "recurrent superficial bladder cancer" might well detect lesions that will do patients no harm.

The well-known limitations of cystoscopy and urinary cytopathology for the detection of urothelial neoplasms have sustained a long-lasting search for more sensitive and specific methods (92,113,141,203). Techniques that require little or no interpretation are preferred, not only because of the anticipation of greater precision but because of lower costs. Almost always, the medium of choice has been urine and the methods have been applied for monitoring patients with a history of previous bladder tumors.

Antibodies. Refinements in immunohistochemistry have facilitated the development of commercially available antibodies to a vast array of substances, ranging from slurries of ground up bladder tumors to specific gene protein products (113,173,203). Among well-characterized antigens, the best known include Lewis X, cytokeratin 20, hyaluronic acid/hyaluronidase, telomerase, uroplakins, thrombomodulin, and p53 protein (112,153,188,192,195, 199). Substances composed of mixtures of (bladder tumor) antigens as well as nuclear matrix proteins that have been associated with bladder neoplasms have become popular (72,77,111,141, 165,204). In most instances, the favored technique for identification has been an antigen-antibody reaction developed with immunoperoxidase, but immunofluorescence, colorimetry, and enzyme-linked immunoabsorbent assays have also been used. Antibodies to tumor-related antigens can be applied to tissue sections to distinguish epithelial cells from stromal cells and to determine the primary site of metastatic cancers. With the possible exception of uroplakins, none of these antigenic substances is specific for urothelial neoplasms, however.

Chromosomes and Genes. Relatively simple methods for detecting aberrations in chromosomal number and more sophisticated techniques for uncovering microsatellite aberrations on chromosomes (especially 9) and mutations in genes (especially *p53*) have been applied to the detection of urothelial neoplasms (114,160, 169,210,225). These approaches have the advantage of identifying the tumor cells themselves rather than by-products of tumor-related changes in the adjacent tissue. Most chromosomal and genetic aberrations are confined to high-grade carcinomas, raising the possibility of epiphenomena. Further, the ability to recognize a single genetically abnormal cell raises questions concerning the point at which early detection has meaningful implications for patient care.

Morphometry. Morphometry has been evaluated as a tool for tumor assessment (71,223). The size, number, and distribution of any particulate cellular component can be quantitated. Using only a few actual measurements, a variety of indices can be calculated. Despite more than two decades of refinements, morphometry has not yet been incorporated into the armamentarium of clinical care.

The volume of data using special techniques to detect urothelial neoplasms has become so weighty that some experts advocate the routine implementation of these methodologies without the rigors of further examination (219). When examined closely for their application to patient care, however, putative markers for the early detection of bladder cancer in urinary specimens have yet to fulfill their promise (69,78,113,182). Most are too sensitive, raising the prospect of a bladder neoplasm in a significant number of patients who either do not have a tumor or whose neoplasm has not developed to the point where its presence can be confirmed by more traditional approaches. Even if they could be made more specific, most of these techniques are best

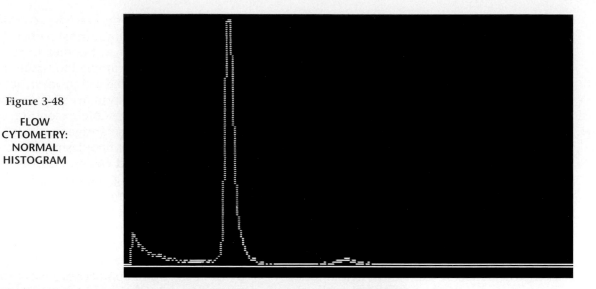

Figure 3-48

FLOW CYTOMETRY: NORMAL HISTOGRAM

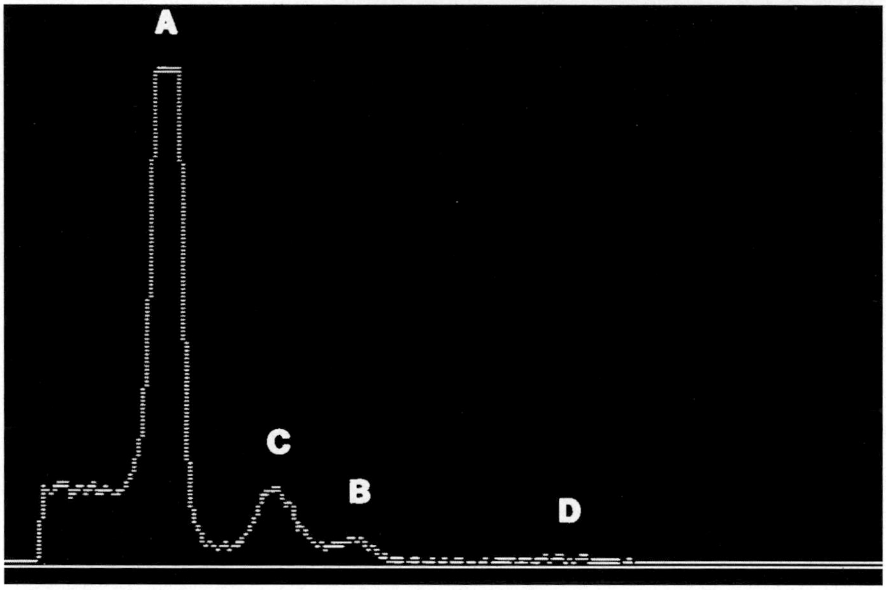

Figure 3-49

FLOW CYTOMETRY: ANEUPLOID HISTOGRAM

A and B mark the normal GIG0 peak and the normal G2M peak, respectively. C and D represent the aneuploid peak and its G2M peak.

suited to the detection of low-grade, noninvasive, papillary neoplasms that are not aggressive and do not require early recognition. Comparisons of data among series are very difficult and no single study has been sufficiently conclusive for general acceptance. The factors that create and maintain a neoplastic state in any individual are extraordinarily complex and cannot be elucidated by the identification of any particular substance at a single point in time.

Cytometry. In contrast to other special techniques, cytometry has come into widespread use for the monitoring of patients with blad-

der neoplasms and for identifying patients with potentially aggressive grade 2 carcinomas of the 1973 WHO system (figs. 3-48–3-50) (222,227). The most popular methods use image analyzers and flow cytometers. Image analyzers process material relatively slowly compared to flow cytometers but offer the advantages of operator interaction and image storage. Flow cytometers can assess large numbers of nuclei in seconds but generally destroy the specimen in the process. Neither method can detect every neoplasm nor can measurements of DNA alone accurately predict the course of the disease

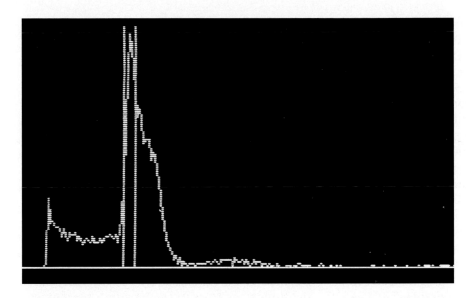

Figure 3-50

FLOW CYTOMETRY: HYPERDIPLOID HISTOGRAM

The diagnostic significance of this type of histogram is controversial. In this case, 62 percent of the cells examined fell outside the normal GIG0 peak and the patient had a urothelial carcinoma of the bladder.

(217). The methodology requires a great deal of operator discretion; it is inaccurate to consider quantitation of DNA content as a totally objective test.

The terminology for expressing DNA ploidy has not been standardized. In general, normal histograms are called diploid or euploid whereas abnormal histograms are labeled aneuploid. Aneuploid histograms are often further subdivided as tetraploid or hypertetraploid when an abnormal amount of DNA is recorded in the 4C position. Histograms with a sloping right shoulder to the G1G0 peak are labeled hyperdiploid (fig. 3-50).

Current terminology in this area can lead to misconceptions. Even though results are expressed in terms of ploidy, the method actually measures total DNA rather than the number of normal chromosomes. Chromosomal abnormalities that do not alter the total amount of DNA cannot be detected in usual preparations. When multiple abnormal peaks occur in DNA histograms, they are often described as different cell lines, although similarities in total DNA can hardly be construed as evidence of genetic lineage.

Used in conjunction with light microscopy, measurements of DNA ploidy can be important in clinical practice (183,213). Whereas tetraploid and hyperdiploid specimens may be benign, essentially all samples containing aneuploid cells are obtained from bladders with neoplasms and almost all of these neoplasms are malignant. Depending upon the classification system, this may be an important factor in separating tumors into groups with different prognoses (180). Using the 1973 WHO classification, for example, the majority of grade 2 transitional cell carcinomas with DNA aneuploidy behave like grade 3 cancers whereas similarly classified neoplasms with DNA diploidy act more like grade 1 tumors. DNA ploidy can be valuable for detecting urothelial neoplasms in cytologic specimens (65,145,176). Using monoclonal antibodies for epithelial differentiation, cytometry can detect malignant elements in specimens having few tumor cells or tumor cells masked by inflammatory debris (108). Knowledge of DNA ploidy may influence the type and extent of treatment, and serve as a predictive factor for patient outcome (125). The precision of available instrumentation is an important factor in quality assurance. In selected cases, the increased level of certainty that a positive histogram brings to a light microscopic interpretation can be important.

Special techniques have been applied to the determination of prognosis. Most often, the question to be addressed is the likelihood of recurrence, even though the development of a new neoplasm is of great importance only when that tumor is high grade or invasive. The risk of future progression, including the likelihood of death from disease, has also been addressed. As with the issue of early detection, expectations for technology in the area of prognostication seem to be higher than the evidence supports.

Long-term observations of the actual effects of prognostic factors are scant and nearly all studies rely on statistics to justify the importance of the results. These statistics can confirm that results are unlikely to have been achieved by chance, but they cannot reveal the importance of the information to patient care and very few caregivers have sufficient expertise to analyze statistics for themselves. Statisticians are aware, for example, that most clinically oriented studies deal with continuous variables and that separating these continuous variables into two categories, based on some arbitrary cut-off point, introduces inaccuracies that might be substantial (137). Statisticians also know that the importance of a p value depends more upon the prior probability of an event than upon the sensitivity and specificity of the methodology (73). Even when the p value is vanishingly low, the results of a study may not be clinically important.

Putative prognostic factors must be assessed with the understanding that biologic interactions among intracellular and extracellular substances are usually interdependent and that ultimately only one of three outcomes can be experienced by patients: 1) apparent cure, i.e., no interval progression, in which the patient is alive with no evidence of disease or dead of other causes at last contact; 2) persistent disease without progression, in which the patient is either alive or dead with disease at last contact; and 3) progressive disease, in which the patient is either dead of disease or alive with disseminated disease unresponsive to medical intervention at last contact.

The clinical value of putative prognostic factors must also be understood in light of the available treatment options. For patients with bladder tumors, these are limited to surgical resection, topical therapy with alkylating agents or bacillus Calmette-Guérin, and systemic chemotherapy for patients with nonresectable cancers. X-ray therapy is not usually employed as a primary modality for treatment in the United States. When treatment options are limited and especially when the effects of treatment, e.g., cystectomy, are life-altering, the question of how information regarding future risk is to be used becomes an important issue.

p53. Perhaps the most vigorously investigated putative prognostic factor is the *p53* gene and its protein product (90,103,117,129,209, 218,236). The gene itself is complex and the expression of the p53 protein is not completely straightforward (98). Many but by no means all abnormalities in the *p53* gene occur at exons 4 to 8, mostly as point mutations rather than deletions. Overexpression of the p53 protein is associated with abnormalities in the gene in only 70 to 80 percent of cases and antibodies detect about 90 percent of gene abnormalities. Nearly all aberrations in *p53* gene expression occur in high-grade carcinomas. When the p53 protein is overexpressed, progression has been documented in 50 percent of cases, compared to a 20 percent progression rate when p53 protein is not detected. Both the *p53* gene and its protein are expressed in nuclei, and when bladder tumors are the substrate, various percentages of positive nuclei have been used to separate patients into positive and negative groups. Often, p53 protein is examined in conjunction with other factors, such as the rate of DNA synthesis and the protein products of other genes.

The results of *p53* gene analysis are confusing and controversial (209). A variety of questions have been addressed. They include the risk of an adverse outcome in patients with urothelial neoplasms that have invaded into the lamina propria; selection of patients with muscle invasive bladder tumors for bladder preservation; the risk of tumor recurrence; and the risk of an adverse outcome after topical therapy. In general, detection of p53 protein in tumor cell nuclei is an unfavorable sign, especially when compared to nondetection in a matched group of cases, but the 20 to 50 percent difference is not considered by most practitioners to be sufficient for patient care decisions. The presence of *p53* gene abnormalities in the initial bladder tumor may correlate with recurrence but does not seem to consistently predict an adverse outcome, once patients have been treated. Considering the number of genetically influenced factors that might interact with *p53*, the clinical value of alterations in this gene or its protein product is likely to be restricted to highly selected cases.

Kinetics. Considering that proliferation is a key event in carcinogenesis, it may seem axiomatic that the rates of DNA synthesis and apoptosis correlate with prognosis. Like other putative prognostic factors, however, the literature is conflicting and claims often do not stand up to critical examination (105). A variety of stimuli cause DNA synthesis in urothelial cells, and the rate of synthesis closely parallels both DNA ploidy and the degree of nuclear anaplasia (grade) (193,220). DNA synthesis and actual cell proliferation are not synonymous (224). DNA synthesis can be determined by cytometry on cell suspensions or by immunohistochemistry on tissue sections. The methods are well established but the value of the results as independent prognostic factors remains to be proved.

The literature on apoptosis and other factors impacting on cell turnover is scant (64,138,142, 215). The term itself is controversial, since it is not possible to determine whether or not the death of a cell has been programmed or has occurred spontaneously. In any case, apoptosis has yet to be accepted as an important prognostic factor. Considering the evidence, it seems unlikely that substances involved in cell cycling will be independent prognostic factors upon which patient care can be based.

The list of putative prognostic factors grows daily. It includes genes, gene products, growth factors, adhesion molecules, tissue inhibitors, and chromosomal aberrations, not to mention assessments that would not be considered among special techniques. Depending upon the experimental design, the variety of factors submitted to multivariate regression analyses, the number of cases in the study, the characteristics of the study population, and the types of statistics employed, a great many factors can be claimed to have independent value for assessing a variety of risks to patients. Some of these risks, e.g., the likelihood of recurrence for a PUNLMP, have minimal impact. Some, e.g., the risk of death from disease if a cystectomy is not performed for a high-grade, muscle invasive carcinoma, are of major significance. If previous experience is any guide, very few of the factors that can be evaluated with special techniques are important in patient care. The complexity is such that computer modeling may be essential to assess the risks with sufficient accuracy for patient care decision-making.

Staging of Urothelial Neoplasms

The most often encountered problem with the staging of a bladder neoplasm is the determination of invasion. The urothelium does not always manifest a well-demarcated stromal interface, even in normal tissues, and the tumor/stromal junction may be further altered by surgery or topical therapy. Pseudovascular spaces surrounding nests of tumor are common. A desmoplastic reaction is not usually present and is not a reliable indicator of invasion when it occurs.

The pathologic assessment of invasion can be daunting and a few guidelines are helpful. In the urinary bladder, invasion and grade are closely linked. Papillomas and PUNLMPs are never invasive and low-grade carcinomas invade in less than 20 percent of cases. In contrast, the majority of high-grade carcinomas are invasive.

Invasion into the lamina propria can be appreciated when tumor cells occur in cords, sheets, or nests that penetrate well below the mucosa. When the neoplastic cells seem to hug the mucosa, they should be more anaplastic than their mucosal counterparts for an interpretation of invasion. An irregular tumor/stromal interface is usually insufficient for an unequivocal interpretation of lamina propria invasion.

Invasion of the muscular wall (detrusor, muscularis propria) is best appreciated when nests of tumor cells insinuate between rounded muscle fascicles. Invasive tumors may seem to carve out the muscle bundles, thus conforming to their contours and preserving a rim of residual muscle tissue. A desmoplastic reaction is not diagnostic but should raise the suspicion of muscle wall invasion. The desmoplastic reaction may be so extensive as to replace large areas of the detrusor muscle, and specimens composed of large, high-grade urothelial carcinomas interspersed with desmoplastic tissue are especially likely to be invasive. Thermocoagulation can mask invasion, especially in transurethral resection of bladder tumors (TURBTs), but remnants of the muscularis propria can usually be discerned. Trichrome stains are not especially helpful and immunohistochemistry is usually not necessary for the determination of invasion.

Staging schemes, like grading systems, are designed to predict future activity by categorizing neoplasms on the basis of their behavior prior to clinical recognition (61). Simple systems with few categories are the easiest to learn and use but convey the least information. Complex systems provide the most data but may be difficult to implement in nonresearch settings. Although intended

Table 3-7

STAGING SYSTEMS FOR BLADDER CANCER[a]

Jewett 1946	Jewett 1952	Marshall 1952	Bladder Cancer Staging (Clinical-Pathologic)		American Joint Cancer Committee 2002[b] Clinical	Pathologic
		0	No tumor in specimen		T0	pT0
			No invasion	- carcinoma in situ		pTis
A	A			- papillary tumor	Ta	pTa
		A	Invasion	- lamina propria	T1	pT1
B	B1	B1		- superficial detrusor muscle	T2	pT2a
	B2	B2		- deep detrusor muscle		pT2b
C	C	C		- paravesical tissue	T3	pT3
				microscopic		pT3a
				macroscopic		pT3b
		D1		- contiguous organs or tissues	T4	pT4
			Metastases	- regional lymph nodes	N1-3 (<2cm, 2-5 cm, >5 cm)	pN1-3
		D2		- distant sites	M1	pM1

[a]Modified from Table 2-9 from Murphy WM. Diseases of the urinary bladder, urethra, ureters, and renal pelves. In: Murphy WM, ed. Urological pathology. Philadelphia: WB Saunders; 1989:85.
[b]The AJCC also uses the following codes: TX, NX, MX meaning items cannot be assessed, and N0, M0 meaning no metastases to lymph nodes or distant sites.

to promote communication by establishing a stable basis for the study of cancer, staging schemes require periodic alterations as new information becomes available. Often, the system is the result of a consensus and should be viewed as "current best practice" rather than a listing based on well-established facts. A comparison of staging systems for bladder cancer is summarized in Table 3-7. The formulation of the American Joint Cancer Committee (AJCC) is recommended (61).

Pathologic Effects of Treatment

An extensive array of regimens have been applied to the treatment of patients with bladder neoplasms: surgery, drugs, attenuated microorganisms, X rays, vitamin analytes, lasers, interferons, immune enhancers, and hyperthermia (170). Most types of treatment produce no or nonspecific morphologic changes in tissues and cells. Nevertheless, the effects of therapy are especially important to the pathologist, who must determine whether changes in treated urothelium represent residual or recurrent neoplasm, or alterations in normal cells caused by the treatment. The literature offers only a little help. Although abundant, it is usually not focused on the tissue and cellular mani-

festations of treated bladders. Assessment of the effects of treatment is often further hindered by incomplete information regarding the health of the patient prior to therapy, the extent of the disease, and the duration of exposure to the regimen. Established treatment modalities that may cause pathologic changes in the bladder are considered in four categories: surgery, chemotherapy, topical bacillus Calmette-Guérin, and radiation therapy.

Surgical procedures disrupt the normal anatomy of the bladder and trigger nonspecific inflammatory responses that may confound the interpretation of subsequent tissue samples. Longstanding inflammation can result in osteoid or bone formation, granulomatous reactions suggestive of infectious disease, and florid stromal proliferations (postoperative spindle cell nodules) suggestive of mesenchymal neoplasms. Epithelial nests trapped in inflammatory tissue may suggest an invasive tumor. Regenerative epithelium can be confused with CIS, especially if it exhibits hyperdiploidy on cytometric histograms (176).

Chemotherapeutic drugs affecting the urinary bladder can be divided into two groups: systemic agents administered primarily for

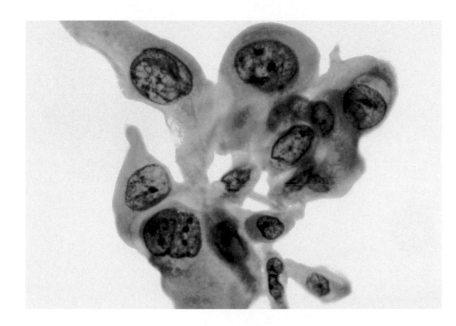

Figure 3-51

EFFECTS OF TOPICAL ALKYLATING AGENTS

This is a characteristic but not a pathognomonic reaction of superficial cells when exposed to agents such as mitomycin C. (Fig. 3-42 from Murphy WM. Urinary cytopathology. Chicago: ASCP Press; 2000:55.)

nonurologic disease but concentrated in urine, and topical chemicals used for prophylaxis or treatment of bladder neoplasms. Among systemic agents, the best studied is cyclophosphamide (Cytoxan). This is an alkylating agent most often given in multidrug cocktails for the treatment of patients with leukemia and lymphoma. It causes a hemorrhagic cystitis that is characterized by denudation of the epithelium with consequent irritative voiding symptoms and gross hematuria (212). Adequate hydration and pretreatment with the acrolein detoxifier 2-mercaptoethane sulfonate (mesna) have greatly decreased the frequency of complications, but the association of cyclophosphamide exposure and bladder cancer is established. Almost all bladder tumors associated with exposure to cyclophosphamide have been carcinomas of high cytologic grade but mesenchymal tumors are well documented (207). These neoplasms have no histologic or cytologic features that distinguish them from similar tumors occurring in patients not exposed to the drug. Cytologic changes characteristic of cyclophosphamide effect have not been established. When cells with abnormal nuclei appear in urinary samples from individuals exposed to cyclophosphamide, the same criteria used to assess any high-grade neoplasm should be used for their evaluation.

Among the topical chemicals instilled for prophylaxis or treatment of bladder tumors, the most effective are the alkylating agents (170). These drugs are active without further metabolism but their mechanism of action is incompletely understood. In vitro, alkylating agents act to prevent DNA replication. The extent to which this occurs in human bladders is complicated by many host-related factors. Pathologic changes are thoroughly documented for triethylene thiophosphoramide (TTP) and mitomycin C (MMC) (178). Both are administered directly into the bladder, where they are in contact with the urothelium for only a few hours. Pathologic changes associated with these drugs include exfoliation of both normal and abnormal urothelial cells resulting in denudation of the bladder, as well as degeneration, multinucleation, and bizarre reactive nuclear changes in superficial cells (fig. 3-51). Although characteristic, none of these alterations is specific for alkylating drugs in general or TTP and MMC in particular. They should not be confounding factors to the accurate interpretation of carcinoma for experienced observers (fig. 3-52). Exfoliation often results in a marked reduction of neoplastic cells in cytologic specimens, a situation that may decrease the effectiveness of cytometry as a monitoring technique (176). TTP and MMC have an abrasive effect on papillary tumors, destroying the tips of papillae and truncating the lesions to the point that they appear flattened or stubby in histologic preparations (see fig. 3-31). Neoplastic cells may persist in Brunn nests (fig. 3-53). It is important to differentiate stubby papillae from irregular

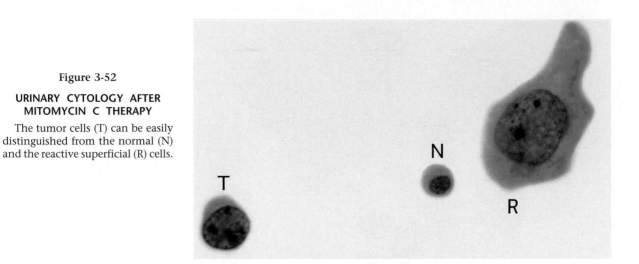

Figure 3-52

URINARY CYTOLOGY AFTER MITOMYCIN C THERAPY

The tumor cells (T) can be easily distinguished from the normal (N) and the reactive superficial (R) cells.

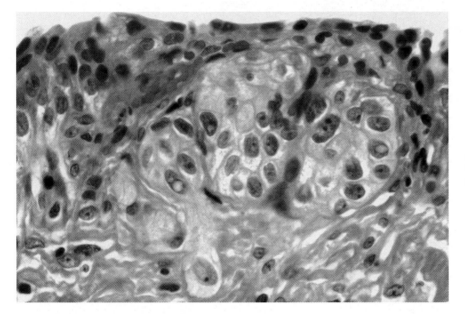

Figure 3-53

NEOPLASTIC CELLS IN BRUNN NESTS AFTER TOPICAL THERAPY

One of the primary concerns of using topical therapy is that the treatment may mask an early invasive event.

areas of CIS or dysplasia, and to recognize residual neoplastic cells in Brunn nests in treated patients since this may constitute the difference between treatment failure (persistent tumor) and success (downgrading).

Topical bacillus Calmette-Guérin (BCG), like TTP and MMC, is instilled directly into the bladder for the prophylaxis and treatment of patients with bladder neoplasms that have not invaded into the muscularis propria (94,121,149, 166). Its efficacy, especially for noninvasive neoplasms, is well established and few systemic complications have been documented, even though the instillate consists of attenuated tubercle bacilli. The mechanism of action is unclear but the

pathologic response is essentially identical to that observed in tuberculous cystitis (fig. 3-54). There is focal denudation of epithelium, with an underlying granulomatous inflammation localized to the lamina propria and sparing of the muscular wall. The granulomatous reaction indicates therapeutic activity of BCG and should be reported. Tubercle bacilli are not easily found in these lesions but their presence does not affect patient care and stains to identify them are not necessary. BCG granulomas are also common in the prostate gland. The cytologic changes associated with BCG are nonspecific and do not confound the interpretation of recurrent or residual carcinoma.

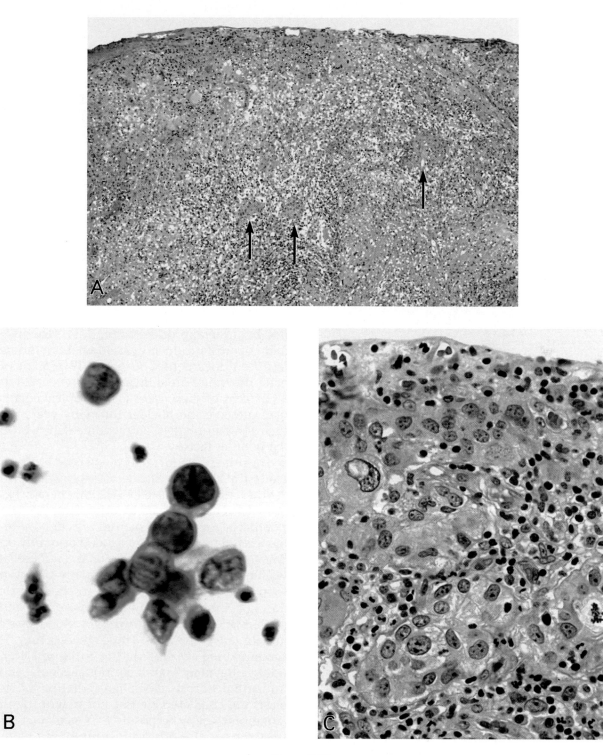

Figure 3-54

GRANULOMATOUS INFLAMMATION SECONDARY TO BACILLUS CALMETTE-GUÉRIN (BCG)

A: Granulomatous inflammation (arrows) indistinguishable from that of primary tuberculosis.

B: High-grade neoplastic cells in a urinary specimen after BCG therapy.

C: The corresponding bladder biopsy with invasive high-grade carcinoma in denuded tissue. (Fig. 3-41 from Murphy WM. Urinary cytopathology; Chicago: ASCP Press; 2000:54.)

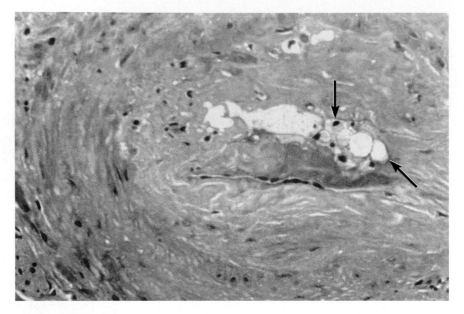

Figure 3-55

**ENDOTHELIAL INJURY
AFTER X-RAY THERAPY**

Exposure to X rays exceeding 20 Gy causes injury to endothelial cells (arrows) as well as to mesenchymal cells.

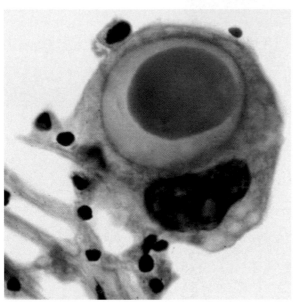

Figure 3-56

**ABNORMAL UROTHELIAL CELLS
AFTER X-RAY THERAPY**

In this case, the X-ray therapy was directed at the patient's prostate cancer.

The apparent effectiveness of topical therapy in rendering bladders cystoscopically free of tumor may engender an unwarranted contentment in both clinicians and patients. High-grade neoplastic cells appearing in urinary samples after treatment are an unfavorable sign that should

not be underappreciated (fig. 3-54). Involvement of prostatic ducts by urothelial carcinoma has been documented in up to 39 percent of patients, and stromal invasion has occurred in 38 percent of these cases (119). Topical agents may preserve the bladder for many years but their long-term effect on outcome depends on many other factors.

The urinary bladder may be exposed to X rays directed at a primary bladder neoplasm or aimed at other pelvic organs (63,157,208). Therapy has been delivered by intralesional implantation and external beam. The mechanism of action on tumors is unknown but may depend primarily on damage to blood vessels (fig. 3-55). Endothelial swelling and necrosis are commonly observed soon after exposure of tissue to therapeutic doses of X rays. Marked mural thickening and hyalinization, with narrowing of blood vessel lumens, are late events. These changes may be accompanied by smoldering inflammation, nonhealing ulcers, lamina proprial edema, and interstitial fibrosis. So-called radiation fibroblasts are characteristic but not diagnostic of radiation therapy. Exposure to X rays may destroy the papillae of a bladder tumor but tends to have less effect on nodular and flat lesions (181). Even relatively small doses can increase the degree of nuclear pleomorphism, thus seeming to increase the tumor grade in histologic sections. In urinary specimens, cells with abundant, often lamellar, acidophilic cytoplasm have been considered evidence of radiation effect (fig. 3-56). As with alkylating agents, these changes should not confound the interpretation of a recurrent or residual neoplasm.

The bladder may be injured by X rays directed toward other pelvic organs (66,157,206). Atypical nuclear changes that occur as reactive alterations in normal urothelial cells have been observed. In addition, several cases of both epithelial and stromal neoplasms have been recorded. In chronically inflamed bladders, irregular islands of benign epithelial cells with abnormal nuclei may be difficult to distinguish from invasive carcinoma until the history is known (66). Urothelia exposed to indirect radiation can manifest changes that mimic CIS but the abundant acidophilic cytoplasm of these lesions in the absence of a prior history of bladder neoplasm is distinguishing (see fig. 3-39).

Urinary cytology is essential for the accurate monitoring of patients after treatment. Residual tumor is often undetectable endoscopically, even when it occurs in areas accessible to the cystoscope. Biopsies sample only a small portion of the urothelium and are often denuded of diagnostic cells. The involvement of Brunn nests, distal ureters, urethra, or prostatic ducts is common and is often detected after a positive cytology has prompted selected site biopsies. The appearance of high-grade neoplastic cells after topical therapy identifies patients who are not responding to their treatment and require other approaches.

SQUAMOUS CELL CARCINOMA

Definition. Squamous cell carcinomas are a group of bladder neoplasms with histologic patterns and cytologic features reminiscent of similar neoplasms of the epidermis. Despite the histologic definition, the term "epidermoid" is not preferred, perhaps because it has been applied to urothelial tumors in the past. As currently defined, squamous cell carcinomas must be sufficiently differentiated to have some combination of individual cell keratinization, keratin pearls, and intercellular bridges. Nonkeratinizing areas of squamous cell carcinomas cannot usually be differentiated from high-grade urothelial neoplasms. The distinction between urothelial carcinoma with squamous differentiation and squamous cell carcinoma is somewhat arbitrary, with most authorities requiring that a squamous cell carcinoma be composed of at least 80 percent squamous elements.

General Features. The majority of squamous cell carcinomas occur in an environment of chronic irritation and chronic inflammation of the urothelium, although a specific history of these findings is often absent from published reports (240,243,245,253,256). In areas where *Schistosoma hematobium* is endemic, the irritation is due to the calcified eggs of the parasites. In nonendemic areas, bladder stones, indwelling catheters, infectious agents, or structural alterations in the bladder provide the stimulus. Chromosomal and genetic aberrations have been observed in squamous tumors and associated urothelia (247,249). These abnormalities have been sought in the same chromosomes as those involved in urothelial carcinomas but seem to occur with different frequencies and tend to be of different types. As with urothelial neoplasms, the role of genes in the pathogenesis of squamous cell carcinoma remains to be elucidated.

Squamous metaplasia is commonly present in the epithelium adjacent to squamous carcinomas but its presence does not necessarily indicate that squamous metaplasia is a precursor (241,251,260). The lack of dysplastic changes in metaplastic lesions adjacent to squamous carcinomas, the low frequency of squamous carcinoma among patients being followed for squamous metaplasia, and the absence of squamous metaplasia in a large percentage of cases of squamous carcinoma militate against this lesion being an obligate phase in the pathogenesis of most tumors.

Squamous cell carcinomas tend to arise insidiously and are difficult to detect even among patients being monitored for dysfunctional bladders. Urinary cytology may be valuable for early detection, especially among high-risk individuals, but the literature suggests that this method has not been widely employed.

Clinical Features. In most series, less than 5 percent of all bladder neoplasms are squamous cell carcinomas, but frequencies of 10 to 15 percent have been reported (245,246,256, 257). Compared to urothelial neoplasms, squamous cell cancers are common in women: the male to female ratio in most series from areas where *S. hematobium* is not endemic is nearly 1 to 1. The disease may occur over a wide age

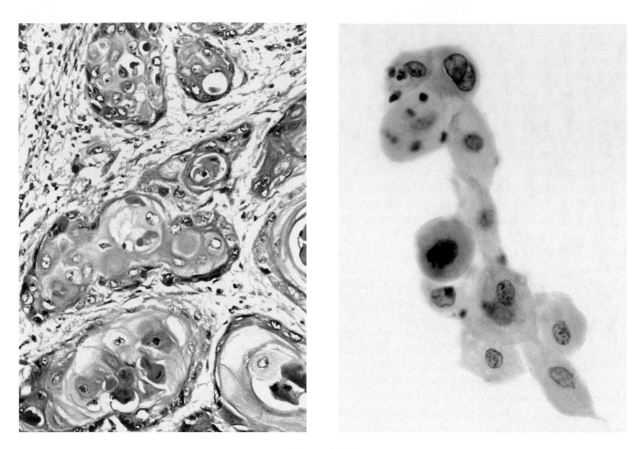

Figure 3-57

SQUAMOUS CELL CARCINOMA

Left: An invasive, keratinizing squamous cell carcinoma.

Right: The corresponding urinary cytology. The malignant cells seem only slightly abnormal. (Fig. 4-2B from Murphy WM. Urinary cytopathology. Chicago: ASCP Press; 2000:74.)

range. Tumors arising de novo are most common in patients aged 60 to 70 years; those arising in parasite-infested areas tend to occur in somewhat younger individuals (248,262). In 70 percent of cases, lesions are detected because of gross hematuria, but at least one third of patients complain of dysuria, nocturia, frequency, or pain. Bacteriuria has been reported in almost 50 percent of patients. At cystoscopy, nodular or plaque-like lesions with a shaggy white surface are often observed. In contrast to urothelial neoplasms, squamous cell carcinomas are often widespread and involve areas other than the bladder base (242,256).

Pathologic Findings. In histologic sections, squamous cell carcinomas arise in the epithelium and infiltrate the underlying tissue in sheets, nests, and islands (figs. 3-57–3-59). It is not uncommon for squamous cell carcinomas

to produce such abundant keratin that a TURBT contains only paucicellular keratinous debris. The pathologist receiving such a specimen should recommend more adequate sampling. Within each tissue configuration, the component cells tend to differentiate toward squamous epithelium reminiscent of epidermis, so that the periphery is composed of rather uniform basal cells which become keratinized as they progress toward the center or the surface. Keratinization of cells at the stromal interface of a squamous cell neoplasm is a sign of invasion and can be an important feature in certain cases. Squamous cell carcinomas must be composed of some combination of well-defined intercellular bridges, individual cell keratinization, and keratin pearls or they are not pure squamous tumors. This requirement excludes very poorly differentiated cancers and may be

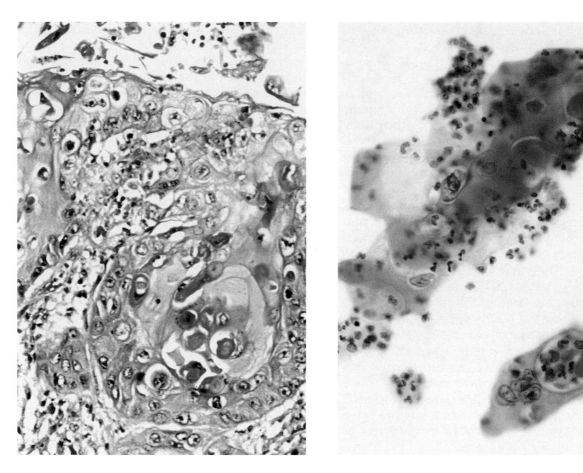

Figure 3-58

SQUAMOUS CELL CARCINOMA

Left: Keratinizing squamous cell carcinoma.
Right: The corresponding urinary cytology contains cells that are difficult to appreciate as malignant.

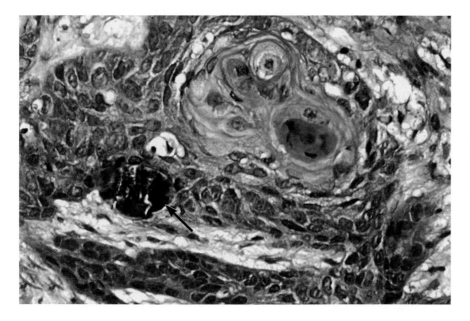

Figure 3-59

**SQUAMOUS
CELL CARCINOMA**

This specimen was from a patient infested with *Schistosoma hematobium*. A calcified ovum (arrow) is present. (Courtesy of Dr. Samir N. Mina, Tanta, Egypt.)

a factor influencing the correlation between grade and prognosis.

In histologic preparations, the cells of squamous cell carcinoma are polygonal, with well-defined borders and amphophilic to acidophilic cytoplasm. Their nuclei are pleomorphic and occasionally bizarre, with irregularly distributed chromatin, which may be either finely or coarsely granular. Prominent nucleoli and mitoses are common. Degenerated cells (dyskeratosis) are characteristic.

Grading of squamous cell carcinoma is based upon the degree of keratinization and published schemes recognize three categories: well, moderately, and poorly differentiated (245, 256,259). The value of this approach is confounded by several factors: most squamous cell carcinomas are large and deeply invasive at diagnosis; the most poorly differentiated cancers lack features of squamous differentiation; and tumors that closely resemble epidermis differ greatly from normal bladder mucosa and cannot be considered well differentiated if the host organ is used as the baseline. These factors probably account for the relatively low predictive value of grading and explain its indifferent acceptance among pathologists.

Squamous carcinoma cells appearing in urinary samples vary considerably in their morphology, and a high index of suspicion is required for detection (252,255). The most characteristic elements are polygonal, fiber-like, or tadpole shaped. They have well-defined cellular borders and amphophilic to acidophilic, occasionally vacuolated cytoplasm. Nuclei are enlarged and slightly pleomorphic, with irregularly distributed chromatin; often, they bulge into the adjacent cytoplasm instead of conforming to its elongated configuration. Nucleoli may be prominent but do not occur in most cells and are often obscured. More poorly differentiated cancers exfoliate cells indistinguishable from those of any high-grade neoplasm. Many neoplastic cells from squamous carcinomas are so well differentiated that they cannot be distinguished from squamous metaplasia, but almost all squamous cancers shed some diagnostic cells in the urine, provided that slight to moderate degrees of nuclear atypia are appreciated as features of malignancy. Degenerative changes are common in these cells and many contain cytoplasmic vacuoles or pyknotic nuclei with condensed chromatin.

Prognosis. Squamous cell carcinomas tend to grow in an expansile fashion and most lesions described in the literature have been large tumors at the time of detection (245,248,256, 259,262). Invasion of the muscular wall is recorded in more than 80 percent of cases. Prognosis is poor but large studies from areas not endemic for parasites are scant. As expected, the stage at detection is the most important prognostic factor. Metastases seem to be a late event. The regional lymph nodes are involved in 10 to 25 percent of patients, with bone and lung being next most frequent sites of metastasis. Overall, reported survival rates have ranged from 25 to more than 50 percent.

Differential Diagnosis. Squamous cell carcinomas must be differentiated from squamous metaplasia, condyloma acuminatum with nuclear atypia, urothelial carcinomas with squamous components, and the verrucous variant. The presence of invasive nests and islands distinguishes squamous carcinoma from benign lesions with nuclear atypia and verrucous carcinoma. Diagnosis in the absence of clear-cut invasion depends primarily on the degree of cellular anaplasia, since in situ squamous neoplasms have not been well defined in morphologic terms. Cases presenting diagnostic dilemmas in this regard are rare. More common is the problem of distinguishing pure squamous cell carcinomas from urothelial lesions with squamous components (see the differential diagnosis of high-grade urothelial carcinoma). The diagnosis depends on the proportion of tumor occupied by the questionable area. Pure squamous cell carcinoma is composed almost entirely of neoplastic tissue differentiated toward keratinizing epithelium. As a practical matter, tumors presenting diagnostic difficulties are usually of high stage, and patients receive similar prognoses and treatments regardless of the name appended to the tumor. Of course, the differential diagnosis of any nonurothelial bladder carcinoma should include metastases and direct extension from cancers of adjacent organs.

Variants of Squamous Cell Carcinoma. *Verrucous Carcinoma.* Squamous cell carcinoma may manifest heterogeneous patterns but the only histologically and clinically distinctive

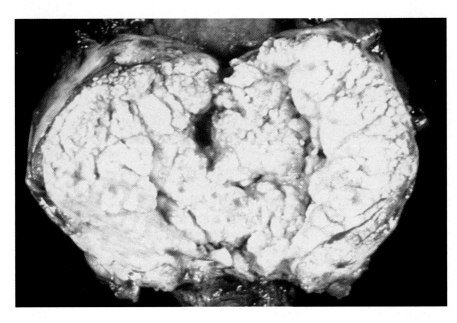

Figure 3-60

VERRUCOUS CARCINOMA OF URINARY BLADDER

In this gross specimen the tumor nearly replaces the urothelium. (Courtesy of Dr. George M. Farrow, Rochester, MN.)

Figure 3-61

VERRUCOUS CARCINOMA

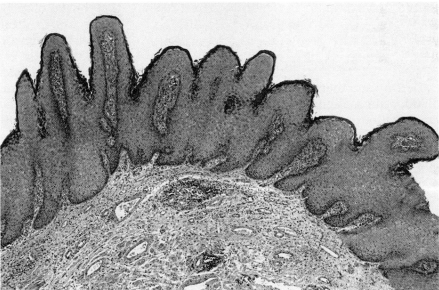

variant is verrucous carcinoma (244,250,260). This lesion is considered among the malignancies primarily because of its potential for widespread local growth. When foci of invasive squamous cell carcinoma occur in a neoplasm that is predominantly verrucous, the most appropriate interpretation is squamous cell carcinoma. Verrucous carcinoma is almost exclusively associated with *S. hematobium* infection and accounts for approximately 3 percent of the bladder cancers arising in areas endemic for the parasite. Rare examples unassociated with schistosomiasis have been recorded in single reports from patients with a condyloma acuminatum, diverticulum, and chronic infection (250,260). Like verrucous carcinomas at other sites, these tumors are indolent growths that spread by direct extension and do not metastasize, but may develop foci of invasive squamous cell carcinoma.

Histologically, verrucous carcinomas of the bladder resemble similar neoplasms at other sites (figs. 3-60, 3-61). Acanthosis with rounded, "pushing" margins is characteristic. Slight cellular atypia may appear at the base or when the lesion is chronically inflamed but cellular anaplasia is not a feature. Mitoses are rare.

Special Techniques. The role of molecular techniques in the diagnosis of squamous cell carcinomas of the urinary bladder remains to be elucidated. Chromosomal evaluation has revealed multiple aberrations, including abnormalities common to high-grade urothelial carcinomas (247,249,254). A large number of squamous cell carcinomas have been examined for DNA ploidy using flow cytometry (258,261); diploid DNA histograms have been recorded in 30 to 40 percent of cases. Most nondiploid tumors have distinct aneuploid peaks rather than the hyperdiploid shoulders often seen in urothelial neoplasms. Aneuploid cancers often have increased synthesizing fractions (S-phase). As expected, both ploidy and S-phase correlate with degree of nuclear anaplasia. Correlations with stage have been less clear.

Staging. Squamous cell carcinomas are staged according to a variety of methods (Table 3-7). The formulation of the AJCC is preferred (239).

ADENOCARCINOMA

Definition. Adenocarcinomas of the urinary bladder are malignant glandular neoplasms, nearly all of which are histologically indistinguishable from similar tumors arising in the colon. Urachal neoplasms are usually included in discussions of bladder adenocarcinomas, primarily because their pathologic features and prognoses are similar. Many authors prefer to separate these tumors, however, since the urachus is not an anatomic component of the adult bladder and not all neoplasms arising in the urachus are glandular.

General Features. The etiology and pathogenesis of adenocarcinoma of the bladder are unknown. Recognizing the close embryologic relationship of the bladder to the hindgut, the absence of intestinal differentiation in normal urothelium, the presence of colonic antigenic factors in bladder and urachal glandular tumors, the frequency of chronic mucosal irritation in association with adenocarcinoma, and the common occurrence of intestinal metaplasia in cancerous bladders, many experts accept the proposition that adenocarcinomas arise through a process of intestinal metaplasia stimulated by chronic irritation (283,287). This theory must be mitigated by the following factors: 1) some bladder adenocarcinomas arise de novo without associated chronic irritation or intestinal metaplasia; 2)adenocarcinomas occurring in patients followed for intestinal metaplasia are rare and not all cancers arising in bladders with intestinal metaplasia are adenocarcinomas; 3) small amounts of intestinal metaplasia, such as occur in cystitis glandularis, have not been proven a risk factor for subsequent malignancies; and 4) significant cellular atypia is uncommon in intestinal metaplasia, even in lesions adjacent to adenocarcinomas (263,265,273). Like squamous cell carcinomas, many adenocarcinomas probably arise as host reactions to long-term mucosal irritation, and intestinal metaplasia is a commonly associated phenomenon. Whether metaplastic changes represent required precursors or concomitant lesions in glandular carcinogenesis is controversial. Most studies suggest that the risk of subsequent carcinoma is related to the degree (and perhaps the duration) of urothelial disturbance as reflected in the amount and distribution of intestinal metaplasia.

Among other factors associated with urothelial adenocarcinoma, exstrophy and persistent urachal remnants are the most common. Exstrophy occurs when the cloacal membrane fails to properly differentiate, leaving the anterior abdominal wall, and thus the anterior bladder wall, undeveloped. Despite a markedly abnormal environment and widespread intestinal metaplasia, adenocarcinoma has been found in less than 10 percent of exstrophied bladders (271). Bladder cancers tend to occur late and are not confined to unrepaired defects, suggesting that carcinogenesis may be aborted and even successful cancerous processes require time to develop and are not totally influenced by changing the mucosal environment to a more normal state.

In contrast to exstrophy, persistence of urachal remnants is a relatively normal condition and adenocarcinomas arising in such remnants, like similar tumors arising at the bladder base, are rare. Among urachal neoplasms, more than 80 percent are adenocarcinomas (269,273). Intestinal metaplasia is not a frequently associated finding although a few cases have arisen in association with cysts and villous adenomas. Adenocarcinomas arising in areas of urachal remnants differ clinically from those occurring at the bladder base, but these

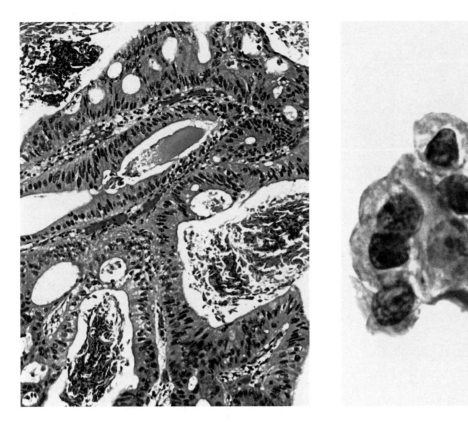

Figure 3-62

ADENOCARCINOMA

Left: These bladder tumors resemble adenocarcinomas of the gastrointestinal tract.
Right: The corresponding urinary cytology.

neoplasms are so similar in their pathology and behavior that they probably do not represent separate entities but a single group of cancers arising at different sites.

Adenocarcinomas, like most other bladder tumors, are usually not detected until patients recognize blood in their urine. Urinary cytology may be an important method for earlier detection but has received little attention in the literature.

Clinical Features. Adenocarcinomas account for less than 2 percent of bladder neoplasms (273,287). The majority (58 to 67 percent) arise at the bladder base, and almost all of the remainder occur in association with urachal remnants. Many clinical features vary with the primary site of the tumor (273). The male to female ratio of nonurachal neoplasms approaches 3 to 1 in contrast to almost 1 to 1 for urachal tumors. Adenocarcinomas may occur in young adults but most patients are middle-aged (mean, approximately 62 years for non-urachal cases; 51 years for urachal cancers). Hematuria is the most common presenting sign, occurring in about 90 percent of patients regardless of the primary site of the tumor. Almost half of the patients with urachal neoplasms complain of irritative bladder symptoms (dysuria, nocturia, frequency, pain) whereas fewer than 15 percent with nonurachal neoplasms have these symptoms. Mucusuria is uncommon. Cystoscopically, bladder adenocarcinomas ordinarily appear as single, nodular tumors that cannot be reliably distinguished from urothelial neoplasms.

Pathologic Findings. Adenocarcinomas of the urinary bladder, regardless of site, may manifest any of the histologic variations that occur in the colon (figs. 3-62–3-64) (273,280). Most tumors are single lesions arising from the bladder mucosa, but rare lesions have extensively infiltrated the bladder wall with little

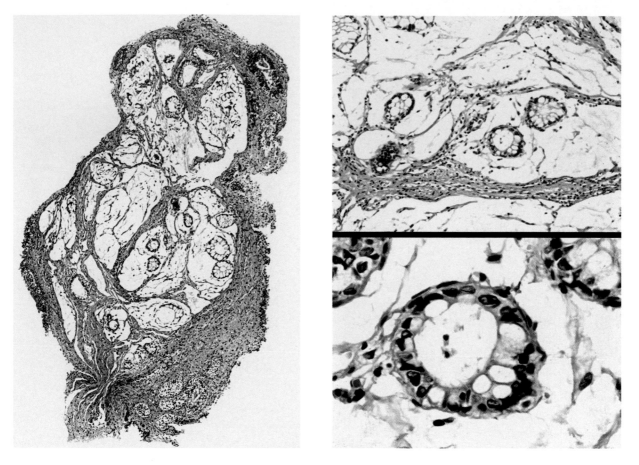

Figure 3-63

ADENOCARCINOMA, MUCINOUS TYPE

Left: Low magnification highlights the predominance of mucinous pools.
Right: Intermediate and high magnifications highlight the cellular component.

Figure 3-64

ADENOCARCINOMA

Intraepithelial mucins (right) are usually readily appreciated in poorly differentiated lesions.

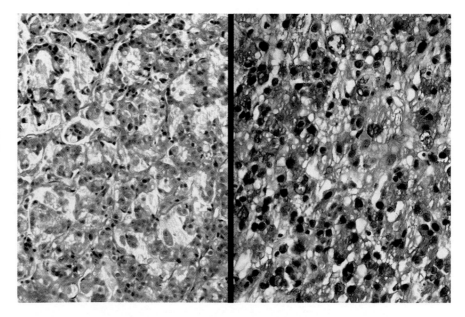

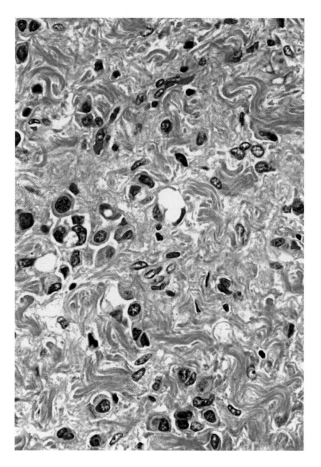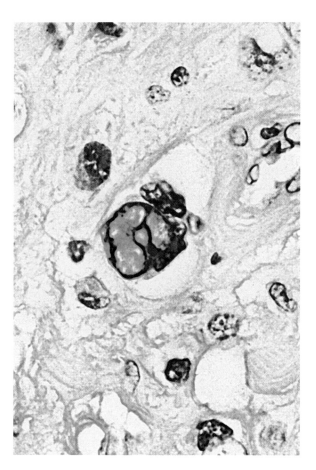

Figure 3-65

ADENOCARCINOMA, SIGNET RING TYPE

Left: The tumor cells in this specimen are almost entirely within the lamina propria and muscular layers. It is common in the bladder for only a few tumor cells to have the classic signet ring appearance.

Right: Cells with intraepithelial mucins are widely scattered (alcian blue).

mucosal involvement. These cancers have no other distinguishing histologic features and histologic subtyping has little significance to the patient, so long as the signet ring pattern is considered an example of poor differentiation rather than a separate histologic entity.

Many authors consider bladder tumors with significant signet ring components to be a distinctive variant rather than a particularly poorly differentiated example of adenocarcinoma (fig. 3-65) (272,274). When pure, these cancers are usually diffusely infiltrating and have the gross characteristics of a linitis plastica. Abnormalities in the urothelium are often difficult to find unless multiple sections are examined. Tumor cells with a characteristic signet ring appearance may react positively for mucins, but mucin pro-

duction is not prominent in many tumors and a paucity of mucin does not affect the interpretation. Pure signet ring carcinomas are often unresectable and the prognosis of patients is correspondingly poor. On the other hand, a few signet ring cells are not uncommon in bladder adenocarcinomas and in those few cases where pure signet ring tumors are of low stage, the prognosis is relatively favorable.

Adenocarcinomas produce colonic-type mucins in various amounts. Paneth cells and argentaffin cells have been identified in a few cases (282). Tumors react to antibodies directed to carcinoembryonic antigens and cytokeratins (273). In rare cases, cells react when exposed to antibodies to prostatic acid phosphatase but bladder adenocarcinomas do not contain cells

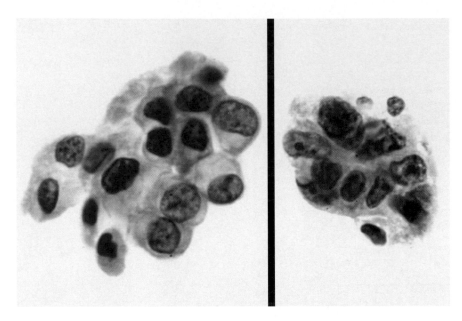

Figure 3-66

ADENOCARCINOMA IN URINARY SPECIMEN

The accurate interpretation of adenocarcinoma in urinary specimens can be challenging, although most tumors are recognized as malignant in cellular samples. Panels represent urinary specimens from two different patients with adenocarcinoma.

reactive for both prostatic acid phosphatase and prostate-specific antigen (270).

Grading of bladder adenocarcinomas has not been well accepted as a prognostic tool by pathologists, perhaps because only patients whose tumors have a significant number of signet ring cells have a distinctly different prognosis, and almost all bladder adenocarcinomas are of high stage at the time of clinical diagnosis. Like all nonurothelial neoplasms, the normal standard for differentiation in adenocarcinoma is difficult to establish since the more a cancer resembles colon, the less differentiated it is if normal bladder is used as a baseline.

With some exceptions, the cells of bladder adenocarcinoma are detectable in urinary samples (fig. 3-66) (276,278). Cancer cells are ordinarily of high cytologic grade but often lack features characteristic of glandular differentiation. Occasionally, adenocarcinomas are so well differentiated that their disaggregated cells cannot be recognized as malignant in cytologic specimens.

Intraepithelial lesions with glandular differentiation are not well characterized, probably owing to the lack of a basal lamina that would distinguish an in situ from a minimally invasive neoplasm. There are rare case reports, but the in situ lesions have been papillary rather than flat, and some are best considered villous variants (266,267, 281). CIS associated with adenocarcinoma is rare and more often of urothelial rather than glandular differentiation (273). Cystitis cystica and cys-

titis glandularis occur in approximately 50 percent of patients with adenocarcinoma located at the bladder base but are uncommon in those with urachal neoplasms. Significant cellular atypia in areas of cystitis is uncommon.

Prognosis. Long-term follow-up is not available for most reported patients with bladder adenocarcinoma. The available literature suggests that the lesions grow locally, primarily into the bladder wall rather than into the lumen. Intramucosal spread is uncommon. Well-documented metastases are infrequently cited even though most patient deaths are considered to be tumor-related. Most reports cite a survival rate of 20 to 40 percent at 5 years for patients with bladder adenocarcinomas, but much of the literature on this subject is dated and the outlook for most current cases may not be quite so grim (273, 279). Prognosis varies with stage, with survival approaching 75 to 100 percent among patients whose tumors are confined to the urinary bladder. Unfortunately, low-stage cancers account for fewer than 30 percent of reported cases. Except for the poor prognosis of patients with signet ring cell tumors, correlation of prognosis with histologic type and grade has not been strong. Patients with urachal tumors tend to have a better short-term survival rate than those with nonurachal cancers, but the overall survival rates at 5 and 10 years are not significantly different. The role of DNA ploidy as well as other putative prognostic factors remains to be established (279,286).

Differential Diagnosis. Adenocarcinomas are characteristic neoplasms that present few differential diagnostic problems. Distinction from invasive colonic cancers or metastases with colonic differentiation cannot be achieved without appropriate clinical information, although exploitation of certain differences in mucins, adhesion molecules, or other factors may prove fruitful (268).

In rare cases, lesions resembling intestinal metaplasia may infiltrate the lamina propria or even the bladder wall (275). Mucinous pools are not uncommon in cases of intestinal metaplasia and their presence in a tissue sample is not diagnostic of adenocarcinoma. The cells of intestinal metaplasia lack nuclear anaplasia and rarely involve the muscularis propria. Nodular areas of cystitis glandularis rich in goblet cells should be considered benign even if the nodules extend into the lamina propria.

Adenocarcinomas must be distinguished from urothelial neoplasms with glandular lumens. This distinction is somewhat arbitrary but not usually difficult if adenocarcinoma is defined as a malignant tumor differentiating toward colonic mucosa. Both lesions contain intracellular and luminal mucins, however, mucins are not abundant in the urothelial lesion and goblet cell formation is not prominent. The "glands" of a urothelial tumor with lumen formation are surrounded by cells with the pseudostratified appearance and superficial cell differentiation of urothelium.

Adenocarcinomas, especially the clear cell variant, must be distinguished from nephrogenic metaplasia. The distinction is rarely a problem, except perhaps in small unrepresentative specimens. It is discussed in the section on tumors of the urethra. Rarely, so-called endocervicosis is a consideration in the differential diagnosis of an adenocarcinoma.

Variants of Adenocarcinoma. Variants of bladder adenocarcinoma are difficult to define. Anecdotal reports, such as adenocarcinoma with hepatoid features, occur sporadically in the literature (285). Signet ring cell cancers could be considered variants but seem better classified among the poorly differentiated adenocarcinomas. Because their location confers slightly different symptoms and short-term prognosis, urachal adenocarcinoma could be considered either as a variant or a separate entity. Villous tumors may contain foci of invasion, thus qualifying as a variant. Even clear cell adenocarcinoma (see section on urethra), often classified as a variant, could be discussed as a separate entity, since these tumors seem to differentiate toward müllerian rather than colonic epithelium and do not, therefore, strictly conform to the definition of a bladder adenocarcinoma.

Special Techniques. DNA ploidy determined by using flow and image cytometry as well as other factors assessed by other techniques have occasionally been investigated in bladder adenocarcinomas (278,285). These methods may increase our understanding but have yet to have a clinical impact.

Staging. The majority of bladder adenocarcinomas have invaded into the muscle wall at the time of diagnosis. Most previous reports used variations of other staging systems but the formulation of the AJCC is currently preferred, although the anatomy of the urachus might require slight alterations, e.g., a reduction in the number of substages applied to invasion of the wall and surrounding structures (Table 3-7) (264,268).

VILLOUS TUMORS

Villous tumors are glandular neoplasms that are histologically indistinguishable from villous and tubulovillous adenomas of the colon (fig. 3-67) (267,269,277,281,284). These neoplasms are difficult to classify, especially since many have foci of carcinoma at the time of detection, and are called adenomas to emphasize their major component and resemblance to colonic lesions. The carcinomatous components may be in situ or invasive, glandular or urothelial. Almost all reports cite well-circumscribed tumors arising at the bladder dome. Many villous adenomas are associated with histologically identifiable urachal remnants or cysts. A few lesions have been associated with exstrophy, cystitis glandularis, chronic mucosal irritation, or even previous urothelial neoplasms. Patients range in age from 18 days to 93 years, with most 40 to 70 years old. The male to female ratio is 2 to 1. Hematuria and mucusuria are the most common presenting signs. Follow-up information is incomplete in most reports, although complete surgical resection was achieved in almost all cases. When a villous adenoma has foci of invasive carcinoma, the prognosis may not be favorable despite radical surgery (284).

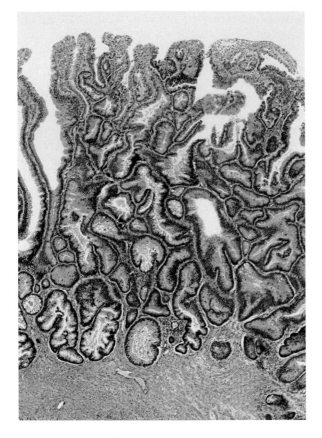

Figure 3-67

**TUBULOVILLOUS ADENOMA
ARISING AT BLADDER DOME**

(Courtesy of Dr. Winfield Morgan, Morgantown, WV.)

POORLY DIFFERENTIATED SMALL CELL CARCINOMA

Definition and General Features. Poorly differentiated carcinomas are a group of malignant neoplasms that differentiate toward epithelium but lack well-formed epithelial structures. Many do not react with cytokeratin cocktails. Some produce polypeptides but neuroendocrine differentiation has been variably documented and is not a requirement for diagnosis. In fact, the list of potential polypeptides that may be produced by poorly differentiated small cell carcinomas is extensive and reactions using broad-spectrum neuroendocrine markers cannot be expected to cover the gamut. Thus, neuroendocrine differentiation is probably never completely excluded in the usual pathologic assessment of these cancers and evalua-

tion for it is of questionable practical value. In rare instances, a tumor lacks so many features of a carcinoma that it is best considered unclassifiable. The temptation to substitute genetic analysis for morphology in such rare cases should be resisted until the database of genetic changes in bladder neoplasms has been more thoroughly analyzed.

The best characterized poorly differentiated carcinoma of the urinary bladder is histologically similar to small cell carcinoma of the lung. It is this lesion that is described in the following section.

The etiology and pathogenesis of poorly differentiated small cell carcinomas of the urinary bladder are unknown but origin via dedifferentiation of neuroendocrine cells seems unlikely. Nearly 50 percent of reported cases have mixed epithelial components, most often urothelial carcinoma (289). Cytologic detection of malignant tumor cells is readily achieved, although accurate typing is not always possible (288).

Clinical Features. Poorly differentiated small cell carcinomas comprise less than 0.5 percent of all bladder neoplasms (289,291–293, 294,296). The clinical features do not differ from those of urothelial carcinomas, even when tumors with mixed epithelial elements are deleted from the evaluation. Paraneoplastic syndromes are distinctly unusual, occurring in less than 5 percent of reported patients. The majority of patients have large, deeply invasive tumors at diagnosis and up to 65 percent either have or soon develop metastases.

Cystoscopically, poorly differentiated small cell carcinomas tend to be polypoid or nodular, often ulcerated masses that cannot be distinguished from other high-grade cancers. They may occur at various locations and are not predominantly localized to the bladder base.

Pathologic Findings. The small cell component of poorly differentiated carcinomas of the bladder is almost always described as histologically indistinguishable from similar cancers arising at other sites (fig. 3-68). It should be noted that pulmonary small cell carcinomas are heterogeneous in both nuclear size and neuroendocrine differentiation (297). Bladder tumors are composed of loosely cohesive sheets of small cells with scant cytoplasm. Necrosis is common. Rarely, nuclei are oat shaped but are commonly polygonal. Nuclear overlapping is

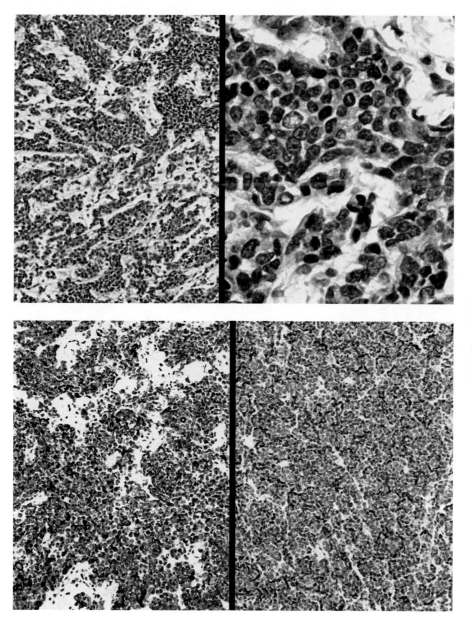

Figure 3-68

POORLY DIFFERENTIATED SMALL CELL CARCINOMA

Top: Low and intermediate magnifications highlight the sheet-like growth pattern of uniform cells.

Bottom: A positive reaction for chromogranin A (left) and a negative reaction for cytokeratin 20 (right).

not a characteristic feature of poorly differentiated small cell carcinomas of the urinary bladder. In optimal preparations, chromatin is coarsely granular and evenly distributed. Nucleoli are usually small or absent but the presence of scattered cells with large nucleoli does not obviate the diagnosis. Mitoses are variable but may be numerous.

Cytologic samples usually contain numerous tumor cells (fig. 3-69). They tend to aggregate in loose clusters and have eccentric nuclei with scant cytoplasm. Chromatin is coarse but evenly dispersed. Nucleoli are usually lacking. The cells of poorly differentiated small cell carcinomas are significantly larger than those of lymphomas. Nonspecific dense core granules have been observed in almost all lesions examined by transmission electron microscopy.

Immunohistochemical studies have recorded variable results (291,297–299). In general, poorly differentiated small cell carcinomas of the bladder react with antibodies to neuron-specific enolase, epithelial membrane antigen, and Cam 5.2. Reactions for polypeptides have

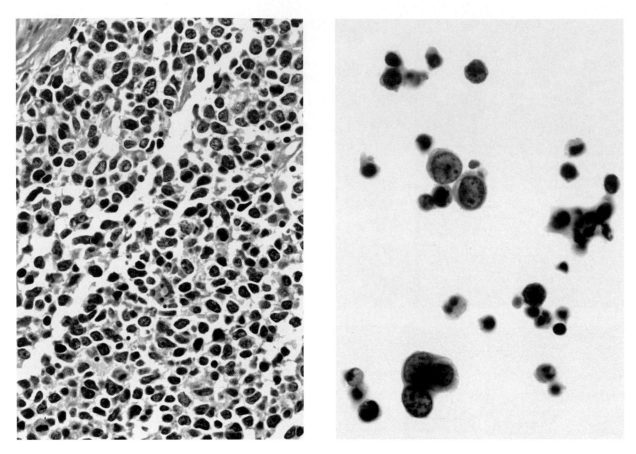

Figure 3-69

POORLY DIFFERENTIATED SMALL CELL CARCINOMA
Left: Histology.
Right: Corresponding urinary cytology.

been sporadic, with synaptophysin offering the greatest chance of positivity. Reactions with cytokeratin cocktails and carcinoembryonic antigens are usually negative.

Prognosis. In contrast to urothelial neoplasms, about 50 percent of reported cases of poorly differentiated small cell carcinomas have been high stage at diagnosis (289). Metastases at or soon after detection occur in up to 65 percent of patients. Like other small cell carcinomas, metastases preferentially involve lymph nodes, liver, and bone. Despite poor differentiation, not all small cell carcinomas of the urinary bladder are fatal (289,291,293,294,296). Survival is directly related to stage at diagnosis and response to treatment. It is apparently not affected by the presence of mixed epithelial elements. When initial tumors are organ-con-

fined, up to 44 percent of reported patients survive, compared to rates of 0 to 19 percent for those with disseminated and locally advanced lesions. Optimal treatment has yet to be determined but most authors favor a multimodality approach (290,295,296). Death from disease ordinarily occurs within 3 years of diagnosis, and unfavorable late events are uncommon.

Differential Diagnosis. Poorly differentiated small cell carcinomas often occur in association with other histologic types of urothelial cancer but any appreciable small cell component is sufficient to place a tumor in this category. Small cell carcinomas can be differentiated from lymphomas and sarcomas by their cell size, cell aggregation, and lack of large nucleoli. Factors associated with fixation and specimen processing can produce histologic appearances

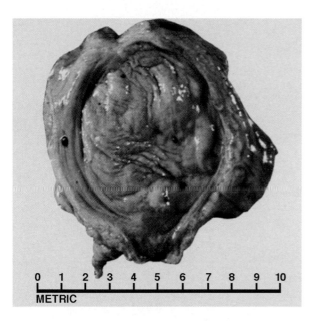

Figure 3-70

METASTATIC MELANOMA IN BLADDER MUCOSA

The patient, a 31-year-old woman, had a cutaneous melanoma approximately 1 year before her death from widespread metastases. (Plate IIIC from Fascicle 31A, 1st Series.)

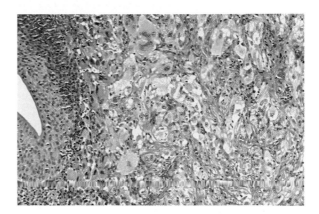

Figure 3-71

MELANOMA IN URINARY BLADDER

that mimic small cell carcinoma so that associated foci of urothelial CIS and immunohistochemical reactions for lymphoid markers, certain cytokeratins, and polypeptides are helpful in diagnosis. Small cell carcinomas metastatic to the bladder cannot be differentiated from primary bladder tumors without appropriate clinical information.

RARE NEOPLASMS

Rarity in the medical literature is an evolving determination. Some lesions, e.g., urothelial carcinoma with spindle cell stroma, are histologically distinctive but essentially a peculiar variation of the carcinoma. Others, e.g., lymphoepithelial (lymphoepithelioma-like) carcinoma, could be similarly categorized but lack urothelial differentiation and seem to have sufficient features to warrant a separate designation. Some authors name nearly every variation separately whereas others prefer a unifying approach. The distinctions between rare and unusual, variant and distinctive entity, often rest upon the judgement of the classifier and can be expected to change with both taste and time.

Carcinoid Tumor

Carcinoid tumors have been reported both as pure lesions and as small components of mixed carcinomas (320). When appearing in the bladder, these neoplasms do not differ from those occurring at other sites. Diagnosis depends primarily upon recognition of the characteristic histologic patterns but can be corroborated with electron microscopy and studies to identify neuroendocrine differentiation. Carcinoid syndrome has not been reported among recorded patients. Despite its rather innocuous histologic appearance, carcinoid tumor of the urinary bladder is not always benign. Three cases with metastases and at least one tumor-related death are recorded. Carcinoid tumor could be construed as a well-differentiated neuroendocrine carcinoma but the significance of polypeptide production by bladder tumors, especially at the poorly differentiated end of the spectrum, is unclear and there seems little to gain by offering an alternative term for a well-established entity.

Melanoma

Primary melanoma has been reported throughout the genitourinary tract, including the bladder (figs. 3-70, 3-71) (304,307,309,318). These tumors do not differ histologically from similar lesions arising in the skin, and extravesical sources of a primary tumor must be excluded before the diagnosis can be confirmed. The pathogenesis is obscure, although melanosis with and without atypia is observed

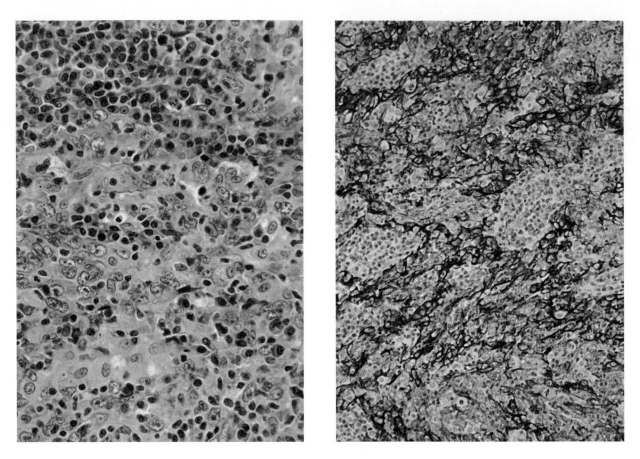

Figure 3-72

LYMPHOEPITHELIAL (LYMPHOEPITHELIOMA-LIKE) CARCINOMA

Left: These bladder tumors are histologically similar to those in the upper respiratory tract.

Right: A positive immunohistochemical reaction for pancytokeratins highlights the epithelial component. (Courtesy of Dr. George Reichel, Lubbock, TX.)

in otherwise normal urothelium as well as in the urothelium adjacent to melanomas (315). Patients are 44 to 81 years of age; the male to female ratio is 1 to 1. Lesions are not localized to the bladder base and not all are pigmented. Nevertheless, immunohistochemical markers for melanomas are positive. The disease has been uniformly fatal in recorded cases.

Lymphoepithelial (Lymphoepithelioma-Like) Carcinoma

Bladder tumors with features reminiscent of lymphoepithelioma of the nasopharynx have been reported as isolated cases and in small series (fig. 3-72) (301,306). The bladder lesions are histologically identical to those in the nasopharynx but since they lack evidence of Epstein-Barr virus, many authors have preferred

the term "lymphoepithelioma-like" to designate them. Lymphoepitheliomatous elements may occur in association with high-grade urothelial carcinomas but the histology of lymphoepithelial carcinoma defines a distinctive entity only when it comprises greater than 50 percent of the tumor. Patients are 59 to 84 years of age; the male to female ratio is close to 2 to 1.

The histologic findings can be confirmed with immunohistochemistry. The lymphoid elements react with panlymphocytic markers and certain B- and T-cell markers. The undifferentiated carcinoma component reacts with pancytokeratin markers. These tumors have invaded muscle at the time of diagnosis. Despite high stage and poor differentiation, the prognosis after surgery, with and without adjuvant therapy, has been extraordinarily favorable.

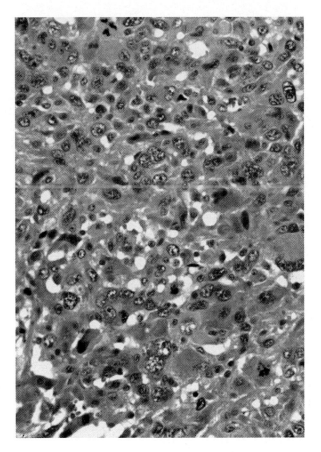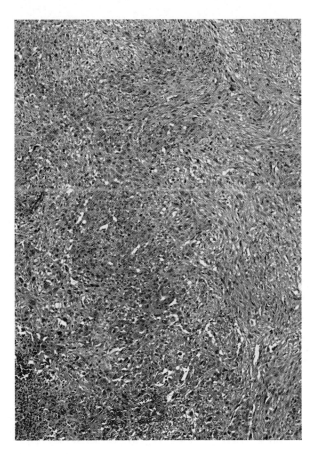

Figure 3-73

GIANT AND SPINDLE CELL CARCINOMA

Large Cell Neuroendocrine Carcinoma

Large cell neuroendocrine carcinoma has been reported in the urinary bladder. Like tumors of similar histology in the lung, the lesions may be either pure or mixed (300,305). If lung lesions are the model, it is very likely that tumors containing components of smaller cells with similar growth patterns but lacking large nucleoli will be recorded in future publications (312). The large neuroendocrine cells react with various polypeptide markers, including chromogranin. Reported cases, whether pure or mixed, have been of high stage and unresponsive to therapy.

Giant and Spindle Cell Carcinoma

This rare, somewhat ill-defined, malignant epithelial neoplasm derives its name from a resemblance to giant cell tumors at other sites (fig. 3-73) (310,314,317,321). Both the large multinucleated cells and the smaller spindle cells con-

tain epithelial markers. The giant cell component is prominent but is usually associated with other poorly differentiated elements, such as high-grade urothelial carcinoma. These tumors should be differentiated from urothelial carcinomas with osteoclast-type giant cells and the equally rare combination of urothelial carcinoma and non-epithelial giant cell tumor of mesenchymal derivation (308,311,322). The prognosis varies, depending on stage at diagnosis and the presence and type of mixed elements.

Plasmacytoid/Lymphomatoid Carcinoma

Isolated reports have described bladder tumors composed of malignant epithelial cells that resemble plasmacytes or lymphocytes by light microscopy but are strongly positive for cytokeratin markers and negative for plasmacyte/lymphocyte markers by immunohistochemistry (316,323). In some instances, the

315

epithelial tumor cells are intermixed with lymphoid elements, either isolated or in small aggregates. In other cases, the tumor cells are the majority of the neoplastic elements. These tumors differ from lymphoepithelial carcinomas in that the tumor cells themselves, rather than a surrounding infiltrate, have lymphoma-like features. Unlike primary plasmacytomas or lymphomas of the bladder, the malignant cells of plasmacytoid/lymphomatoid carcinomas do not produce or contain gamma globulins or light chains. Plasmacytoid/lymphomatoid carcinoma can be distinguished from melanoma immunohistochemically. Bone marrow, peripheral blood, and serum studies are unremarkable. The prognosis has not been completely determined but some tumors are inoperable at diagnosis.

Rhabdoid Tumor

Rhabdoid tumor is a somewhat controversial malignant neoplasm in the bladder, but even if cases describing lesions with mixed histology are excluded, at least two tumors with features nearly identical to those of rhabdoid renal neoplasms can be accepted (302,313). They presented in patients aged 6 and 14 years and both were high stage. The characteristic pathologic features of childhood renal rhabdoid tumors were confirmed. The case reports did not include long-term follow-up.

Basaloid (Basaloid Squamous) Carcinoma

A single case of a bladder tumor with features reminiscent of basaloid carcinoma of the upper aerodigestive tract has been described and illustrated (319). The authors considered this tumor to be a variant of squamous cell carcinoma. The patient was a woman who had undergone multiple major surgical procedures and reconstructions of her urethra and bladder neck.

This list of rare neoplasms encompasses nearly all of the well-documented lesions of which we are aware but is probably not all-inclusive. No doubt other rare neoplasms have been observed in the urinary bladder. We have seen a lipid-rich carcinoma, for example, and are cognizant of a letter to the editor citing a primitive neuroectodermal tumor (PNET) documented by the presence of the WTS/FLI-1 fusion transcript (303).

METASTASES TO URINARY BLADDER

Extravesical tumors usually involve the urinary bladder by direct extension from adjacent pelvic organs such as the prostate gland, uterine cervix, and rectum. Given the appropriate history, pathologic interpretation is not usually difficult, but extravesical cancers can mimic urothelial malignancies. Prostatic carcinomas can arise in the bladder from ectopic tissue and colon cancers cannot be distinguished from primary bladder adenocarcinomas histologically. Metastases from distant sites are rare and are almost always associated with widely disseminated disease (328). Metastatic lesions may originate from unlikely sites and histologic types. Metastatic melanomas and lymphomas are frequently cited in the literature (331). A wide variety of malignancies have been observed. These include cancers of the stomach, breast, prostate, lung, kidney, pancreas, testis, appendix, ovary, uterus, gallbladder, liver, and even tongue (324–330,332–335). Many cases are found at autopsy but patients may present with symptoms related to the metastatic bladder tumor. The urothelium is usually spared in metastatic disease, a situation that provides an important clue to the diagnosis. Bladder involvement by lesions that appear glandular or poorly differentiated but do not involve the urothelium suggests metastatic disease.

NONEPITHELIAL NEOPLASMS

Mesenchymal Neoplasms

Definition and General Features. Mesenchymal neoplasms are tumors differentiating toward muscle, nerve, bone, cartilage, fat, fibrous tissue, or blood vessels. They account for less than 1 percent of all bladder neoplasms and may be histologically benign or malignant. The etiology and pathogenesis are unknown.

Clinical Features. As with other bladder neoplasms, most patients with mesenchymal tumors are male. An origin in the bladder usually produces hematuria and may result in dysuria or a palpable pelvic mass. In many cases, the tumor occupies more than one pelvic organ and the site of origin is difficult to determine. Large tumors may obstruct the urethra or ureter, and renal failure is a frequent serious complication. Mesenchymal tumors are ordinarily detected by

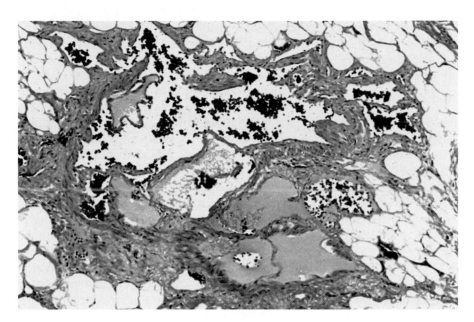

Figure 3-74

HEMANGIOMA OF URINARY BLADDER

This patient had clinical signs of Klippel-Trenaunay syndrome.

pelvic examination and cystoscopy rather than cytology or radiography. Most present as polypoid growths with intact or focally ulcerated mucosal surfaces. Both benign and malignant tumors tend to grow locally. Dissemination in malignant lesions is usually a late event.

Pathologic Findings. Mesenchymal neoplasms of the urinary bladder do not differ pathologically from similarly classified tumors arising at other sites, and the pathologist confronted with such a case should consult a recent reference devoted to soft tissue tumors for details of histology, ultrastructure, immunohistochemistry, and molecular biology. Almost all histologic variations of mesenchymal tumors have been recorded as primary bladder lesions. The older literature cites fibroma, osteoma, mesenchymoma, ganglioneuroma, granular cell tumor, adenofibroma, hemangiopericytoma, and fibrosarcoma, but it is likely that some of the designations of these tumors would be changed were they to be encountered today (366,385). More recently cited benign neoplasms include hemangioma, solitary fibrous tumor, leiomyoma, lymphangioma, neurofibroma and neurofibromatosis, lipoma, xanthoma, spindle cell tumor with features of gastrointestinal stromal tumor (GIST), aggressive angiomyxoid tumor, angiomyolipoma, and clear cell myomelanocytic tumor (341,344,345,347,350,351,358,369,371, 375,378,384). Malignant tumors include rhabdomyosarcoma, leiomyosarcoma, angiosar-

coma, osteosarcoma, chondrosarcoma, malignant fibrous histiocytoma, and adenosarcoma (346,353,359,361,367,368,372,381,383). Mesenchymal tumors are rare in the urinary bladder and only those that are the most common, have peculiar features, or present especially difficult differential diagnostic problems are discussed.

Hemangioma

Hemangiomas of the bladder are generally considered congenital anomalies, although almost 50 percent are detected in adults (344, 384). Their importance is magnified in the bladder because transurethral resections have occasionally resulted in severe hemorrhage. Gross hematuria is the most frequent presenting sign, although bladder lesions may be discovered in patients with cutaneous, perineal, and genital hemangiomas. Vascular lesions of the bladder often occur in patients who have the Klippel-Trenaunay syndrome (port-wine hemangiomas, varicose veins, soft tissue and bone hemihypertrophy) (357). Patients are from 5 weeks to 76 years of age. Lesions are usually single but may be multiple and occur anywhere in the bladder wall. They vary from a few millimeters to 10 cm in greatest dimension but many have nonspecific features cystoscopically. Histologically, most hemangiomas are of the cavernous type (fig. 3-74).

Accurate interpretation is not difficult once the pathologist is mentally attuned to search for such rare lesions. Hemangiomas are differentiated from telangiectasias by their growth pattern, from arteriovenous malformations by lack of arterial structures, and from angiosarcomas by lack of significant endothelial atypia.

Solitary Fibrous Tumor

Solitary fibrous tumors, histologically indistinguishable from lesions arising in the pleura, have been recorded in the bladder and other pelvic organs (347,385). Men, aged 50 to 67 years, are affected. Even though the tumors tend to be large, patients may be asymptomatic and the tumor detected incidently. Reported lesions react with CD34. Recurrence has not been reported after cystectomy.

Leiomyoma

Leiomyomas are benign neoplasms that occur with equal frequency in men and women (361,369). Patients are 22 to 78 years of age. Most patients have symptoms, even though many tumors are small. The histologic features are characteristic of similar tumors occurring at other sites but the rarity of these lesions should raise the possibility of a well-differentiated leiomyosarcoma. Clinically corroborated criteria for the pathologic distinction of leiomyoma from well-differentiated leiomyosarcoma are not well established but it seems prudent to adopt a conservative approach to diagnosis and treatment. Lesions that are not well circumscribed, are focally necrotic, or have readily identifiable mitoses are suspects for adverse behavior (361). The presence of any abnormal mitoses should probably result in an interpretation of malignancy. On the other hand, bizarre or symplastic nuclei in the absence of other abnormal features should not alter the interpretation. Immunohistochemistry is not particularly helpful for accurate interpretation.

Myosarcoma

Definition and General Features. The most common mesenchymal tumors of the urinary bladder manifest features of muscle differentiation and are considered myosarcomas (346,349, 359,362,374,384). These neoplasms constitute less than 0.5 percent of all bladder tumors. In children, they are classified as *rhabdomyosarcomas* because some of the primitive cells of which they are composed have features of skeletal muscle differentiation (349). These bladder tumors have been observed in association with congenital anomalies of the brain and nephroblastomas. A few have occurred in fetuses.

Clinical Features and Pathologic Findings in Children. Rhabdomyosarcomas in children most often affect boys (sex ratio, 3 to 1). They grow as polypoid masses which may obstruct the urinary outflow. When this configuration resembles a bunch of grapes, the term *botryoid sarcoma* has been used (fig. 3-75).

Histologically, rhabdomyosarcomas characteristically have a "cambium" layer of compressed rhabdomyoblasts immediately beneath an intact urothelium. Masses of stellate, round, and spindle cells occupy an edematous stroma rich in hyaluronic acid (fig. 3-76). The cytoplasm of the rhabdomyoblasts is scanty and cross striations are very difficult to identify in untreated cases. Tumor cells react weakly or not at all with antibodies to myoglobin, in contrast to a more diffuse and robust reaction with antibodies to desmin and actin (359). Treatment often increases the number of recognizable myoblasts but seems to have little effect on the immunohistochemistry.

Rhabdomyosarcomas grow locally and recur if inadequately excised. Survival is increasingly favorable, with a 10-year survival rate of about 90 percent; several patients are alive more than 20 years after treatment. Initial low tumor stage, an exophytic (botryoid) growth pattern, an embryonal rather than an alveolar histology, and both maturation as well as decreased cellularity after multimodality treatment are favorable prognostic factors.

Clinical Features and Pathologic Findings in Adults. Myosarcomas in adults generally have features of smooth muscle differentiation and are classified as *leiomyosarcomas* (361,362, 374,379,384). Patients of all ages are affected but most are 40 to 60 years old. Men predominate in a ratio of 3 to 2. The tumors are often poorly circumscribed and invasive, with ulcerated surfaces (figs. 3-77, 3-78). These cancers do not differ histologically from similar lesions at other sites except that the myxoid variant is reported with increasing frequency. They are highly cellular with variable numbers of mitoses. Necrosis is common. Immunohistochemical reactions for actins are positive in 65 to 80 percent of cases but reactions for desmin are

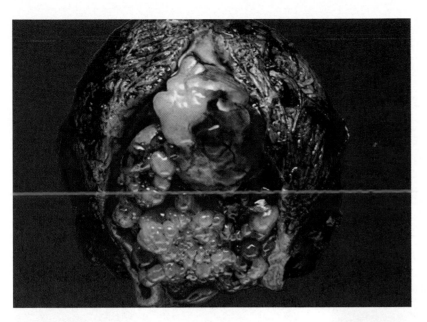

Figure 3-75

RHABDOMYOSARCOMA, BOTRYOID TYPE

The reference to a bunch of grapes is apropos. (Courtesy of Dr. George M. Farrow, Rochester, MN.)

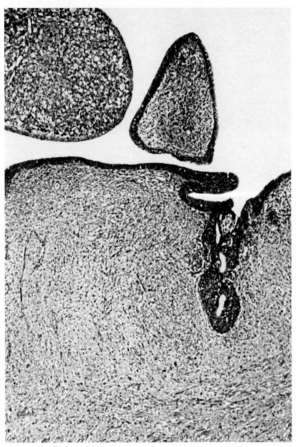

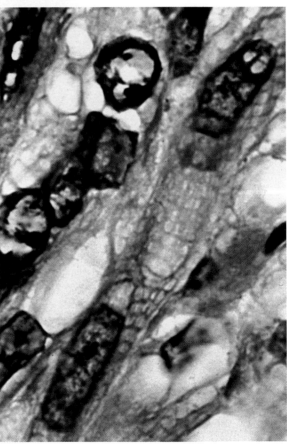

Figure 3-76

RHABDOMYOSARCOMA

Left: Polypoid surface of a rhabdomyosarcoma arising in the bladder of a child.
Right: High magnification reveals cells with cross striations. (Courtesy of Dr. David Parham, Little Rock, AR.)

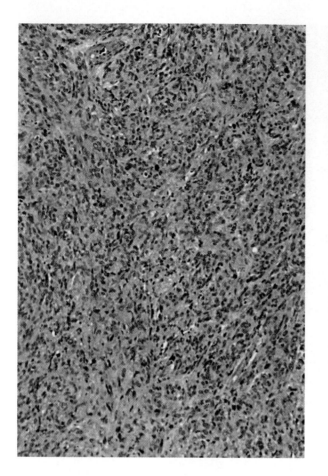
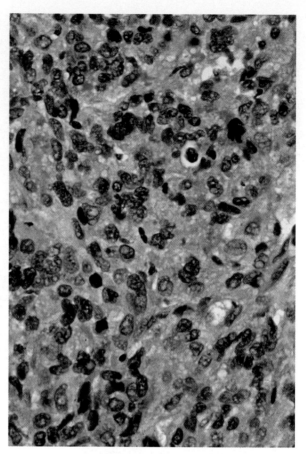

Figure 3-77

LEIOMYOSARCOMA

often negative. A few tumors react with antibodies to c-kit (361).

Adult myosarcoma tends to grow locally but has a higher frequency of metastases than its childhood counterpart. The dismal prognosis reported in the older literature has been only slightly improved in more recent series; progressive disease occurs in more than 50 percent of patients, with death from disease in nearly as many (338,361).

Leiomyosarcomas are differentiated from sarcomatoid urothelial carcinomas by their lack of malignant epithelial islands and negative reactions for cytokeratins. Differentiation from pseudosarcomatous fibromyxoid tumor (inflammatory pseudotumor) is straightforward as long as the leiomyosarcoma has the characteristic nuclear pleomorphism, high cellularity, necrosis, and abnormal mitoses. In the few

cases in which these features are lacking, especially with the myxoid variant, accurate assessment can be more daunting. In such cases, immunohistochemistry is usually of little help, unless the lesion is more than focally positive for desmin. Necrosis at the tumor-smooth muscle interface and abnormal mitoses are the most reliable diagnostic features of a leiomyosarcoma that lacks significant nuclear pleomorphism. Doubtful cases are best considered low-grade neoplasms and treated accordingly.

Pheochromocytoma (Paraganglioma)

Pheochromocytoma is the most common designation for a paraganglioma arising in the urinary bladder (343,354,365,366,373,384). These tumors comprise less than 0.1 percent of all bladder neoplasms. Rare cases are associated with neurofibromatosis, urothelial carcinoma, and

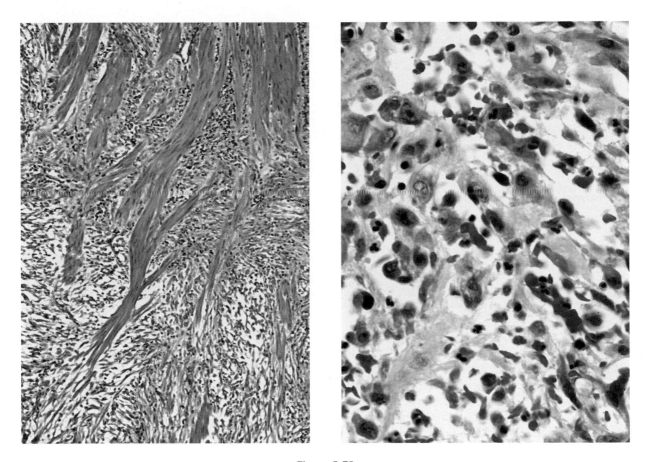

Figure 3-78

LEIOMYOSARCOMA, MYXOID TYPE

Left: Destruction of muscle fascicles at the tumor-muscle interface is one of the features distinguishing this lesion from a pseudosarcomatous fibromyxoid tumor (inflammatory pseudotumor).

Right: Nuclear pleomorphism and intralesional necrosis are other distinguishing features.

renal cell carcinoma, but bladder pheochromocytomas have not been observed as part of the multiple endocrine neoplasia syndrome.

Patients are 10 to 78 years of age (mean, 42 years), and young women are more often affected. Hematuria is a common complaint but more than 50 percent of recorded patients experience symptoms that can be directly related to the release of catecholamines from their tumors. Discomfort is associated with a full bladder or voiding. The most characteristic symptom complex is the "micturition attack," consisting of bursting headache, anxiety, tremulousness, pounding sensation, blurred vision, sweating, and even syncope. Hypertension is observed in most individuals. Catecholamines or their metabolites are elevated in the serum or urine

of at least 50 percent of patients examined for these substances.

Pheochromocytomas, unlike many other bladder tumors, are not necessarily localized to the bladder base but occur anywhere in the organ. Most are single lesions measuring only a few millimeters in greatest dimension, but multiple and large tumors are recorded. Small aggregates of paraganglionic cells occurring in the lamina propria may be mistaken for Brunn nests.

Histologically, pheochromocytomas usually assume the characteristic zellballen pattern but fibrous and ganglioneuromatous arrangements are observed (fig. 3-79). Vascular invasion is recorded. Cells tend to be round with amphophilic to acidophilic cytoplasm and ovoid nuclei. Occasional bizarre nuclei, such as seen in other

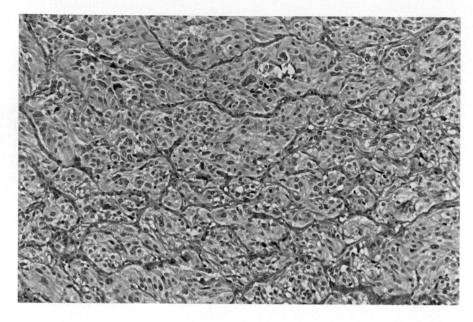

Figure 3-79

PHEOCHROMOCYTOMA

(Courtesy of Dr. Albert S. Hollingsworth, Anderson, SC.)

neuroendocrine neoplasms, may be present. Mitoses are uncommon. Occasional foci of neuroblast-like cells occur. Tumor cells react with antibodies to chromogranin and synaptophysin as well as S-100 protein, and are negative for cytokeratins. Other substances identified in these tumors include adrenocorticotropin (ACTH), calcitonin, gastrin, glucagon, serotonin, somatostatin, vasoactive intestinal polypeptide, and glial fibrillary acidic protein (366). Interestingly, pheochromocytomas tend to be aneuploid (343). Ultrastructurally, dense core granules are common.

The behavior of pheochromocytomas cannot be accurately predicted from pathologic examination alone. Multiple recurrences, nuclear anaplasia, vascular invasion, abnormal DNA ploidy, and an invasive growth pattern may identify patients at increased risk but none of these features are highly predictive of future progression. Nevertheless, 5 to 18 percent of reported bladder pheochromocytomas have metastasized.

Lymphoma

Bladder involvement has been documented in 10 to 25 percent of lymphomas and leukemias but lymphoid neoplasms arising primarily in the urinary bladder are rare (336,339, 355,363,370,384). The disease is usually detected in middle-aged women undergoing cystoscopy for nonspecific urinary symptoms but may present as a pelvic mass.

Grossly, bladder lymphomas usually appear as discrete tumors rather than diffuse infiltrates. Most are large masses centered in the dome or lateral walls. Histologically, infiltrating sheets of uniform cells surrounding and separating, rather than destroying, muscle fascicles are characteristic (fig. 3-80). Cytologic features do not differ from those of lymphomas at other sites. Well-differentiated lymphocytic lymphomas of B-cell type are the most common, although T-cell, mucosa-associated lymphoid tissue (MALT) type, poorly differentiated lymphocytic, large cell, and even sarcomatous and signet ring varieties have been observed (339,342, 352,363,376). A single case of primary Hodgkin disease of the bladder is well documented (360).

The prognosis of patients with primary bladder lymphoma is favorable, with many alive and well several years after treatment. Prolonged survival probably reflects the low grade and stage of most tumors.

Well-differentiated lymphocytic lymphomas of the urinary bladder pose few differential diagnostic problems to knowledgeable observers once systemic disease is excluded. There appears to be no relationship to follicular cystitis, and pseudolymphoma of the bladder is not well documented. More poorly differentiated lymphomas can be distinguished from small cell cancers by suitable immunohistochemical reactions for polypeptides, cytokeratins, and leukocytes.

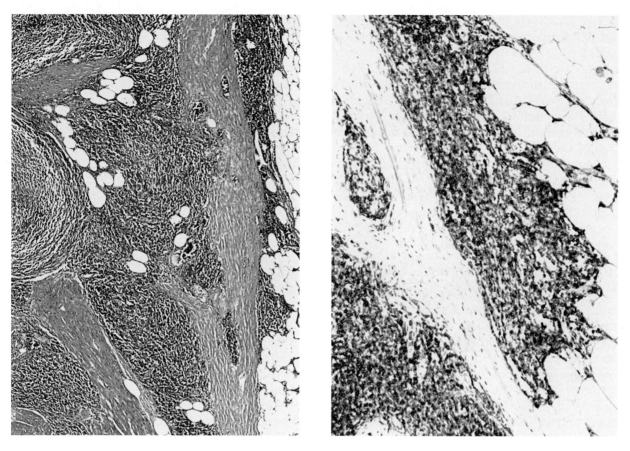

Figure 3-80

MUCOSA-ASSOCIATED LYMPHOID TISSUE (MALT) LYMPHOMA INVOLVING URINARY BLADDER

Left: Lymphomas commonly infiltrate the interstitium of the bladder, preserving the muscle bundles of the detrusor.
Right: Positive immunohistochemical reaction for CD43.

Plasmacytoma

Plasmacytomas arising in the urinary bladder are rare and all information concerning these neoplasms is derived from case reports (348,384, 386). The few recorded patients are both men and women ranging in age from 39 to 89 years. Signs and symptoms are nonspecific. Like plasmacytomas at other extramedullary sites, these lesions look and act more like solid tumors than lymphoproliferative neoplasms. Depending on size and cellular activity, monoclonal immunoglobulins may occur in the serum and urine; this finding should not necessarily indicate disseminated disease in the case of an unresected tumor. Plasmacytomas may present as single or multiple nodular masses in the bladder wall.

Histologically, a wide range of mature and immature forms, including giant and multi-nucleated cells, occur. Immunoglobulins A and G as well as both kappa and lambda light chains have been documented in individual cases. Although often difficult to identify immunohistochemically in paraffin-embedded tissue, the presence of immunoglobulins is an important distinguishing feature, especially since plasmacytomas can resemble various poorly differentiated cancers when examined using routine histologic preparations.

The prognosis is favorable. Recurrences are reported but no patient died of a plasmacytoma arising in the bladder.

Germ Cell Tumors

Germ cell tumors arising in the urinary bladder include choriocarcinoma, dermoid cyst, teratoma, and yolk sac tumor (356,366,377,384). Most reports describe choriocarcinomatous elements arising in association with a high-grade urothelial carcinoma but pure lesions have been recorded (337,356,364,371). Most patients with choriocarcinomatous foci are men and the women are postmenopausal. The prognosis is guarded, with survival in recently reported cases; nevertheless, nearly all reported patients with more than a few months of follow-up have died of their disease.

Dermoid cysts have been described in the bladders of women 30 to 49 years of age (340, 384). These tumors do not differ clinically or histologically from their ovarian counterparts. There are isolated case reports of teratoma and yolk sac tumor (374,380,382).

NON-NEOPLASTIC TUMOROUS CONDITIONS

Non-neoplastic tumorous conditions constitute a vast array of lesions described under various names by individuals with diverse views on the nature of disease. Some tumorous lesions are common and others rare. A few are not really tumors, in the sense of a space-occupying mass, but require discussion because they have features that raise the suspicion of a neoplasm. These lesions are briefly described primarily for the sake of completeness. More thorough discussions can be found in texts not limited to the pathology of bladder tumors.

Condyloma Acuminatum-Squamous Cell Papilloma

Condyloma acuminatum is a characteristic proliferation of squamous cells that is highly associated with molecular evidence of past or present infection with human papillomavirus (HPV) (393,400,452). Bladder involvement ordinarily occurs by direct extension from urethral lesions. Primary condyloma acuminatum of the urinary bladder is exceedingly rare.

The lesion does not differ histologically from similar tumors at other sites. Using sophisticated techniques that detect the presence of a few gene copies or previously imprinted RNA, viral DNA of HPV subtypes 6 and 11, but not 16 and 18, are demonstrated in primary bladder condylomas. Structural viral antigens, on the other hand, are rarely observed.

Condyloma acuminatum may be distinguished from squamous cell papilloma in histologic preparations if the presence of typical koilocytes is required for the diagnosis of the former and a single, small lesion is required for the recognition of the latter. These lesions are very similar, however, and their relationship is unclear. Moderate nuclear atypia may occur in both lesions but areas of cellular anaplasia are not present. Grading the degree of nuclear atypia is unlikely to be helpful and might provoke unwarranted treatment, since the propensity of condylomas to progress to carcinomas is not well documented for primary bladder lesions. Condyloma acuminatum and squamous cell papilloma are distinguished from verrucous carcinoma primarily by the extent of bladder involvement, since none of these lesions has unequivocally invasive margins and all lack significant cellular anaplasia.

Metaplasia

Metaplastic lesions of the urinary bladder are of three basic types: squamous, intestinal, and nephrogenic. Osseous, cartilaginous, and myeloid metaplasias also occur but are rare. Metaplastic changes can be considered reflections of a deranged urothelial response to injurious stimuli. They are often associated with structural defects and sources of chronic irritation. It is not uncommon for various types of metaplasia to coexist, and for metaplasias to coexist with proliferative reactions of Brunn nests. The risk for subsequent cancer among patients with metaplasia is low and tends to vary with the type of metaplasia, and its duration and extent.

Squamous Metaplasia. Squamous metaplasia describes the replacement of normal urothelium with an epithelium composed of stratified squamous cells (fig. 3-81). Lesions resembling vaginal epithelium (sometimes called "trigonitis" clinically) are so common in women that many authors consider this change to be normal (450). The vaginal type of squamous metaplasia arises de novo. It is usually not associated with chronic irritation and is associated with little or no risk for subsequent carcinoma (449).

The keratinizing type of squamous metaplasia (leukoplakia) is of more concern. The lesion is usually associated with sources of chronic irritation and occurs more commonly in men (389). It is especially frequent in bladders with chronic indwelling catheters, stones, or calcified parasite eggs. Considerable cellular atypia, especially

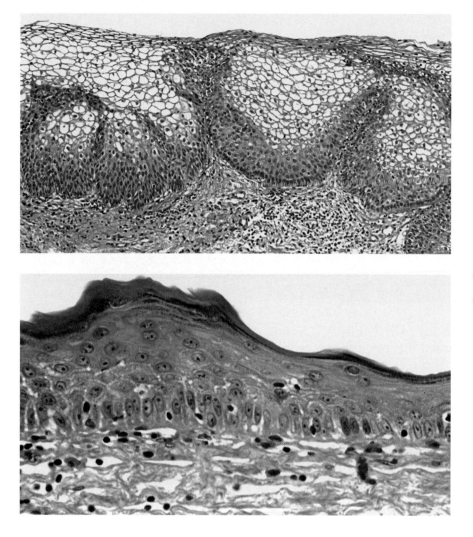

Figure 3-81

SQUAMOUS METAPLASIA OF URINARY BLADDER

Top: The nonkeratinizing (vaginal) type.

Bottom: The keratinizing (leukoplakia) type.

in the basilar layers, may occur and persist for long periods of time without the development of invasive carcinoma. Grading the degree of nuclear atypia in such cases is likely to introduce a degree of interpretive complexity that is unwarranted by the frequency of documented progression of squamous metaplasia to carcinoma. If experience with the grading of other intraepithelial lesions can serve as a guide, low-grade lesions will have poor reproducibility among pathologists and high-grade lesions will pose significant therapeutic problems for a group of patients whose prognosis is at best uncertain. It is important to note that the degree of intraepithelial atypia required for a pathologic diagnosis of squamous cell carcinoma in situ has not been determined. Foci of anaplastic nuclear change in the absence of in-

vasive carcinoma are distinctly unusual in squamous metaplasia of the urinary bladder. Nodular and papillary squamous lesions suggestive of condyloma acuminatum or squamous cell papilloma may develop in the urinary bladder, especially among patients with sources of chronic irritation.

Intestinal Metaplasia. Intestinal metaplasia is often used to describe the presence of isolated or aggregated goblet cells in proliferations of Brunn nests, but the term is more usefully employed to define replacement of urothelium by colonic mucosa (fig. 3-82) (398,407,447,452). The intestinal glands ordinarily lack cellular atypia and are confined to the area of the former urothelium. Involvement of the lamina propria may occur, occasionally with mucinous pools that lack epithelial cells, but the muscularis

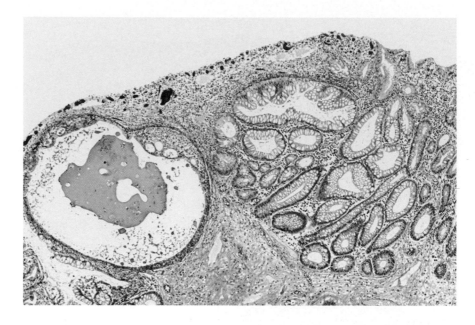

Figure 3-82

INTESTINAL METAPLASIA

propria is spared. Rarely, extensive areas of urothelium are replaced by intestinal mucosa, the most extreme examples occurring in exstrophy. Adenomatous changes and Paneth cells have been observed (392). The mucins of intestinal metaplasia are not diagnostically distinguishing, nor are they risk factors for subsequent carcinoma (388,391). Carcinomas are recorded among patients presenting with intestinal metaplasia but the risk is low (398).

Nephrogenic Metaplasia (Nephrogenic Adenoma). Nephrogenic metaplasia is a peculiar reactive process that results in papillary and tubular growths reminiscent of immature urothelial or metanephric structures (fig. 3-83) (402,409, 428,431). Despite the common appellation "adenoma," the evidence favoring a neoplasm is fragmentary (402,426). Certain lesions share lectin expression with fetal renal tubules or exhibit the same restriction in X chromosome expression as found in allografted kidneys, but the virtual absence of completely de novo lesions and the fluctuation of nephrogenic lesions with recurrent urinary tract infections are decidedly uncharacteristic of a neoplasm. Like squamous and intestinal metaplasia, nephrogenic changes are almost always associated with sources of chronic irritation of the urothelium, such as recurrent infections of the bladder. They are also common in diverticula and at sites of previous surgery. Considering the available evidence, it seems best to include these lesions

among the metaplasias, recognizing that they represent a peculiar form of the genre.

The papillary component of nephrogenic metaplasia is usually mistaken for a urothelial carcinoma cystoscopically and the pathology transmittal form can be expected to contain the clinical impression of "bladder cancer." Histologically, foci of nephrogenic metaplasia replace the urothelium and ordinarily involve the lamina propria; the muscularis propria is spared. The lesion is distinguished by the presence of a single layer of cytologically bland cuboidal cells that line the stalks and tubules. Significant nuclear atypia is unusual in nephrogenic metaplasia and focal even when present. Limited analyses of chromosomes has revealed monosomy 9 and trisomy 7 in this completely benign lesion (446).

When nephrogenic metaplasia occurs in diverticula and at previous surgical sites, e.g., after transurethral resections, the lesions usually lack the papillary component and are composed solely of tubules. Such lesions may resemble prostatic carcinomas but can be distinguished by their histologic pattern and lack of prostatic antigens in immunohistochemical reactions. They may resemble the nested variant of urothelial carcinoma but have only a single layer of cells rather than cystic degeneration of a nest. They may produce mucins and resemble a signet ring carcinoma but can be distinguished by a thickened basal lamina as well as the absence of nuclear atypia. They

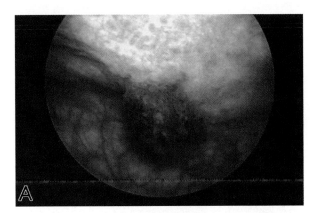

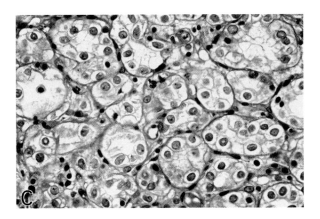

Figure 3-83

NEPHROGENIC METAPLASIA

A: Cystoscopically, these lesions resemble papillary neoplasms. (Courtesy of Dr. Mark S. Soloway, Miami, FL.)

B: The papillary component. (Fig. 146 from Murphy WM. Atlas of bladder carcinoma. Chicago: ASCP Press; 1986:126.)

C: The tubular component resembles a well-differentiated prostatic carcinoma.

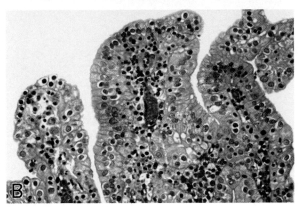

may resemble a capillary hemangioma but can be distinguished by positive reactions for cytokeratins. Nephrogenic metaplasia can be distinguished from clear cell adenocarcinoma by its lack of widespread nuclear anaplasia and lack of muscle invasion (453). Despite a tendency to recur, nephrogenic metaplasia is not a significant risk factor for subsequent carcinoma.

Inflammation

The urinary bladder may manifest a complex array of reactions to a variety of injurious stimuli. Pathologic lesions often poorly correlate with clinical disease even though their morphology may be distinctive. Inflammatory reactions seem to be host dependent, since the same stimulus can cause different lesions and different stimuli often result in the same lesions among individual patients. Many reactive processes have been termed "cystitis," even though most such lesions lack a significant component of leukocytic infiltration and some represent hyperplastic or metaplastic alterations of normal structures. The nodular lesions categorized

as cystitis are different from other types of inflammation and are discussed separately. Lesions described in this section include postoperative spindle cell nodule, inflammatory pseudotumor, malakoplakia, and granulomas that arise primarily in the urinary bladder.

Postoperative Spindle Cell Nodule. This increasingly recognized myofibroblastic proliferation arises within a few months of a previous surgical procedure at the surgical site (415, 435,452). Most lesions involve the genital tract of women and the periurethral prostatic tissue of men. Postoperative spindle cell nodules (PSCN) of the urinary bladder are usually small (less than 1 cm), poorly defined nodules occurring in men. Histologically, these lesions resemble nodular fasciitis and inflammatory pseudotumor (fig. 3-84). Characteristic changes include interlacing fascicles of spindle cells, areas rich in thin-walled blood vessels, and a sparse but uniformly distributed polymorphous leukocytic infiltrate. Mitoses may be numerous but are not atypical. Myxoid areas are often present. Infiltration of the detrusor muscle

327

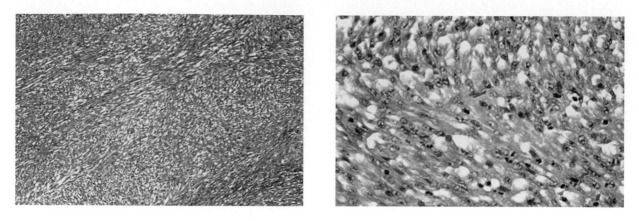

Figure 3-84

POSTOPERATIVE SPINDLE CELL NODULE

Left: A typical lesion with interlacing fascicles of myofibroblastic tissue.

Right: At high magnification, the cells are uniform and intermixed with inflammatory elements. (Courtesy of Dr. Charles Slonaker, Gulfport, MS.)

may occur but necrosis at the invading margin is not a feature of PSCN. Immunohistochemical and ultrastructural studies confirm myofibroblastic differentiation but positive reactions to cytokeratins have also been recorded (448).

Inflammatory Pseudotumor (Pseudosarcomatous Fibromyxoid Tumor). This is a nodular reaction of myofibroblasts which differs from PSCN primarily in the absence of a history of previous surgery (403,416,437,445,452). The name is misleading in that the lesions are tumors in the sense of space-occupying masses but an inflammatory etiology or pathogenesis has not been proven. The designation pseudosarcomatous fibromyxoid tumor is somewhat more accurate and both names are in use. Most lesions are observed in the female genital tract but reported patients with primary bladder lesions are of both sexes. Lesions occur over a wide age range, including children and the elderly, but most patients are middle-aged women. Gross hematuria is the predominant presenting sign. In contrast to PSCN, these lesions range from 2 to 8 cm in greatest dimension and the myxoid component is so prominent as to suggest a "tissue culture" appearance (fig. 3-85). Tumor cells in the few cases examined are diploid (421). The infiltrative growth pattern, histology, ultrastructure, immunohistochemistry, and clinical course of inflammatory pseudotumors are similar to PSCNs.

PSCNs and inflammatory pseudotumors probably represent similar processes despite differences in clinical presentation and variations in pathology among individual cases. Their histologic resemblance to benign myofibroblastic proliferations at other sites and their failure to progress even after incomplete resection strongly support a reactive process, even though these lesions have an invasive growth pattern and occasional tumors recur. In most situations, differentiation from malignant spindle cell tumors, including myxoid sarcomatoid carcinoma, is not difficult, but it may not be possible to exclude a myxoid leiomyosarcoma in every case. Immunohistochemistry is not helpful in the differential diagnosis (397). The distinction between benign and malignant tumors rests primarily on the nuclear pleomorphism, abnormal mitoses, and necrosis of the detrusor muscle characteristic of sarcomas. Underinterpretation of equivocal tumors should be avoided but may make little difference to the patient so long as the lesion can be completely resected. It is likely that patients with myxoid leiomyosarcomas that are so histologically innocuous that they cannot be distinguished from an inflammatory pseudotumor have a favorable outcome anyway.

Malakoplakia. Malakoplakia is a peculiar host reaction to chronic infection that is stimulated by an inability to completely metabolize certain bacteria. It is manifested by the accumulation of histiocytes and other inflammatory elements

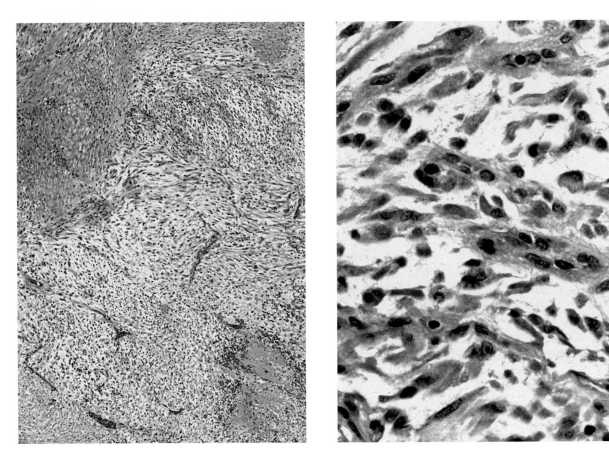

Figure 3-85

INFLAMMATORY PSEUDOTUMOR (PSEUDOSARCOMATOUS FIBROMYXOID TUMOR)

Left: The tumor-muscle interface is sharply demarcated and any necrotic areas are superficial.

Right: The myofibroblastic cells have an architectural pattern reminiscent of a tissue culture. Numerous mitoses are usual in these lesions. (Courtesy of Dr. George M. Farrow, Rochester, MN.)

in plaques or nodules (399). The bladder is the most common site but lesions are recognized throughout the genitourinary system as well as in many other organs. Reported patients range in age from 6 weeks to 96 years, and are more often women than men.

Malakoplakia occurs predominantly in the lamina propria. Sheets of histiocytes intermixed with variable numbers of lymphocytes, plasma cells, neutrophils, and eosinophils are characteristic (fig. 3-86). These lesions are often classified as granulomatous, although neither granulomas nor giant cells are usually present histologically. The diagnosis rests upon the identification of Michaelis-Gutmann bodies, i.e., mineralized intracellular or extracellular particles often consisting of a central core of partially digested bacteria coated with iron and calcium phosphate

(427). Histologically, Michaelis-Gutmann bodies appear as target or ring-like structures that react with periodic acid–Schiff and other reagents.

Xanthogranulomatous Inflammation. Xanthogranulomatous inflammation is usually associated with the kidney but also occurs in the urinary bladder (394,444). Interestingly, most cases are associated with the urachus. Histologically, the lesions resemble malakoplakia but lack Michaelis-Gutmann bodies and tend to have Touton-type giant cells. Granuloma formation is not characteristic.

Isolated case reports of primary bladder granulomas are recorded. These are inflammatory lesions of diverse histologic composition which may elicit signs and symptoms suggesting bladder disease or present clinically as discrete bladder tumors. They include paravesical suture

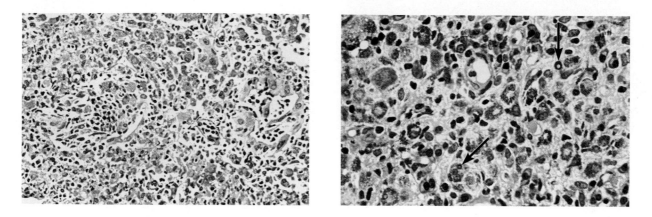

Figure 3-86

MALAKOPLAKIA

Left: Although the term means plaque-like, the depth of lesions eroding the bladder mucosa may be variable in microscopic sections.

Right: The target-shaped Michaelis-Gutmann bodies (arrows) are prominent (periodic acid–Schiff stain).

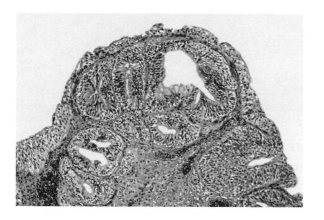

Figure 3-87

CYSTITIS GLANDULARIS

granulomas, occurring after herniorrhaphy; granulomatous reactions resembling rheumatoid nodules, appearing after transurethral resections; tubercular granulomas secondary to BCG treatment; and reparative granulomas in association with urothelial carcinoma (424,452, 454). Most reviews cite single cases of plasma cell granuloma and sarcoidosis (422,440). Fungal granulomas, parasitic tumors, and gummas have also been recorded (412–414)

"Cystitis"

A variety of hyperplasias, metaplasias, and reactive processes have been labeled "cystitis." Some are poorly defined in histopathologic terms whereas others are histologically characteristic but clinically unimportant. These lesions may produce symptoms and often appear to the cystoscopist as discrete abnormalities. Accurate pathologic assessment is required to exclude a neoplasm.

Cystitis Glandularis et Cystica. Cystitis glandularis is a proliferation of Brunn nests most likely resulting from injury to the bladder mucosa (411,450,452). The "glands" consist of layers of basal and intermediate urothelial cells lined by superficial urothelial cells that have been compressed into columnar shapes (fig. 3-87). The "cysts" arise from obstruction of the pores of Brunn nests. Superficial urothelial cells secrete and store small amounts of mucin and this material commonly accumulates in the lumens of the gland-like structures. Some authors prefer the term *proliferative cystitis* to describe lesions composed entirely of urothelial cells, reserving the term cystitis glandularis for lesions with focal goblet cell transformation. Rarely, the cells of cystitis glandularis may be markedly atypical in the absence of previous or coincident bladder cancer. Florid examples of cystitis glandularis et cystica may form nodular masses in the lamina propria (fig. 3-88). Such lesions have been considered either variants of inverted papilloma or hamartoma by some authors (423). Cystitis glandularis et cystica is distinguished from the nested type of urothelial carcinoma primarily by its nodular, noninfiltrative growth pattern

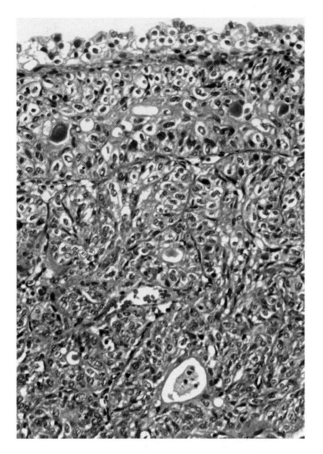

Figure 3-88

FLORID CYSTITIS GLANDULARIS

(Courtesy of Dr. Brian Montgomery, Fairhope, AL.)

and the accumulation of luminal mucins. Well-documented cases of adenocarcinoma associated with cystitis glandularis et cystica are rare and this lesion is not considered a risk factor for subsequent bladder cancer.

Cystitis Follicularis. Cystitis follicularis describes the appearance of lymphoid follicles within the lamina propria. The lymphoid tissue is histologically unremarkable but the attenuated overlying urothelium often develops slight to moderate cellular atypia (fig. 3-89) (452). These lesions have been associated with urinary tract infection, especially with *Salmonella* sp. They can be seen after BCG therapy but the association may be coincidental.

Bullous Cystitis. Bullous cystitis is a term coined by cystoscopists to describe an edematous bladder mucosa (fig. 3-90) (452). Edema of the lamina propria is a nonspecific finding but has been associated with recurrent neoplasms as well as reactions to radiation therapy. Most often, edema results from chronic irritation, e.g., from an indwelling catheter. The lesion may represent part of a spectrum of changes that include polypoid/papillary cystitis and fibroepithelial polyp.

Polypoid/Papillary Cystitis. The term polypoid or papillary cystitis is ordinarily used to describe a histologic lesion composed of normal or slightly reactive urothelium covering a focally fibrotic lamina propria (fig. 3-91). Such

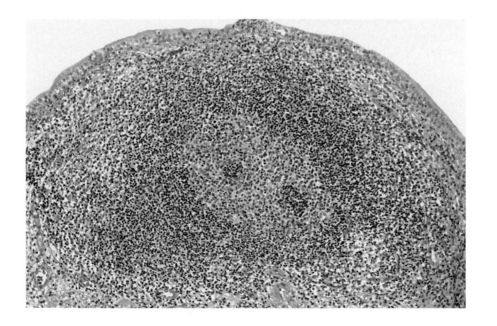

Figure 3-89

CYSTITIS FOLLICULARIS

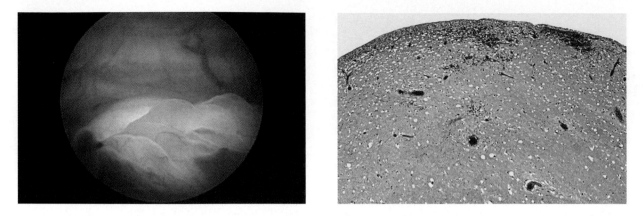

Figure 3-90

BULLOUS CYSTITIS

Left: Cystoscopic appearance. (Courtesy of Dr. Mark S. Soloway, Miami, FL.)
Right: Histologic features of bullous cystitis.

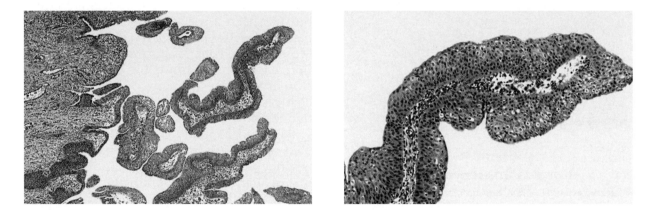

Figure 3-91

POLYPOID/PAPILLARY CYSTITIS

Left: Low magnification highlights the papillae with broad stalks.
Right: If inadequately sampled, such lesions may be confused with a urothelial papilloma.

configurations are often mistaken for neoplasms cystoscopically. When the fibrosis is particularly well developed, the lesion can be construed as a fibroepithelial polyp. The association of this rare lesion with Beckwith-Wiedemann syndrome suggests that it may be a separate entity rather than a variant of polypoid cystitis (450,452).

Like similar lesions elsewhere, the cores of polypoid/papillary lesions may have numerous, occasionally bizarre, stellate giant cells and focal muscle fibers, suggesting a hamartomatous tumor. Polypoid/papillary cystitis may occur in bladders treated for urothelial carcinomas, and

close scrutiny of abnormal nuclei in the stroma of polypoid lesions is required to exclude the rare invasive carcinoma that may be lurking there. The lesions may represent part of a spectrum that includes bullous cystitis.

Emphysematous Cystitis. Emphysematous cystitis is a term used by cystoscopists to describe gas-filled spaces in the bladder wall (436,452). The lesions usually result from collections of gas produced by microorganisms, most commonly *Escherichia coli* and *Enterobacter aerogenes*. Many patients are diabetics with neurogenic bladders.

Interstitial Cystitis. Interstitial cystitis is a rare chronic disease defined primarily by its

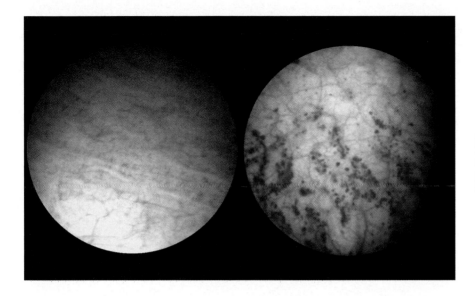

Figure 3-92

INTERSTITIAL CYSTITIS

Cystoscopic appearance before (left) and after (right) distension. Note the glomerulations, punctate hemorrhages in the lamina propria. (Courtesy of Dr. Mark S. Soloway, Miami, FL.)

symptoms and the reaction of the bladder to hydrodistension under anesthesia (396,401, 419,425,433,434). The disease may occur in children but nearly all reported patients are middle-aged Caucasian women (mean age, 44 years). Patients complain of frequency, dysuria, and abdominal pain relieved by voiding, all of many months' duration. By definition, the cause of the symptoms is unknown; infection must be specifically excluded. Although not life-threatening and often not associated with progressive destruction of bladder tissue, interstitial cystitis tends to be persistent, debilitating, and not particularly amenable to treatment.

The bladder capacity is often reduced and when the organ is distended under anesthesia, two types of reactions are observed. In the milder, so-called nonulcer form of the disease, where the bladder capacity is greater than 400 mL, glomerulations and fissures occur in the urothelium only after a second distension (fig. 3-92). In the severe, so-called ulcer form, where the capacity is less than 400 mL, the fissures occur at the initial distension.

The diagnosis of interstitial cystitis cannot be made from the pathologic findings. In fact, the changes in the tissue specimens tend to be less severe than either the symptoms or the cystoscopic findings imply (401). In patients with the nonulcer form of the disease, the most characteristic changes are fissuring of the urothelium with focal hemorrhage in the adjacent lamina propria (fig. 3-93). Edema and a slight lympho-

cytic infiltrate may be present but are confined to the lamina propria, are not necessarily perineural or perivascular, and do not involve the muscularis propria. Mast cells are not an important histologic feature. The trigone is not involved. Pathologic changes apparently do not progress over time, suggesting that the two forms of interstitial cystitis actually represent two separate diseases with similar symptoms.

In the severe (ulcer) form, the characteristic pathologic changes are wedge-shaped ulcers complete with chronic and organizing inflammation at their bases (fig. 3-93). Inflammation is more intense than with the nonulcer type, and may include plasma cells and mast cells. Leukocytes may accumulate around nerves and vessels in the interstitium between the fascicles of the muscularis propria but the infiltration tends to be slight and the muscle itself is spared. As with the nonulcer form of the disease, mast cell counts are not helpful, the changes are predominantly in the lamina propria, and the trigone is not involved.

The major contribution of pathology to patients with a clinical diagnosis of interstitial cystitis is to corroborate the clinical impression by excluding infection, CIS, and other chronic bladder processes that lack the histologic features of interstitial cystitis. Laboratory studies can exclude infections. CIS can be excluded by the examination of multiple urinary and tissue specimens. Other chronic bladder diseases are suspected when the pathologic changes involve

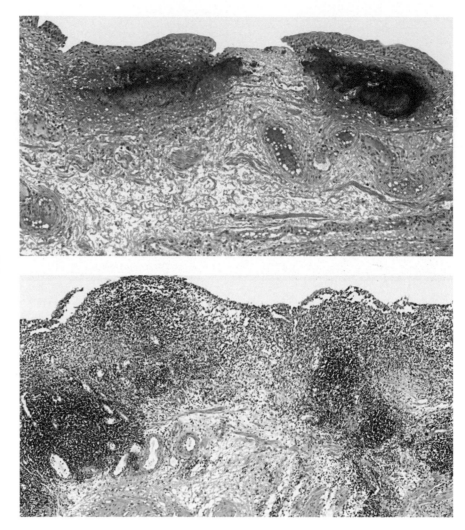

Figure 3-93

INTERSTITIAL CYSTITIS

Top: Nonulcerative type.
Bottom: Ulcerative (Hunner's ulcer) type. (Courtesy of Dr. Sonny L. Johansson, Omaha, NE.)

the trigone, are transmural, manifest necrosis of the muscularis propria, or fail to fissure or ulcerate the urothelium.

Eosinophilic Cystitis. Eosinophilic cystitis is difficult to recognize as a distinctive entity (391, 417,420,441). Nearly all reports are anecdotal and the presence of large numbers of eosinophils is recorded in association with every type of bladder disease as well as after surgery. Neither the symptoms, the cystoscopic findings, nor the pathologic changes are particularly distinguishing. Most patients lack eosinophilia in blood or urine. The term might be useful in situations where patients complain of irritative voiding (dysuria, pain, frequency) and manifest chronic changes in their bladder biopsies. The most important pathologic changes are transmural inflammation with or without fi-

brosis, focal necrosis of the muscularis propria, and lack of mucosal ulcers. Eosinophils are present in variable numbers. In no case should an interpretation of eosinophilic cystitis be influenced primarily by the presence of large numbers of eosinophils.

Amyloid

Amyloid describes the presence of amyloid fibrils and associated ground substances in the urinary bladder. The disease is nearly always primary rather than systemic, and is most often of type A lambda (406,410). Patients present with gross hematuria, often associated with nodular mucosal lesions misinterpreted clinically as carcinoma. Amyloid involving the urinary bladder characteristically occurs as large masses of acidophilic proteinaceous material associated with hemorrhage in the lamina propria (figs. 3-94, 3-95). Vascular involvement occurs but is not usually prominent. The diagnosis is easily confirmed once the condition is suspected and it is prudent to perform reactions for amyloid in any case where amorphous acidophilic material occurs in the lamina propria. As in many conditions involving attenuation of the urothelium, atypical epithelial changes may occur. These may assume unwarranted significance if too much emphasis is placed upon a clinical diagnosis of carcinoma and the amyloid deposition is overlooked.

Cysts, Rests, Choristomas, Hamartomas, and Vascular Lesions

Cysts. Most bladder cysts are urachal. Persistent urachal remnants are most likely a normal phenomenon and clinically important only when complicated by infection, neoplasia, or cystic dilatation (404). Urachal cysts are ordinarily small, multilocular, asymptomatic structures which occur anywhere along the urachal tract as well as within the bladder (fig. 3-96). Depending on size, urachal cysts are lined by urothelium or cuboidal, flat, or atrophic cells. Cysts and sinuses of apparent müllerian and urothelial derivation are also recorded (439,452).

Endometriosis and Endocervicosis. Cystic and solid lesions lined by müllerian-type epithelium are recorded in the bladder wall (387, 395,405,430,442,443,452). Estrogen seems to be required and nearly all reported patients are premenopausal women; the men are on estrogens for prostate cancer. The lesions most likely arise through implantation, sometimes facilitated by surgery. Any type of müllerian epithelium may predominate and it is tempting to recognize different types with separate names like endometriosis, endocervicosis, and even endosalpingiosis. Endometriosis tends to be more histologically homogeneous than endocervicosis, in which the lining cells can be flat, cuboidal, or ciliated (figs. 3-97, 3-98). Rarely, cancers arise in association with vesical endometriosis (387,442).

Ectopic Prostate. Ectopic prostatic tissue ordinarily presents as a polypoid mass at the bladder base (452). Histologic recognition is not difficult and is confirmed using immunohistochemical reactions for prostatic antigens. Similar lesions occur after transurethral resections

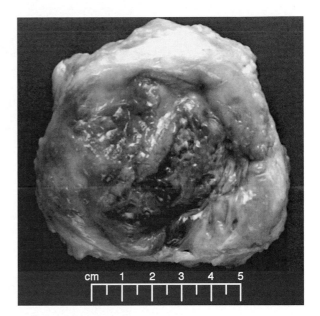

Figure 3-94

AMYLOID IN URINARY BLADDER

(Courtesy of Dr. George M. Farrow, Rochester, MN.)

and probably represent regrowths of adenomatous prostatic tissue into defects caused by the surgery. Diagnostic problems occasionally arise when the prostatic tissue contains a few glands or arises at bladder sites distant from the prostate (429).

Paraganglionic Tissue. Rarely, prominent paraganglionic tissue occurs in the bladder (452). These areas may cause diagnostic concern to the unwary, especially if the hyperplastic cells are seen in a small biopsy specimen. Accurate interpretation can be facilitated using immunohistochemical reactions.

Extramedullary Hematopoiesis. Tumors composed of hematopoietic cells may occur in various organs, including the urinary bladder (418). A history of a myeloproliferative disorder should be sought but is not essential to accurate pathologic interpretation.

Hamartomas. Hamartomas are described in the urinary bladder (390,432,452). Almost all occur in children. Nodular accumulations of Brunn glands, with or without metaplasia, are so predominant that the correct classification of these lesions becomes controversial. Certain cases of fibroepithelial polyp may represent hamartomatous malformations (451).

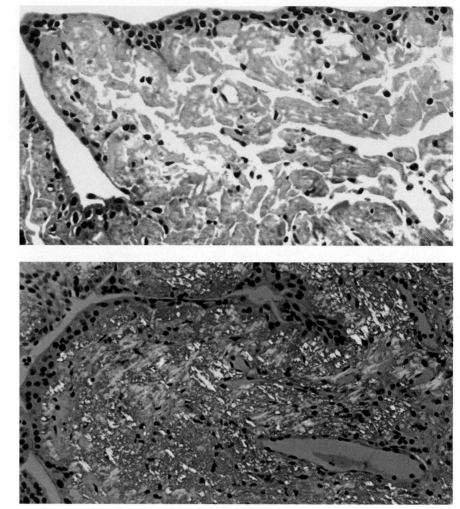

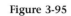
Figure 3-95

**AMYLOID IN
URINARY BLADDER**

Top: In contrast to other organs, the amyloid in a urinary bladder commonly accumulates as large masses in the lamina propria rather than in the walls of blood vessels.

Bottom: Congo red reaction exposed to polarized light.

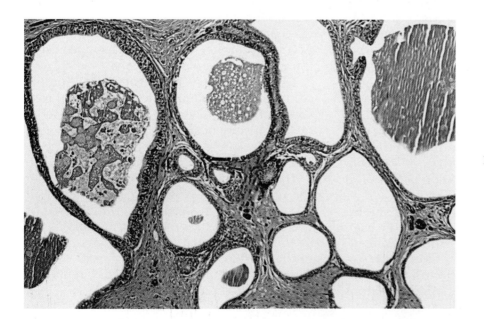

Figure 3-96

URACHAL CYST

(Courtesy of Dr. Lawrence Parrott, Camden, SC.)

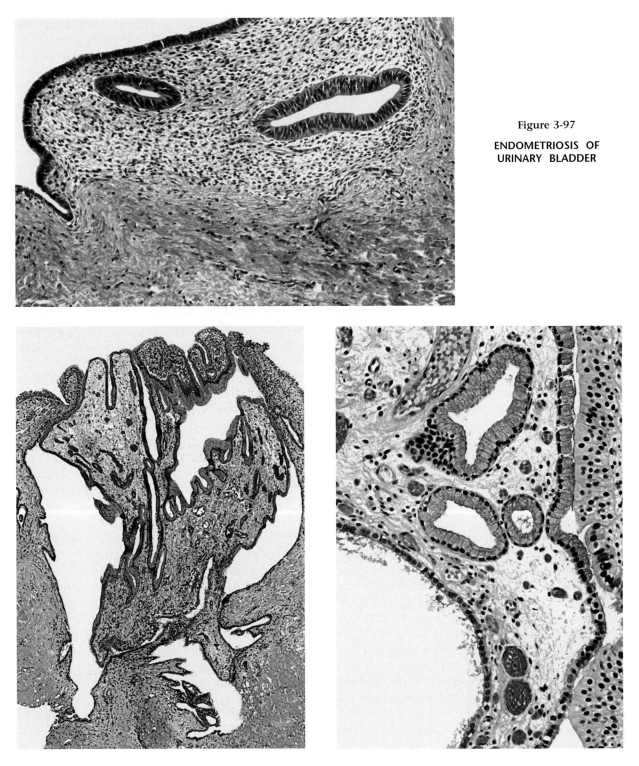

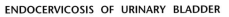

Figure 3-97

ENDOMETRIOSIS OF URINARY BLADDER

Figure 3-98

ENDOCERVICOSIS OF URINARY BLADDER

Left: Low magnification highlights the cysts.

Right: The lining of the glands varies from columnar and mucinous to flat or cuboidal. (Courtesy of Dr. John Pedersen, Melbourne, Australia.)

Vascular Lesions. Rarely, non-neoplastic vascular lesions present as masses in the bladder. On cystoscopic examination, these lesions may be recognized as vascular or confused with a neoplasm. Among the more exotic examples are polyarteritis nodosa and so-called caliber persistent artery (408,438).

TREATMENT OF BLADDER NEOPLASMS

The literature on the treatment of bladder tumors is a work in progress and a detailed exposition of the subject is beyond the scope of this atlas. Despite periodic publications of consensus statements and guidelines, there seems to be no standard approach to treatment in the United States, much less the world. The effects of certain therapies on bladder tissue have been previously discussed and illustrated (see Pathologic Effects of Treatment). This section summarizes general principles of the subject, primarily so that pathologists can become aware of the implications of their interpretations. The discussion applies primarily to urothelial neoplasms, since they comprise nearly 90 percent of all bladder tumors.

The generally recognized treatment options for patients with bladder tumors are limited to: surveillance after transurethral excision; topical therapy after transurethral excision; radical surgery; X-ray therapy; and chemotherapy. Immunotherapy can be included if BCG and interferons are thought to act via immune mechanisms (455).

Surveillance is appropriate for the management of patients presenting with low-grade (papilloma, PUNLMP, low-grade carcinoma, transitional cell carcinoma grade 1), noninvasive urothelial neoplasms, so long as the tumors are small and focal. Follow-up is (or should be) directed toward early recognition of high-grade or invasive neoplasms, not for the detection of recurrent low-grade, noninvasive tumors. Surveillance is justified by the low risk of progression among these patients: less than 10 percent in most studies.

Topical therapy is ordinarily employed for the treatment of so-called superficial bladder cancer (all grades of noninvasive or lamina propria invasive neoplasms). It is most efficacious for urothelial CIS. Low-grade noninvasive neoplasms may be treated if they are multiple, large, or not particularly amenable to complete re-

section. A variety of agents are used, most are alkylating drugs or BCG (456,462). Combinations that include interferon-alpha are popular among some clinicians (458). Since the index tumor is almost always excised, the goal of treatment is to prevent the growth of new neoplasms, some of which might be progressive. Topical therapy is widely accepted for the treatment of noninvasive carcinomas but is more controversial for invasive tumors, the majority of which are also high grade (459). The controversy deepens when patients fail to respond to the initial course. Since the distal ureters, prostatic urethra, and paraurethral prostatic glands are minimally exposed to topical drugs, progression may occur while the bladder itself remains tumor free (461). Complications of topical therapy are minimal in competent hands.

Radical surgery is most often used for tumors that have invaded into the muscularis propria but are clinically confined to the bladder. It may be appropriate when superficial lesions are unmanageable with other forms of treatment or for the eradication of locally advanced cancers (460). Ordinarily, the specimen includes the bladder, segments of distal ureters, and selected regional lymph nodes, plus, depending on the patient's sex, all or part of the urethra, prostate gland, and seminal vesicles. The goals of surgery are to cure and to obtain information relating to prognosis. The lack of effective adjuvant therapy, however, limits the usefulness of the latter. As expected, radical surgery is associated with a higher rate of short- and long-term complications than surveillance and topical therapy (457). Complications are manageable and well within acceptable limits. The increasing popularity of continent diversions has augmented patients' assessments of their quality of life.

X-ray therapy (XRT) used as a single modality is not popular as primary treatment for most bladder tumors, at least in the United States (461, 463,464). This approach seems to be most effective for papillary tumors that can be excised surgically. The size of the bladder and the lack of efficacy of XRT for flat lesions severely limit its usefulness in prophylaxis. Still, complete eradication of invasive, localized bladder tumors can be achieved in some cases. In the United States, XRT is primarily employed as neoadjuvant therapy in selected protocols or used in combination with other modalities for patients with advanced disease. Long-term bladder preservation can be achieved but the percentage of patients who benefit from multimodality therapy has varied in published reports.

Chemotherapy is used for the treatment of advanced disease (465). The most popular regimens comprise combinations of agents including cisplatin, doxorubicin, vinblastine, and methotrexate. These "cocktails" tend to be poorly tolerated and other types of chemotherapeutic drugs are gaining favor (466). Complete remissions are recorded but the identification of residual carcinoma after systemic chemotherapy may require a diligent search through multiple tissue sections. The value of chemotherapy seems to be primarily palliative.

The treatment of bladder tumors is complicated by many factors, including patient preference, tolerance, and acceptance of the modality as well as the vagaries of individual host-tumor interaction. Essentially all reported cohorts are composed of individuals with variable susceptibilities to their tumors and reactions to the treatment. Thus, any particular regimen may seem efficacious, depending on patient selection if not the potential of the therapy itself. The complexities tend to confound the analysis of small cohorts with short follow-up, i.e., the majority of published reports.

URINARY DIVERSIONS

Urinary diversions using portions of intestine are used in both children and adults for the treatment of congenital anomalies, dysfunctional bladders, and bladder neoplasms (468, 471,472,475,477). They may be crafted to enlarge the capacity of the bladder (augmentation), channel urine into an artificial reservoir while a more functional bladder is being constructed or after cystectomy for cancer (conduit), or create a new bladder by anastomosis directly to the urethra after cystectomy for cancer (neobladder). Depending upon the goal, portions of colon or ileum may be preferred. Complications depend upon the nature of the primary disease, patient age, and the type of conduit (467,468,470,473,474). Colonic conduits are associated with an increased frequency of intestinal adenocarcinomas but a low frequency of reflux and stenosis. Ileal conduits rarely develop primary intestinal neoplasms but commonly reflux. Even so, renal failure is recorded in less than 10 percent of cases and decreased renal function in less than 30 percent. Augmentation cystoplasties have the highest rate of neoplasms, primarily adenocarcinomas and adenomas arising on the bladder side of the anastomosis. In most cases, neoplasms are detected years after the surgery. Nearly all are urothelial or adenocarcinomas but carcinoid tumors and even metastatic melanoma are recorded (469,478).

Pathologically, the epithelium of intestinal conduits is usually chronically inflamed, atrophic, and partially denuded (475). Ileal conduits are especially prone to colonization by *Candida* sp but lack well-formed Peyer patches. Urinary diversions are best monitored using urinary cytology, especially since almost all malignancies occurring in these structures are of high cytologic grade (fig. 3-99) (476,479). Malignant cells in urinary specimens are best detected using procedures that include direct smears after centrifugation, since the high mucin content of intestinal secretions tends to inhibit dispersion of cells. In contrast to bladder specimens, neoplastic elements appearing in urinary diversion specimens are often more degenerated. They must be further differentiated from the abundant aggregates of intestinal cells ordinarily present in these samples. Aggregates of intestinal cells often resemble papillary structures and can be a confounding factor for interpretation, especially since many urinary diversion specimens are labeled simply "urine." Frequent monitoring using urinary cytology should detect neoplasms before they become large, and most urothelial carcinomas are both focal and in situ. Multiple sections may be required to achieve a histologic correlation.

PROCEDURES FOR PATHOLOGIC EXAMINATION

Standardization of pathologic procedures for the processing and reporting of bladder neoplasms has received a good deal of emphasis by the leadership of organized pathology (481,485, 487). Many recommend that pathology reports be rendered in the form of a list, lest the pathologist forget an important bit of information.

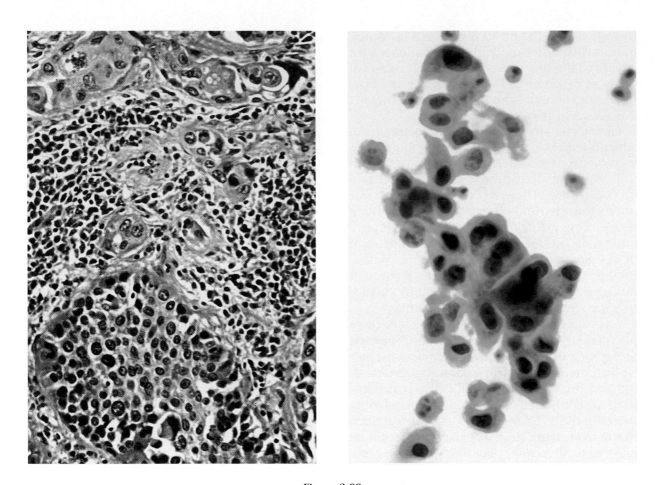

Figure 3-99

UROTHELIAL CARCINOMA OF RENAL PELVIS FOLLOWING CYSTECTOMY

Left: High-grade tumor cells in an ileal conduit specimen.
Right: Urothelial carcinoma, high grade, of renal pelvis.

Standardization of pathology reports, initially couched in terms of guidelines, are gradually being transformed into requirements (486).

Bladder Biopsy

Bladder biopsies are ordinarily obtained to establish a definitive diagnosis of a bladder neoplasm. They are best collected using a "cold cup" cutting forceps but many cystoscopists are tempted to use an electrically heated instrument. Bladder biopsy specimens tend to round up in fluids, so that the mucosa covers most of the underlying tissue and orientation at the epithelial-stromal interface is not a significant problem. The orientation of deeper tissues (e.g., wisps of muscle fibers and thick-walled blood vessels in the lamina propria) is more problematic but of little significance.

The gross inspection of bladder biopsy specimens is not particularly revealing. They can be measured in one dimension to document the amount of tissue received but they need not be weighed. The entire specimen should be submitted for histologic examination; sectioning at the cutting board is not usually necessary. In most practices, phosphate buffered formalin is the fixative of choice but zinc formalin produces better cellular detail without a significant impact upon the laboratory. Picric acid–based fixatives are even better for light microscopy but are more difficult to use and are probably not suitable for practices with relatively small volumes. The exact number of sections necessary to uncover all significant pathologic abnormalities in a biopsy has not been firmly established, but most practices prepare sections at two or three levels of the paraffin block. Long ribbons of sections on a slide are not recommended, two sections per slide being sufficient. On the other hand, representative sections of the tissue between levels should be kept unstained in case immunohistochemical reactions are required after the H&E-stained sections have been examined. Expending the block in an effort to be thorough is not necessary and not recommended.

There is a high degree of conformity among practitioners in their assessment of bladder biopsies (484). Neoplasms are analyzed for their histologic type; grading is only required for urothelial neoplasms. The presence and depth of invasion must be determined: the layers of the bladder are mucosa, lamina propria, and muscularis propria. As previously discussed, a muscularis mucosae similar to that in the gastrointestinal tract does not exist as a continuous anatomic structure in the urinary bladder and attempts to substage on the basis of remnants of this structure are inaccurate. Still, urothelial carcinomas that abut the muscularis propria seem to behave more like pT2 lesions whereas invasive tumors that hug the mucosa seem to behave more like noninvasive neoplasms. It is important to mention the presence or absence of muscularis propria (muscular wall) in all cases of neoplasms, whether or not the portion of muscular wall is actually attached to the tumor. Since there is no superficial muscle layer in the bladder and the superficial half of the muscular wall thickness has prognostic implications in addition to muscularis propria involvement, the use of the term "deep muscle" to denote the muscularis propria tends to be confusing to clinicians. Despite the clinical emphasis on documenting the presence or absence of muscular wall in bladder specimens, as many as 25 percent of biopsies of bladder neoplasms do not contain portions of muscular wall (483). It is not really necessary to remark upon the presence or absence of muscular wall in biopsies where the neoplasm is CIS but most authors recommend it for the sake of completeness.

Invasion of endothelial-lined spaces is usually difficult to assess in bladder biopsies. Most of the apparent spaces containing nests of tumor cells at the epithelial-stromal interface are actually artifacts (see fig. 3-17) (482). Often, the urothelium in a bladder biopsy is denuded. In such cases, the interpretation of "denudation" is more appropriate than "negative" or "chronic inflammation."

The only essential information required when a pathologist interprets a bladder biopsy as neoplastic is the histologic type of tumor (and whatever variant might be present), its grade (if urothelial), its depth of invasion (including presence or absence of muscular wall), and the presence or absence of invasion of endothelial-lined spaces. CIS is important if the lesion is separate from a papillary or nodular tumor or (rarely) the papillary or nodular tumor is low grade. Grading nonurothelial neoplasms of the bladder seems potentially misleading, but forms a part of the AJCC requirements (480). Pathologists should be aware that they are communicating with both very knowledgeable and relatively unsophisticated individuals, and the language of the report should be clear to both groups. Pathologic nuances (e.g., urothelial carcinoma with spindle cell stroma) that have no significance for patient care can be confusing and should not be included in the interpretation. The diagnosis can be amplified in a comment if necessary. Pathologic information can be communicated in a variety of ways but it should be clear to anyone reading a pathologist's report that the results represent a medical consultation and not a series of observations. The term "interpretation" should appear frequently in such documents.

Transurethral Resection

TURBTs are almost always performed for the removal of a mass, and the mass is ordinarily a neoplasm. In contrast to bladder biopsies, electrocautery is usually employed and significant amounts of the tissue are thermocoagulated. The amount of tissue is documented by weighing the specimen and measuring the largest piece of tissue in one dimension. Expressing the amount of tissue as an aggregate is much less accurate, since the size of the aggregate depends upon how tightly the examiner compresses the tissue. In general, all of the specimen should be submitted, with one section being prepared from each block. Recommendations for histologic examination and reporting are similar to those for bladder biopsies containing neoplasms. It is important to remember that fat may occur in both the lamina propria and in the muscularis propria so that the presence of fat in a TURBT does not necessarily indicate that a completely transmural resection has occurred (see fig. 3-2).

Cystectomy

Cystectomies are nearly always performed for the treatment of known bladder neoplasms when both the type and grade have already been determined. Specimens are ordinarily received fresh. Depending on the patient's sex, they may include segments of the ureters and the entire urethra (women) or segments of ureters, a segment of urethra, the prostate gland, and seminal vesicles (men). Selected regional lymph nodes are submitted separately. Gross examination should include a complete description of all organs received as well as appropriate measurements. There is very little value in weighing the specimen and it is not necessary to completely ink it. The paravesical fat is best dissected and examined fresh; very few if any lymph nodes should be found. The specimen can then be opened anteriorly and pinned to a board for overnight fixation. After fixation, a diagram documenting further dissection can be constructed according to the following guidelines (fig. 3-100).

• Transect the distal urethra and any associated organs transversely at a point approximately 1 cm from the specimen margin rather than attempting to obtain an en face section of the distal urethral margin. The portion of urethra thus obtained should be sectioned in the sagittal plane so that the urethral specimen margin can be examined microscopically at multiple intervals. In men, these sections also include a significant portion of the prostatic ducts for assessment of neoplastic involvement. The surgical margin is easily distinguished from the dissection incision in microscopic sections.

• Sample all bladder tumors and surgical defects to include at least one section from the deepest extent of the lesion and one section of the margin for each centimeter in greatest dimension of the defect or tumor.

• Take random samples of normal-appearing areas of mucosa (CIS has adverse prognostic implications).

• Section the ureteral margins on each side as well as the intramural ureters. In many

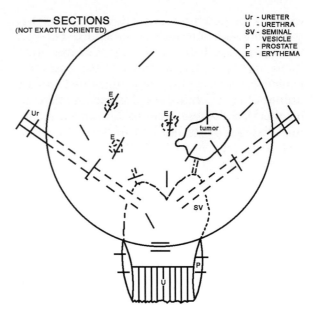

Figure 3-100

GROSS DISSECTION OF CYSTECTOMY SPECIMEN

cases, the distal ureters have been separately submitted for frozen section.

• Breadloaf and examine the remaining prostate gland, sampling any grossly visible lesions or at least one block from the periphery of each side. These sections augment those taken with the distal urethra. Prostatic carcinomas are commonly found in cystoprostatectomy specimens but they are usually small and of low grade. Further, they are completely excised. If a prostatic carcinoma is found, the periphery of the gland can be subsequently examined for extraprostatic extension (capsular penetration) and specimen margin involvement.

The histologic examination and reporting of cystectomy specimen findings are essentially the same as what is recommended for biopsies and TURBTs. In addition, the level of invasion of the muscular wall should be reported in terms of greater than or less than 50 percent of its thickness. If the prostate gland is involved by urothelial carcinoma, it is important to distinguish between stromal invasion and ductular involvement only. It is also important to report CIS in the urethra or ureters. Extension of a bladder carcinoma to the specimen margins is rare but should be reported and localized, as should tumor involvement of any and all organs received. Since radical cystectomies tend to be complex specimens, clarity in reporting can be achieved if the interpretations are rendered by organ rather than simply listed. For example, in men, the organs include: urinary bladder, segment of urethra, segments of ureters, prostate gland, and seminal vesicles.

The lymph nodes received with a radical cystectomy specimen can be examined using fairly standard techniques. Sections should be taken at right angles to the long axes of nodes large enough to require dissection, i.e., greater than 0.2 cm in greatest dimension. One section per block is sufficient. Immunohistochemical reactions to detect micrometastases are not recommended (489). Metastases to regional lymph nodes are unusual in radical cystectomy specimens and their effect on prognosis is controversial, especially with currently available adjuvant therapy.

Frozen Section

Frozen sections for the pathologic evaluation of bladder tumors are primarily employed at the time of radical cystectomy. An intraoperative interpretation of regional lymph nodes may occasionally be requested. After freeing the nodes from external fat, they should be sectioned at 1- to 2-mm intervals across their long axes. Representative sections can be examined but microscopic assessment of the entire specimen is usually not onerous.

Most often, samples of the distal ureters are received for frozen section. A cross section of the specimen is most beneficial, making no attempt to shave the specimen margins. Invasive carcinoma is rare in these tissues and intraepithelial lesions are uncommon. In fact, the practice of freezing distal ureters has been discouraged (488). An intraoperative interpretation of dysplasia or atypia in distal ureters is of little or no help, and pathologists should limit their diagnostic repertoire to carcinoma (almost always CIS) and no carcinoma.

The urethra rapidly retracts after resection and attempts to evaluate the distal urethral margin during surgery are not recommended. On occasion, the distal part of a cystoprostatectomy specimen may be assessed by frozen section for the presence of prostatic tissue.

PROGNOSTIC FACTORS

The study of prognostic factors for human neoplasms will remain incomplete and very likely unfulfilling until methods to analyze the host, rather than only the tumor, are developed. In the meantime, a bewildering array of chromosomes, genes, gene products, enzymes, cell cycle and other inhibitors, adhesion molecules, growth factors, and as yet unknown substances with putative prognostic value fill the literature. Any attempt to catalogue them would be futile, as more accumulate each day. Factors with proven or traditionally respected prognostic value have been discussed with each tumor type, briefly summarized in the section on Special Techniques, and will not be reiterated here.

It is extraordinarily difficult to compile data on the actual outcomes of large groups of patients presenting with bladder neoplasms and it is essentially impossible to identify factors that influence the course of any particular individual's disease (485). Therefore, investigators extrapolate from short-term follow-up or devise surrogate endpoints like recurrence, change in grade, or change in depth of invasion. The effect of any particular prognostic factor is usually determined at only one point in time, even though human neoplasia is generally recognized to be a dynamic process. Only occasionally is the factor compared to other factors in a controlled trial and it is almost never evaluated in terms of its statistically documented benefits to patients, taking into account the very limited treatment options available.

The term "prognostic factor" sometimes means a predictor of patient outcome and sometimes means a predictor of response to treatment. At other times, it may be used to predict the concomitant presence of an adverse condition like metastatic disease. Usually, studies touting the importance of prognostic factors are retrospective so that the outcome is already known and it is difficult to separate the influence of the factor from an epiphenomenon. In some situations, e.g., studies of CIS, patients are selected because of a lesion that developed during the course of follow-up for a more prognostically serious neoplasm such as invasive high-grade urothelial carcinoma. It is important to reiterate in this regard that no matter the number of factors reputed to have independent prognostic value, only three outcomes are available to patients: cure, progression, or persistence of disease without progression.

It is likely that much of the prognosis for any individual is determined by the time the neoplasm is detected, otherwise why would grade and stage be consistently important. More than half of patients presenting with a PUNLMP, for example, never develop another pathologically documented urothelial neoplasm. In contrast, 25 to 50 percent of patients presenting with a high-grade urothelial carcinoma die of their disease and even those without progression have a reduced life-span. Medical intervention can influence the course of bladder tumors in many cases so that even well-accepted prognostic factors may not be predictive in cohorts that respond to treatment (480a). The complexity of the subject is daunting and not likely to be resolved in an environment that seems to address the issue one protein at a time.

Individual practices may introduce unique protocols, and pathologic interpretations that are integral to these should be provided. In most practices, the information shown in Table 3-8 should appear in the pathology report when appropriate to the specimens being evaluated.

Table 3-8

PATHOLOGY REPORT INFORMATION

Bladder Biopsies and TURBTs[a]
 Type of neoplasm and variants (if present)
 Grade
 Depth of invasion: none, lamina propria, muscularis propria (muscular wall)
 Presence or absence of muscularis propria
 Presence of invasion of endothelial-lined spaces

Cystectomy
 Everything for biopsies and TURBTs plus
 Depth of invasion: more or less than half the muscle wall thickness
 CIS if NOT contiguous with a papillary or nodular high-grade carcinoma
 Extravesical extension
 Involvement of prostatic ducts and glands
 Involvement of prostatic stroma
 CIS in the urethra
 CIS in the ureters

[a]TURBT = Transurethral resection of a bladder tumor; CIS = carcinoma in situ.

REFERENCES

Normal Anatomy

1. Baskin LS, Sutherland RS, Thomson AA, Hayward SW, Cunha GR. Growth factors and receptors in bladder development and obstruction. Lab Invest 1996;75:157–66.

2. Cohen MB, Griebling TL, Ahaghotu CA, Rokhlin OW, Ross JS. Cellular adhesion molecules in urologic malignancies. Am J Clin Pathol 1997;107:56–63.

3. Edwards BF, Rossitto PV, Baker WC, et al. Transitional cell cytokeratins as a second parameter in flow cytometry of bladder cancer. World J Urol 1987;5:123–6.

4. Fradet Y, Cordon-Cardo C, Whitmore WF Jr, Melamed MR, Old LJ. Cell surface antigens of human bladder tumors: definition of tumor subsets by monoclonal antibodies and correlation with growth characteristics. Cancer Res 1986;46:5183–8.

5. Hang L, Wullt B, Shen Z, Karpman D, Svanborg C. Cytokine repertoire of epithelial cells lining the human urinary tract. J Urol 1998;159:2185–92.

6. Keep JC, Piehl M, Miller A, Oyasu R. Invasive carcinomas of the urinary bladder. Am J Clin Pathol 1989;91:575–9.

7. Kissane JM. Development and structure of the urogenital system. In: Murphy WM, ed. Urological pathology. Philadelphia: WB Saunders; 1997:10–16.

8. Koss LG. Tumors of the urinary bladder. Supplement. Atlas of Tumor Pathology, 2nd Series, Fascicle 11. Washington, D.C.: Armed Forces Institute of Pathology; 1985:S1–3.

9. Limas C, Lange P. A, B, H antigen detectability in normal and neoplastic urothelium: influence of methodologic factors. Cancer 1982;49:2476–84.

10. Messing EM. Clinical implications of the expression of epidermal growth factor receptors in human transitional cell carcinoma. Cancer Res 1990;50:2530–7.

11. Philip AT, Amin MB, Tamboli P, Lee TJ, Hill CE, Ro JY. Intravesical adipose tissue: a quantitative study of its presence and location with implications for therapy and prognosis. Am J Surg Pathol 2000;24:1286–90.

12. Platz CE, Cohen MB, Jones MP, Olson DB, Lynch CF. Is microstaging of early invasive cancer of the urinary bladder possible or useful? Mod Pathol 1996;11:1035–9.
13. Reuter VE. Urinary bladder and ureter. In: Sternberg SS, ed. Histology for pathologists. New York: Raven Press; 1992:709–19.
14. Russell PJ, Brown JL, Grimmond SM, Raghavan D. Molecular biology of urological tumours. Br J Urol 1990;65:121–30.
15. Wu XR, Lin JH, Walz T, et al. Mammalian uroplakins. A group of highly conserved urothelial differentiation-related membrane proteins. J Biol Chem 1994;269:13716–24.

Classification

16. Broders AC. Epithelioma of the genito-urinary organs. Ann Surg 1922;75:574–604.
17. Eble JN, Sauter G, Epstein JI, Sesterhenn IA, eds. World Health Organization Classification of Tumours. Pathology and genetics of tumours of the urinary system and male genital organs. IARC Press: Lyon; 2004.
18. Epstein JI, Amin MB, Reuter VR, Mostofi FK. The World Health Organization/International Society of Urological Pathology consensus classification of urothelial (transitional cell) neoplasms of the urinary bladder. Bladder Consensus Conference Committee. Am J Surg Pathol 1998;22:1435–48.
19. Koss LG. Tumors of the urinary bladder. Atlas of Tumor Pathology, 2nd Series, Fascicle 11. Washington, D.C.: Armed Forces Institute of Pathology; 1975.
20. Malmstrom PU, Busch C, Norlen BJ. Recurrence, progression and survival in bladder cancer. A retrospective analysis of 232 patients with 5-year follow-up. Scand J Urol Nephrol 1987;21:185–95.
21. Miller A, Mitchell JP, Brown NJ. The Bristol Bladder Tumour Registry. Br J Urol 1969;41(Suppl):1–64.
22. Mostofi FK, Davis CJ, Sesterhenn IA, et al. Histological typing of urinary bladder tumours. International histological classification of tumours, 2nd ed. Springer, Berlin: World Health Organization; 1999.
23. Mostofi FK, Sobin LH, Torloni H. Histological typing of urinary bladder tumours. International histological classification of tumours, No. 10. Geneva: World Health Organization; 1973.

Bladder Neoplasia

24. Boyd PJ, Burnand KG. Site of bladder-tumour recurrence. Lancet 1974;2:1290–2.
25. Chaturvedi V, Li L, Hodges S, et al. Superimposed histologic and genetic mapping of chromosome 17 alterations in human bladder neoplasia. Oncogene 1997;14:2059–70.
26. Cheng L, Gu J, Ulbright TW, et al. Precise microdissection of human bladder carcinomas reveals divergent tumor subclones in the same tumor. Cancer 2002;94:104–10.
27. Chetsanga C, Malmstrom PU, Gyllensten U, Moreno-Lopez J, Dinter Z, Pettersson U. Low incidence of human papillomavirus type 16 DNA in bladder tumor detected by the polymerase chain reaction. Cancer 1992;69:1208–11.
28. Chowaniec J. Aetiology: epidemiological and experimental considerations. In: Skrabanek P, Walsh A, eds. Bladder cancer, Vol 60. Geneva: UICC Technical Report Series; 1981:118–43.
29. Cohen SM, Shirai T, Steineck G. Epidemiology and etiology of premalignant and malignant urothelial changes. Scand J Urol Nephrol Suppl 2000;205:105–15.
30. Cordon-Cardo C, Cote RJ, Sauter G. Genetic and molecular markers of urothelial premalignancy and malignancy. Scand J Urol Nephrol Suppl 2000;205:82–93.
31. Czerniak B, Chaturvedi V, Li L, et al. Superimposed histologic and genetic mapping of chromosome 9 in progression of human bladder neoplasia: implications for a genetic model of multistep urothelial carcinogenesis and early detection of urinary bladder cancer. Oncogene 1999;18:1185–96.
32. Droller MJ. Transitional cell cancer: upper tracts and bladder. In: Walsh PC, Gittes RF, Perlmutter AD, Stamey TA, eds. Campbell's urology, 5th ed. Philadelphia: WB Saunders; 1986:1343–440.
33. El-Bolkainy MN, Tawfik HN, Kamel IA. Histopathologic classification of carcinomas in the schistosomal bladder. In: El-Bolkainy MN, Chu EW, eds. Detection of bladder cancer associated with schistosomiasis. Cairo: Al-Ahram Press; 1981:106–23.
34. Farber E, Rubin H. Cellular adaptation in the origin and development of cancer. Cancer Res 1991;51:2751–61.
35. Jemal A, Tirvari RC, Murray T, et al. Cancer statistics, 2004. CA Cancer J Clin 2004;54:8–29.
36. Jordan AM, Weingarten J, Murphy WM. Transitional cell neoplasms of the urinary bladder. Can biologic potential be predicted from histologic grading? Cancer 1987;60;2766–74.
37. Kaubisch S, Lum BL, Reese J, Freiha F, Torti FM. Stage T1 bladder cancer: grade is the primary determinant for risk of muscle invasion. J Urol 1991;146:28–31.
38. Koss LG. Diagnostic cytology and its histopathologic bases. Vol 2, 4th ed. Philadelphia: JB Lippincott; 1992:890–933.
39. Koss LG, Melamed MR, Kelly RE. Further cytologic and histologic studies of bladder lesions in workers exposed to para-aminodiphenyl: progress report. J Natl Cancer Inst 1969;43:233–43.

40. Kroft SH, Oyasu R. Urinary bladder cancer: mechanisms of development and progression. Lab Invest 1994;71:158–74.

41. Li M, Cannizzaro LA. Identical clonal origin of synchronous and metachronous low-grade, noninvasive papillary transitional cell carcinomas of the urinary tract. Hum Pathol 1999;30:1197–200.

42. Mostofi FK, Sobin LH, Torloni H. Histological typing of urinary bladder tumours. International Classification of Tumours, No. 10. Geneva: World Health Organization; 1973.

43. Murphy WM. Diseases of the urinary bladder, urethra, ureters, and renal pelves. In: Murphy WM, ed. Urological pathology. Philadelphia: WB Saunders; 1997:64–98.

44. Murphy WM. Urinary cytopathology. Chicago: ASCP Press; 2000.

45. Murphy WM, Busch C, Algaba F. Intraepithelial lesions of urinary bladder: morphologic considerations. Scand J Urol Nephrol Suppl 2000;205:67–81.

46. Murphy WM, Nagy GK, Rao MK, et al. "Normal" urothelium in patients with bladder cancer: a preliminary report from the National Bladder Cancer Collaborative Group A. Cancer 1979;44:1050–58.

47. Murphy WM, Soloway MS. Developing carcinoma (dysplasia) of the urinary bladder. Pathol Annu 1982;17(Pt 1):197–217.

48. Nowell PC. Cancer, chromosomes, and genes. Lab Invest 1992;66:407–17.

49. Paiss T, Wohr G, Hautmann RE, et al. Some tumors of the bladder are polyclonal in origin. J Urol 2002;167:718–23.

50. Plna K, Hemminki K. Familial bladder cancer in the National Swedish Family Cancer Database. J Urol 2001;166:2129–33.

51. Prout GR Jr, Wesley MN, Greenberg RS, et al. Bladder cancer: race differences in extent of disease at diagnosis. Cancer 2000;89:1349–58.

52. Rew DA. Tumour biology, chaos and non-linear dynamics. Eur J Surg Oncol 1999;25:86–9.

53. Shinka T, Sawada Y, Morimoto S, Fujinaga T, Nakamura J, Ohkawa T. Clinical study on urothelial tumors of dye workers in Wakayama City. J Urol 1991;146:1504–07.

54. Sidransky D, Frost P, Von Eschenbach A, Oyasu R, Preisinger AC, Vogelstein B. Clonal origin of bladder cancer. N Engl J Med 1992;326:737–40.

55. Silverberg E, Holleb AI. Cancer statistics, 1971. CA Cancer J Clin 1971;21:13–31.

56. Spruck CH 3rd, Ohneseit PF, Gonzalez-Zulueta M, et al. Two molecular pathways to transitional cell carcinoma of the bladder. Cancer Res 1994;54:784–8.

57. Strohman R. Epigenesis: the missing beat in biotechnology? Biotechnology 1994;12:156–64.

58. Yossepowitch O, Dalbagni G. Transitional cell carcinoma of the bladder in young adults: presentation, natural history and outcome. J Urol 2002;168:61–6.

Urothelial (Transitional Cell) Neoplasms

59. Alroy J, Miller AW 3rd, Coon JS 4th, James KK, Gould VE. Inverted papilloma of the urinary bladder. Cancer 1980;46:64–70.

60. Alsheikh A, Mohamedali Z, Jones E, Masterson J, Gilks CB. Comparison of the WHO/ISUP classification and cytokeratin 20 expression in predicting the behavior of low-grade papillary urothelial tumors. World Health Organization/International Society of Urologic Pathology. Mod Pathol 2001;14:267–72.

61. American Joint Committee on Cancer (AJCC). Manual for staging of cancer, 6th ed. Philadelphia: Lippincott-Raven; 2002:335–40.

62. Amin MB, Ro JY, el-Sharkawy T, et al. Micropapillary variant of transitional cell carcinoma of the urinary bladder. Histologic pattern resembling ovarian papillary serous carcinoma. Am J Surg Pathol 1994;18:1224–32.

63. Antonakopoulos GN, Hicks RM, Berry RJ. The subcellular basis of damage to the human urinary bladder induced by irradiation. J Pathol 1984;143:103–16.

64. Arends MJ, Wyllie AH. Apoptosis: mechanisms and roles in pathology. Int Rev Exp Pathol 1991;32:223–54.

65. Badalament RA, Hermansen DK, Kimmel M, et al. The sensitivity of bladder wash flow cytometry, bladder wash cytology, and voided cytology in the detection of bladder carcinoma. Cancer 1987;60:1423–7.

66. Baker PM, Young RH. Radiation-induced pseudocarcinomatous proliferations of the urinary bladder: a report of 4 cases. Hum Pathol 2000;31:678–83.

67. Baschinsky D, Chen JH, Vadmal MS, Lucas JG, Bahnson RR, Niemann TH. Carcinosarcoma of the urinary bladder—an aggressive tumor with diverse histogenesis. A clinicopathologic study of 4 cases and review of the literature. Arch Pathol Lab Med 2000;124:1172–8.

68. Bastacky S, Ibrahim S, Wilczynski SP, Murphy WM. The accuracy of urinary cytology in daily practice. Cancer 1999;87:118–28.

69. Belair CD, Yeager TR, Lopez PM, Reznikoff CA. Telomerase activity: a biomarker of cell proliferation, not malignant transformation. Proc Natl Acad Sci U S A 1997;94:13677–82.

70. Bergkvist A, Ljungqvist A, Moberger G. Classification of bladder tumours based on the cellular pattern. Preliminary report of a clinical-pathological study of 300 cases with a minimum follow-up of eight years. Acta Chir Scand 1965;130:371–8.

71. Blomjous CE, Schipper NW, Vos W, Baak JP, de Voogt HJ, Meijer CJ. Comparison of quantitative and classic prognosticators in urinary bladder carcinoma. A multivariate analysis of DNA flow cytometric, nuclear morphometric and clinicopathological features. Virchows Arch A Pathol Anat Histopathol 1989;415:421–8.

72. Boman H, Hedelin H, Holmang S. Four bladder tumor markers have a disappointingly low sensitivity for small size and low grade recurrence. J Urol 2002;167:80–3.

73. Browner WS, Newman TB. Are all significant P values created equal? The analogy between diagnostic tests and clinical research. JAMA 1987;257:2459–63.

74. Campo E, Algaba F, Palacin A, Germa R, Sole-Balcells FJ, Cardesa A. Placental proteins in high-grade urothelial neoplasms. An immunohistochemical study of human chorionic gonadotropin, human placental lactogen, and pregnancy-specific beta-1-glycoprotein. Cancer 1989;63:2497–504.

75. Carbin BE, Ekman P, Gustafson H, Christensen NJ, Silfversward C, Sandstedt B. Grading of human urothelial carcinoma based on nuclear atypia and mitotic frequency. II. Prognostic importance. J Urol 1991;145:972–6.

76. Caro DJ, Tessler A. Inverted papilloma of the bladder: a distinct urological lesion. Cancer 1978;42:708–13.

77. Casella R, Huber P, Blochlinger A, et al. Urinary level of nuclear matrix protein 22 in the diagnosis of bladder cancer: experience with 130 patients with biopsy confirmed tumor. J Urol 2000;164:1926–8.

78. Cassel A, Rahat MA, Lahat N, Lindenfeld N, Mecz Y, Stein A. Telomerase activity and cytokeratin 20 as markers for the detection and followup of transitional cell carcinoma: an unfulfilled promise. J Urol 2001;166:841–4.

79. Chan TY, Epstein JI. In situ adenocarcinoma of the bladder. Am J Surg Pathol 2001;25:892–9.

80. Chaturvedi V, Li L, Hodges S, et al. Superimposed histologic and genetic mapping of chromosome 17 alterations in human bladder neoplasia. Oncogene 1997;14:2059–70.

81. Chen SS, Chen KK, Lin AT, et al. The significance of tumour grade in predicting disease progression in stage Ta transitional cell carcinoma of the urinary bladder. Br J Urol 1996;78:209–12.

82. Cheng L, Cheville JC, Neumann RM, Bostwick DG. Flat intraepithelial lesions of the urinary bladder. Cancer 2000;88:625–31.

83. Cheng L, Cheville JC, Neumann RM, Bostwick DG. Natural history of urothelial dysplasia of the bladder. Am J Surg Pathol 1999;23:443–7.

84. Cheng L, Cheville JC, Neumann RM, et al. Survival of patients with carcinoma in situ of the urinary bladder. Cancer 1999;85:2469–74.

85. Cheng L, Darson M, Cheville JC, et al. Urothelial papilloma of the bladder. Clinical and biologic implications. Cancer 1999;86:2098–101.

86. Cheng L, Neumann RM, Bostwick DG. Papillary urothelial neoplasms of low malignant potential. Clinical and biological implications. Cancer 1999;86:2102–8.

87. Cheng L, Weaver AL, Leibovich BC, et al. Predicting the survival of bladder carcinoma patients treated with radical cystectomy. Cancer 2000;88:2326–32.

88. Cheville JC, Wu K, Sebo TJ, et al. Inverted urothelial papilloma: is ploidy, MIB-1 proliferative activity, or p53 protein accumulation predictive of urothelial carcinoma? Cancer 2000;88:632–6.

89. Chu P, Wu E, Weiss LM. Cytokeratin 7 and cytokeratin 20 expression in epithelial neoplasms: a survey of 435 cases. Mod Pathol 2000;13:962–72.

90. Cina SJ, Lancaster-Weiss KJ, Lecksell K, Epstein JI. Correlation of Ki-67 and p53 with the new World Health Organization/International Society of Urological Pathology Classification System for Urothelial Neoplasia. Arch Pathol Lab Med 2001;125:646–51.

91. Cookson MS, Herr HW, Zhang ZF, Soloway S, Sogani PC, Fair WR. The treated natural history of high risk superficial bladder cancer: 15-year outcome. J Urol 1997;158:62–7.

92. Cordon-Cardo C, Cote RJ, Sauter G. Genetic and molecular markers of urothelial premalignancy and malignancy. Scand J Urol Nephrol Suppl 2000;205:82–93.

93. Czerniak B, Chaturvedi V, Li L, et al. Superimposed histologic and genetic mapping of chromosome 9 in progression of human urinary bladder neoplasia: implications for a genetic model of multistep urothelial carcinogenesis and early detection of urinary bladder cancer. Oncogene 1999;18:1185–96.

94. Davis JW, Sheth SI, Doviak MJ, Schellhammer PF. Superficial bladder carcinoma treated with bacillus Calmette-Guerin: progression-free and disease specific survival with minimum 10-year followup. J Urol 2002;167:494–501.

95. Delladetsima J, Antonakopoulos GN, Dapolla V, Kittas C. Intraepithelial lumina in urothelial bladder neoplasms. A histochemical, immunohistochemical and electron microscopy study. APMIS 1989;97:406–12.

96. Dirnhofer S, Koessler P, Ensinger C, Feichtinger H, Madersbacher S, Berger P. Production of trophoblastic hormones by transitional cell carcinoma of the bladder: association to tumor stage and grade. Hum Pathol 1998;29:377–82.

97. Donhuijsen K, Schmidt U, Richter HJ, Leder LD. Mucoid cytoplasmic inclusions in urothelial carcinomas. Hum Pathol 1992;23:860–4.

98. Downing SR, Jackson P, Russell PJ. Mutations within the tumour suppressor gene p53 are not confined to a late event in prostate cancer progression: a review of the evidence. Urol Oncol 2001;6:103–10.

99. Drew PA, Furman J, Civantos F, Murphy WM. The nested variant of transitional cell carcinoma: an aggressive neoplasm with innocuous histology. Mod Pathol 1996;9:989–94.

100. Drew PA, Murphy WM, Kubilis PS, Areford M. Can androgen deprivation therapy with leuprolide be predicted from histology alone? If not, why not? J Urol 1997;157:2201–5.

101. Eble JN, Young RH. Stromal osseous metaplasia in carcinoma of the bladder. J Urol 1991;145: 823–5.

102. Epstein JI, Amin MB, Reuter VR, Mostofi FK. The World Health Organization/International Society of Urological Pathology consensus classification of urothelial (transitional cell) neoplasms of the urinary bladder. Am J Surg Pathol 1998;22:1435–48.

103. Esrig D, Elmajian D, Groshen S, et al. Accumulation of nuclear p53 and tumor progression in bladder cancer. N Engl J Med 1994;331:1259–64.

104. Esrig D, Freeman JA, Elmajian DA, et al. Transitional cell carcinoma involving the prostate with a proposed staging classification for stromal invasion. J Urol 1996;156:1071–6.

105. Farber E. Cell proliferation as a major risk factor for cancer: a concept of doubtful validity. Cancer Res 1995;55:3759–62.

106. Farrow GM, Utz DC. Observations on microinvasive transitional cell carcinoma of the urinary bladder. Clinics Oncol 1982;1:609–15.

107. Farrow GM, Utz DC, Rife CC. Morphological and clinical observations of patients with early bladder cancer treated with total cystectomy. Cancer Res 1976;36:2495–501.

108. Feitz WF, Beck HL, Smeets AW, et al. Tissue-specific markers in flow cytometry of urological cancers: cytokeratins in bladder carcinoma. Int J Cancer 1985;36:349–56.

109. Friedell GH, Mcauley RL. Untreated bladder cancer: 31 autopsy cases. J Urol 1968;100:293–6.

110. Genega EM, Hutchinson B, Reuter VE, Gaudin PB. Immunophenotype of high-grade prostatic adenocarcinoma and urothelial carcinoma. Mod Pathol 2000;13:1186–91.

111. Giannopoulos A, Manousakas T, Gounari A, Constantinides C, Choremi-Papadopoulou H, Dimopoulos C. Comparative evaluation of the diagnostic performance of the BTA stat test, NMP22 and urinary bladder cancer antigen for primary and recurrent bladder tumors. J Urol 2001;166:470–5.

112. Golijanin D, Shapiro A, Pode D. Immunostaining of cytokeratin 20 in cells from voided urine for detection of bladder cancer. J Urol 2000;164:1922–5.

113. Grossman HB, Schmitz-Drager B, Fradet Y, Tribukait B. Use of markers in defining urothelial premalignant and malignant conditions. Scand J Urol Nephrol Suppl 2000;205:94–104.

114. Halling KC, King W, Sokolova IA, et al. A comparison of BTA stat, hemoglobin dipstick, telomerase and Vysis Uro vysion assays for the detection of urothelial carcinoma in urine. J Urol 2002;167:2001–6.

115. Hashimoto Y, Asamoto M, Futakuchi M, Okamura T, Kohri K, Shirai T. Immunohistochemical demonstration of p53 protein nuclear accumulation in preneoplastic and neoplastic lesions of the human urinary bladder. J Urol Pathol 1996;5:21–7.

116. Helpap B, Kollermann J. Assessment of basal cell status and proliferative patterns in flat and papillary urothelial lesions: a contribution to the new WHO classification of urothelial tumors of the urinary bladder. Hum Pathol 2000;31:745–50.

117. Herr HW, Bajorin DF, Scher HI, Cordon-Cardo C, Reuter VE. Can p53 help select patients with invasive bladder cancer for bladder preservation? J Urol 1999;161:20–3.

118. Herr HW, Bochner BH, Dalbagni G, Donat SM, Reuter VE, Bajorin DF. Impact of the number of lymph nodes retrieved on outcome in patients with muscle invasive bladder cancer. J Urol 2002;167:1295–8.

119. Herr HW, Donat SM. Prostatic tumor relapse in patients with superficial bladder tumors: 15-year outcome. J Urol 1999;161:1854–7.

120. Herr HW, Donat SM, Bajorin DF. Bladder cancer, the limits of surgical excision—when/how much? Urol Oncol 2001;6:221–4.

121. Herr HW, Wartinger DD, Fair WR, Oettgen HF. Bacillus Calmette-Guerin therapy for superficial bladder cancer: a 10-year followup. J Urol 1992;147:1020–3.

122. Holmang S, Andius P, Hedelin H, Wester K, Busch C, Johansson SL. Stage progression in Ta papillary urothelial tumors: relationship to grade, immunohistochemical expression of tumor markers, mitotic frequency and DNA ploidy. J Urol 2001;165:1124–30.

123. Holmang S, Hedelin H, Anderstrom C, Holmberg E, Busch C, Johansson SL. Recurrence and progression in low grade papillary urothelial tumors. J Urol 1999;162:702–7.

124. Holtzman NA, Marteau TM. Will genetics revolutionize medicine? N Engl J Med 2000;343: 141–4.

125. Hug EB, Donnelly SM, Shipley WU, et al. Deoxyribonucleic acid flow cytometry in invasive bladder carcinoma: a possible predictor for successful bladder preservation following transurethral surgery and chemotherapy-radiotherapy. J Urol 1992;148:47–51.

126. Ikegami H, Iwasaki H, Ohjimi Y, Takeuchi T, Ariyoshi A, Kikuchi M. Sarcomatoid carcinoma of the urinary bladder: a clinicopathologic and immunohistochemical analysis of 14 patients. Hum Pathol 2000;31:332–40.

127. Iles RK, Chard T. Human chorionic gonadotropin expression by bladder cancers: biology and clinical potential. J Urol 1991;145:453–8.

128. Izadifar V, de Boer WI, Muscatelli-Groux B, Maille P, van der Kwast TH, Chopin DK. Expression of transforming growth factor beta 1 and its receptors in normal human urothelium and human transitional cell carcinomas. Hum Pathol 1999;30:372–7.

129. Jahnson S, Karlsson MG. Tumor mapping of regional immunostaining for p21, p53, and mdm2 in locally advanced bladder carcinoma. Cancer 2000;89:619–29.

130. Johansson SL, Borghede G, Holmang S. Micropapillary bladder carcinoma: a clinicopathological study of 20 cases. J Urol 1999;161:1798–802.

131. Jones EC, Young RH. Myxoid and sclerosing sarcomatoid transitional cell carcinoma of the urinary bladder: a clinicopathologic and immunohistochemical study of 25 cases. Mod Pathol 1997;10:908–16.

132. Jordan AM, Weingarten J, Murphy WM. Transitional cell neoplasms of the urinary bladder. Can biological potential be predicted from histologic grading? Cancer 1987;60:2766–74.

133. Kanno J, Sakamoto A, Washizuka M, Kawai T, Kasuga T. Malignant mixed mesodermal tumor of bladder occurring after radiotherapy for cervical cancer: report of a case. J Urol 1985;133:854–6.

134. Kaubisch S, Lum BL, Reese J, Freiha F, Torti FM. Stage T1 bladder cancer: grade is the primary determinant for risk of muscle invasion. J Urol 1991;146:28–31.

135. Kaufmann O, Volmerig J, Dietel M. Uroplakin III is a highly specific and moderately sensitive immunohistochemical marker for primary and metastatic urothelial carcinomas. Am J Clin Pathol 2000;113:683–7.

136. Kaye KW, Lange PH. Mode of presentation of invasive bladder cancer: reassessment of the problem. J Urol 1982;128:31–3.

137. Keegan PE, Matthews JN, Lunec J, Neal DE. Statistical problems with "optimal" thresholds in studies of new prognostic factors in urology. BJU Int 2000;85:392–7.

138. King ED, Matteson J, Jacobs SC, Kyprianou N. Incidence of apoptosis, cell proliferation and bcl-2 expression in transitional cell carcinoma of the bladder: association with tumor progression. J Urol 1996;155:316–20.

139. Klan R, Huland E, Baisch H, Huland H. Sensitivity of urinary quantitative immunocytology with monoclonal antibody 486 P3/12 in 241 unselected patients with bladder carcinoma. J Urol 1991;145:495–7.

140. Kondylis FI, Demirci S, Ladaga L, Kolm P, Schellhammer PF. Outcomes after intravesical bacillus Calmette-Guerin are not affected by substaging of high grade T1 transitional cell carcinoma. J Urol 2000;163:1120–3.

141. Konety BR, Getzenberg RH. Urine based markers of urological malignancy. J Urol 2001;165:600–11.

142. Korkolopoulou P, Christodoulou P, Konstantinidou AE, Thomas-Tsangli E, Kapralos P, Davaris P. Cell cycle regulators in bladder cancer: a multivariant survival study with emphasis on p27Kip1. Hum Pathol 2000;31:751–60.

143. Koss LG. Diagnostic cytology and its histopathologic bases. Vol 2, 4th ed. Philadelphia: JB Lippincott; 1992:890–1017.

144. Koss LG. Mapping of the urinary bladder: its impact on the concepts of bladder cancer. Hum Pathol 1979;10:533–48.

145. Koss LG, Wersto RP, Simmons DA, Deitch D, Herz F, Freed SZ. Predictive value of DNA measurements in bladder washings. Comparison of flow cytometry, image cytophotometry, and cytology in patients with a past history of urothelial tumors. Cancer 1989;64:916–24.

146. Kotliar SN, Wood CG, Schaeffer AJ, Oyasu R. Transitional cell carcinoma exhibiting clear cell features. A differential diagnosis for clear cell adenocarcinoma of the urinary tract. Arch Pathol Lab Med 1995;119:79–81.

147. Kunze E, Schauer A, Schmitt M. Histology and histogenesis of two different types of inverted urothelial papillomas. Cancer 1983;51:348–58.

148. Lam KY. Chondroid and osseous metaplasia in carcinoma of the bladder: report of two cases and review of literature. J Urol Pathol 1995;3:255–61.

149. Lamm DL, van der Meijden PM, Morales A, et al. Incidence and treatment of complications of bacillus Calmette-Guerin intravesical therapy in superficial bladder cancer. J Urol 1992;147:596–600.

150. Larsen MP, Steinberg GD, Brendler CB, Epstein JI. Use of Ulex europaeus agglutinin I (UEAI) to distinguish vascular and "pseudovascular" invasion in transitional cell carcinoma of bladder with lamina propria invasion. Mod Pathol 1990;3:83–8.

151. Leblanc B, Duclos AJ, Benard F, et al. Long-term followup of initial Ta grade 1 transitional cell carcinoma of the bladder. J Urol 1999;162:1946–50.

152. Lebret T, Bohin D, Kassardjian Z, et al. Recurrence, progression and success in stage Ta grade 3 bladder tumors treated with low dose bacillus Calmette-Guerin instillations. J Urol 2000;163:63–7.

153. Lokeshwar VB, Obek C, Pham HT, et al. Urinary hyaluronic acid and hyaluronidase: markers for bladder cancer detection and evaluation of grade. J Urol 2000;163:348–56.

154. Lokeshwar VB, Soloway MS. Current bladder tumor tests: does their projected utility fulfill clinical necessity? J Urol 2001;165:1067–77.

155. Lopez-Beltran A, Pacelli A, Rothenberg HJ, et al. Carcinosarcoma and sarcomatoid carcinoma of the bladder: clinicopathological study of 41 cases. J Urol 1998;159:1497–503.

156. Mahadevia PS, Alexander JE, Rojas-Corona R, Koss LG. Pseudosarcomatous stromal reaction in primary and metastatic urothelial carcinoma. A source of diagnostic difficulty. Am J Surg Pathol 1989;13:782–90.

157. Maier U, Ehrenbock PM, Hofbauer J. Late urological complications and malignancies after curative radiotherapy for gynecological carcinomas: a retrospective analysis of 10,709 patients. J Urol 1997;158:814–7.

158. Malik S, Murphy WM. Monitoring patients for bladder neoplasms: what can be expected of urinary cytology consultations in clinical practice. Urology 1999;54:62–6.

159. Malmstrom PU, Busch C, Norlen BJ. Recurrence, progression and survival in bladder cancer. A retrospective analysis of 232 patients with greater than or equal to 5-year follow-up. Scand J Urol Nephrol 1987;21:185–95.

160. Mao L. Genetic alterations as clonal markers for bladder cancer detection in urine. J Cell Biochem Suppl 1996;25:191–6.

161. Maranchie JK, Bouyounes BT, Zhang PL, O'Donnell MA, Summerhayes IC, DeWolf WC. Clinical and pathological characteristics of micropapillary transitional cell carcinoma: a highly aggressive variant. J Urol 2000;163:748–51.

162. McKenney JK, Desai S, Cohen C, Amin MB. Discriminatory immunohistochemical staining of urothelial carcinoma in situ and non-neoplastic urothelium: an analysis of cytokeratin 20, p53, and CD44 antigens. Am J Surg Pathol 2001;25:1074–8.

163. Melamed MR, Voutsa NG, Grabstald H. Natural history and clinical behavior of in situ carcinoma of the human urinary bladder. 1964. CA Cancer J Clin 1993;43:348–70.

164. Melicow MM. Histological study of vesical urothelium intervening between gross neoplasms in total cystectomy. J Urol 1952;68:261–79.

165. Mian C, Pycha A, Wiener H, Haitel A, Lodde M, Marberger M. Immunocyt: a new tool for detecting transitional cell cancer of the urinary tract. J Urol 1999;161:1486–9.

166. Morales A. Long-term results and complications of intracavitary bacillus Calmette-Guerin therapy for bladder cancer. J Urol 1984;132:457–9.

167. Mostofi FK, Davis CJ, Sesterhenn IA, et al. Histological typing of urinary bladder tumours. International histological classification of tumours, 2nd ed. Berlin: World Health Organization; 1999.

168. Mostofi FK, Sobin LH, Torloni H. Histological typing of urinary bladder tumours. International Classification of Tumours, No. 10. Geneva: World Health Organization; 1973.

169. Mourah S, Cussenot O, Vimont V, et al. Assessment of microsatellite instability in urine in the detection of transitional-cell carcinoma of the bladder. Int J Cancer 1998;79:629–33.

170. Murphy WM. Diseases of the urinary bladder, urethra, ureters, and renal pelves. In: Murphy WM, ed. Urological pathology. Philadelphia: WB Saunders; 1997:64–98.

171. Murphy WM. Media hype in the medical literature: what's a doctor to do? J Urol 2000;163:916–8.

172. Murphy WM. Urinary cytopathology. Chicago: ASCP Press; 2000.

173. Murphy WM, Beckwith JB, Farrow GM. Tumors of the kidney, bladder, and related urinary structures. Atlas of Tumor Pathology, 3rd Series, Fascicle 11. Washington, DC: Armed Forces Institute of Pathology; 1994:233–9.

174. Murphy WM, Busch C, Algaba F. Intraepithelial lesions of urinary bladder: morphologic considerations. Scand J Urol Nephrol Suppl 2000;205:67–81.

175. Murphy WM, Chandler RW, Trafford RM. Flow cytometry of deparaffinized nuclei compared to histological grading for the pathological evaluation of transitional cell carcinomas. J Urol 1986;135:694–7.

176. Murphy WM, Emerson LD, Chandler RW, Moinuddin SM, Soloway MS. Flow cytometry versus urinary cytology in the evaluation of patients with bladder cancer. J Urol 1986;136:815–9.

177. Murphy WM, Nagy GK, Rao MK, et al. "Normal" urothelium in patients with bladder cancer: a preliminary report from the National Bladder Cancer Collaborative Group A. Cancer 1979;44:1050–8.

178. Murphy WM, Soloway MS, Finebaum PJ. Pathological changes associated with topical chemotherapy for superficial bladder cancer. J Urol 1981;126:461–4.

179. Murphy WM, Takezawa K, Maruniak NA. Interobserver discrepancy using the 1998 World Health Organization/International Society of Urologic Pathology classification of urothelial neoplasms: practical choices for patient care. J Urol 2002;168:968–72.

180. Neulander E, Kaneti J, Chaimovitz C, Sion-Vardy N, Douvdevani A. Deoxyribonucleic acid ploidy and the clinical pattern of grade 2 superficial bladder cancer. J Urol 1997;157:1254–9.

181. Neumann MP, Limas C. Transitional cell carcinomas of the urinary bladder. Effects of preoperative irradiation on morphology. Cancer 1986;58:2758–63.

182. Neves M, Ciofu C, Larousserie F, et al. Prospective evaluation of genetic abnormalities and telomerase expression in exfoliated urinary cells for bladder cancer detection. J Urol 2002;167:1276–81.

183. Norming U, Nyman CR, Tribukait B. Comparative histopathology and deoxyribonucleic acid flow cytometry of random mucosal biopsies in untreated bladder carcinoma. J Urol 1991;145:1164–8.

184. Okamura K, Miyake K, Koshikawa T, Asai J. Growth fractions of transitional cell carcinomas of the bladder defined by the monoclonal antibody Ki-67. J Urol 1990;144:875–8.

185. Oliai BR, Kahane H, Epstein JI. A clinicopathologic analysis of urothelial carcinomas diagnosed on prostate needle biopsy. Am J Surg Pathol 2001;25:794–801.

186. Olsen LH, Overgaard S, Frederiksen P, et al. The reliability of staging and grading of bladder tumours. Impact of misinformation on the pathologist's diagnosis. Scand J Urol Nephrol 1993;27:349–53.

187. Ooms EC, Anderson WA, Alons CL, Boon ME, Veldhuizen RW. Analysis of the performance of pathologists in the grading of bladder tumors. Hum Pathol 1983;14:140–3.

188. Orlando C, Gelmini S, Selli C, Pazzagli M. Telomerase in urological malignancy. J Urol 2001;166:666–73.

189. Orozco RE, Martin AA, Murphy WM. Carcinoma in-situ of the urinary bladder. Clues to host involvement in human carcinogenesis. Cancer 1994;74:115–22.

190. Orozco RE, Vander Zwaag R, Murphy WM. The pagetoid variant of urothelial carcinoma in situ. Hum Pathol 1993;24:1199–202.

191. Paez A, Coba JM, Murillo N, et al. Reliability of the routine cytological diagnosis in bladder cancer. Eur Urol 1999;35:228–32.

192. Parker DC, Folpe AL, Bell J, et al. Potential utility of uroplakin III, thrombomodulin, high molecular weight cytokeratin, and cytokeratin 20 in noninvasive, invasive, and metastatic urothelial (transitional cell) carcinomas. Am J Surg Pathol 2003;27:1–10.

193. Pfister C, Lacombe L, Vezina MC, et al. Prognostic value of the proliferative index determined by Ki-67 immunostaining in superficial bladder tumors. Hum Pathol 1999;30:1350–5.

194. Pich A, Chiusa L, Formiconi A, Galliano D, Bortolin P, Navone R. Biologic differences between noninvasive papillary urothelial neoplasms of low malignant potential and low-grade (grade 1) papillary carcinomas of the bladder. Am J Surg Pathol 2001;25:1528–33.

195. Pode D, Golijanin D, Sherman Y, Lebensart P, Shapiro A. Immunostaining of Lewis X in cells from voided urine, cytopathology and ultrasound for noninvasive detection of bladder tumors. J Urol 1998;159:389–93.

196. Prout GR Jr, Griffin PP, Daly JJ, Heney NM. Carcinoma in situ of the urinary bladder with and without associated vesical neoplasms. Cancer 1983;52:524–32.

197. Raab SS, Slagel DD, Jensen CS, et al. Low-grade transitional cell carcinoma of the urinary bladder: application of select cytologic criteria to improve diagnostic accuracy [corrected]. Mod Pathol 1996;9:225–32.

198. Reuter VR, Epstein JI, Amin MB, et al. A newly illustrated synopsis of the World Health Organization/International Society of Urological Pathology (WHO/ISUP) consensus classification of urothelial (transitional-cell) neoplasms of the urinary bladder. J Urol Pathol 1999;11:1–27.

199. Righi E, Rossi G, Ferrari G, et al. Does p53 immunostaining improve diagnostic accuracy in urine cytology? Diagn Cytopathol 1997;17:436–9.

200. Ro JY, Ayala AG, Wishnow KI, Ordonez NG. Sarcomatoid bladder carcinoma: clinicopathologic and immunohistochemical study on 44 cases. Surg Pathol 1988;1:359–74.

201. Robertson AJ, Beck JS, Burnett RA, et al. Observer variability in histopathological reporting of transitional cell carcinoma and epithelial dysplasia in bladders. J Clin Pathol 1990;43:17–21.

202. Rosai J. The continuing role of morphology in the molecular age. Mod Pathol 2001;14:258–60.

203. Ross JS, Cohen MB. Ancillary methods for the detection of recurrent urothelial neoplasia. Cancer 2000;90:75–86.

204. Sanchez-Carbayo M, Ciudad J, Urrutia M, Navajo JA, Orfao A. Diagnostic performance of the urinary bladder carcinoma antigen ELISA test and multiparametric DNA/cytokeratin flow cytometry in urine voided samples from patients with bladder carcinoma. Cancer 2001;92:2811–9.

205. Schade RO, Swinney J. The association of urothelial abnormalities with neoplasia: a 10-year followup. J Urol 1983;129:1125–6.

206. Sella A, Dexeus FH, Chong C, Ro JY, Logothetis CJ. Radiation therapy-associated invasive bladder tumors. Urology 1989;33:185–8.

207. Seo IS, Clark SA, McGovern FD, Clark DL, Johnson EH. Leiomyosarcoma of the urinary bladder: 13 years after cyclophosphamide therapy for Hodgkin's disease. Cancer 1985;55:1597–603.

208. Shipley WU, Kaufman SD, Prout GR Jr. Intraoperative radiation therapy in patients with bladder cancer. A review of techniques allowing improved tumor doses and providing high cure rates without loss of bladder function. Cancer 1987;60:1485–8.

209. Smith ND, Rubenstein JN, Eggener SE, Kozlowski JM. The p53 tumor suppressor gene and nuclear protein: basic science review and relevance in the management of bladder cancer. J Urol 2003;169:1219–28.

210. Smith SD, Wheeler MA, Plescia J, Colberg JW, Weiss RM, Altieri DC. Urine detection of survivin and diagnosis of bladder cancer. JAMA 2001;285:324–8.

211. Spruck CH 3rd, Ohneseit PF, Gonzalez-Zulueta M, et al. Two molecular pathways to transitional cell carcinoma of the bladder. Cancer Res 1994;54:784–8.

212. Stillwell TJ, Benson RC Jr. Cyclophosphamide-induced hemorrhagic cystitis. A review of 100 patients. Cancer 1988;61:451–7.

213. Stockle M, Tanke HJ, Mesker WE, Ploem JS, Jonas U, Hohenfellner R. Automated DNA-image cytometry: a prognostic tool in infiltrating bladder carcinoma? World J Urol 1987;5:127–32.

214. Summers DE, Rushin JM, Frazier HA, Cotelingam JD. Inverted papilloma of the urinary bladder with granular eosinophilic cells. An unusual neuroendocrine variant. Arch Pathol Lab Med 1991;115:802–6.

215. Suwa Y, Takano Y, Iki M, et al. Cyclin D1 protein overexpression is related to tumor differentiation, but not to tumor progression or proliferative activity, in transitional cell carcinoma of the bladder. J Urol 1998;160:897–900.

216. Talbert ML, Young RH. Carcinomas of the urinary bladder with deceptively benign-appearing foci. A report of three cases. Am J Surg Pathol 1989;13:374–81.

217. Tetu B, Allard P, Fradet Y, Roberge N, Bernard P. Prognostic significance of nuclear DNA content and S-phase fraction by flow cytometry in primary papillary superficial bladder cancer. Hum Pathol 1996;27:922–6.

218. Tetu B, Fradet Y, Allard P, Veilleux C, Roberge N, Bernard P. Prevalence and clinical significance of HER/2neu, p53 and Rb expression in primary superficial bladder cancer. J Urol 1996;155:1784–8.

219. Titus K. Bladder markers gunning for green light. CAP Today 2002;16:32,42,46,50,52,54.

220. Tong YC, Monson FC, Erika B, Levin RM. Effects of acute in vitro overdistension of the rabbit urinary bladder on DNA synthesis. J Urol 1992;148:1347–50.

221. Tosoni I, Wagner U, Sauter G, et al. Clinical significance of interobserver differences in the staging and grading of superficial bladder cancer. BJU Int 2000;85:48–53.

222. Tribukait B. Flow cytometry in surgical pathology and cytology of tumors of the genitourinary tract. In: Koss LG, Coleman DV, eds. Advances in clinical cytology. Vol II. New York: Masson; 1984:163–89.

223. van der Poel HG, Boon ME, van Stratum P, et al. Conventional bladder wash cytology performed by four experts versus quantitative image analysis. Mod Pathol 1997;10:976–82.

224. van Oijen MG, Medema RH, Slootweg PJ, Rijksen G. Positivity of the proliferation marker Ki-67 in noncycling cells. Am J Clin Pathol 1998;110:24–31.

225. Vet JA, Hessels D, Marras SA, et al. Comparative analysis of p53 mutations in bladder washings and histologic specimens. Am J Clin Pathol 1998;110:647–52.

226. Wagner U, Sauter G, Moch H, et al. Patterns of p53, erbB-2, and EGF-r expression in premalignant lesions of the urinary bladder. Hum Pathol 1995;26:970–8.

227. Wheeless LL, Badalament RA, de Vere White RW, Fradet Y, Tribukait B. Consensus review of the clinical utility of DNA cytometry in bladder cancer. Report of the DNA Cytometry Concensus Conference. Cytometry 1993;14:478–81.

228. Wick MR, Brown BA, Young RH, Mills SE. Spindle-cell proliferations of the urinary tract. An immunohistochemical study. Am J Surg Pathol 1988;12:379–89.

229. Witjes JA, Umbas R, Debruyne FM, Schalken JA. Expression of markers for transitional cell carcinoma in normal bladder mucosa of patients with bladder cancer. J Urol 1995;154:2185–9.

230. Wood DP Jr, Montie JE, Pontes JE, Levin HS. Identification of transitional cell carcinoma of the prostate in bladder cancer patients: a prospective study. J Urol 1989;142:83–5.

231. Young RH. Carcinosarcoma of the urinary bladder. Cancer 1987;59:1333–9.

232. Young RH, Eble JN. Unusual forms of carcinoma of the urinary bladder. Hum Pathol 1991;22:948–65.

233. Young RH, Zukerberg LR. Microcystic transitional cell carcinomas of the urinary bladder. A report of four cases. Am J Clin Pathol 1991;96:635–9.

234. Zamecnik M. Urothelial carcinoma of the bladder with foci of yolk sac tumor. J Urol Pathol 1999;11:161–70.

235. Zieger K, Wolf H, Olsen PR, Hojgaard K. Long-term survival of patients with bladder tumours: the significance of risk factors. Br J Urol 1998;82:667–72.

236. Zlotta AR, Noel JC, Fayt I, et al. Correlation and prognostic significance of p53, p21 WAF1/CIP1 and Ki-67 expression in patients with superficial bladder tumors treated with bacillus Calmette-Guerin intravesical therapy. J Urol 1999;161:792–8.

237. Zuk RJ, Rogers HS, Martin JE, Baithun SI. Clinicopathological importance of primary dysplasia of bladder. J Clin Pathol 1988;41:1277–80.

238. Zukerberg LR, Armin AR, Pisharodi L, Young RH. Transitional cell carcinoma of the urinary bladder with osteoclast-type giant cells: a report of two cases and review of the literature. Histopathology 1990;17:407–11.

Squamous Cell Carcinoma

239. American Joint Committee on Cancer (AJCC). Manual for staging of cancer, 6th ed. Philadelphia: Lippincott-Raven; 2002;335–40.

240. Bejany DE, Lockhart JL, Rhamy RK. Malignant vesical tumors following spinal cord injury. J Urol 1987;138:1390–2.

241. Benson RC Jr, Swanson SK, Farrow GM. Relationship of leukoplakia to urothelial malignancy. J Urol 1984;131:507–11.

242. Costello AJ, Tiptaft RC, England HR, Blandy JP. Squamous cell carcinoma of bladder. Urology 1984;22:234–6.

243. El-Bolkainy MN, Mokhtar NM, Ghoneim MA, Hussein MH. The impact of schistosomiasis on the pathology of bladder carcinoma. Cancer 1981;48:2643–8.

244. el-Sebai I, Sherif M, el-Bolkainy MN, Mansour MA, Ghoneim MA. Verrucous squamous carcinoma of bladder. Urology 1974;4:407–10.

245. Faysal MH. Squamous cell carcinoma of the bladder. J Urol 1981;126:598–9.

246. Friedell GH, Bell JR, Burney SW, Soto EA, Tiltman AJ. Histopathology and classification of urinary bladder carcinoma. Urol Clin North Am 1976;3:53–70.

247. Ghaleb AH, Pizzolo JG, Melamed MR. Aberrations of chromosomes 9 and 17 in bilharzial bladder cancer as detected by fluorescence in situ hybridization. Am J Clin Pathol 1996;106:234–41.

248. Ghoneim MA, el-Mekresh MM, el-Baz MA, el-Attar IA, Ashamallah A. Radical cystectomy for carcinoma of the bladder: critical evaluation of the results in 1,026 cases. J Urol 1997;158:393–9.

249. Gonzalez-Zulueta M, Shibata A, Ohneseit PF, et al. High frequency of chromosome 9p allelic loss and CDKN2 tumor suppressor gene alterations in squamous cell carcinoma of the bladder. J Natl Cancer Inst 1995;87:1383–93.

250. Horner SA, Fisher HA, Barada JH, Eastman AY, Migliozzi J, Ross JS. Verrucous carcinoma of the bladder. J Urol 1991;145:1261–3.

251. Kerley SW, Persons DL, Fishback JL. Human papillomavirus and carcinoma of the urinary bladder. Mod Pathol 1991;4:316–9.

252. Koss LG. Tumors of the urinary tract and prostate in urinary sediment. In: Diagnostic cytology and its histopathologic bases, 4th ed. Philadelphia: JB Lippincott; 1992:964.

253. Locke JR, Hill DE, Walzer Y. Incidence of squamous cell carcinoma in patients with long-term catheter drainage. J Urol 1985;133:1034–5.

254. Lundgren R, Elfving P, Heim S, Kristoffersson U, Mandahl N, Mitelman F. A squamous cell bladder carcinoma with karyotypic abnormalities reminiscent of transitional cell carcinoma. J Urol 1989;142:374–6.

255. Murphy WM. Urinary cytopathology. Chicago: ASCP Press; 2000:72–5.

256. Rundle JS, Hart AJ, McGeorge A, Smith JS, Malcolm AJ, Smith PM. Squamous cell carcinoma of bladder. A review of 114 patients. Br J Urol 1982;54:522–6.

257. Schroder LE, Weiss MA, Hughes C. Squamous cell carcinoma of bladder: an increased incidence in blacks. Urology 1986;28:288–91.

258. Shaaban AA, Tribukait B, el-Bedeiwy AF, Ghoneim MA. Characterization of squamous cell bladder tumors by flow cytometric deoxyribonucleic acid analysis: a report of 100 cases. J Urol 1990;144:879–83.

259. Tannenbaum SI, Carson CC 3rd, Tatum A, Paulson DF. Squamous carcinoma of urinary bladder. Urology 1983;22:597–9.

260. Walther M, O'Brien DP 3rd, Birch HW. Condylomata acuminata and verrucous carcinoma of the bladder: case report and literature review. J Urol 1986;135:362–5.

261. Winkler HZ, Nativ O, Hosaka Y, Farrow GM, Lieber MM. Nuclear deoxyribonucleic acid ploidy in squamous cell bladder cancer. J Urol 1989;141:297–302.

262. Zaghloul MS. Distant metastasis from bilharzial bladder cancer. Cancer 1996;77:743–9.

Adenocarcinoma and Villous Tumor

263. Abenoza P, Manivel C, Fraley EE. Primary adenocarcinoma of urinary bladder. Clinicopathologic study of 16 cases. Urology 1987;29:9–14.

264. American Joint Committee on Cancer (AJCC). Manual for staging of cancer, 6th ed. Philadelphia: Lippincott-Raven; 2002:335–40.

265. Bullock PS, Thoni DE, Murphy WM. The significance of colonic mucosa (intestinal metaplasia) involving the urinary tract. Cancer 1987;59:2086–90.

266. Chan TY, Epstein JI. In situ adenocarcinoma of the bladder. Am J Surg Pathol 2001;25:892–9.

267. Daroca PJ Jr, Mackenzie F, Reed RJ, Keane JM. Primary adenovillous carcinoma of the bladder. J Urol 1976;115:41–5.

268. Eble JN. Abnormalities of the urachus. In:Young RH, ed. Pathology of the urinary bladder. New York: Churchill Livingstone; 1989:234–5.

269. Eble JN, Hull MT, Rowland RG, Hostetter M. Villous adenoma of the urachus with mucusuria: a light and electron microscopic study. J Urol 1986;135:1240–4.

270. Epstein JI, Kuhajda FP, Lieberman PH. Prostate-specific acid phosphatase immunoreactivity in adenocarcinomas of the urinary bladder. Hum Pathol 1986;17:939–42.

271. Goyanna R, Emmett JL, McDonald JR. Exstrophy of the bladder complicated by adenocarcinoma. J Urol 1951;65:391–400.

272. Grignon DJ, Ro JY, Ayala AG, Johnson DE. Primary signet-ring cell carcinoma of the urinary bladder. Am J Clin Pathol 1991;95:13–20.

273. Grignon DJ, Ro JY, Ayala AG, Johnson DE, Ordonez NG. Primary adenocarcinoma of the urinary bladder. A clinicopathologic analysis of 72 cases. Cancer 1991;67:2165–72.

274. Holmang S, Borghede G, Johansson SL. Primary signet ring cell carcinoma of the bladder: a report on 10 cases. Scand J Urol Nephrol 1996;31:145–8.

275. Jacobs LB, Brooks JD, Epstein JI. Differentiation of colonic metaplasia from adenocarcinoma of urinary bladder. Hum Pathol 1997;28:1152–7.

276. Koss LG. Tumors of the urinary tract and prostate in urinary sediment. In: Diagnostic cytology and its histopathologic bases, 4th ed. Philadelphia: JB Lippincott; 1992:934–1017.

277. Miller DC, Gang DL, Gavris V, Alroy J, Ucci AA, Parkhurst EC. Villous adenoma of the urinary

bladder: a morphologic or biologic entity? Am J Clin Pathol 1983;79:728–31.

278. Murphy WM. Urinary cytopathology. Chicago: ASCP Press; 2000:72–9.

279. Nakanishi K, Kawai T, Suzuki M, Torikata C. Prognostic factors in urachal adenocarcinoma. A study in 41 specimens of DNA status, proliferating cell-nuclear antigen immunostaining, and argyrophilic nucleolar-organizer region counts. Hum Pathol 1996;27:240–7.

280. Newbould M, McWilliam LJ. A study of vesical adenocarcinoma, intestinal metaplasia and related lesions using mucin histochemistry. Histopathology 1990;17:225–30.

281. O'Brien AM, Urbanski SJ. Papillary adenocarcinoma in situ of bladder. J Urol 1985;134:544–6.

282. Pallesen G. Neoplastic Paneth cells in adenocarcinoma of the urinary bladder: a first case report. Cancer 1981;47:1834–7.

283. Pantuck AJ, Bancila E, Das KM, et al. Adenocarcinoma of the urachus and bladder expresses a unique colonic epithelial epitope: an immunohistochemical study. J Urol 1997;158:1722–7.

284. Seibel JL, Prasad S, Weiss RE, Bancila E, Epstein JI. Villous adenoma of the urinary tract: a lesion frequently associated with malignancy. Hum Pathol 2002;33:236–41.

285. Sinard J, Macleay L Jr, Melamed J. Hepatoid adenocarcinoma in the urinary bladder. Unusual localization of a newly recognized tumor type. Cancer 1994;73:1919–25.

286. Song J, Farrow GM, Lieber MM. Primary adenocarcinoma of the bladder: favorable prognostic significance of deoxyribonucleic acid diploidy measured by flow cytometry. J Urol 1990;144:1115–8.

287. Wang HL, Lu DW, Yerian LM, et al. Immunohistochemical distinction between primary adenocarcinoma of the bladder and secondary colorectal adenocarcinoma. Am J Surg Pathol 2001;25:1380–7.

Poorly Differentiated Small Cell Carcinoma

288. Ali SZ, Reuter VE, Zakowski MF. Small cell neuroendocrine carcinoma of the urinary bladder. A clinicopathologic study with emphasis on cytologic features. Cancer 1997;79:356–61.

289. Angulo JC, Lopez JI, Sanchez-Chapado M, et al. Small cell carcinoma of the urinary bladder: a report of two cases with complete remission and a comprehensive literature review with emphasis on therapeutic decisions. J Urol Pathol 1996;5:1–19.

290. Bastus R, Caballero JM, Gonzalez G, et al. Small cell carcinoma of the urinary bladder treated with chemotherapy and radiotherapy: results in five cases. Eur Urol 1999;35:323–6.

291. Blomjous CE, Vos W, De Voogt HJ, Van der Valk P, Meijer CJ. Small cell carcinoma of the urinary bladder. A clinicopathologic, morphometric, immunohistochemical, and ultrastructural study of 18 cases. Cancer 1989;64:1347–57.

292. Christopher ME, Seftel AD, Sorenson K, Resnick MI. Small cell carcinoma of the genitourinary tract: an immunohistochemical, electron microscopic and clinicopathological study. J Urol 1991;146:382–8.

293. Grignon DJ, Ro JY, Ayala AG, et al. Small cell carcinoma of the urinary bladder. A clinicopathologic analysis of 22 cases. Cancer 1992;69:527–36.

294. Holmang S, Borghede G, Johansson SL. Primary small cell carcinoma of the bladder: a report of 25 cases. J Urol 1995;153:1820–2.

295. Lohrisch C, Murray N, Pickles T, Sullivan L. Small cell carcinoma of the bladder: long-term outcome with integrated chemoradiation. Cancer 1998;86:2346–52.

296. Mackey JR, Au HJ, Hugh J, Venner P. Genitourinary small cell carcinoma: determination of clinical and therapeutic factors associated with survival. J Urol 1998;159:1624–9.

297. Marchevsky AM, Gal AA, Shah S, Koss MN. Morphometry confirms the presence of considerable nuclear size overlap between "small cells" and "large cells" in high-grade pulmonary neuroendocrine neoplasms. Am J Clin Pathol 2001;116:466–72.

298. Ordonez NG, Khorsand J, Ayala AG, Sneige N. Oat cell carcinoma of the urinary tract. An immunohistochemical and electron microscopic study. Cancer 1986;58:2519–30.

299. Podesta AH, True LD. Small cell carcinoma of the bladder. Report of five cases with immunohistochemistry and review of the literature with evaluation of prognosis according to stage. Cancer 1989;64:710–4.

Rare Neoplasms

300. Abenoza P, Manivel C, Sibley RK. Adenocarcinoma with neuroendocrine differentiation of the urinary bladder. Clinicopathologic, immunohistochemical, and ultrastructural study. Arch Pathol Lab Med 1986;110:1062–6.

301. Amin MB, Ro JY, Lee KM, et al. Lymphoepithelioma-like carcinoma of the urinary bladder. Am J Surg Pathol 1994;18:466–73.

302. Carter RL, McCarthy KP, al-Sam SZ, Monaghan P, Agrawal M, McElwain TJ. Malignant rhabdoid tumour of the bladder with immunohistochemical and ultrastructural evidence suggesting histiocytic origin. Histopathology 1989;14:179–90.

303. Colecchia M, Dagrada GP, Poliani PL, Pilotti S. Immunophenotypic and genotypic analysis of a case of primary peripheral primitive neuroectodermal tumour (pPNET) of the urinary bladder. Histopathology 2002;40:108–9.

304. De Torres I, Fortuno MA, Raventos A, Tarragona J, Banus JM, Vidal MT. Primary malignant melanoma of the bladder: immunohistochemical study of a new case and review of the literature. J Urol 1995;154:525–7.

305. Hailemariam S, Gaspert A, Komminoth P, Tamboli P, Amin M. Primary, pure, large-cell neuroendocrine carcinoma of the urinary bladder. Mod Pathol 1998,11:1016–20.

306. Holmang S, Borghede G, Johansson SL. Bladder carcinoma with lymphoepithelioma-like differentiation: a report of 9 cases. J Urol 1998;159:779–82.

307. Ironside JW, Timperley WR, Madden JW, Royds JA, Taylor CB. Primary melanoma of the urinary bladder presenting with intracerebral metastases. Br J Urol 1985;57:593–4.

308. Kitazawa M, Kobayashi H, Ohnishi Y, Kimura K, Sakurai S, Sekine S. Giant cell tumor of the bladder associated with transitional cell carcinoma. J Urol 1985;133:472–5.

309. Kojima T, Tanaka T, Yoshimi N, Mori H. Primary malignant melanoma of the urinary bladder. Arch Pathol Lab Med 1992;116:1213–6.

310. Koss LG. Tumors of the urinary bladder. Atlas of Tumor Pathology, 2nd Series, Fascicle 11. Washington, D.C.: Armed Forces Institute of Pathology; 1975:46–52.

311. Lidgi S, Embon OM, Turani H, Sazbon AI. Giant cell reparative granuloma of the bladder associated with transitional cell carcinoma. J Urol 1989;142:120–2.

312. Marchevsky AM, Gal AA, Shah S, Koss MN. Morphometry confirms the presence of considerable nuclear size overlap between "small cells" and "large cells" in high-grade pulmonary neuroendocrine neoplasms. Am J Clin Pathol 2001;116:466–72.

313. McBride JA, Ro JY, Hicks J, Ordonez NG, Raney RB, Ayala AG. Malignant rhabdoid tumor of the bladder in an adolescent: case report and discussion of extrarenal rhabdoid tumor. J Urol Pathol 1994;2:255–63.

314. O'Connor RC, Hollowell CM, Laven BA, Yang XJ, Steinberg GD, Zagaja GP. Recurrent giant cell carcinoma of the bladder. J Urol 2002;167:1784.

315. Rossen K, Petersen MM. Simple melanosis of the bladder. J Urol 1999;161:1564.

316. Sahin AA, Myhre M, Ro JY, Sneige N, Dekmezian RH, Ayala AG. Plasmacytoid transitional cell carcinoma. Report of a case with initial presentation mimicking multiple myeloma. Acta Cytol 1991;35:277–80.

317. Serio G, Zampatti C, Ceppi M. Spindle and giant cell carcinoma of the urinary bladder: a clinico-pathological light microscopic and immunohistochemical study. Eur J Urol 1995;75:167–72.

318. Tainio HM, Kylmala TM, Haapasalo HK. Primary malignant melanoma of the urinary bladder associated with widespread metastases. Scand J Urol Nephrol 1999;33:406–7.

319. Vakar-Lopez F, Abrams J. Basaloid squamous cell carcinoma occurring in the urinary bladder. Arch Pathol Lab Med 2000;124:455–9.

320. Walker BF, Someren A, Kennedy JC, Nicholas EM. Primary carcinoid tumor of the urinary bladder. Arch Pathol Lab Med 1992;116:1217–20.

321. Young RH, Eble JN. Unusual forms of carcinoma of the urinary bladder. Hum Pathol 1991;22:948–65.

322. Zukerberg LR, Armin AR, Pisharodi L, Young RH. Transitional cell carcinoma of the urinary bladder with osteoclast-type giant cells: a report of two cases and a review of the literature. Histopathology 1990;17:407–11.

323. Zukerberg LR, Harris NL, Young RH. Carcinomas of the urinary bladder simulating malignant lymphoma. A report of five cases. Am J Surg Pathol 1991;15:569–76.

Metastases to Urinary Bladder

324. Berger Y, Nissenblatt M, Salwitz J, Lega B. Bladder involvement in metastatic breast carcinoma. J Urol 1992;147:137–9.

325. Chen KT, Spaulding RW. Appendiceal carcinoma masquerading as primary bladder carcinoma. J Urol 1991;145:821–2.

326. Ferris DO, Beare JB. Wilms' tumor: report of a case with unusual postoperative metastasis. Staff Meet Mayo Clin Proc 1947;22:94–8.

327. Franks ME, Konety BR, Bastacky S, Gritsch HA. Hepatocellular carcinoma metastatic to the bladder after liver transplantation. J Urol 1999;162:799–800.

328. Goldstein AG. Metastatic carcinoma to the bladder. J Urol 1967;98:209–15.

329. Mai KT, Ford JC, Morash C, Gerridzen R. Primary and secondary prostatic adenocarcinoma of the urinary bladder. Hum Pathol 2001;32:434–40.

330. Sim SJ, Ro JY, Ordonez NG, Park YW, Kee KH, Ayala AG. Metastatic renal cell carcinoma to the bladder: a clinicopathologic and immunohistochemical study. Mod Pathol 1999;12:351–5.

331. Sufrin G, Keogh B, Moore RH, Murphy GP. Secondary involvement of the bladder in malignant lymphoma. J Urol 1977;118:251–3.

332. Viddeleer AC, Lycklama a Nijeholt GA, Beekhuis-Brussee JA. A late manifestation of testicular seminoma in the bladder of a renal transplant recipient: a case report. J Urol 1992;148(2 Pt 1):401–2.

333. Voytek TM, Ro JY, El-Nagger AK, et al. Metastatic ovarian granulosa cell tumor to urinary bladder mimicking primary transitional cell carcinoma: a case report with immunohistochemical, electron microscopic, DNA flow cytometric, and interphase cytogenetic studies. J Urol Pathol 1996;4:57–67.

334. Young RH. Unusual variants of primary bladder carcinoma and secondary tumors of the bladder. In: Young RH, ed. Pathology of the urinary bladder. New York: Churchill Livingstone; 1989:128–30.

335. Young RH, Johnston WH. Serous adenocarcinoma of the uterus metastatic to the urinary bladder mimicking primary bladder neoplasia. A report of a case. Am J Surg Pathol 1990;14:877–80.

Nonepithelial Neoplasms

336. Abraham NZ, Maher TJ, Hutchison RE. Extranodal monocytoid B-cell lymphoma of the urinary bladder. Mod Pathol 1993;6:145–9

337. Abratt RP, Temple-Camp CR, Pontin AR. Choriocarcinoma and transitional cell carcinoma of the bladder—a case report and review of the clinical evolution of the disease in reported cases. Eur J Surg Oncol 1989;15:149–53.

338. Ahlering TE, Weintraub P, Skinner DG. Management of adult sarcomas of the bladder and prostate. J Urol 1988;140:1397–9.

339. Al-Maghrabi J, Kamel-Reid S, Jewett M, Gospodarowicz M, Wells W, Banerjee D. Primary low-grade B-cell lymphoma of mucosa-associated lymphoid tissue type arising in the urinary bladder: report of 4 cases with molecular genetic analysis. Arch Pathol Lab Med 2001;125:332–6.

340. Cauffield EW. Dermoid cysts of the bladder. J Urol 1956;75:801–4.

341. Cesarani F, Garretti L, Denegri F, Valente G, Rossetti SR. Sonographic appearance of aggressive angiomyxoma of the bladder. J Clin Ultrasound 1999;27:399–401.

342. Chaitin BA, Manning JT, Ordonez NG. Hematologic neoplasms with initial manifestations in lower urinary tract. Urology 1984;23:35–42.

343. Cheng L, Leibovich BC, Cheville JC, et al. Paraganglioma of the urinary bladder: can biologic potential be predicted? Cancer 2000;88:844–52.

344. Cheng L, Nascimento AG, Neumann RM, et al. Hemangioma of the urinary bladder. Cancer 1999;86:498–504.

345. Cheng L, Scheithauer BW, Leibovich BC, Ramnani DM, Cheville JC, Bostwick DG. Neurofibroma of the urinary bladder. Cancer 1999;86:505–13.

346. Coffin CM, Rulon J, Smith L, Bruggers C, White FV. Pathologic features of rhabdomyosarcoma before and after treatment: a clinicopathologic and immunohistochemical analysis. Mod Pathol 1997;10:1175–87.

347. Corti B, Carella R, Gabusi E, D'Errico A, Martorana G, Grigioni W. Solitary fibrous tumor of the urinary bladder with expression of bcl-2, CD34, and insulin-growth factor type II. Eur Urol 2001;39:484–8.

348. De Bruyne R, Peters O, Goossens A, Braeckman J, Denis LJ. Primary IgG-lambda immunocytoma of the urinary bladder. Eur J Surg Oncol 1987;13:361–4.

349. Dehner LP. Pathology of the urinary bladder in children. In: Young RH, ed. Pathology of the urinary bladder. New York: Churchill Livingstone; 1989:179–211.

350. De Siati M, Visona A, Shah J, Franzolin N. Angiomyolipoma of the bladder wall. J Urol 2000;163:901–2.

351. Eggener SE, Hairston J, Rubenstein JN, Gonzalez CM. Bladder lipoma. J Urol 2001;166:1395.

352. Forrest JB, Saypol DC, Mills SE, Gillenwater JY. Immunoblastic sarcoma of the bladder. J Urol 1983;130:350–1.

353. Ghalayini IF, Bani-Hani IH, Almasri NM. Osteosarcoma of the urinary bladder occurring simultaneously with prostate and bowel carcinomas: report of a case and review of the literature. Arch Pathol Lab Med 2001;125:793–5.

354. Grignon DJ, Ro JY, Mackay B, et al. Paraganglioma of the urinary bladder: immunohistochemical, ultrastructural, and DNA flow cytometric studies. Hum Pathol 1991;22:1162–9.

355. Guthman DA, Malek RS, Chapman WR, Farrow GM. Primary malignant lymphoma of the bladder. J Urol 1990;144:1367–9.

356. Hanna NH, Ulbright TM, Einhorn LH. Primary choriocarcinoma of the bladder with the detection of isochromosome 12p. J Urol 2002;167:1781.

357. Hockley NM, Bihrle R, Bennett RM 3rd, Curry JM. Congenital genitourinary hemangiomas in a patient with the Klippel-Trenaunay syndrome: management with the neodymium: YAG laser. J Urol 1989;141:940–1.

358. Lasota J, Carlson JA, Miettinen M. Spindle cell tumor of urinary bladder serosa with phenotypic and genotypic features of gastrointestinal stromal tumor. Arch Pathol Lab Med 2000;124:894–7.

359. Leuschner I, Harms D, Mattke A, Koscielniak E, Treuner J. Rhabdomyosarcoma of the urinary bladder and vagina: a clinicopathologic study with emphasis on recurrent disease: a report from the Kiel Pediatric Tumor Registry and the German CWS Study. Am J Surg Pathol 2001;25:856–64.

360. Marconis JT. Primary Hodgkin's (paragranulomatous type) disease of the bladder. J Urol 1959;81:275–81.

361. Martin SA, Sears DL, Sebo TJ, Lohse CM, Cheville JC. Smooth muscle neoplasms of the urinary bladder: a clinicopathologic comparison of leiomyoma and leiomyosarcoma. Am J Surg Pathol 2002;26:292–300.

362. Mills SE, Bova GS, Wick MR, Young RH. Leiomyosarcoma of the urinary bladder. A clinicopathologic and immunohistochemical study of 15 cases. Am J Surg Pathol 1989;13:480–9.

363. Mourad WA, Khalil S, Radwi A, Peracha A, Ezzat A. Primary T-cell lymphoma of the urinary bladder. Am J Surg Pathol 1998;22:373–7.

364. Morton KD, Burnett RA. Choriocarcinoma arising in transitional cell carcinoma of bladder: a case report. Histopathology 1988;12:325–8.

365. Moyana TN, Kontozoglou T. Urinary bladder paragangliomas. An immunohistochemical study. Arch Pathol Lab Med 1988;112:70–2.

366. Murphy WM. Diseases of the urinary bladder, urethra, ureters, and renal pelves. In: Murphy WM, ed. Urological pathology. Philadelphia: WB Saunders; 1997:106–11.

367. Navon JD, Rahimzadeh M, Wong AK, Carpenter PM, Ahlering TE. Angiosarcoma of the bladder after therapeutic irradiation for prostate cancer. J Urol 1997;157:1359–60.

368. Oesterling JE, Epstein JI, Brendler CB. Myxoid malignant fibrous histiocytoma of the bladder. Cancer 1990;66:1836–42.

369. Oh-Oka H, Gotoh A, Hanioka K, Okada H. Leiomyoma of the urinary bladder causing tamponade. Scand J Urol Nephrol 1998;32:420–1.

370. Ohsawa M, Aozasa K, Horiuchi K, Kanamaru A. Malignant lymphoma of bladder. Report of three cases and review of the literature. Cancer 1993;72:1969–74.

371. Pan CC, Yu IT, Yang AH, Chiang H. Clear cell myomelanocytic tumor of the urinary bladder. Am J Surg Pathol 2003;27:689–2.

372. Pierson C, Nassar H, Sakr W, Banerjee R, Grignon D. Primary malignant fibrous histiocytoma of the urinary bladder: a case report and review of the literature. J Urol Pathol 1999;11:195–205.

373. Pinto KJ, Jerkins GR. Bladder pheochromocytoma in a 10-year-old girl. J Urol 1997;158:583–4.

374. Pollack AD. Malignant teratoma of the urinary bladder: report of a case. Am J Pathol 1936;12:561–8.

375. Pycha A, Klinger CH, Reiter WJ, Schroth B, Haitel A, Latal D. Von Recklinghausen neurofibromatosis with urinary bladder involvement. Urology 2001;58:106.

376. Siegel RJ, Napoli VM. Malignant lymphoma of the urinary bladder. A case with signet-ring cells simulating urachal adenocarcinoma. Arch Pathol Lab Med 1991;115:635–7.

377. Sievert K, Weber EA, Herwig R, Schmid H, Roos S, Eickenberg HU. Pure primary choriocarcinoma of the urinary bladder with long-term survival. Urology 2000;56:856.

378. Skopelitou A, Mitselou A, Gloustianou G. Xanthoma of the bladder associated with transitional cell carcinoma. J Urol 2000;164:1303–4.

379. Swartz DA, Johnson DE, Ayala AG, Watkins DL. Bladder leiomyosarcoma: a review of 10 cases with 5-year follow-up. J Urol 1985;133:200–2.

380. Taylor G, Jordan M, Churchill B, Mancer K. Yolk sac tumor of the bladder. J Urol 1983;129:591–4.

381. Torenbeek R, Blomjous CE, Meijer CJ. Chondrosarcoma of the urinary bladder: report of a case with immunohistochemical and ultrastructural findings and review of the literature. Eur Urol 1993;23:502–5.

382. Vance RP, Geisinger KR, Randall MB, Marshall RB. Immature neural elements in immature teratomas. An immunohistochemical and ultrastructural study. Am J Clin Pathol 1988;90:397–11.

383. Vara AR, Ruzics EP, Moussabeck O, Martin DC. Endometrioid adenosarcoma of the bladder arising from endometriosis. J Urol 1990;143:813–5.

384. Walker AN, Mills SE, Young RH. Mesenchymal and miscellaneous other primary tumors of the urinary bladder. In: Young RH, ed. Pathology of the urinary bladder. New York: Churchill Livingstone; 1989:139–78.

385. Westra WH, Grenko RT, Epstein J. Solitary fibrous tumor of the lower urogenital tract: a report of five cases involving the seminal vesicles, urinary bladder, and prostate. Hum Pathol 2000;31:63–8.

386. Yang C, Motteram R, Sandeman TF. Extramedullary plasmacytoma of the bladder: a case report and review of literature. Cancer 1982;50:146–9.

Non-Neoplastic Tumorous Conditions

387. al-Izzi MS, Horton LW, Kelleher J, Fawcett D. Malignant transformation in endometriosis of the urinary bladder. Histopathology 1989;14:191–8.

388. Barsotti P, Crescenzi A, Mingazzini PL, De Matteis A. Mucus-secreting lesions of the urinary tract: histochemical observations. J Urol Pathol 1993;1:135–43.

389. Benson RC Jr, Swanson SK, Farrow GM. Relationship of leukoplakia to urothelial malignancy. J Urol 1984;131:507–11.

390. Billis A, Lima AC, Queiroz LS, Cia EM, Oliveira ER, Pinto W Jr. Adenoma of bladder in siblings with renal dysplasia. Urology 1980;16:299–302.

391. Brown EW. Eosinophilic granuloma of the bladder. J Urol 1960;83:665–8.

392. Bullock PS, Thoni DE, Murphy WM. The significance of colonic mucosa (intestinal metaplasia) involving the urinary tract. Cancer 1987;59:2086–90.

393. Cheng L, Leibovich BC, Cheville JC, et al. Squamous papilloma of the urinary tract is unrelated to condyloma acuminata. Cancer 2000;88:1679–86.

394. Chung MK, Seol MY, Cho WY, Seo HK, Kim JS. Xanthogranulomatous cystitis associated with suture material. J Urol 1998;159:981–2.

395. Clement PB, Young RH. Endocervicosis of the urinary bladder. A report of six cases of a benign mullerian lesion that may mimic adenocarcinoma. Am J Surg Pathol 1992;16:533–42.

396. Close CE, Carr MC, Burns MW, et al. Interstitial cystitis in children. J Urol 1996;156:860–2.

397. Cook JR, Dehner LP, Collins MH, et al. Anaplastic lymphoma kinase (ALK) expression in the inflammatory myofibroblastic tumor: a comparative immunohistochemical study. Am J Surg Pathol 2001;25:1364–71.

398. Corica FA, Husmann DA, Churchill BM, et al. Intestinal metaplasia is not a strong risk factor for bladder cancer: study of 53 cases with long-term follow-up. Urology 1997;50:427–31.

399. Damjanov I, Katz SM. Malakoplakia. Pathol Annu 1981;16(Pt 2):103–26.

400. Del Mistro A, Koss LG, Braunstein J, Bennett B, Saccomano G, Simons KM. Condylomata acuminata of the urinary bladder. Natural history, viral typing, and DNA content. Am J Surg Pathol 1988;12:205–15.

401. Denson MA, Griebling TL, Cohen MB, Kreder KJ. Comparison of cystoscopic and histological findings in patients with suspected interstitial cystitis. J Urol 2000;164:1908–11.

402. Devine P, Ucci AA, Krain H, et al. Nephrogenic adenoma and embryonic kidney tubules share PNA receptor sites. Am J Clin Pathol 1984;81:728–32.

403. Dietrick DD, Kabalin JN, Daniels GF Jr, Epstein AB, Fielding IM. Inflammatory pseudotumor of the bladder. J Urol 1992;148:141–4.

404. Eble JN. Abnormalities of the urachus. In: Young RH, ed. Pathology of the urinary bladder. New York: Churchill Livingstone; 1989:213–44.

405. Edmondson JD, Vogeley KJ, Howell JD, Koontz WW, Koo HP, Amaker B. Endosalpingiosis of bladder. J Urol 2002;167:1401–2.

406. Ehara H, Deguchi T, Yanagihara M, Yokota T, Uchino F, Kawada Y. Primary localized amyloidosis of the bladder: an immunohistochemical study of a case. J Urol 1992;147:458–60.

407. Erturk E, Erturk E, Sheinfeld J, Davis RS. Metaplastic cystitis complicated with Von Brunn nests, cystitis cystica, and intestinal type of glandular metaplasia. Urology 1988;32:165–7.

408. Fischer AH, Wallace VL, Keane TE, Clarke HS. Two cases of vasculitis of the urinary bladder: diagnostic and pathogenetic considerations. Arch Pathol Lab Med 1998;122:903–6.

409. Friedman NB, Kuhlenbeck H. Adenomatoid tumors of the bladder reproducing renal structures (nephrogenic adenomas). J Urol 1950;64:657–70.

410. Fujihara S, Glenner GG. Primary localized amyloidosis of the genitourinary tract: immunohistochemical study on eleven cases. Lab Invest 1981;44:55–60.

411. Goldstein AM, Fauer RB, Chinn M, Kaempf MJ. New concepts on formation of Brunn's nests and cysts in urinary tract mucosa. Urology 1978;11:513–7.

412. Gourlay WA, Chiu A, Montessori VC, Dunn IJ. Urinary filariasis presenting as bladder pseudotumors. J Urol 1999;161:603–4.

413. Guermazi A, de Kerviler E, Welker Y, Zagdanski AM, Desgrandchamps F, Frija J. Pseudotumoral vesical actinomycosis. J Urol 1996;156:2002–3.

414. Harold DL, Koff SA, Kass EJ. Candida albicans "fungus ball" in bladder. Urology 1977;9:662–3.

415. Huang WL, Ro JY, Grignon DJ, Swanson D, Ordonez NG, Ayala AG. Postoperative spindle cell nodule of the prostate and bladder. J Urol 1990;143:824–6.

416. Iczkowski KA, Shanks JH, Gadaleanu V, et al. Inflammatory pseudotumor and sarcoma of urinary bladder: differential diagnosis and outcome in thirty-eight spindle cell neoplasms. Mod Pathol 2001;14:1043–51.

417. Itano NM, Malek RS. Eosinophilic cystitis in adults. J Urol 2001;165:805–7.

418. Iyengar V, Smith DK, Jablonski DV, Gallivan MV. Extramedullary hematopoiesis in the urinary bladder in a case of agnogenic myeloid metaplasia. J Urol Pathol 1993;1:419–23.

419. Johansson SL. In consultation. Interstitial cystitis. Mod Pathol 1993;6:738–42.

420. Johansson SL, Smout MS, Taylor RJ. Eosinophilic cystitis associated with symptomatic ureteral involvement: a report of two cases. J Urol Pathol 1993;1:69–77.

421. Jones EC, Clement PB, Young RH. Inflammatory pseudotumor of the urinary bladder. A clinicopathological, immunohistochemical, ultrastructural, and flow cytometric study of 13 cases. Am J Surg Pathol 1993;17:264–74.

422. Jufe R, Molinolo AA, Fefer SA, Meiss RP. Plasma cell granuloma of the bladder: a case report. J Urol 1984;131:1175–6.

423. Kunze E, Schauer A, Schmitt M. Histology and histogenesis of two different types of inverted urothelial papillomas. Cancer 1983;51:348–58.

424. Lidgi S, Embon OM, Turani H, Sazbon AI. Giant cell reparative granuloma of the bladder associated with transitional cell carcinoma. J Urol 1989,142.120–2.

425. Lynes WL, Flynn SD, Shortliffe LD, Stamey TA. The histology of interstitial cystitis. Am J Surg Pathol 1990;14:969–76.

426. Mazal PR, Schaufler R, Altenhuber-Muller R, et al. Derivation of nephrogenic adenomas from renal tubular cells in kidney-transplant recipients. N Engl J Med 2002;347:653–9.

427. McClurg FV, D'Agostino AN, Martin JH, Race GJ. Ultrastructural demonstration of intracellular bacteria in three cases of malakoplakia of the bladder. Am J Clin Pathol 1973;60:780–8.

428. McIntire TL, Soloway MS, Murphy WM. Nephrogenic adenoma. Urology 1987;29:237–41.

429. Morey AF, Kreder KJ, Wikert GA, Cooper G, Dresner ML. Ectopic prostate tissue at the bladder dome. J Urol 1989;141:942–3.

430. Nazeer T, Ro JY, Tornos C, Ordonez NG, Ayala AG. Endocervical type glands in the urinary bladder: a clinicopathologic study of six cases. Hum Pathol 1996;816–20.

431. Oliva E, Young RH. Nephrogenic adenoma of the urinary tract: a review of the microscopic appearance of 80 cases with emphasis on unusual features. Mod Pathol 1995;8:722–30.

432. Park C, Kim H, Lee YB, Song JM, Ro JY. Hamartoma of the urachal remnant. Arch Pathol Lab Med 1989;113;1393–5.

433. Peeker R, Fall M. Toward a precise definition of interstitial cystitis: further evidence of differences in classic and nonulcer disease. J Urol 2002;167:2470–2.

434. Propert KJ, Schaeffer AJ, Brensinger CM, Kusek JW, Nyberg LM, Landis JR. A prospective study of interstitial cystitis: results of longitudinal followup of the interstitial cystitis data base cohort. The International Cystitis Data Base Study Group. J Urol 2000;163:1434–9.

435. Proppe KH, Scully RE, Rosai J. Postoperative spindle cell nodules of genitourinary tract resembling sarcomas: a report of eight cases. Am J Surg Pathol 1984;8:101–8.

436. Quint HJ, Drach GW, Rappaport WD, Hoffman CJ. Emphysematous cystitis: a review of the spectrum of disease. J Urol 1992;147:134–7.

437. Ro JY, el-Nagger AK, Amin MB, Sahin AA, Ordonez NG, Ayala AG. Pseudosarcomatous fibromyxoid tumor of the urinary bladder and prostate: immunohistochemical, ultrastructural, and DNA flow cytometric analysis of nine cases. Hum Pathol 1993;24:1203–10.

438. Roberts PF. Vascular anomaly of the urinary bladder resembling calibre persistent artery: report of three cases. J Urol Pathol 2000;13:95–103.

439. Steele AA, Byrne AJ. Paramesonephric (mullerian) sinus of urinary bladder. Am J Surg Pathol 1982;6:173–6.

440. Tammela T, Kallioinen M, Kontturi M, Hellstrom P. Sarcoidosis of the bladder: a case report and literature review. J Urol 1989;141:608–9.

441. Thijssen A, Gerridzen RG. Eosinophilic cystitis presenting as invasive bladder cancer: comments on pathogenesis and management. J Urol 1990;144:977–9.

442. Vara AR, Ruzics EP, Moussabeck O, Martin DC. Endometrioid adenosarcoma of the bladder arising from endometriosis. J Urol 1990;143:813–5.

443. Vercellini P, Meschia M, De Giorgi O, Panazza S, Cortesi I, Crosignani PG. Bladder detrusor endometriosis: clinical and pathologic implications. J Urol 1996;155:84–6.

444. Walther M, Glenn JF, Vellios F. Xanthogranulomatous cystitis. J Urol 1985;134:745–6.

445. Watanabe K, Baba K, Saito A, Hoshi N, Suzuki T. Pseudosarcomatous fibromyxoid tumor and myosarcoma of the urogenital tract. Arch Pathol Lab Med 2001;125:1070–3.

446. Weiner H, Mian C, Pycha A, et al. Numerical chromosomal aberrations in nephrogenic adenoma of the bladder (abstract). Acta Cytol 1997;41:1223.

447. Wells M, Anderson K. Mucin histochemistry of cystitis glandularis and primary adenocarcinoma of the urinary bladder. Arch Pathol Lab Med 1985;109:59–61.

448. Wick MR, Brown BA, Young RH, Mills SE. Spindle-cell proliferations of the urinary tract. An immunohistochemical study. Am J Surg Pathol 1988;12:379–89.

449. Widran J, Sanchez R, Gruhn J. Squamous metaplasia of the bladder: a study of 450 patients. J Urol 1974;112:479–82.

450. Wiener DP, Koss LG, Sablay B, Freed SZ. The prevalence and significance of Brunn's nests, cystitis cystica and squamous metaplasia in normal bladders. J Urol 1979;122:317–21.

451. Williams MP, Ibrahim SK, Rickwood AM. Hamartoma of the urinary bladder in an infant with Beckwith-Wiedemann syndrome. Br J Urol 1990;65:106–7.

452. Young RH. Non-neoplastic epithelial abnormalities and tumorlike lesions. In: Young RH, ed. Pathology of the urinary bladder. New York: Churchill Livingstone; 1989:1–64.

453. Young RH, Scully RE. Nephrogenic adenoma. A report of 15 cases, review of the literature, and comparison with clear cell adenocarcinoma of the urinary tract. Am J Surg Pathol 1986;10:268–75.

454. Zilberman M, Laor E, Moriel E, Reid RE, Farkas A. Paravesical granulomas masquerading as bladder neoplasms: late complications of inguinal hernia repair. J Urol 1990;143:489–91.

Treatment

455. Broghammer EL, Ratliff TL. Immunotherapy of urologic tumors: principles and progress. Urol Oncol 2002;7:45–56.

456. Davis JW, Sheth SI, Doviak MJ, Schellhammer PF. Superficial bladder carcinoma treated with bacillus Calmette-Guerin: progression-free and disease specific survival with minimum 10-year followup. J Urol 2002;167:494–501.

457. Gerharz EW, Weingartner K, Dopatka T, Kohl UN, Basler HD, Riedmiller HN. Quality of life after cystectomy and urinary diversion: results of a retrospective interdisciplinary study. J Urol 1997;158:778–85.

458. Glashan RW. A randomized controlled study of intravesical alpha-2b-interferon in carcinoma in situ of the bladder. J Urol 1990;144:658–61.

459. Herr HW, Donat SM. Prostatic tumor relapse in patients with superficial bladder tumors: 15-year outcome. J Urol 1999;161:1854–7.

460. Herr HW, Sogani PC. Does early cystectomy improve the survival of patients with high risk superficial bladder tumors? J Urol 2001;166:1296–9.

461. Holmang S, Hedelin H, Borghede G, Johansson SL. Long-term followup of a bladder carcinoma cohort: questionable value of radical radiotherapy. J Urol 1997;157:1642–6.

462. Kurth K, Tunn U, Ay R, et al. Adjuvant chemotherapy for superficial transitional cell bladder carcinoma: long-term results of a European Organization for Research and Treatment of Cancer randomized trial comparing doxorubicin, ethoglucid and transurethral resection alone. J Urol 1997;158:378–84.

463. Petrovich Z, Jozsef G, Brady LW. Radiotherapy for carcinoma of the bladder: a review. Am J Clin Oncol 2001;24:1–9.

464. Retz M, Lehmann J, Trocha C, et al. Long term follow-up of combined radiochemotherapy for locally advanced bladder carcinoma. Cancer 2000;89:1089–94.

465. Thrasher JB, Crawford ED. Current management of invasive and metastatic transitional cell carcinoma of the bladder. J Urol 1993;149:957–72.

466. von der Maase H. Current and future perspectives in advanced bladder cancer: is there a new standard? Semin Oncol 2002;29(suppl 3):3–14.

Urinary Diversions

467. Barrington JW, Fulford S, Griffiths D, Stephenson TP. Tumors in bladder remnant after augmentation enterocystoplasty. J Urol 1997;157:482–6.

468. Filmer RB, Spencer JR. Malignancies in bladder augmentations and intestinal conduits. J Urol 1990;143:671–8.

469. Frese R, Doehn C, Baumgartel M, Holl-Ulrich K, Jocham D. Carcinoid tumor in an ileal neobladder. J Urol 2001;165:522–3.

470. Gregoire M, Kantoff P, DeWolf WC. Synchronous adenocarcinoma and transitional cell carcinoma of the bladder associated with augmentation: case report and review of the literature. J Urol 1993;149:115–8.

471. Hautmann RE, de Petriconi R, Gottfried HW, Kleinschmidt K, Mattes R, Paiss T. The ileal neobladder: complications and functional results in 363 patients after 11 years of followup. J Urol 1999;161:422–8.

472. Helander KG, Ahren C, Philipson BM, Samuelsson BM, Ojerskog BO. Structure of mucosa in continent ileal reservoirs 15 to 19 years after construction. Hum Pathol 1990;21:1235–8.

473. Husmann DA, Spence HM. Current status of tumor of the bowel following ureterosigmoidoscopy: a review. J Urol 1990;144:607–10.

474. Iseki M, Tsuda N, Hayashi T, et al. Multifocal villous adenomas of the anastomotic area following ileocystoplasty: a case report and literature review. J Urol Pathol 2000;12:29–37.

475. Murphy WM. Diseases of the urinary bladder, urethra, ureters, and renal pelves. In: Murphy WM, ed. Urological pathology. Philadelphia: WB Saunders; 1997:131–4.

476. Murphy WM. Urinary cytopathology. Chicago: ASCP Press; 2000:62–5.

477. Stein R, Fisch M, Stockle M, Demirkesen O, Hohenfellner R. Colonic conduit in children: protection of the upper urinary tract 16 years later? J Urol 1996;156:1146–50.

478. Theodorescu D, Older RA, Sorenson EJ. Metastatic melanoma presenting as an ileal conduit filling defect. J Urol 2001;166:1393–4.

479. Watarai Y, Satoh H, Matubara M, et al. Comparison of urine cytology between the ileal conduit and Indiana pouch. Acta Cytol 2000;44:748–51.

Procedures for Pathologic Examination

480. American Joint Committee on Cancer (AJCC). Manual for staging of cancer, 6th ed. Philadelphia: Lippincott-Raven; 2002:335–40.

480a. Dalbagni G, Genega E, Hashibe M, et al. Cystectomy for bladder cancer: a contemporary series. J Urol 2001;165:1111–6.

481. Hammond EH, Henson DE, et al. Practice protocol for the examination of specimens removed from patients with carcinoma of the urinary bladder, ureter, renal pelvis, and urethra. Arch Pathol Lab Med 1996;120:1103–10.

482. Larsen MP, Steinberg GD, Brendler CB, Epstein JI. Use of Ulex europaeus agglutinin I (UEAI) to distinguish vascular and "pseudovascular" invasion in transitional cell carcinoma of bladder with lamina propria invasion. Mod Pathol 1990;3:83–8.

483. Maruniak NA, Takezawa K, Murphy WM. Accurate pathological staging of urothelial neoplasms requires better cystoscopic sampling. J Urol 2002;167:2404–7.

484. Murphy WM. ASCP survey on anatomic pathology examination of the urinary bladder. Am J Clin Pathol 1994;102:715–23.

485. Murphy WM. Diseases of the urinary bladder, urethra, ureters, and renal pelves. In: Murphy WM ed. Urological pathology. Philadelphia: WB Saunders; 1997:71–3, 96–8.

486. Murphy WM. The evolution of the anatomic pathologist from medical consultant to information specialist. Am J Surg Pathol 2002;26:99–102.

487. Recommendations for the reporting of urinary bladder specimens containing bladder neoplasms. Association of Directors of Anatomic and Surgical Pathology. Am J Clin Pathol 1996;106:568–70.

488. Schoenberg MP, Carter HB, Epstein JI. Ureteral frozen section analysis during cystectomy: a reassessment. J Urol 1996;155:1218–20.

489. Yang XJ, Lecksell K, Epstein JI. Can immunohistochemistry enhance the detection of micrometastases in pelvic lymph nodes from patients with high-grade urothelial carcinoma of the bladder? Am J Clin Pathol 1999;112:649–53.

4 TUMORS OF THE URETHRA

NORMAL ANATOMY

The urethra develops from the caudal portion of the urogenital sinus (1,49). In females, failure of the genital swellings to fuse and growth of the genital tubercle result in a short organ that empties into a vestibule shared with the vagina. The mature female urethra is lined predominantly with squamous epithelium and receives ducts from multiple paraurethral glands (Skene glands), homologues of the prostatic glands in the male (50). The mucosa is surrounded by a thick muscular wall that contains scanty erectile tissue. In males, the growth of the genital tubercle and fusion of the genital swellings produce an elongated urethra, which becomes surrounded by the prostate gland and fuses with the phallic ectoderm to form prostatic, membranous, and penile portions. The prostatic and membranous parts of the mature male urethra are lined predominantly by urothelium but areas of prostatic epithelium are frequent in the prostatic portion. Pseudostratified columnar and squamous epithelia appear in the penile portion.

The urothelial cells of the normal urethra are more compact and have less cytoplasmic clearing than those of the urinary bladder. In usual histologic preparations, their nuclei seem larger, with slightly more granular chromatin. Whether these changes reflect normal development or acquired alterations is unclear but they are important when the urethral mucosa is evaluated for dysplastic (atypical hyperplastic) changes. Paired bulbourethral glands (Cowper glands), the male homologue of Bartholin glands, form adjacent to the membranous urethra and empty into the bulbous urethra through discrete ducts. Tubular paraurethral glands (glands of Littré) lubricate the penile urethra at multiple sites along its course. Regardless of location, these accessory urethral glands are rich in mucus-secreting cells. The posterior prostatic portion of the male urethra is elevated by the utricle (uterus masculinus) and terminal portions of the ejaculatory ducts, which together form the verumontanum (colliculus seminalis). Depending on its location, the male urethra is surrounded by the musculature of the bladder neck, the prostate gland, the urogenital diaphragm (external sphincter), or the corpus spongiosum.

EPITHELIAL NEOPLASMS

Definition and General Features. Epithelial neoplasms of the urethra are almost exclusively carcinomas (37). If squamous cell papilloma is considered an inflammatory reaction similar to condyloma acuminatum, benign epithelial neoplasms are rare. The literature concerning urethral neoplasms is almost identical to that for bladder lesions. It suggests that carcinomas arising in the urethra differ from those originating in the urinary bladder in only a few respects: lower incidence; higher frequency in women; greater percentage of high-grade invasive tumors; greater percentage of squamous cell carcinomas; greater likelihood of high stage at diagnosis; and poorer prognosis (14,17,30,59). The etiology, pathogenesis, methods of detection and monitoring, histologic classification, and staging of urethral cancers are essentially the same as for their bladder counterparts (see previous chapter and Tables 4-1, 4-2) (59). Reactions to therapy as well as non-neoplastic epithelial atypias have been less thoroughly studied in the urethra than in the bladder but are probably essentially the same. Therefore, this section will not reiterate the information discussed and illustrated in the previous chapter but will concentrate on neoplasms for which urethral occurrence is associated with features of special interest. Those neoplasms are carcinoma in situ, clear cell adenocarcinoma, and melanoma.

Clinical Features. Primary carcinomas of the urethra comprise less than 1 percent of all urothelial neoplasms. Patients are usually

Table 4-1

NEOPLASMS OF THE URETHRA

Epithelial Neoplasms
    Squamous cell carcinoma
    Urothelial (transitional cell) carcinoma
    Adenocarcinoma
        Enteric – all types
        Clear cell
    Adenoid cystic carcinoma
    Adenosquamous carcinoma
    Poorly differentiated small cell carcinoma
        Neuroendocrine carcinoma
    Cloacogenic carcinoma
    Carcinoma in situ
        Primary
        Secondary
    Carcinoid tumor

Melanoma

Lymphoma

Plasmacytoma

Mesenchymal Neoplasms
    Leiomyoma
    Hemangioma
    Sarcoma–most common types

Yolk Sac Tumor

Non-neoplastic Tumorous Conditions
    Condyloma acuminatum
    Polyps
    Caruncle

Table 4-2

STAGING OF URETHRAL NEOPLASMS: AMERICAN JOINT COMMITTEE ON CANCER[a]

TX	Primary tumor cannot be assessed
T0	No tumor
Ta	Noninvasive tumor (papillary, polypoid, verrucous)
Tis	Carcinoma in situ
T1	Invasion of subepithelial connective tissue
T2	Invasion of: corpus spongiosum / periurethral muscle / prostate gland
T3	Invasion of: corpus cavernosum / extraprostatic tissue / anterior vagina / bladder neck
T4	Invasion of other adjacent organs
NX	Regional lymph nodes cannot be assessed
N0	No regional lymph node metastases
N1	One nodal metastasis, ≤ 2.0 cm
N2	Multiple nodal metastases or one metastasis, > 2.0 cm
MX	Distant metastases cannot be assessed
M0	No distant metastases
M1	Distant metastases

[a]AJCC Cancer staging manual, 6th ed. New York: Springer; 2002:341–6.

women (male to female ratio, 1 to 4) with a mean age of 60 years (14,17). Sex has an effect on the frequency of different histologic types of carcinoma, with most adenocarcinomas occurring in women. In men, the majority of urethral carcinomas are squamous cell and involve the penile portion of the organ. Chronic irritation, urethral stricture, urethral diverticula, and chronic infections from sexually transmitted organisms have been considered predisposing factors. Human papillomavirus (HPV) activity has been demonstrated in the neoplastic cells of rare patients (33). Bladder cancer is a commonly associated condition and more than a few cases reported as urethral carcinoma represent secondary involvement by multifocal carcinoma in situ of the bladder (3,15,27). A bleeding urethral mass is the most common presenting complaint in women; obstruction is most often observed in men. Patients of both sexes may have dysuria, suprapubic pain, and discharge.

Pathologic Findings. Histologically, epithelial neoplasms of the urethra are almost all squamous cell, urothelial, or adenocarcinomas, although other types have been reported (fig. 4-1) (23,24,25,51,59). The histologic subtype varies with the location of the lesion. Distal urethral tumors are usually squamous cell carcinoma in both men and women. More proximal carcinomas tend to be urothelial or adenocarcinomas. In women, the lesions often occupy the entire urethra; in men, over 75 percent of primary urethral carcinomas occur in the membranous and penile regions.

Prognosis. Regardless of sex, urethral carcinomas tend to grow locally (14,17,28). Metastases to distant organs are unusual but preferentially involve lymph nodes when present. The prognosis for patients with proximal urethral tumors is poor, with a median survival time of less than 2 years and death from disease occurring in more than 50 percent. Carcinomas arising in the penile urethra are associated with a more

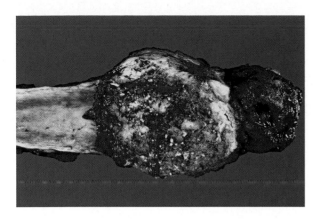 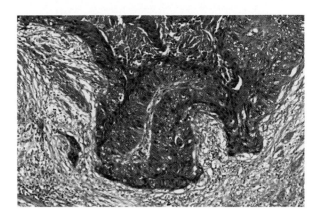

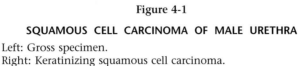

Figure 4-1

SQUAMOUS CELL CARCINOMA OF MALE URETHRA

Left: Gross specimen.
Right: Keratinizing squamous cell carcinoma.

favorable prognosis, perhaps because their location allows complete surgical resection prior to dissemination.

Differential Diagnosis. The differential diagnosis of primary urethral tumors follows the guidelines established for bladder neoplasms. Most carcinomas present no diagnostic problems. Primary ductal prostatic carcinomas commonly present as papillary lesions in the urethra. Careful examination reveals the uniform nuclei; the finely granular, evenly distributed chromatin; and the prominent nucleoli characteristic of high-grade prostatic carcinomas. Immunohistochemical reactions for prostatic antigens can be used if necessary.

Carcinoma in Situ

Carcinoma in situ (CIS) in the urethra, like the bladder, is urothelial; squamous and glandular types have not been defined. CIS rarely occurs as a primary urethral neoplasm but has been documented in about 10 percent of urethras following cystoprostatectomy for bladder cancer, where the urethra has been left in situ (11,15,16,58). The histology of urethral CIS does not differ from that of CIS in other urothelial-lined organs; rarely, the CIS may take the so-called pagetoid form (3).

Interest in urethral CIS stems from its occurrence after cystoprostatectomy for bladder cancer (11,15,16,22,23). If the entire urethra is not removed at the time of radical surgery, patho-

logic evaluation of the resected portion is essential to subsequent patient care. Patients having CIS in the urethra, prostatic ducts, or the grossly uninvolved bladder mucosa are at especially high risk for subsequent involvement of the residual urethra (11,15).

The best current method for monitoring the penile urethra after cystoprostatectomy is urethral wash cytopathology (fig. 4-2) (16,37). The tumor cells in urethral washings may be more poorly preserved than similar elements in bladder washings but can be distinguished by their eccentricity, high nuclear-cytoplasmic ratios, pleomorphism, and granular chromatin. Neoplastic cells in specimens obtained at periodic intervals from asymptomatic patients signal the presence of focal CIS. These lesions are rarely detectable at subsequent urethroscopy, and biopsy confirmation prior to complete urethrectomy is usually not possible. The urethral mucosa in urethrectomy specimens is ordinarily markedly denuded. In such cases, the neoplasm can be expected to be focal CIS, usually present only in paraurethral glands.

Considering the major surgery that is provoked by a positive urethral wash interpretation and the paucity of residual neoplasm in the histologic specimens, a conservative approach to pathologic diagnosis is warranted. On the other hand, it seems unnecessary to process serial sections of the entire penile urethrectomy specimen to reconfirm focal CIS when

365

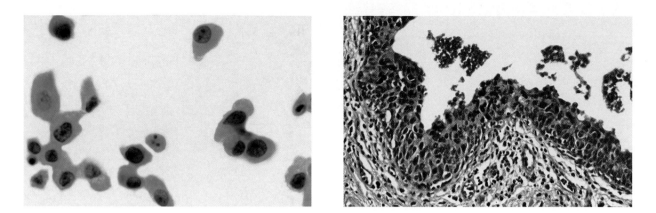

Figure 4-2

CARCINOMA IN SITU OF URETHRAL STUMP

Left: High-grade urothelial neoplasm in urethral washing.
Right: Carcinoma in situ.

the diagnosis of malignancy has been made cytopathologically. Paradoxically, both our own experience and that of others indicate that the prognosis of patients is not improved by urethrectomy, at least over the short term (22,23). Our experience indicates that the value of monitoring with urethral wash cytopathology rests in the stratification of patients into prognostic groups: those having positive results have a statistically greater risk of an adverse outcome than those with negative findings. In addition, urethral neoplasms that cause gross hematuria or a palpable mass, in contrast to those detected cytologically in asymptomatic individuals, are often invasive, and patients have a correspondingly poorer prognosis (11,58).

Clear Cell Adenocarcinoma

Definition and General Features. Various histologic types of adenocarcinoma occur in the urethra but the only one of special interest in a discussion of urethral pathology is the clear cell type. This is a relatively rare tumor with distinctive histogenetic and histologic features (8,12,39,40). Cases have been reported in the bladder but are most frequent in the female urethra, where they may arise in paraurethral ducts or diverticula. Unlike other urethral carcinomas, an association with sources of chronic irritation is not strong. The histologic features are most reminiscent of clear cell adenocarcinoma of the uterus or vagina, and most authors favor a müllerian differentiation, if not derivation. Histologic changes suggestive of endometriosis, or mesonephric or nephrogenic differentiation also occur but derivation from these sources has been rejected by most experts.

Clinical Features. Reported patients with clear cell adenocarcinoma range in age from 22 to 83 years (mean, 57 years) and almost all are women. Most cancers arise at paraurethral sites. Gross hematuria, dysuria, suprapubic pain, and discharge are the usual presenting complaints and a visible mass is present in nearly every case.

Pathologic Findings. The pathology of clear cell adenocarcinoma is distinctive (fig. 4-3). Tumors are composed predominantly of sheets of uniform, ovoid cells with moderately well-defined borders and amphophilic to acidophilic cytoplasm. Papillary, tubular, and even cystic areas are common, and all may be partially lined by "hobnailed" cells. A single layer of neoplastic cells usually lines the papillae or tubules. Clear cells rich in glycogen are characteristic but are rarely the predominant element, in our experience. Small amounts of luminal mucin and some psammoma bodies have been observed. The nuclei of the clear cells tend to be round and uniform, with slightly irregular borders, finely granular and evenly distributed chromatin, and prominent nucleoli. Mitoses are readily found. Cytologic and ultrastructural studies have confirmed the histologic findings. The immunohistochemical findings have varied

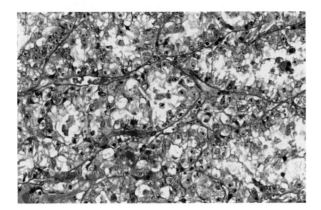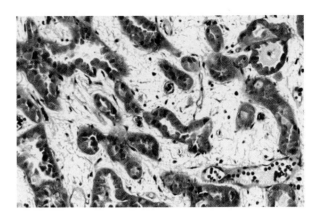

Figure 4-3

CLEAR CELL ADENOCARCINOMA OF URETHRA
Left: Clear cell pattern.
Right: Hobnail cells in tubular pattern.

in reported studies. Most tumors react with pancytokeratins and CA125. Some react with cytokeratins 7 and 20, S-100 protein, carcinoembryonic antigen, CA19.9, and Leu M1. Reactions for prostatic antigens are almost uniformly negative.

Prognosis. The prognosis of patients with clear cell adenocarcinoma is unclear. Most reported patients have been treated with radical surgery but followed for less than 5 years. Metastases have occurred in at least 15 percent of patients; death from disease has been recorded in 25 to 30 percent. Tumor-related deaths have occurred after apparently adequate surgical excision and after many years of follow-up.

Differential Diagnosis. Clear cell adenocarcinoma must be differentiated from other types of adenocarcinoma, mesonephric carcinoma, nephrogenic metaplasia, and metastatic carcinomas. The histologic pattern of sheets, papillae, and tubules without significant mucin distinguishes these tumors from other urothelial adenocarcinomas. Mesonephric carcinoma is a controversial tumor which may not exist as a separate entity and is almost always difficult to confirm. The hobnailed pattern suggestive of this lesion is common to other neoplasms, has never predominated in reported cases of clear cell adenocarcinoma, and cannot be considered strong evidence of mesonephric differentiation. Further, clear cell adenocarcinomas tend to arise at anterior and posterior sites rather than at the lateral locations expected of

a tumor arising in mesonephric remnants. Nephrogenic metaplasia is histologically similar to clear cell adenocarcinoma and it is possible that nephrogenic and clear cell patterns differentiate simultaneously. Clear cell adenocarcinoma has not been observed among the numerous patients followed for nephrogenic metaplasia. Cellular anaplasia is rare in nephrogenic metaplasia and never occurs in large portions of the lesion. Metastatic carcinomas, especially from kidney or prostate gland, may be difficult to distinguish from clear cell adenocarcinoma on histologic grounds alone. Radiographic studies may be required in selected cases.

Melanoma

The urethra is the most common site of primary melanoma in the genitourinary tract (20, 43). The etiology and pathogenesis are unknown. Melanomas are more common in women (male to female ratio, 1 to 2.6) and occur in blacks as well as whites. Most patients are 50 to 70 years of age (mean, 64 years). Lesions usually occur in the distal urethra where they may produce symptoms of dysuria or hematuria. Lesions in the urethra may be secondary to melanomas of the glans penis or labia. The pathology does not differ from that of melanoma at other body sites, except that a significant proportion of the tumors may be amelanotic and melanomas can be papillary or spindled (59). Most urethral melanomas are localized at diagnosis. Even so, prognosis is poor, with few patients surviving more than 5 years.

Figure 4-4

CONDYLOMA ACUMINATUM OF PENILE URETHRA
A: Low magnification.
B: Koilocytotic change.
C: Nuclei harboring human papilloma virus (HPV) type 16.

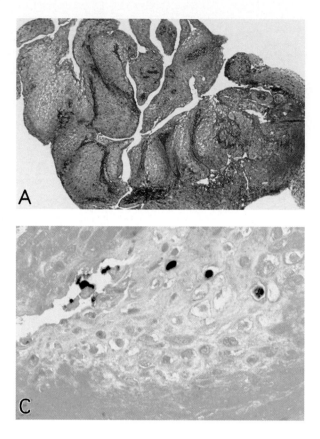

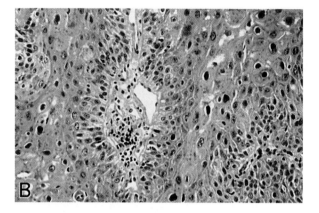

OTHER URETHRAL NEOPLASMS

A variety of neoplasms of the urethra have been reported as individual cases. They include carcinoid tumor, cloacogenic carcinoma, villous adenoma, rhabdomyosarcoma, lymphoma, plasmacytoma, granular cell tumor, hemangioma, leiomyoma, intravascular angiomatosis (Masson's angiomatosis), neuroendocrine carcinoma, and adenosquamous carcinoma (19, 21,25,35,37,41,52,53,57). The pathology of these lesions is characteristic of each type of tumor and does not differ from that of similar neoplasms at other body sites.

NON-NEOPLASTIC TUMOROUS CONDITIONS

Condyloma Acuminatum

Condyloma acuminatum is an inflammatory reaction manifested by a proliferation of squamous epithelium. The urethra is ordinarily involved by direct extension from lesions arising at adjacent sites, but primary urethral condylomas occur. Evidence of infection with HPV can be demonstrated in almost every case and it is generally accepted that condylomata acuminata are caused by infection with HPV. Using sophisticated techniques to detect gene copies, HPV type 6 or 11 is most commonly identified; a few lesions contain other types (6,32). In contrast to the almost universal evidence of viral exposure, many lesions fail to manifest viral structural antigens and even when present, these antigens occur in only a tiny percentage of the cells examined (38). Condyloma acuminatum rarely coexists with, and does not appear to be a direct precursor of, cancer.

Condyloma acuminatum is common, especially in men, where it accounts for up to 30 percent of tumorous lesions of the urethra (14). Most patients are 20 to 40 years of age. Lesions grow slowly and are often asymptomatic. Multiplicity and recurrence are common.

The pathologic features of condyloma acuminatum do not differ from those of similar lesions arising elsewhere (fig. 4-4). Condylomas may be either papillary or flat, and characteristically manifest koilocytotic areas. Significant

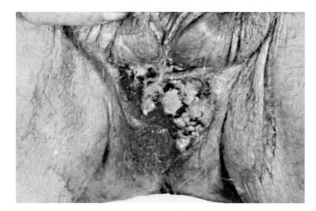 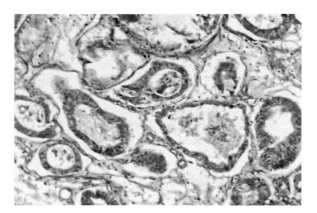

Figure 4-8

CARCINOMA OF COWPER'S GLAND

Left: Clinical appearance. (Fig. 266 from Fascicle 8, 2nd Series.)
Right: Adenocarcinoma. (Fig. 267 from Fascicle 8, 2nd Series.)

cells (18). They are variable in number and size, and secrete a seromucinous fluid into the urethra at multiple sites along its course. Paraurethral glands in females (Skene glands) are homologues of prostatic tissue, as judged by their expression of prostatic antigens (50). In males, paraurethral glands describe those structures arising in the penile urethra (glands of Littré). Bulbourethral glands (Cowper glands) are paired seromucinous organs arising from the urogenital sinus that become embedded in the urogenital diaphragm of males. In contrast to paraurethral glands, these structures are larger and more discrete, and empty into the bulbous urethra via well-formed ducts.

Tumors of these accessory urethral glands are predominantly cysts and adenocarcinomas (34, 37,45). Syringoceles of the ducts have also been reported (4). With the exception of clear cell adenocarcinoma and caruncle, most accessary gland lesions arise in the bulbourethral glands and are rare. Given their size and variable distribution, it is not surprising that the sites of origin of tumors attributed to the paraurethral glands are difficult to confirm. Cysts are lined with urothelial, pseudostratified columnar, and squamous epithelium. The most common neoplasm is clear cell adenocarcinoma in women (48). Mucus-secreting adenocarcinoma has also been reported (45).

The site of origin of bulbourethral gland tumors is somewhat easier to establish (36,37). Cysts may be either congenital or acquired (42). Congenital cysts are attributed to developmental fusion of, and acquired cysts to inflammatory obstruction of, the bulbourethral ducts. Carcinomas are less common than cysts. These neoplasms may remain localized for prolonged periods, eventually causing symptoms related to urethral obstruction or painful defecation. Histologically, primary bulbourethral gland neoplasms are mucus-secreting adenocarcinomas or adenoid cystic carcinomas; urothelial CIS rarely extends into Cowper's gland ducts (fig. 4-8) (36,46). The prognosis is unclear, especially since large tumors in this region are difficult to confirm as bulbourethral and many cases were reported before the advent of modern treatment and life support techniques.

REFERENCES

1. Altemus AR, Hutchins GM. Development of the human anterior urethra. J Urol 1991;146:1085–93.
2. Baroudy AC, O'Connell JP. Papillary adenoma of the prostatic urethra. J Urol 1984;132:120–2.
3. Begin LR, Deschenes J, Mitmaker B. Pagetoid carcinomatous involvement of the penile urethra in association with high-grade transitional cell carcinoma of the urinary bladder. Arch Pathol Lab Med 1991;115:632–5.
4. Bevers RF, Abbekerk EM, Boon TA. Cowper's syringocele: symptoms, classification and treatment of an unappreciated problem. J Urol 2000;163:782–4.
5. Davis BL, Robinson DG. Diverticula of the female urethra: assay of 120 cases. J Urol 1970;104:850–3.
6. Del Mistro A, Braunstein JD, Halwer M, Koss LG. Identification of human papillomavirus types in male urethral condylomata acuminata by in situ hybridization. Hum Pathol 1987;18:936–40.
7. Downs RA. Congenital polyps of the prostatic urethra. A review of the literature and report of two cases. Br J Urol 1970;42:76–85.
8. Drew PA, Murphy WM, Civantos F, Speights VO. The histogenesis of clear cell adenocarcinoma of the lower urinary tract. Case series and review of the literature. Hum Pathol 1996;27:248–52.
9. Duckett JW, Snow BW. Disorders of the urethra and penis. In: Walsh PC, Gittes RF, Perlmutter AD, Stamey TA, eds. Campbell's urology, 5th ed. Philadelphia: WB Saunders; 1986;2000–30.
10. Elbadawi A, Malhoski WE, Frank IN. Mucinous urethral caruncle. Urology 1978;12:587–90.
11. Freeman JA, Esrig D, Stein JP, Skinner DG. Management of the patient with bladder cancer: urethral recurrence. Urol Clin North Am 1994;21:645–51.
12. Gilcrease MZ, Delgado R, Vuitch F, Albores-Saavedra J. Clear cell adenocarcinoma and nephrogenic adenoma of the urethra and urinary bladder: a histopathologic and immunohistochemical comparison. Hum Pathol 1998;29:1451–6.
13. Gonzalez MO, Harrison ML, Boileau MA. Carcinoma in diverticulum of female urethra. Urology 1985;26:328–32.
14. Grabstald H. Proceedings: Tumors of the urethra in men and women. Cancer 1973;32:1236–55.
15. Hardeman SW, Soloway MS. Urethral recurrence following radical cystectomy. J Urol 1990;144:666–9.
16. Hickey DP, Soloway MS, Murphy WM. Selective urethrectomy following cystoprostatectomy for bladder cancer. J Urol 1986;136:828–30.
17. Hopkins SC, Nag SK, Soloway MS. Primary carcinoma of male urethra. Urology 1984;23:128–33.
18. Huffman JW. The detailed anatomy of the paraurethral ducts in the adult human female. Am J Obstet Gynecol 1948;55:86–101.
19. Kageyama S, Ueda T, Kushima R, Sakamoto T. Primary adenosquamous cell carcinoma of the male distal urethra: magnetic resonance imaging using a circular surface coil. J Urol 1997;158:1913–4.
20. Kim CJ, Pak K, Hamaguchi A, et al. Primary malignant melanoma of the female urethra. Cancer 1993;71:448–51.
21. Kitamura H, Umehara T, Miyake M, Shimizu T, Kohda K, Ando M. Non-Hodgkin's lymphoma arising in the urethra of a man. J Urol 1996;156:175–6.
22. Knapik JA, Murphy WM. Urethral wash cytopathology for monitoring patients after cystoprostatectomy with urinary diversion. Cancer 2003;99:352–6.
23. Lin DW, Herr HW, Dalbagni G. Value of urethral wash cytology in the retained male urethra after radical cystoprostatectomy. J Urol 2003;169:961–3.
24. Loo KT, Chan JK. Colloid adenocarcinoma of the urethra associated with mucosal in situ carcinoma. Arch Pathol Lab Med 1992;116:976–7.
25. Lucman L, Vadas G. Transitional cloacogenic carcinoma of the urethra. Cancer 1973;31:1508–10.
26. Madden NP, Turnock RR, Rickwood AM. Congenital polyps of the posterior urethra in neonates. J Pediatr Surg 1986;21:193–4.
27. Mahadevia PS, Koss LG, Tar IJ. Prostatic involvement in bladder cancer. Prostate mapping in 20 cystoprostatectomy specimens. Cancer 1986;58:2096–102.
28. Mayer R, Fowler JE Jr, Clayton M. Localized urethral cancer in women. Cancer 1987;60:1548–51.
29. McIntire TL, Soloway MS, Murphy WM. Nephrogenic adenoma. Urology 1987;29:237–41.
30. Medeiros LJ, Young RH. Nephrogenic adenoma arising in urethral diverticula. A report of five cases. Arch Pathol Lab Med 1989;113:125–8.
31. Meis JM, Ayala AG, Johnson DE. Adenocarcinoma of the urethra in women. A clinicopathologic study. Cancer 1987;60:1038–52.
32. Melchers WJ, Schift R, Stolz E, Lindeman J, Quint WG. Human papillomavirus detection in urine samples from male patients by the polymerase chain reaction. J Clin Microbiol 1989;27:1711–4.
33. Mevorach RA, Cos LR, di Sant'Agnese PA, Stoler M. Human papillomavirus type 6 in grade I transitional cell carcinoma of the urethra. J Urol 1990;143:126–8.
34. Miller EV. Skene's duct cyst. J Urol 1984;131:966–7.

35. Mira JL, Fan G. Leiomyoma of the male urethra: a case report and review of the literature. Arch Pathol Lab Med 2000;124:302–3.

36. Mostofi FK, Price EB Jr. Tumors of the male genital system. Atlas of Tumor Pathology, 2nd Series, Fascicle 8. Washington, D.C.: Armed Forces Institute of Pathology; 1973:263–6.

37. Murphy WM. Diseases of the urinary bladder, urethra, ureters, and renal pelves. In: Murphy WM, ed. Urological pathology. Philadelphia: WB Saunders; 1997:119–22.

38. Murphy WM, Fu YS, Lancaster WD, Jenson AB. Papillomavirus structural antigens in condyloma acuminatum of the male urethra. J Urol 1983;130:84–5.

39. Oliva E, Amin MB, Jimenez R, Young RH. Clear cell carcinoma of the urinary bladder: a report and comparison of four tumors of mullerian origin and nine of probable urothelial origin with discussion of histogenesis and diagnostic problems. Am J Surg Pathol 2002;26:190–7.

40. Oliva E, Young RH. Clear cell adenocarcinoma of the urethra: a clinicopathologic analysis of 19 cases. Mod Pathol 1996;9:513–20.

41. Raju GC, Roopnarinesingh A, Woo J. Villous adenoma of female urethra. Urology 1987;29:446–7.

42. Redman JF, Rountree GA. Pronounced dilatation of Cowper's gland duct manifest as a perineal mass: a recommendation for management. J Urol 1988;139:87–8.

43. Sanders TJ, Venable DD, Sanusi ID. Primary malignant melanoma of the urethra in a black man: a case report. J Urol 1986;135:1012–4.

44. Schinella R, Thurm J, Feiner H. Papillary pseudotumor of the prostatic urethra: proliferative papillary urethritis. J Urol 1974;111:38–40.

45. Silverman ML, Eyre RC, Zinman LA, Corsson AW. Mixed mucinous and papillary adenocarcinoma involving male urethra, probably originating in periurethral glands. Cancer 1981;47:1398–402.

46. Small JD, Albertsen PC, Graydon RJ, Ricci A Jr, Sardella WV. Adenoid cystic carcinoma of Cowper's gland. J Urol 1992;147:699–701.

47. Smith VC, Boone TB, Truong LD. Collagen polyp of the urinary tract: a report of two cases. Mod Pathol 1999;12:1090–3.

48. Spencer JR, Brodin AG, Ignatoff JM. Clear cell adenocarcinoma of the urethra: evidence for origin within periurethral ducts. J Urol 1990;143:122–5.

49. Tanagho EA. Anatomy of the lower urinary tract. In: Walsh PC, Retik AB, Stamey TA, Vaughan ED Jr, eds. Campbell's urology, 6th ed. Philadelphia: WB Saunders: 1992:50–4.

50. Tepper SL, Jagirdar J, Heath D, Geller SA. Homology between the female paraurethral (Skene's) glands and the prostate. Immunohistochemical demonstration. Arch Pathol Lab Med 1984;108:423–5.

51. Tran KP, Epstein JI. Mucinous adenocarcinoma of urinary bladder type arising from the prostatic urethra. Distinction from mucinous adenocarcinoma of the prostate. Am J Surg Pathol 1996;20:1346–50.

52. Uchida K, Fukuta F, Ando M, Miyake M. Female urethral hemangioma. J Urol 2001;166:1008.

53. Vadmal MS, Steckel J, Teichberg S, Hajdu SI. Primary neuroendocrine carcinoma of the penile urethra. J Urol 1997;157:956–7.

54. Vasudevan P, Stein AM, Pinn VW, Rao CN. Primary amyloidosis of urethra. Urology 1981;17:181–3.

55. Walker AN, Mills SE. Papillary and polypoid tumors of the prostatic urethra. In: Damjanov I, Cohen AH, Mills SE, Young RH, eds. Progress in reproductive and urinary tract pathology. New York: Field & Wood Medical Publishers, Inc; 1989:113–37.

56. Walther HW. Caruncle of the urethra in the female with special reference to the importance of histological examination in the differential diagnosis. J Urol 1943;50:380–8.

57. Witjes JA, De Vries JD, Schaafsma HE, Bogman MJ, Barentsz JO, Corten RL. Extramedullary plasmacytoma of the urethra: a case report. J Urol 1991;145:826–8.

58. Wolinska WH, Melamed MR, Schellhammer PF, Whitmore WF Jr. Urethral cytology following cystectomy for bladder carcinoma. Am J Surg Pathol 1977;1:225–34.

59. Young RH, Srigley JR, Amin MB, Ulbright TM, Cubilla AL. Tumors of the prostate gland, seminal vesicles, male urethra, and penis. Atlas of Tumor Pathology, Fascicle 28, 3rd Series. Washington, DC: Armed Forces Institute of Pathology; 2000;367–402.

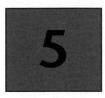

5 TUMORS OF THE URETERS AND RENAL PELVES

NORMAL ANATOMY

The ureters and renal pelves form by elongation and branching of diverticular outgrowths from the mesonephric ducts (47,58). Initial branches are absorbed by dilatation of the advancing ureters to form the renal pelves, but later branches are retained as renal calyces and terminal portions of the collecting ducts. The mature structures function as conduits for the passage of urine. Each is lined by a folded epithelium supported by a lamina propria and surrounded by a muscular wall with a fibrous adventitia.

The structural components of the ureter and renal pelvis are similar to those of the urinary bladder, but certain features deserve further elaboration. Except for its distal portion, the wall of the ureter consists of interlacing bundles of smooth muscle that are not arranged into distinct longitudinal and circular layers (29). When portions of the ureteral wall appear in surgical resection specimens of adjacent organs, this lack of organization may be a source of diagnostic difficulty, especially when the ureteral mucosa is not present. In contrast to the bladder, the mucosa of the upper collecting system is normally arranged in folds, creating crypts from which rounded aggregates of cells may be avulsed into urinary specimens during catheterization or ureteroscopy. These "papillary" clusters may cause diagnostic confusion in the cytologic evaluation of low-grade urothelial tumors if too much emphasis is placed on papillary aggregation as a sign of neoplastic growth. The nuclei of urothelial cells from the upper collecting system are larger and more irregular than their bladder counterparts. These features also occur in dysplasia, and both normal and slightly reactive ureteral mucosa can be easily confused with dysplastic epithelium, especially in frozen section specimens taken at the time of cystectomy for bladder cancer. Considering the embryologic development of the renal collecting ducts, it is not surprising that urothelium extending into them may be a possible con-

founding factor to determining the origin of small glandular neoplasms arising in this area.

Almost all tumors and variants, including rare lesions, that have been previously described in the urinary bladder and urethra have been recorded in the ureters or renal pelves (8,53). Neoplasms arising in these structures differ very little from their bladder counterparts and are only briefly summarized.

EPITHELIAL NEOPLASMS

Definition and General Features. Epithelial neoplasms arising in the ureters and renal pelves are uncommon lesions whose clinical behavior and pathologic features have remained essentially unchanged over the past half century (8,18,25,35,41,51,53). Age, sex ratio, and frequency of histologic types do not differ significantly from those of similar tumors arising in the bladder. Important variations from bladder neoplasms include: a lower frequency of all types; a stronger association with certain types of chemical agents, such as phenacetin; a stronger association with obstruction to urinary outflow; a decreased value of cytology and endoscopy for detection and monitoring; and an increased frequency of synchronous or metachronous urothelial neoplasms at other sites.

The etiologic and pathogenetic factors that influence the development of upper collecting system neoplasms are similar to those described for the bladder. Associations with phenacetin abuse, Balkan nephropathy, and Lynch's syndrome II seem particularly strong (34,36,45,59). Urothelial carcinomas of the upper collecting system that manifest microsatellite instability at selected sites are associated with the nonpolyposis colorectal cancer syndrome (10). There is a history of infection or urinary stones in 15 to 20 percent of patients (25). Urothelial neoplasms of the upper collecting system are frequently associated with similar lesions at other sites. Renal pelvic and ureteral tumors occur simultaneously in 6 to 38 percent of patients, and

50 percent of patients with upper collecting system lesions have subsequent bladder tumors.

Clinical Features. Epithelial neoplasms of the upper collecting system may be primary or arise following the detection and treatment of a bladder neoplasm. Primary neoplasms constitute less than 5 percent of all urothelial tumors (8,18,25,27,35,51,53). They are recorded in patients of all ages, most commonly in men aged 50 to 70 years. Any part of the system may be involved but the distal third of the ureter and the extrarenal portion of the renal pelvis are most commonly affected. Single lesions are the rule, although multiple tumors are not rare. Signs and symptoms are nonspecific: most patients have hematuria (90 percent) or flank pain (20 percent). Upper tract neoplasms can be recognized by urinary cytology and endoscopy, but most tumors are localized by radiography (7,31,53).

Pathologic Findings. Epithelial neoplasms arising in the ureters and renal pelves do not differ pathologically from those of the bladder (figs. 5-1–5-3). All histologic types, including inverted papilloma and rare variants of carcinoma, are recorded with similar frequencies, and the nomenclature applied to bladder tumors has traditionally been adopted for similar neoplasms of the upper collecting system (1,8,9, 11–13,15,21,39,40,50,53,54,61,64,68). Immunohistochemical findings and DNA ploidy are similar (2,26,28,54,55,57).

Grading classifications are the same as for tumors of the urinary bladder but staging systems developed for bladder lesions have been slightly modified to apply to similar tumors arising in the upper collecting system (3). Pathologic T3 tumors in the renal pelvis are those that have invaded either through the muscularis propria or into the renal parenchyma. Involvement of renal collecting ducts without parenchymal invasion does not alter the stage. Pathologic T3 tumors in the ureter are those that have invaded through the muscularis propria; pathologic T4 tumors are those that have invaded adjacent organs or have invaded through the renal parenchyma into perirenal fat. Reactions to therapy and the features of epithelial atypias are difficult to study in the ureters and renal pelves, and current knowledge in this regard is fragmentary.

Prognosis. Like bladder tumors, upper collecting system neoplasms grow initially by extension into adjacent structures. While not considered invasion, involvement of the distal renal collecting ducts is common, especially by high-grade carcinomas (46). Metastases usually involve regional structures, including lymph nodes, peritoneum, and liver (7). Metastases to the upper collecting system generally involve the ureters and arise from cancers of the kidney, breast, and lymph nodes (16).

Considering that a significant percentage of upper urinary tract tumors are invasive at detection and that the literature states that nearly 50 percent of these have invaded the muscularis propria, the overall prognosis is surprisingly favorable (27,51). The most important prognostic factors in multivariate analyses are stage, patient age, and type of treatment. Survival among patients with treated pTa/pTis lesions is 100 percent and even patients with pT2 tumors can expect a survival rate of 75 percent.

When upper urinary tract neoplasms arise following cystectomy for bladder carcinoma, the features and expectations are less favorable (6,48). Overall, the incidence of neoplasms remains low, at 2 to 4 percent, but has been reported as high as 21 percent among patients with bladder-sparing treatment regimens (30). Upper tract tumors appearing in patients followed for previous bladder carcinomas tend to be of higher stage (up to 58 percent pT3) and are more often bilateral (31 percent) than neoplasms occurring as the patients' primary tumors at these sites. The prognosis is poor, with 40 to 68 percent of patients succumbing to their disease and few individuals remaining tumor free during follow-up.

Differential Diagnosis. The guidelines for the differential diagnosis of epithelial neoplasms arising in the ureters and renal pelves are similar to those for lesions arising in the bladder. Certain tumors of the renal pelvis must be distinguished from carcinomas of the renal collecting ducts (38). In addition to location, renal pelvic neoplasms are more solid and the urothelial type is often accompanied by an in situ component. Collecting duct carcinomas tend to be accompanied by dysplastic changes in adjacent renal tubules but this is not as reliable a feature for diagnosis as the occurrence of urothelial CIS.

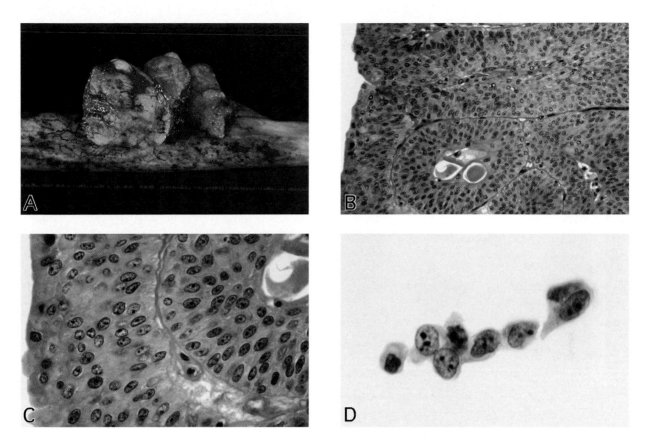

Figure 5-1

UROTHELIAL CARCINOMA, LOW GRADE, OF URETER

A: Gross specimen.
B: Urothelial carcinoma, low grade.
C: High magnification.
D: Corresponding ureteral washing.

OTHER NEOPLASMS

A variety of nonepithelial neoplasms are observed in the ureters and renal pelves. These tumors do not differ histologically from similar lesions at other body sites. They include hemangioma, hemangiomyoma, leiomyoma, neurofibroma, leiomyosarcoma, angiosarcoma, choriocarcinoma, and Wilms' tumor (4,17,36, 44,56,60,62,65–67,69).

NON-NEOPLASTIC TUMOROUS CONDITIONS

Polyp

Polyps of the ureters and renal pelves are usually acquired rather than congenital (8,14,19, 53,70). Few cases are associated with predisposing conditions although many etiologic factors have been proposed. Most polyps are hamartomatous growths that tend to arise in the proximal portions of the left ureter of men. Single tumors are the rule, but multiple or branched lesions are observed (fig. 5-4). Signs and symptoms occur if the ureter is obstructed.

Pathologically, polyps grow as intraluminal lesions and consist of a broad core of loose connective tissue covered by normal or denuded urothelium. The connective tissue core may be rich in smooth muscle, collagen, or blood vessels, and may even contain small numbers of lipid-laden macrophages. The composition of the stalk is variable but there is no evidence that the nature of the polyp is altered by the relative proportion of blood vessels, smooth muscle, or connective tissue comprising its core.

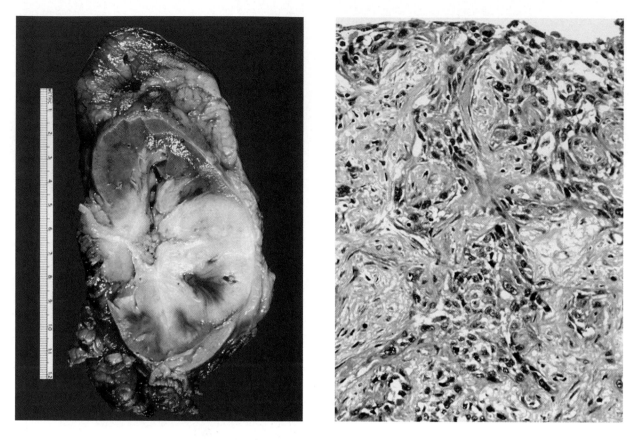

Figure 5-2

UROTHELIAL CARCINOMA, HIGH GRADE, OF RENAL PELVIS
Left: Gross specimen.
Right: Urothelial carcinoma, high grade.

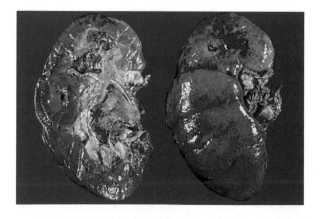
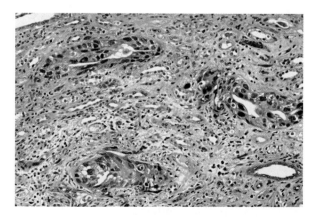

Figure 5-3

UROTHELIAL CARCINOMA WITH INVOLVEMENT OF COLLECTING DUCTS
Left: Gross specimen.
Right: Collecting duct involvement.

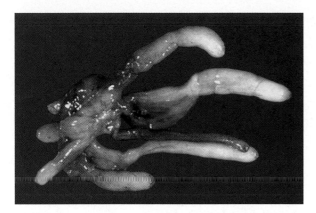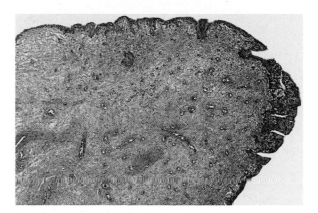

Figure 5-4

FIBROEPITHELIAL POLYP OF URETER

This fibroepithelial polyp of the ureter was removed from a 12-year-old boy with gross hematuria who was found to have delayed renal emptying. The gross specimen on the left is illustrated by the fibrovascular core covered with urothelium on the right.

Retroperitoneal Fibrosis

Retroperitoneal fibrosis is an inflammatory process that must often be considered in the differential diagnosis of ureteral tumors (5,8,53). Most cases are of unknown etiology, although a close association with ergot compounds such as methysergide has been documented. The disease develops insidiously, eventuating in a dense fibrosis that causes medial deviation of the ureters and ureteral obstruction. Depending upon the stage of disease, the fibrosis may not be the predominant component in a biopsy specimen. A nonspecific pattern of chronic inflammation often occurs. Perhaps more importantly, any condition that attenuates urothelium may cause dysplastic epithelial changes, mimicking those of CIS on rare occasions.

A wide range of non-neoplastic tumorous conditions are recorded in the ureters and renal pelves. Most lesions are described in single case reports, with or without a review of the literature. These lesions do not differ pathologically from similar conditions occurring at other body sites. They include amyloidosis, endometriosis, nephrogenic metaplasia, schistosomal infection producing ureteritis cystica, ectopic ureter presenting as an abdominal mass, mycetoma, plasma cell granuloma, hamartoma, hematoma (Antopol-Goldman lesion), cholesteatoma, paraffinoma, and inflammatory pseudotumor (11,20,22–24,32,33,37,42,43,49,52,63).

REFERENCES

1. Akhtar M, Aslam M, Lindstedt E, Pesti T, Kovacs G. Osteoclast-like giant cell tumor of renal pelvis. J Urol Pathol 1999:11:181–93.

2. al-Abadi H, Nagel R. Transitional cell carcinoma of the renal pelvis and ureter: prognostic relevance of nuclear deoxyribonucleic acid ploidy studied by slide cytometry: an 8-year survival time study. J Urol 1992;148:31–7.

3. American Joint Committee on Cancer. Manual for staging of cancer, 6th ed. New York: Springer; 2002:329–34.

4. Anderson JB, Lee JJ, Hancock RA, Black SR. Hemangioma of the kidney pelvis. J Urol 1953;70:869–73.

5. Baker LR, Mallinson WJ, Gregory MC, et al. Idiopathic retroperitoneal fibrosis. A retrospective analysis of 60 cases. Br J Urol 1987;60:497–503.

6. Balaji KC, McGuire M, Grotas J, Grimaldi G, Russo P. Upper tract recurrences following radical cystectomy: an analysis of prognostic factors, recurrence pattern and stage at presentation. J Urol 1999:162:1603–6.

7. Batata MA, Whitmore WF, Hilaris BS, Tokita N, Grabstald H. Primary carcinoma of the ureter: a prognostic study. Cancer 1975;35:1626–32.

8. Bennington JL, Beckwith JB. Tumors of the kidney, renal pelvis, and ureter. Atlas of Tumor Pathology, 2nd Series, Fascicle 12. Washington, D.C.: Armed Forces Institute of Pathology; 1975:243–336.

9. Blacher EJ, Johnson DE, Abdul-Karim FW, Ayala AG. Squamous cell carcinoma of renal pelvis. Urology 1985;25:124–6.

10. Blaszyk H, Wang L, Dietmaier W, et al. Upper tract urothelial carcinoma: a clinicopathologic study including microsatellite instability analysis. Mod Pathol 2002;15:790–7.

11. Bradford JA, Ireland EW, Giles WB. Ureteric endometriosis: 3 case reports and a review of the literature. Aust N Z J Obstet Gynaecol 1989;29:421–4.

12. Byard RW, Bell ME, Alkan MK. Primary carcinosarcoma: a rare cause of unilateral ureteral obstruction. J Urol 1987;137:732–3.

13. Chalik YN, Wieczorek R, Grasso M. Lymphoepithelioma-like carcinoma of the ureter. J Urol 1998;159:503–4.

14. Chang HH, Ray P, Ockuly E, Guinan P. Benign fibrous ureteral polyps. Urology 1987;30:114–8.

15. Chen KT, Workman RD, Flam MS, DeKlotz RJ. Carcinosarcoma of renal pelvis. Urology 1983;22:429–31.

16. Cohen WM, Freed SZ, Hasson J. Metastatic cancer to the ureter: a review of the literature and case presentations. J Urol 1974;112:188–9.

17. Coup AJ. Angiosarcoma of the ureter. Br J Urol 1988;62:275–6.

18. Das AK, Carson CC, Bolick D, Paulson DF. Primary carcinoma of the upper urinary tract. Effect of primary and secondary therapy on survival. Cancer 1990;66:1919–23.

19. de Jonge JP, von Kortzfleisch D, Blessing MH, Stoker W. Fibroepithelioma of the renal pelvis. Urol Int 1988;43:56–9.

20. Eisenberg RL, Hedgcock MW, Shanser JD. Aspergillus mycetoma of the renal pelvis associated with ureteropelvic junction obstruction. J Urol 1977;118:466–7.

21. Essenfeld H, Manivel JC, Benedetto P, Albores-Saavedra J. Small cell carcinoma of the renal pelvis: a clinicopathological, morphological and immunohistochemical study of 2 cases. J Urol 1990;144(2 Pt 1):344–7.

22. Finan BF, Mollitt DL, Golladay ES, Redman JF. Giant ectopic ureter presenting as abdominal mass in infant. Urology 1987;30:246–7.

23. Fitko R, Gallagher L, Gonzalez-Crussi F, Oyasu R. Urothelial leiomyomatous hamartoma of the kidney. Am J Clin Pathol 1991;95:481–3.

24. Freedberg LE, Stables DP, Bloustein PA, Donohue R. Cholesteatoma of renal pelvis. Urology 1977;10:263–5.

25. Grabstald H, Whitmore WF, Melamed MR. Renal pelvic tumors. JAMA 1971;218:845–54.

26. Hall L, Faddoul A, Saberi A, Edson M. The use of the red cell surface antigen to predict the malignant potential of transitional cell carcinoma of the ureter and renal pelvis. J Urol 1982;127:23–5.

27. Hall MC, Womack S, Sagalowsky AI, Carmody T, Erickstad MD, Roehrborn CG. Prognostic factors, recurrence, and survival in transitional cell carcinoma of the upper urinary tract: a 30-year experience in 252 patients. Urology 1998;52:594–601.

28. Han AC, Duszak R Jr. Coexpression of cytokeratins 7 and 20 confirms urothelial carcinoma presenting as an intrarenal tumor. Cancer 1999;86:2327–30.

29. Hanna MK, Jeffs RD, Sturgess JM, Barkin M. Ureteral structure and ultrastructure. Part I. The normal human ureter. J Urol 1976;116:718–24.

30. Herr HW, Cookson MS, Soloway SM. Upper tract tumors in patients with primary bladder cancer followed for 15 years. J Urol 1996;156:1286–7.

31. Huffman JL, Bagley DH, Lyon ES, Morse MJ, Herr HW, Whitmore WF Jr. Endoscopic diagnosis and treatment of upper-tract urothelial tumors. A preliminary report. Cancer 1985;55:1422–8.

32. Itoh H, Namiki M, Yoshioka T, Itatani H. Plasma cell granuloma of the renal pelvis. J Urol 1982;127:1177–8.

33. Jakse G, Mikuz G. Nephrogenic adenoma of the ureter. Eur Urol 1983;9:60–2.

34. Johansson S, Angervall L, Bengtsson U, Wahlqvist L. Uroepithelial tumors of the renal pelvis associated with abuse of phenacetin-containing analgesics. Cancer 1974;33:743–53.

35. Kakizoe T, Fujita J, Murase T, Matsumoto K, Kishi K. Transitional cell carcinoma of the bladder in patients with renal pelvic and ureteral cancer. J Urol 1980;124:17–9.

36. Kao VC, Graff PW, Rappaport H. Leiomyoma of the ureter. A histologically problematic rare tumor confirmed by immunohistochemical studies. Cancer 1969;24:535–42.

37. Kelleher J, Wilson S, Witherow RO. Paraffinoma of the ureter. Br J Urol 1987;59:92–3.

38. Kennedy SM, Merino MJ, Linehan WM, Roberts JR, Robertson CN, Neumann RD. Collecting duct carcinoma of the kidney. Hum Pathol 1990;21:449–56.

39. Kobayashi S, Ohmori M, Akaeda T, Ohmori H, Miyaji Y. Primary adenocarcinoma of the renal pelvis. Report of two cases and brief review of literature. Acta Pathol Jpn 1983;33:589–97.

40. Kvist E, Lauritzen AF, Bredesen J, Luke M, Sjolin KE. A comparative study of transitional cell tumors of the bladder and upper urinary tract. Cancer 1988;61:2109–12.

41. Kyriakos M, Royce RK. Multiple simultaneous inverted papillomas of the upper urinary tract. A case report with a review of ureteral and renal pelvic inverted papillomas. Cancer 1989;63:368–80.

42. Leroy X, Copin MC, Graziana JP, Wacrenier A, Gosselin B. Inflammatory pseudotumor of the renal pelvis. A report of 2 cases with clinicopathologic and immunohistochemical study. Arch Pathol Lab Med 2000;124:1209–12.

43. Levitt S, Waisman J, deKernion J. Subepithelial hematoma of the renal pelvis (Antopol-Goldman lesion): a case report and review of the literature. J Urol 1984;131:939–41.

44. Loomis RC. Primary leiomyosarcoma of the kidney: report of a case and review of the literature. J Urol 1972;107:557–60.

45. Lynch HT, Ens JA, Lynch JF. The Lynch syndrome II and urological malignancies. J Urol 1990;143:24–8.

46. Mahadevia PS, Karwa GL, Koss LG. Mapping of urothelium in carcinomas of the renal pelvis and ureter. A report of nine cases. Cancer 1983;51:890–7.

47. Maizels M. Normal development of the urinary tract. In: Walsh PC, Gittes RF, Pearlmutter AD, Stamey TA, eds. Campbell's urology. 5th ed. Philadelphia: WB Saunders; 1986:1638–64.

48. Millan-Rodriguez F, Chechile-Toniolo G, Salvador-Bayarri J, Huguet-Perez J, Vicente-Rodriguez J. Upper urinary tract tumors after primary superficial bladder tumors: prognostic factors and risk groups. J Urol 2000;164:1183–7.

49. Miller R, Bowley NB. Localized amyloidosis of the ureter. J Urol 1984;131:112–3.

50. Molinie V, Pouchot J, Vinceneux P, Barge J. Osteoclastoma-like giant cell tumor of the renal pelvis associated with papillary transitional cell carcinoma. Arch Pathol Lab Med 1997;121:162–6.

51. Munoz JJ, Ellison LM. Upper tract urothelial neoplasms: incidence and survival during the last 2 decades. J Urol 2000;164:1523–5.

52. Murphy MN, Alguacil-Garcia A, MacDonald RG. Primary amyloidosis of renal pelvis with duplicate collecting system. Urology 1986;27:470–3.

53. Murphy WM. Diseases of the urinary bladder, urethra, ureters, and renal pelves. In: Murphy WM, ed. Urological pathology. Philadelphia: WB Saunders; 1997:127–31.

54. Nativ O, Winkler HZ, Reiman HM Jr, Lieber MM. Squamous cell carcinoma of the renal pelvis: nuclear deoxyribonucleic acid ploidy studied by flow cytometry. J Urol 1990;144:23–6.

55. Nemoto R, Hattori K, Sasaki A, Miyanaga N, Koiso K, Harada M. Estimations of the S phase fraction in situ in transitional cell carcinoma of the renal pelvis and ureter with bromodeoxyuridine labelling. Br J Urol 1989;64:339–44.

56. Ogata S, Mizoguchi H, Arita M, Sakamoto S, Ogata J. A case of hemangiomyoma of the ureter in a child. Eur Urol 1985;11:355–6.

57. Oldbring J, Hellsten S, Lindholm K, Mikulowski P, Tribukait B. Flow DNA analysis of the characterization of carcinoma of the renal pelvis and ureter. Cancer 1989;64:2141–5.

58. Osathanondh V, Potter EL. II. Development of human kidney as shown by microdissection: renal pelvis, calyces, and papillae. Arch Pathol 1963;76:277–89.

59. Petronic VJ, Bukurov NS, Djokic MR, et al. Balkan endemic nephropathy and papillary transitional cell tumors of the renal pelvis and ureters. Kidney Int 1991;34(Suppl):S77–9.

60. Ravich A. Neurofibroma of the ureter: report of a case with operation and recovery. Arch Surg 1935;30:442–8.

61. Ross DG, D'Amato NA. Papillary mucinous cystadenoma of probable renal pelvic origin in a horseshoe kidney. Arch Pathol Lab Med 1985;109:954–5.

62. Rushton HG, Sens MA, Garvin AJ, Turner WR Jr. Primary leiomyosarcoma of the ureter: a case report with electron microscopy. J Urol 1983;129:1045–6.

63. Saad SM, Hanafy HM. Bilharzial (schistosomal) ureteritis cystica. Urology 1974;4:261–6.

64. Tajima Y, Aizawa M. Unusual renal pelvic tumor containing transitional cell carcinoma, adenocarcinoma, and sarcomatoid elements (so-called sarcomatoid carcinoma of the renal pelvis). A case report and review of the literature. Acta Pathol Jpn 1988;38:805–14.

65. Uchida M, Watanabe H, Mishina T, Shimada N. Leiomyoma of the renal pelvis. J Urol 1981;125:572–4.

66. Uhlir K. Hemangioma of the ureter. J Urol 1973;110:647–9.

67. Vahlensieck W Jr, Riede U, Wimmer B, Ihling C. Beta-human chorionic gonadotropin-positive extragonadal germ cell neoplasia of the renal pelvis. Cancer 1991;67:3146–9.

68. Vang R, Abrams J. A micropapillary variant of transitional cell carcinoma arising in the ureter. Arch Pathol Lab Med 2000;124:1347–8.

69. Weinberg AG, Currarino G, Hurt GE Jr. Botryoid Wilms' tumor of the renal pelvis. Arch Pathol Lab Med 1984;108:147–8.

70. Wolgel CD, Parris AC, Mitty HA, Schapira HE. Fibroepithelial polyp of renal pelvis. Urology 1982;19:436–9.

Index*

The Kidney

*Numbers in boldface indicate table and figure pages.

The Ureters and Renal Pelves